MRI of the Pelvis
A Text Atlas

MRI of the Pelvis

A Text Atlas

Hedvig Hricak, MD
Professor of Radiology and Urology
University of California
San Francisco, CA

Bernadette M Carrington, MRCP, FRCR
Visiting Assistant Professor, Radiology
University of California
San Francisco, CA

APPLETON & LANGE
Norwalk, Connecticut/San Mateo, California

MARTIN DUNITZ

Library of Congress Cataloging-in-Publication Data
Hricak, Hedvig.
    MRI of the pelvis: a text atlas/Hedvig Hricak.
    Bernadette M. Carrington.
        p.   cm.
    Includes index.
    ISBN 0-8385-6527-1.— ISBN 1-85317-027-5
    1. Pelvis — Magnetic resonance imaging. 2. Pelvis —
Magnetic resonance imaging — Atlases. I. Carrington.
Bernadette M. II. Title.
        [DNLM : 1. Magnetic Resonance Imaging — methods
        — atlases. 2. Pelvis — anatomy & histology — atlases.
        3. Pelvis — pathology — atlases. WE 17 H872m]
    RC946.H75   1991
    617.b.b — dc20
    DN1.M/DLO
    For Library of Congress.   91-4531
                                                          CIP

Notice: Our knowledge in clinical sciences is constantly
changing. As new information becomes available, changes
in treatment and in the use of drugs become necessary. The
author(s) and the publisher of this volume have taken care
to make certain that the doses of drugs and schedules of
treatment are correct and compatible with the standards
generally accepted at the time of publication. The reader is
advised to consult carefully the instruction and information
material included in the package insert of each drug or
therapeutic agent before administration. This advice is
especially important when using new or infrequently used
drugs.

Composition by Scribe Design, Gillingham, Kent
Origination by Toppan Printing, Singapore
Printed and bound by Toppan Printing, Singapore

Contents

Foreword

Magnetic resonance imaging (MRI) was introduced into the array of diagnostic imaging techniques in 1981. Similar to the initial clinical experience with computed tomography, MRI was applied almost exclusively for the diagnosis of diseases of the brain. Recognizing and accepting the limitations of MRI for body imaging, a few institutions pursued the exploration and further refinement of the technique for imaging of the body. Because the limitations of respiratory and cardiovascular motion were less severe than in the upper abdomen and chest, the value of the technique in the pelvis was recognized early by a few workers and then slowly accepted around the world. Certainly, Dr Hricak was one of the first investigators to recognize and enthusiastically pursue the capabilities of MRI for the diagnosis of disease of the male and female pelvis. Early papers stressed the advantages of multiple imaging planes and improved contrast resolution as important for advancing the diagnosis of disease in this region, especially for the diagnosis and staging of pelvic malignancies.

Dr Hricak initiated a continuous evaluation of the role of MRI for the diagnosis of pelvic disease. Her experience with MRI in this region of the body has been gathered over eight years so the richness and depth of description of MRI for the panoply of pelvic disease is invaluable for both the student and experi-enced radiologist. The precise and elaborate descrip-tion of pelvic anatomy and the presentation of it with high quality images reflect this long-term interest in radiologic–pathologic correlations.

Although this book started as an atlas of the pelvis, it has developed into a comprehensive treatise on MRI of the pelvis. While the book emphasizes that anatomy is the trellis upon which diagnoses by MRI rest, it also strongly emphasizes the importance of the proper utilization of the other multifaceted aspects of MRI such as the manipulation of differential contrast between normal and pathologic tissues using T1 and T2 relaxation times, MR contrast media, and varia-tions of imaging techniques.

Drs Hricak and Carrington have succinctly con-veyed a substantial amount of information and experi-ence on this topic. It is indeed fortunate that this book has become available as interest in MR imaging of the pelvis is increasing, and knowledge of anatomy and of the MR manifestations of disease are essential for the correct interpretation that will ensure continued acceptance.

Charles B Higgins, MD
Professor and Vice Chairman of Radiology
Chief, Magnetic Resonance Imaging
University of California, San Francisco

Preface

Magnetic resonance, with its advantages of superior soft tissue contrast resolution, multiplanar imaging and a wealth of techniques which increase the sensitivity for detecting tissue abnormalities with no known biologic or genetic ill effects, is a superb approach for examining the pelvis. This application is gaining in importance as the various treatment approaches become increasingly dependent on precise anatomic information. Magnetic resonance imaging (MRI) shows particular promise in the accurate staging of pelvic cancer when decisions on whether to perform local excision, radical resection, radiation therapy or chemotherapy are often guided by morphologic findings such as the stage of the disease, tumor size and depth of penetration. In the past, such information could only be obtained by exploratory laparotomy.

This book has been written to familiarize radiologists, gynecologists, urologists and general surgeons, as well as medical, surgical and radiation oncologists, with modern MRI of the pelvis obtained with the latest techniques—suppressing motion, enhancing contrast resolution, and the intravenous application of gadolinium-DTPA contrast medium. Guided by the premise that even the most detailed verbal description is no substitute for an image as a means of conveying visual concepts, the book is illustrated with over 1100 images, and where complicated anatomic relationships need to be simplified, by schematic drawings. It may be assumed that all the images were taken on a 1.5T unit unless otherwise indicated in the caption.

As MRI is not the only imaging modality currently employed for depicting pelvic disease, the indications, advantages and disadvantages of this technique compared to other techniques, such as ultrasound, computed tomography or conventional studies (eg intravenous pyelography and barium enema) are discussed and examples are included. The text is arranged to provide detailed embryologic, anatomic, pathologic and imaging information, giving the necessary background for understanding the MR image in the light of pathology. Chapters on MRI techniques, on biologic effects of MR and on the use of contrast media have been included to provide an essential base for understanding how optimal MR images are obtained. Contraindications for the use of this technique are also discussed. It is hoped that the technical background for MRI will be used as a guide for designing individualized programs for specific situations, as the 'cookbook' approach does not utilize many of the advantages of this method. We hope that we have succeeded in achieving our goal, as the use of MRI in the pelvis, when properly performed, can be of great benefit to patients.

The authors would like to take this opportunity to acknowledge and express gratitude to the many individuals without whose help it would have been difficult or impossible to achieve the publication of this book.

First, we wish to thank Dr Leon Kaufman whose contributions made clinical MRI possible and who served as an inspiration in conveying the capabilities that this technique possesses. Dr Lawrence Crooks helped immensely by giving expert advice on techniques and clarifying many of the intricate concepts of MRI, the nature and origin of artifacts and approaches to minimize them. Drs Wilbert Chew and Michael Moseley gave unselfishly of their expertise to make this book technically correct and clear. Drs Eduardo Secaf and Kostaki Bis were untiring helpers and critics, and provided constant encouragement. Our administrative assistants, Johnette Coleman, Sheila Momaney, Steven Miller, Elizabeth Ruyle and Shirley Semingran were tireless in helping with the production of the manuscript. Katherine Pitcoff was essential in helping us express our ideas in an effective and concise fashion. The beautiful and valuable drawings were made by Paul Stempen from whom we learned much. Mary Banks, Alison Campbell and Jacky Alderson of Martin Dunitz Publishers helped in the initiation and completion of the book. Our young colleagues, clinical instructors in the MRI section, helped with their suggestions. We are also grateful to our clinical colleagues in urology, gynecology, surgery and radiation oncology for their input.

Thus, this book is in many ways a team effort, and we thank all concerned for helping create the ambiance at the University of California at San Francisco that was conducive to and indispensable for this book to be born.

HH
BMC

Acknowledgments

Some of the illustrations reproduced in this book have been used in previously published cases as follows:

Chapter 5
Demas BE, Hricak H, Jaffe RB, Uterine MR imaging: effects of hormonal stimulation, *Radiology* (1986) 159:123–6; Carrington BM, Hricak H, Nuruddin RR, MRI evaluation of Müllerian duct anomalies, accepted by *Radiology*; Hricak H, Tscholakoff D, Heinrichs L et al, Uterine leiomyomas: correlation of MR, histopathologic findings and symptoms, *Radiology* (1986) 158:385–91; Hricak H, Stern JL, Fisher MR et al, Endometrial carcinoma staging by MR imaging, *Radiology* (1987) 162:297–305; Shapeero LH, Hricak H, Mixed Müllerian sarcoma of the uterus: MR imaging findings, *AJR* (1989) 153:317–19; Hricak H, Chang YCF, Cann CE et al, Cervical incompetence: preliminary evaluation with MR imaging, *Radiology* (1990) 174:821–6; Hricak H, Lacey CG, Sandles LG et al, Invasive cervical carcinoma: comparison of MR imaging and surgical findings, *Radiology* (1988) 166:623–31; Chang YCF, Hricak H, Thurnher S et al, Evaluation of the vagina by magnetic resonance imaging: Part II Neoplasm, *Radiology* (1988) 169:569–71.

Chapter 6
Dooms GC, Hricak H, Tscholakoff D, Adnexal structures: MR imaging, *Radiology* (1986) 158:639–46; Arrivé L, Hricak H, Martin MC, Pelvic endometriosis: MR imaging, *Radiology* (1989) 171:687–92; Stevens S, Hricak H, Carrington BM et al, Detection and characterization of ovarian lesions at 1.5T using gadolinium-DTPA, submitted to *Radiology*.

Chapter 7
McCarthy SM, Filly RA, Stark DD et al, Obstetrical magnetic resonance imaging: fetal anatomy, *Radiology* (1985) 154:427–32; McCarthy SM, Stark DD, Filly RA et al, Obstetrical magnetic resonance imaging: maternal anatomy, *Radiology* (1985) 154:421–5; Hricak H, Demas BE, Braga CA et al, Gestational trophoblastic neoplasm of the uterus: MR assessment, *Radiology* (1986) 161:11–16.

Chapter 8
Thurnher S, Hricak H, Tanagho EA, Müllerian duct cyst: diagnosis with MR imaging, *Radiology* (1988) 167:631–6; Nuruddin RN, Hricak H, McClure RD et al, Magnetic resonance imaging of the seminal vesicles, *AJR* (in press); Hricak H, Editorial on imaging prostate carcinoma, *Radiology* (1988) 169:569–71; Hricak H, Dooms GC, Jeffrey RB et al, Prostate carcinoma: staging by clinical asssessment, CT and MR imaging, *Radiology* (1987) 162:331–6.

Chapter 9
Nuruddin RN, Hricak H, McClure RD et al, Magnetic resonance imaging of the seminal vesicles, submitted to *AJR*; Hricak H, Dooms GC, Jeffrey RB et al, Prostate carcinoma: staging by clinical assessment, CT and MR imaging, *Radiology* (1987) 162:331–6; Sugimura K, Carrington B, Quivey J et al, Postirradiation changes in the pelvis: assessment with MR imaging, *Radiology* (1990) 175:805–13; Thurnher S, Hricak H, Tanagho EA, Müllerian duct cyst: diagnosis with MR imaging, *Radiology* (1988) 167:631–6.

Chapter 10
Thurnher S, Hricak H, Pobiel R et al, Imaging the testis: comparison between MR imaging and US, *Radiology* (1988) 167:631–6; Fritzsche PJ, Hricak H, Kogan BA et al, Undescended testis: value of MR imaging, *Radiology* (1987) 164:169–73; Chew W, Hricak H, McClure RD, The assessment of human testicular function by ^{31}P MRS. Presented at the 73rd Scientific Assembly of the Radiologic Society of North America, Nov 29–Dec 4, 1987, *Radiology* (in press); Semelka R, Anderson M, Hricak H, Prosthetic testicle: appearance at MR imaging, *Radiology* (1989) 173(2):561–2.

Chapter 11
Hricak H, Marotti M, Gilbert TJ et al, Normal penile anatomy and abnormal penile conditions: evaluation with MR imaging, *Radiology* (1988) 169:683–90.

Chapter 12
Hricak H, Secaf E, Buckley D et al, MRI in female urethra, *Radiology* (in press); Fisher MR, Hricak H, Tanagho EA, Urinary bladder MR imaging. II Neoplasm, *Radiology* (1985) 157:471–7.

Chapter 13
Sugimura K, Carrington BM, Quivey JM et al, Postirradiation changes in the pelvis: assessment with MR imaging, *Radiology* (1990) 175:805–13.

Chapter 14
Sugimura K, Carrington BM, Quivey JM et al, Postirradiation changes in the pelvis: assessment with MR imaging, *Radiology* (1990) 175:805–13; Arrivé L, Chang YCF, Hricak H et al, Radiation-induced uterine changes: MR imaging, *Radiology* (1989) 170:55–8.

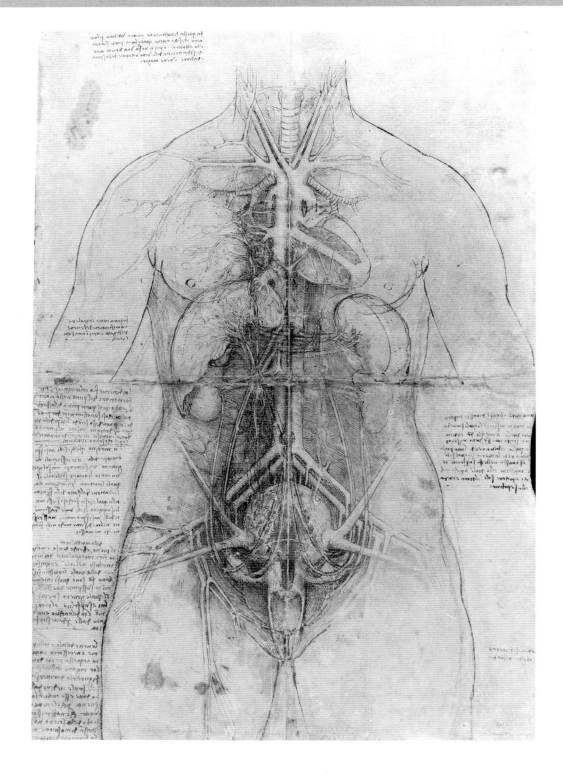

'Knowledge of the structure of the body is only a preparation for knowledge of the form'

Situs viscerum, Leonardo Da Vinci

1
Technical Considerations

Hedvig Hricak

Physical principles of MRI

Magnetic resonance imaging (MRI) is a nonionizing, computer-based technique which provides cross-sectional images. The underlying physical principles are founded in the fact that in a strong external magnetic field, nuclei with an odd number of protons or neutrons have a magnetic moment and will align with the external field.[1] Theoretically, imaging can be carried out with any atom which has a magnetic moment. However, because hydrogen is abundant in the human body, MRI is currently conducted almost exclusively with hydrogen nuclei (protons). By applying a specific (Larmor) radiofrequency (RF) pulse to the aligned protons, their magnetic moment can be flipped out of alignment with the main magnetic field. After the RF pulse is turned off, the protons gradually realign with the external magnetic field. While doing so, they emit energy at a frequency proportional to the field, and this energy can be detected and is the MR signal used to form the image.[1-3] Since the Larmor frequency is directly related to the strength of the magnetic field, spatial information can be obtained by shaping the main magnetic field with relatively small gradient fields in a known way, such that the given frequency can be equated with protons at a given point in space.

The MR image is produced by the application of many sets of RF pulses. Each pulse flips the protons through a known angle relative to the direction of the main magnetic field (eg, a 90° pulse flips aligned protons to a right angle with the main field). The time interval between the sets of RF pulses is called the **repetition time (TR)**. The time interval between the initial RF pulse in a sequence and the acquisition of the emitted RF pulse from the sample is called the **echo delay time (TE)**.

The physical characteristics of small volumes of tissue, called voxels, are translated by the computer into a two-dimensional image composed of pixels. On the MR image, the pixel **signal intensity** is influenced by both intrinsic, patient-related parameters (such as density of mobile hydrogen nuclei, T1 and T2 magnetic relaxation times, and motion) and extrinsic, instrument-related parameters (such as magnetic field strength, type of image acquisition, and choice of TR and TE acquisition parameters). The **T1 relaxation time** represents the time needed for protons to realign with the external magnetic field after having been tilted or flipped by an RF pulse. **T2 relaxation time** represents the time needed for protons to dephase with one another after the cessation of an RF pulse.[1-6] **T2★**, similar to T2, value reflects the time for nuclei that are resonating in phase to decay into random phase, but also has dependence on magnetic field inhomogeneity.

The resolving power of an MR image, often referred to as **image quality**, is a machine-determined ability to discriminate a lesion from its background.[7] In MRI, the resolving power of the image depends on signal-to-noise ratio, spatial resolution and tissue contrast. All three parameters—signal-to-noise ratio, spatial resolution and contrast resolution—are in part dependent on instrumentation. The vast array of options offered in MR instruments necessitates an understanding of the general principles of instrumentation.

Instrumentation

The following general components of an MR imaging system are illustrated in Figure 1.1:[8,9]

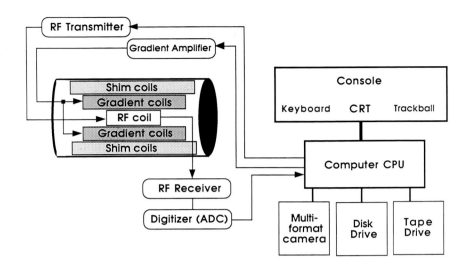

Figure 1.1

Schematic drawing of an MR imaging system. (CRT)–cathode ray tube; (CPU)–central processing unit; (ADC)–analog to digital converter.

(1) A **magnet** which generates the main external field (B_0).

(2) **Magnetic field gradients** which spatially encode the image information.

(3) **Radiofrequency coils** used for the transmission of RF pulses (the B_1 field) and for the reception of signals.

(4) The **computer** system controls the electronics of the MR system—the RF receiver, the RF transmitter, and the gradient power supplies. The computer system is also responsible for processing, display and storage of the resultant digital images.

(5) **Shimming coils** or iron which provide field homogeneity.

(6) **Ancillary devices** including consoles, RF and magnetic shielding, sliding table, and positioning devices and camera.

The magnet (the B_0 field)

The magnet needs to be large enough for a person to be positioned within the homogeneous portion of its field. Two important properties of magnets are the strength of the B_0 and the homogeneity of the field over the imaged volume. The strength of the magnetic field directly governs the intensity of the MR signal received. Field homogeneity influences the image quality. B_0 inhomogeneity of only a few parts per million (ppm) leads to noticeable shading of the MR image, especially when gradient-recall-echo (GRE) sequence is used. Any greater inhomogeneity of the B_0 field causes spatial distortion. A shimming procedure to improve homogeneity is therefore essential. **Shim coils** are electromagnetic coils which, by adjusting the amount of current passing through them, improve B_0 field homogeneity. The shimming coils can be located either within the bore of the magnet along with field gradient and RF coils, or incorporated into the main magnet.

Types of magnets

There are four types of magnets used in MRI devices: (1) permanent; (2) resistive; (3) hybrid; and (4) superconducting.

Permanent magnets Permanent magnets do not require electric power, have negligible fringe field, and have a field orientation transverse to the bore. Strength is presently limited to approximately 0.3 Tesla (T) for a 1 m bore magnet. Permanent magnets may weigh from 6 to 100 tons, depending on field strength. New materials are being investigated to increase field strength and/or reduce weight. In addition, advances are being made in the design of ultra-low magnetic field (0.03–0.1 T) imagers.

Resistive magnets Resistive magnets are air core magnets created by wrapping wire into coils around a bore. Although relatively inexpensive, resistive magnets require a great deal of electric power to run, and cooling, usually with circulating water, is also necessary. With present technology the field strength of resistive magnets is limited to about 0.2 T. The field homogeneity of these magnets, like that of permanent magnets, is sensitive to temperature.

Hybrid magnets These magnets are an attempt to combine the advantages of permanent and resistive magnets. They usually contain an iron core surrounded by electromagnets. They are lighter than permanent magnets and field strengths of 0.4 T have been achieved. Cooling is necessary, and field homogeneity is again sensitive to temperature changes.

Superconducting magnets Magnet coils made of nyobium titanium cooled with liquid helium (to 4.2 Kelvin) can conduct an electric current without resistance. Once started, superconducting magnets require no additional energy. Fields of 2 T, and even 4 T, have been achieved in full bore imagers. These devices have high field homogeneity and stability. Requirements for siting and cooling of these high field superconducting magnets are expensive, but they vary between the manufacturers.

Magnetic field gradients

Field gradients along the three orthogonal axes are fundamental to spatially encoding image information. Additional gradients along oblique axes can be achieved by combining the orthogonal gradients.[9] There are three important features of magnetic field gradients. First, the maximum gradient **amplitude**, or change in the magnetic field per unit of distance, expressed in Tesla/meter, limits the minimum slice thickness and affects the best achievable resolution. Second, uniformity of **slope** along the gradient axis also affects image quality; nonuniformity causes distortions. Finally, the '**rise time**', or the time for the gradient to be powered from zero to full amplitude, affects the speed at which echoes can be elicited.

Gradients are powered only during certain times of a pulse sequence. When gradients are switched on and off, electric eddy currents are induced in the magnet. These currents generate their own magnetic fields and produce image distortion. Self-shielded gradients are used to overcome this problem.[9]

Radiofrequency coils

Radiofrequency coils act as a broadcasting antenna, emitting RF pulses constituting the B_1 field at the proton Larmor frequency. Imagers may either have two RF antennas, one to transmit and one to receive, or a single antenna which can be switched between the transmit and receive modes. Signal amplifiers are an essential part of the RF system.

The size of the coil and the filling factor of the area of interest affect signal-to-noise ratio (see below). Most pelvic images are acquired with saddle-shaped or solenoid-whole body receiver coils. A surface coil improves signal-to-noise ratio, but its use is limited to superficial locations. The depth of penetration with a surface coil is proportional to its radius. Because the surface coil improves signal-to-noise ratio, it allows thinner slices without increasing imaging time. Low signal-to-noise ratio is usually compensated for by averaging several excitations (increasing NEX), but this maneuver increases imaging time.

The computer system

A modern MR system has several computers linked by a communications network. The mode of partitioning varies with the instrument used, but, in general, the computer has a main memory unit directly accessed by central processing units. The memory must be large enough to contain multiple data sets as well as operating software. In addition, an array processor is needed for speedy image reconstruction. Long-term memory storage is provided by tape or disk.

Ancillary devices

Console

A 'user friendly' design for the console adds to operating efficiency.

Radiofrequency shielding

The weak RF signal may be disturbed by interfering RF sources in the environment, for example, TV, radio, paging units, etc, and some form of insulation through RF shielding is required. RF shielding is usually incorporated in the walls, ceilings, and floor of the scan room and consists of copper or specially treated aluminum alloys.

Magnetic shielding

Magnetic shielding is needed not only to prevent disturbances to electric devices outside of the scan room, but also to preserve homogeneity of the field, which could be disturbed by large moving metallic objects such as cars or trucks.[8,9] There are three approaches to magnetic shielding. In the first approach, **external shielding** with iron is used to absorb the magnetic force. External shielding has to

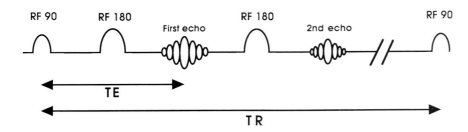

Figure 1.2

Pulse sequence for spin-echo imaging. (TE)–echo time; (TR)–repetition time.

be custom designed to meet the requirements of the individual site and magnet. The field strength outside the room must be 5 Gauss or less to meet Food and Drug Administration guidelines. In the second approach, **self-shielded magnets** have the shield incorporated into the device itself, by special designs individualized by the manufacturer for a particular model. This approach usually reduces external shielding requirements, but does not eliminate them. The third approach is **active shielding**, based on setting up an opposing external magnetic field diminishing other shielding needs.

Image acquisition (pulse sequence technique)

The MRI gray scale can be manipulated by the use of different image acquisition techniques. Slice selective excitations, frequency encoding, phase encoding, and image reconstruction are similar for all signal acquisitions. The type of signal acquisition does not affect spatial resolution. Contrast resolution, however, varies with different signal acquisitions. Techniques applied to pelvic imaging include spin-echo sequences,[10] fat saturation spin-echo sequences,[11] inversion recovery sequences,[12] and gradient-echo sequences.[9]

Spin-echo (SE) sequences

At present, spin echo (SE) is considered the standard technique for imaging the pelvis. In SE imaging an initial 90° RF pulse is followed by a 180° RF pulse. Subsequent 180° RF pulses are used for acquisition of multiple echoes, as shown in Figure 1.2. The TR for SE imaging is always longer than the time required for both excitation and signal detection in a single slice (TE). Therefore, the remaining time within each TR interval may be used for either excitation and detection in other slices (as in a multislice technique), or for additional 180° RF pulses applied to the same slice to obtain multiple echo images. As long as the number of multiple echoes and the number of slices desired is not longer than the TR of the sequence, there is no penalty. If there are too many multiple echoes, however, then the number of slices must be reduced. If it is necessary to maintain the length of coverage (number of slices) then the number of multiple echoes has to be decreased.

The effect of acquisition parameters on signal intensity of spin-echo images is illustrated in the following formula:

$$I = N(H)f(v)(1-e^{-TR/T1})e^{-TE/T2}$$

In this formula, N(H) is the MR visible mobile proton density, f(v) is an unspecified functional flow and e is the base of natural logarithms. This equation indicates that hydrogen density, T1, and T2 relaxation values influence the signal intensity relative to TR and TE (the instrument sequence parameters).

Fat saturation spin-echo (fatsat SE) sequences

Fat saturation spin-echo sequences differ from regular spin-echo sequences in that the magnetic moment of fat is saturated (zeroed) prior to the slice selective 90° RF pulse. The relative signal intensity of nonfat containing tissues is the same as on a standard spin-echo image. However, because there is no signal from fat (which is the brightest tissue on a conventional SE

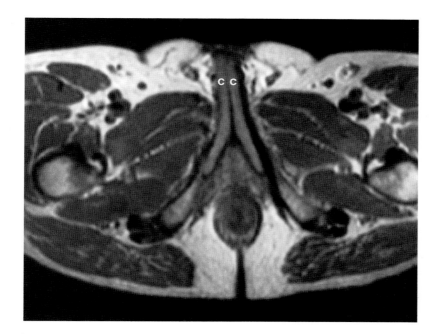

a

Figure 1.3

Conventional spin-echo (**a**) and fat saturation spin-echo (**b**) images through the male pelvis at the level of the corpora cavernosa (1.5 T; TR 2500/TE 20; 256 × 192; NEX 2; FOV 36; slice thickness 5 mm). The corpora cavernosa (cc) appear of higher signal intensity on the fat saturation image compared to the conventional spin echo, but signal intensity measurements are identical. Suppression of fat in the ischial bone marrow (open arrowhead), resulting in marrow of lower signal intensity, facilitates the differentiation of the corpora cavernosa, ischiocavernosus muscle (arrows) and ischium.

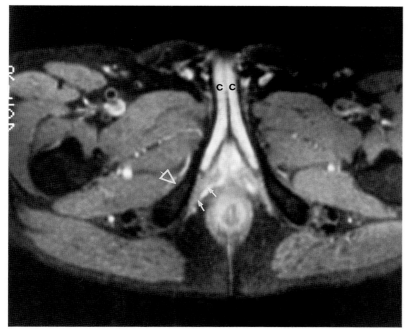

b

image), the computer gray scale is automatically readjusted. This results in a different visual impression of signal intensity, as shown in Figure 1.3. Because the bright signal from fat is removed, motion artifacts are less prominent and the signal-to-noise ratio is improved as seen in Figure 1.4. Signal intensity in a fatsat SE image is governed by the same equation as that for a standard SE sequence. At present, fat saturation SE sequences can be operator-dependent, and when improperly executed, can result not only in an uneven fat saturation but can cause water saturation as well, as seen in Figure 1.5.

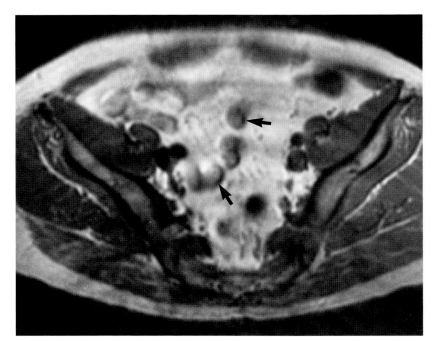

a

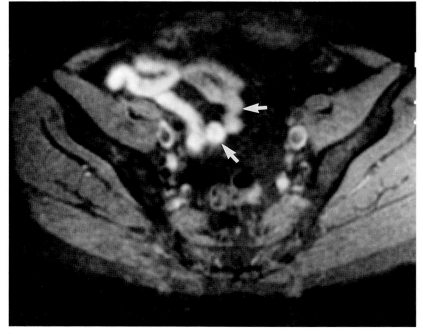

b

Figure 1.4

Noise suppression effect of fat saturation (1.5 T; TR 2500/TE 20; 256 × 192; NEX 2; FOV 36; slice thickness 5 mm): conventional spin-echo image (**a**), fat saturation spin-echo image (**b**). Delineation of small bowel (arrows) is improved on the fat saturation image.

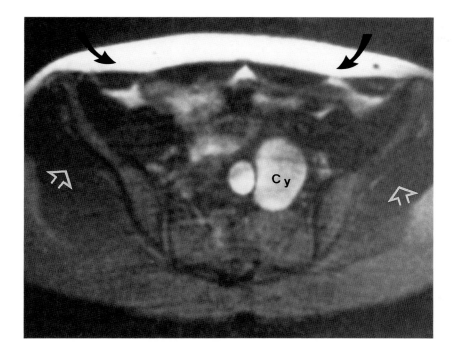

a

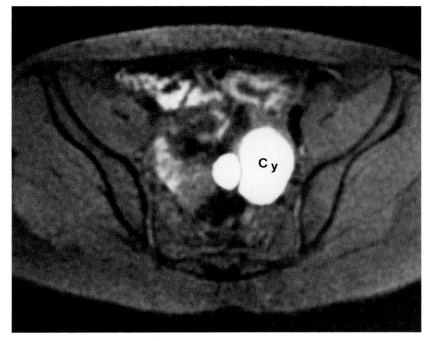

b

Figure 1.5

Operator dependence of fat saturation technique. Both (**a**) and (**b**) have the same scan parameters (TR 700/TE 15; 256 × 192; NEX 2; FOV 36; slice thickness 5 mm). (**a**) When improperly executed (center frequency not set on fat), not all fat tissue will saturate (curved arrows) and even water saturation may result as seen by lower signal intensity of the muscle (open arrowheads). Respiratory artifacts through the ovarian cysts (Cy) are pronounced. (**b**) Properly performed study, center frequency set on fat.

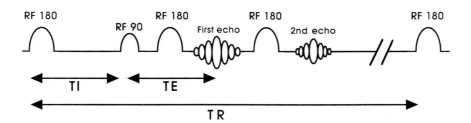

Figure 1.6

Pulse sequence for inversion recovery imaging. (TI)–inversion time; (TE)–echo time; (TR)–repetition time.

Inversion recovery (IR) sequences

Inversion recovery sequences can be used for obtaining heavily T1-weighted images. As shown in Figure 1.6, the initial RF pulse in this technique is 180°, and it is followed by a 90° RF pulse and the signal obtained. The period of time between the two pulses, which allows for magnetization recovery, is called inversion time (TI).

Signal intensities on inversion recovery images differ from those on spin-echo images. The initial 180° pulse flip inverts the nuclei around the zero line. During the time TI the nuclei are relaxing so that the following 90° pulse excites nuclei at different levels, emphasizing TI tissue differences.

Inversion recovery is a tailored sequence used to the best advantage where inherent tissue contrast variables are limited, for example, brain or liver (the only required tissue difference is lesion versus normal tissue). In such a clinical setting, the choice of TI will govern the signal intensity of the tissue to be studied. The equation for choosing the TI is $\ln(2) \times$ T1 of the tissue to be studied (to be of very low signal intensity). The recommended choice of TR for the IR sequence is long in order to allow full remagnetization (T1 recovery) to occur. The use of short TR reduces the advantages of IR and such images are similar to T1-weighted SE (see Figure 1.7). The disadvantage of IR sequences is that the inclusion of TI limits the number of slices obtained, so for large area coverage, increased imaging time is a problem.

In the pelvis, the number of tissue variables is considerably greater than in the liver or brain, making the use of IR in the pelvis limited. As illustrated in Figure 1.8 with a long TR, if the TI of 320 is chosen, because T1 of the muscle on 1.5 T is 600 msec, this sequence will affect muscle signal intensity (void of signal). If, however, with the same TR/TE parameters, the TI is 100 msec (T1 of the fat on 1.5 T is 180 msec), the intensity of the fat will be mostly affected, while the muscle and urine now demonstrate higher signal intensity.

Gradient-recall-echo (GRE) sequences

As shown in Figure 1.9, gradient-recall-echo (GRE) sequences do not employ a 180° RF pulse, and the initial RF pulses can be changed to any angle of 90° or less. Following the initial slices' selective RF pulse the application of a magnetic field gradient dephases the nuclei, and reversal of the same gradient rephases them, creating an echo.

Gradient-recall-echo images are more susceptible than spin-echo images to magnetic field inhomogeneity and presence of motion. Therefore, artifacts such as those caused by metallic implants (Figure 1.10) or motion (Figure 1.11) are more pronounced. In addition, in gradient-echo sequences the signal intensity for a given TE is a function of the T2* value rather than the T2 value, emphasizing tissues with short T2*. In addition to TR and TE parameters, the signal intensity per pixel also depends on the angle of the RF pulse chosen. As illustrated in Figure 1.12, on scans performed with the same TE value, low angle values increased T2-weighting whereas high angle values increased T1-weighting. As seen in Figure 1.13, at very short TR values, regardless of the angle, the image appears to be T2 over T1-weighted, so that the tissues with long T2 values, such as liquids, appear bright.

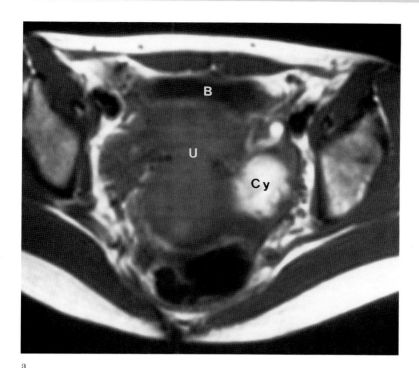

a

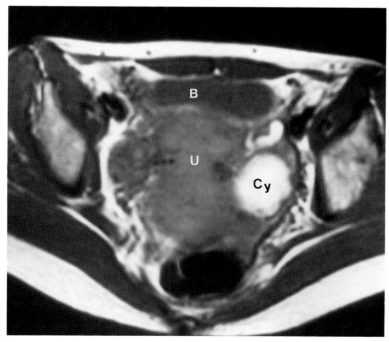

b

Figure 1.7

Inversion recovery sequence with a short TR. Transaxial image of female pelvis: (**a**) spin-echo TR 600/TE 20 (slice thickness 5 mm; FOV 36; matrix 256 × 192; NEX 2: identical for both sequences); (**b**) inversion recovery TR 600/TE 20; TI 50. On the inversion recovery image with a very short TR and TI the signal intensity ratio stays similar to spin echo. There is no benefit to this set of IR parameters. The disadvantage, however, is the smaller number of slices. (B)–bladder; (U)–uterus; (Cy)–hemorrhagic cyst.

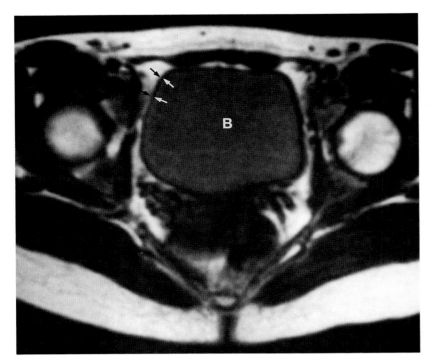

a

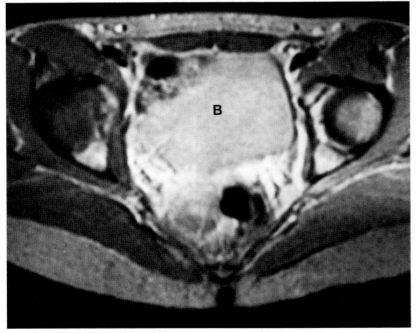

b

Figure 1.8

Inversion recovery with a long TR. Transaxial images of female pelvis: (**a**) inversion recovery TR 1500/TE 20; TI 320; (**b**) inversion recovery TR 1500/TE 20; TI 100. Altering TI affects signal intensity so in image (**a**) muscle is of low signal intensity and the muscle–fat interface is accentuated as shown at the bladder wall–fat interface (arrows). In (**b**), with TI of 100, muscle and urine are of higher signal intensity while fat is nulled. (B)–bladder.

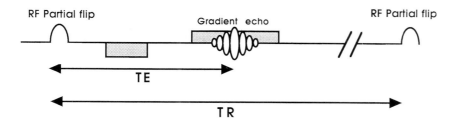

Figure 1.9

Pulse sequence for gradient-recall-echo image. (TE)–echo time; (TR)–repetition time.

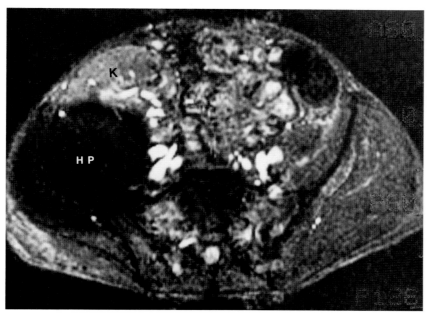

a

Figure 1.10

Hip prosthesis with increased artifacts on gradient-recall-echo image. Artifact due to metal hip prosthesis (HP) is more pronounced on (**a**) gradient-recall-echo image (TR 33/TE 13; angle 70°) than on (**b**) spin-echo image (TR 2000/TE 20). The visualization of the transplant kidney (K) is obscured on the GRE image.

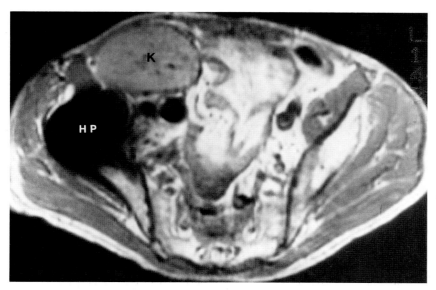

b

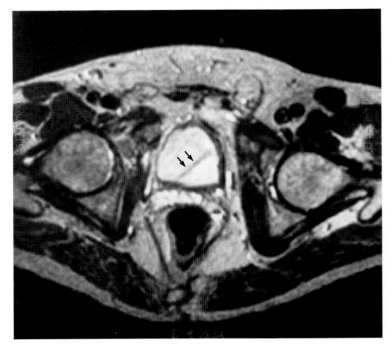

a

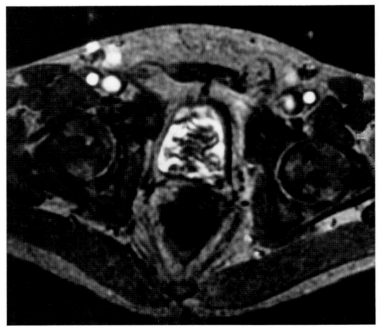

b

Figure 1.11

Motion artifact due to urine 'jet' phenomenon (**a**) 1.5 T with 5 mm slice thickness. T2-weighted spin-echo image (TR 2500/TE 70) (**b**) GRE image (TR 33/TE 13; angle 70°). Turbulence in bladder due to urine 'jet' entering from the ureteric orifice seen as low signal intensity line (arrows) on the T2-weighted image. The effect of turbulence is more pronounced on the GRE image, resulting in a large heterogeneous artifact within the bladder.

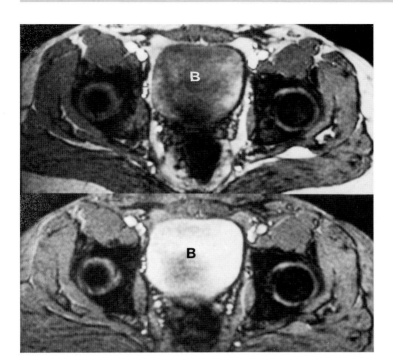

Figure 1.12

The effect of high (90°) (top image) and low (20°) (bottom image) angle on tissue signal intensity. TR (300) and TE (20) were kept constant. High angle values (top) increase T1-weighted sensitivity resulting in urine (B) of lower signal intensity, while lower angle values (bottom) increase T2-weighted sensitivity, resulting in urine (B) of higher signal intensity.

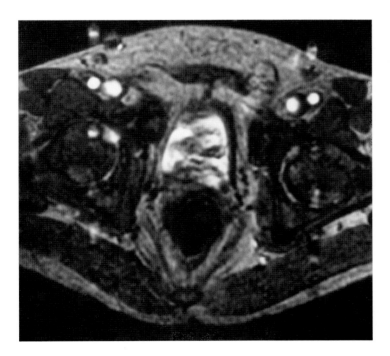

Figure 1.13

GRE sequence with an angle of 90° but short TR (33) demonstrates that despite a large flip angle, the very short TR causes T2 over T1-weighting and tissue with an inherent high T2/T1 ratio, eg urine appears of high signal intensity. Note that a difference in angle of only 20° between Figures 1.11b and 1.13 causes no appreciable difference in signal intensity.

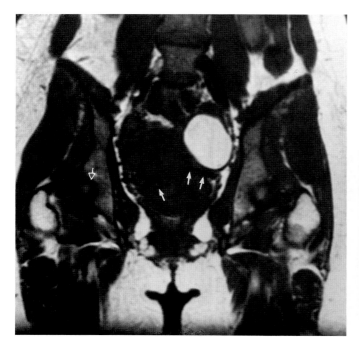

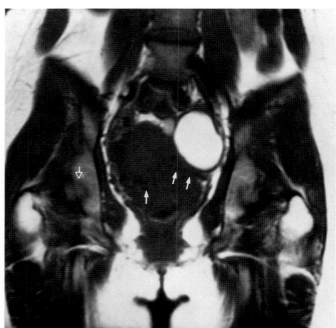

a   b

Figure 1.14

Effect of slice thickness on signal-to-noise level and spatial resolution (TR 500 msec, TE 20 msec, matrix 256 × 192, NEX 2, FOV 32 cm). The slice thickness of image (**a**) was 4 mm, and of image (**b**), 10 mm. By increasing the slice thickness, the signal-to-noise ratio is improved resulting in a smoother image, but the spatial resolution is decreased as exemplified by the indistinct uterine vessels (small arrows) and the pronounced partial volume effect, making the femoral head indistinct on the 10 mm section but clearly seen on the 4 mm section (open arrow).

Image quality

Three factors influence the quality of the images acquired by any sequencing technique: (1) signal-to-noise ratio (SNR); (2) spatial resolution; and (3) contrast resolution. Signal-to-noise ratio affects the 'graininess' of an image, spatial resolution refers to the sharpness of the boundaries between tissues, and contrast resolution refers to the differences in signal intensity among varying tissues. There are many factors which affect these three elements, and these can be manipulated alone or in combination to achieve optimal choices regarding parameter selection and imaging acquisition time. The number of averages (NEX) affects only SNR. However, matrix size, slice thickness, and field-of-view affect both SNR and spatial resolution. For example, increasing the matrix size decreases signal-to-noise ratio, but increases spatial resolution. Increasing the field-of-view, on the other hand, increases the signal-to-noise ratio, but decreases spatial resolution. Attempts to decrease acquisition time usually result in decreased signal-to-noise ratio. Acquisition time can be calculated using the following simple equation:

number of slices × matrix size in phase encoding direction × NEX × TR

Understanding these trade-offs is essential in designing optimal imaging sequences.

Signal-to-noise ratio (SNR)

The intensity of a given pixel in an MR image reflects the amplitude of MR signal received from the corresponding voxel. There is, however, a noise factor inherent in the acquisition of the signal and the quality of the final MR image depends on the ratio of the

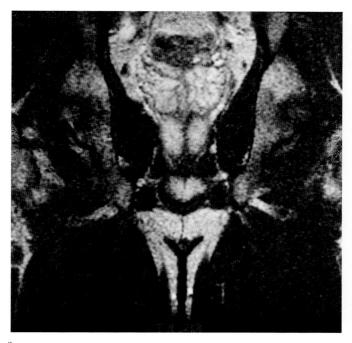

a

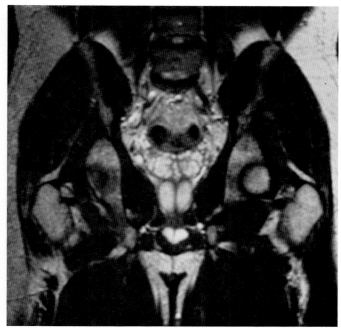

b

Figure 1.15

Effect on signal-to-noise ratio of changing field-of-view (1.5 T; TR 2500/TE 70; matrix 256 × 192; NEX 2; slice thickness 5 mm). (**a**) Field-of-view 24 cm. (**b**) Field-of-view 36 cm.

Increasing the field-of-view results in higher signal-to-noise ratio and the image is less grainy. However, the penalty is a decrease in spatial resolution.

signal amplitude to that of noise (the signal-to-noise ratio). Both extrinsic factors (related to field strength and to operator-controlled instrument parameters) and intrinsic factors (patient-related parameters such as proton density, T1 and T2 values, and movement) affect the SNR.

Extrinsic instrument parameters affecting SNR include field strength, TR, TE, slice thickness, number of excitations (NEX), field-of-view, and matrix size. The larger the external field (B_0) the higher the signal-to-noise ratio. The SNR also rises with the length of TR. As shown in Figures 1.14 and 1.15, increased slice thickness (Figure 1.14) and increased field-of-view in the phase encoding direction (Figure 1.15) both produce increases in the SNR. The SNR also rises with the square root of the number of signal acquisitions (for example, doubling the SNR requires four times the NEX), as illustrated in Figure 1.16. Increasing TE or spatial resolution, on the other hand, results in a reduction of the signal-to-noise ratio.

Intrinsic (patient-related) parameters such as proton density and T1 and T2 relaxation time affect the signal part of the signal-to-noise ratio. Movement—cardiac, respiratory, vascular, gastrointestinal (peristalsis), or voluntary—increases the noise part of the signal-to-noise ratio.

Spatial resolution

Spatial resolution depends on three instrument-controlled parameters: (1) matrix size; (2) slice thickness; and (3) field-of-view. In general, increases in slice thickness or in the field-of-view decrease spatial resolution; and increases in the matrix size increase the spatial resolution. Increasing slice thickness decreases spatial resolution by decreasing the ability to discern small elements and increasing the artifact from partial volume averaging, as seen in Figure 1.14. Increasing

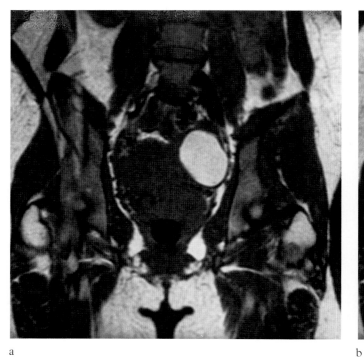

a

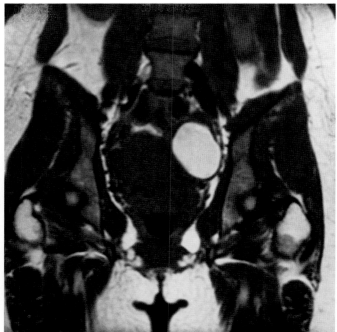

b

Figure 1.16

Effect on signal-to-noise ratio by changing NEX. Doubling the signal-to-noise ratio by increasing NEX from 1 on image (**a**), to 4 on image (**b**), and keeping all the other imaging parameters equal (SE TR 500/TE 20, matrix 256 × 192, FOV 32 cm, slice thickness 4 mm). By increasing the number of excitations, the signal-to-noise ratio improves, resulting in a smoother image (**b**), but there is a time penalty (1:43 minutes for image (**a**) versus 6:27 minutes for image (**b**)).

---

the field-of-view while keeping the matrix size constant increases the voxel size, which results in a decrease in spatial resolution, as illustrated in Figure 1.15. Increasing the matrix size, from 256 × 128 to 256 × 256 for example, doubles the number of views and decreases voxel size by a factor of 2. This maneuver doubles the spatial resolution in the phase encoding direction of the image. Using the same principle as shown in Figure 1.17, increasing the matrix size concomitantly with decreasing the field-of-view will result in improved spatial resolution, and if the number of NEX is also increased, the loss of signal-to-noise will be compensated for.

Contrast resolution

Contrast resolution is the ability to discern differences in tissue signal intensity. Because MR signal intensity is a function of patient-related parameters as well as instrument parameters, tissue contrast can be manipulated by selection of imaging parameters.[13] As illustrated in Figure 1.18, changing TR and TE parameters on a spin-echo sequence can be used to demonstrate how manipulating imaging parameters changes signal intensity and influences contrast resolution.

Images acquired with short TR and TE times, called **T1-weighted images**, emphasize the differences

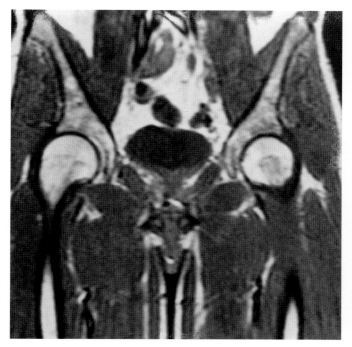

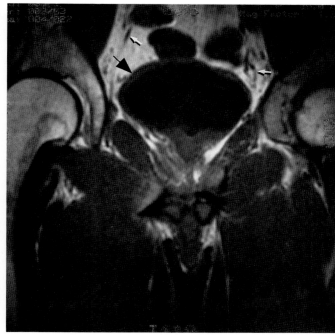

a

b

Figure 1.17

Effect of increased number of excitations, increased matrix size and decreased field-of-view (1.5 T; TR 600/TE 20; slice thickness 4 mm): (**a**) matrix 256 × 128, FOV 36, NEX 1; (**b**) matrix 256 × 192, FOV 24, NEX 2. Image (**b**) has better spatial resolution because of a smaller field-of-view and increased matrix, in addition to better signal-to-noise ratio because of doubling the number of excitations. This allows improved visualization of the bladder wall (large arrow), perivesical tissue and branches of the internal iliac vessels (black and white small arrows).

between T1 tissue relaxation times, as seen in Figure 1.18a. Signal intensity on these T1-weighted images is directly related to the degree of magnetization. Tissues with short T1 values, such as fat, demonstrate high signal intensity because of the rapid rate of magnetization recovery after an RF pulse. Tissues with longer T1 relaxation times, such as urine or muscle, demonstrate low signal intensity because of their slower rate of magnetization recovery. As illustrated in Figure 1.18b, the shorter the T1, the greater the percentage of the magnetization factor that returns in the longitudinal plane before the next pulse, and, therefore, the more signal will be generated.

If the TR value is long enough, more than four times the T1 value of the tissue being studied, there is almost complete T1 relaxation recovery between repetitions. If the TE is kept short (much less than the T2 value), an image acquired with long TR reflects differences in proton density, and is referred to as a **proton density image** (Figure 1.18c).

When both the TR and TE values are long, differences in T2 tissue relaxation times are emphasized, as depicted in Figure 1.18d, and the image is referred to as a **T2-weighted image.** This occurs because as the TE lengthens there is loss of coherence in the transverse plane and the signal intensity

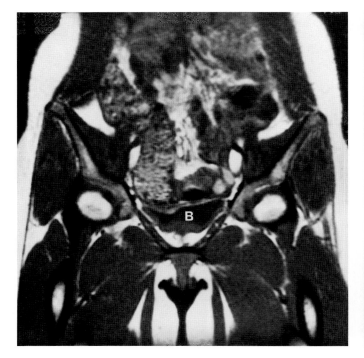

a

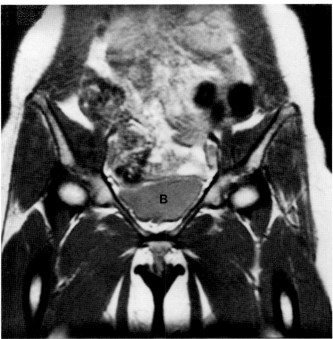

c

b

Figure 1.18

Tissue contrast resolution as a function of TR and TE instrument parameters; 1.5 T. (**a**) T1-weighted image. (**b**) Schematic drawing illustrating the relation between signal intensity and TR for tissues with a short (eg, fat) or long (eg, urine, muscle) T1 value.

(**c**) Proton density image. (**d**) T2-weighted image. (**e**) Schematic drawing illustrating the relation between signal intensity and TE for tissues with short (eg, muscle) and long (eg, urine) T2 value. (B)–bladder.

---

decreases exponentially. On a T2-weighted image the signal from every tissue decays, which is why a T2-weighted image has a lower signal-to-noise level than a proton density image with the same TR. Tissues with short T2 values decay faster than those with long T2 values, as illustrated in Figure 1.18e. For example, the signal from muscle, which characteristically has a very short T2 value, decays quickly and muscle images with low signal intensity on T2-weighted scans. The signal from urine, on the other hand, which has a long T2

value, decays relatively slowly, and urine images with high signal intensity on these scans (Figure 1.18d).

Tissue that appears dark regardless of the TR/TE selection generally has low hydrogen content, long T1, and short T2 relaxation values; or is in motion during signal acquisition. Tissues with a low hydrogen density include calcified tissues, cortical bone, and air. Tissue with a long T1 value and a short T2 value, such as muscle, images with low signal intensity on both T1- and T2-weighted images (Figures 1.18a and

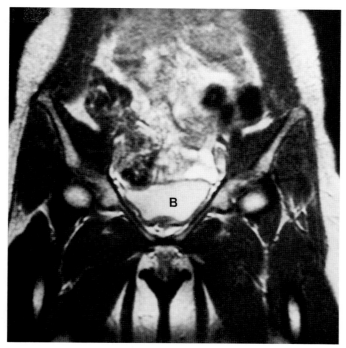

d

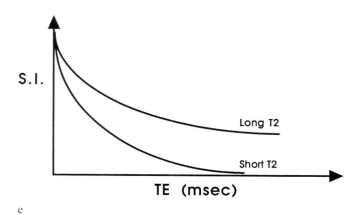

e

orientation, and the presence or absence of turbulence (see also the discussion of vascular motion artifact below).

Artifacts

Chemical-shift artifact

Although the majority of the MR signal comes from the hydrogen nuclei of water molecules, lipid protons in fatty tissue also contribute. Because fat and water protons do not resonate at the same frequency (fat protons resonate at a frequency 3 ppm higher than water), the difference between the two creates a 'chemical-shift artifact'.[16] The chemical-shift artifact is always seen along the readout (frequency encoded) axis relative to water, as seen in Figures 1.19, 1.20 and 1.21.

The absolute frequency difference depends on the strength of the main magnetic field. For example, at 0.35 T (15 megahertz [MHz] resonating frequency), a 3 ppm chemical shift results in fat resonating at a frequency 45 hertz (Hz) higher than water. At 1.5 T (64 MHz frequency), however, fat resonates at a frequency 192 Hz higher than water. Assuming that all instrument parameters are the same, the frequency difference due to the chemical shift between fat and water is comparable to the frequency difference across 2.4 pixels at 1.5 T and only half a pixel at 0.35 T. In addition to being more noticeable at higher magnetic fields, the chemical-shift artifact is also increased when the strength of the gradient field is reduced. Therefore, when MR systems of the lower or medium magnetic field strengths use weaker gradients with consequent increase in signal-to-noise ratio, acquired images will suffer from increased chemical-shift artifact,[17] as seen in Figure 1.21. Changing the bandwidth at any magnetic field strength affects chemical-shift artifact.[17] The effect of different bandwidth at 1.5 T is seen in Figure 1.22.

1.18d). Tissue with a relatively short T1 value and a long T2 value, such as fat, images with high signal intensity on both T1- and T2-weighted scans (Figures 1.18a and 1.18d). Tissue with a long TR and a long T2, such as urine, images with low signal intensity on T1-weighted images and high signal intensity on T2-weighted images. The signal intensity of flowing blood is a complex problem which, in spite of many studies, is still not fully understood.[14,15] It is affected by TR, TE, velocity of flow, direction of flow relative to slice

Motion artifact

Cardiac, respiratory, vascular, gastrointestinal (peristalsis), or voluntary patient motion cause artifacts in magnetic resonance imaging.[17,18] It is essential to understand and recognize motion artifacts in order to avoid diagnostic errors. Physiologic motion results in increased noise, increased edge blurring, and streak artifacts. Motion artifact is more pronounced in MR imaging than in CT because the MRI sampling process is relatively long. The sampling process is especially

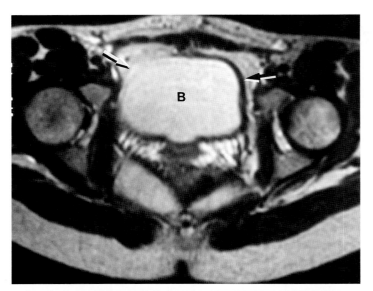

Figure 1.19

Chemical-shift artifact at 1.5 T (T2-weighted image TR 2000/ TE 60). The chemical-shift artifact causes the left lateral bladder wall to appear abnormally thickened and of low signal intensity (arrow), with corresponding high signal intensity causing the right bladder wall to appear to be absent (arrow). (B)–bladder.

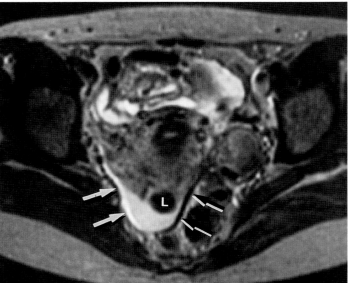

Figure 1.20

Example of chemical-shift artifact at the interface between fluid in the cul-de-sac and adjacent extraperitoneal fat (arrows). (L)–leiomyoma. (1.5 T, TR 2000/TE 60).

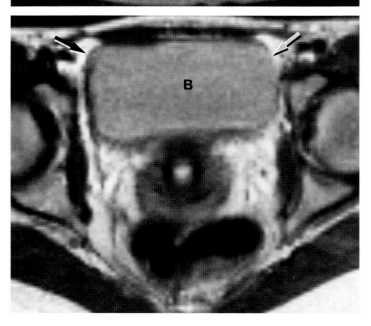

Figure 1.21

Chemical shift at 0.35 T. At medium field strength, chemical-shift artifact at the bladder/fat interface (arrows) is pronounced due to the use of weaker gradients. Note that the polarity of the readout gradient is opposite to Figure 1.19. (B)– bladder.

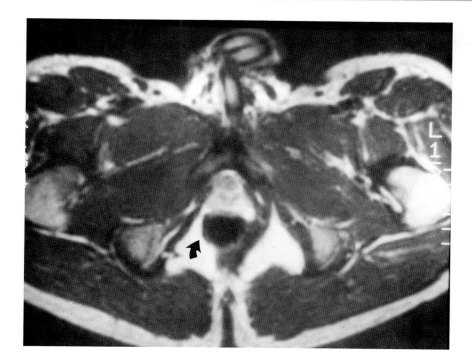

a

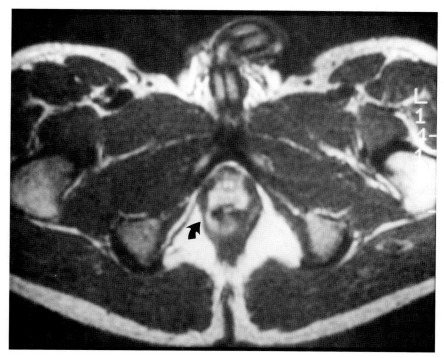

b

Figure 1.22
Change in thickness of chemical-shift artifact (1.5 T) as a function of change in bandwidth at 1.5 T. (**a**) Narrow bandwidth—pronounced chemical-shift artifact (arrow). (**b**) Wide bandwidth—chemical-shift artifact less pronounced (arrow).

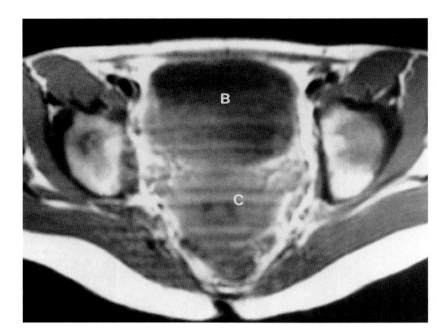

Figure 1.23

Respiratory motion artifact in the pelvis at the level of the cervix (C) degrading image quality. (B)–bladder.

long (on the order of minutes) in the phase encoding direction, and that is where motion artifacts are most common. Of the types of motion mentioned above, cardiac motion does not usually affect pelvis imaging, and cardiac gating is not necessary.

Respiratory motion

Respiratory motion is transmitted to the pelvis via abdominal muscles and bowel, and does affect pelvic images, as shown in Figure 1.23. The resulting artifacts are increased noise and edge blurring, seen in the phase encoding direction. **Respiratory gating** or **respiratory compensation** is necessary to improve the image quality.[18] The improved overall image resolution achieved by applying respiratory compensation is shown in Figure 1.24. In the respiratory compensation technique, motion artifact is reduced by continuous monitoring of the respiratory cycle via a signal from a pressure transducer placed around the patient's abdomen. Compensation is then applied to phase encoding to minimize brightness variation. Respiratory compensation is favored over respiratory gating, because the selection of TR is considerably constrained in the latter.

Vascular motion

Vascular motion—blood flow—is faster than respiratory motion, and the time between the excitation pulse and detection is sufficient for the blood protons to experience a substantial displacement, causing a **phase mismatch**. In a phase mismatch, protons moving at different velocities have different phases at the time of the spin echo. This causes loss (**flow void**) due to phase disbursing within the voxel. Because blood flow velocities vary throughout the cardiac cycle, phase mismatches can cause ghosting in the phase encoding direction if the phase shift varies from view to view. Flow artifacts are particularly prominent on axial images, where much of the intraluminal signal intensity is from so-called '**flow-related enhancement**'. This phenomenon is a function of the slice location and the direction of the flow relative to the order in which the slices are excited. If flow runs into the advancing slices, even the inner slice can have substantial flow-related enhancement.

The phase ghosting artifact can be eliminated by the use of **spatial presaturation (SAT)** or **flow compensation technique**.[19,20] In SAT, saturation is achieved by applying an RF pulse before the slice selection, flipping the moving spins into the transverse plane,

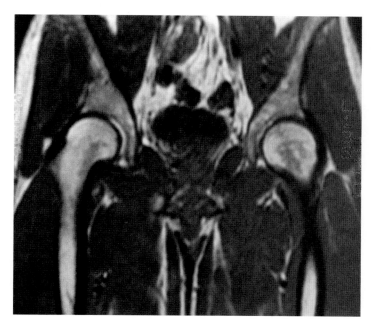

a

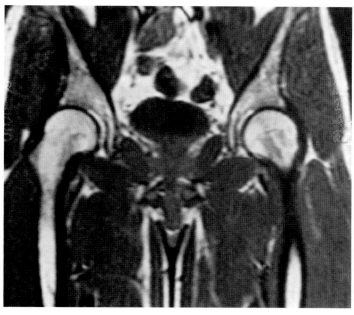

b

Figure 1.24

Respiratory motion (1.5 T; TR 600/TE 20; NEX 1; matrix 256 × 128; slice thickness 5 mm). (**a**) No respiratory compensation. (**b**) Respiratory compensation. Use of respiratory compensation markedly improves image quality.

and then applying a gradient pulse to dephase them. By applying SAT, the moving spins are saturated before they enter the imaging volume, thus suppressing the flow-related enhancement effect. Because the moving spins have no signal, the technique is also helpful in distinguishing between patent and obstructed vessels. SAT provides a complete flow void in patent vessels as seen in Figure 1.25a. One of the drawbacks of SAT is that it increases excitation time, and reduces the number of slices per unit of time.

Flow compensation, or **gradient moment nulling**, is achieved by applying extra gradient pulses so that the phase at the time of the echo delay is exactly zero for both moving and stationary spins. As a result, vessels

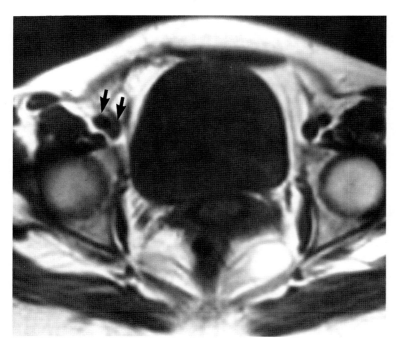

a

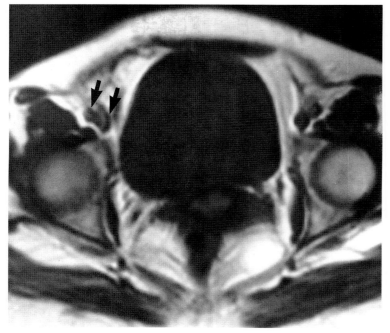

b

Figure 1.25

Compensation for flow-related artifacts (1.5 T, TR 500/TE 30). (**a**) Spatial presaturation (SAT). (**b**) Flow compensation (flow comp). The use of SAT provides a flow void in patent vessels (arrows), while the use of flow comp results in medium signal intensity in the vessel lumen (arrows). The latter precludes differentiation between flowing blood and thrombus.

image with high signal intensity in plane flow or moderate intensity in density flow perpendicular to the imaging plane. Although flow compensation improves image quality by decreasing motion artifacts, the bright signal of the vessels may mask a vascular obstruction, precluding differentiation between flow-ing blood and thrombus as seen in Figure 1.25b. The flow compensation technique also requires an increase in the minimum TE, since the additional balancing gradients require an extra five milliseconds. This translates to a minimum TE of 30 milliseconds when flow compensation is used.

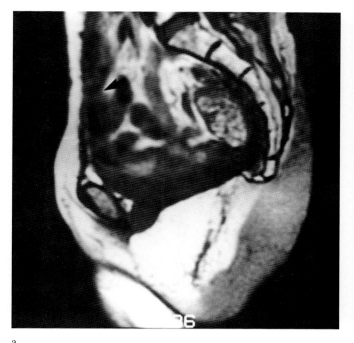

a

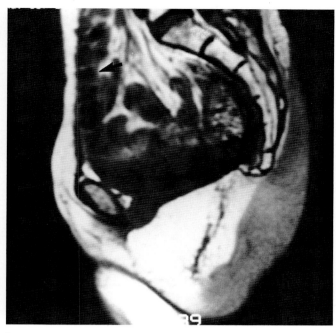

b

Figure 1.26

Use of glucagon to decrease motion artifacts due to peristalsis. (**a**) Without glucagon. (**b**) After 1 mg glucagon intramuscularly. Following the glucagon injection, details of the bowel wall (arrows) are better visualized.

Figure 1.27

Bowel and flow motion causing artifact in phase-encoding direction on coronal image through bladder (TR 2500, TE 20). The image degradation results in blurring of the bladder dome (B) compared to its inferior portion where the bladder wall is clearly seen (arrows).

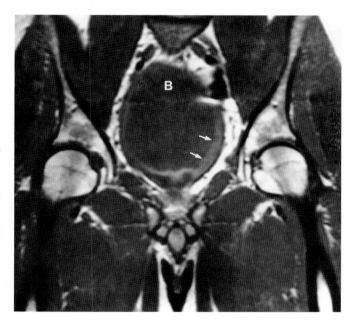

Peristalsis

Gastrointestinal motion causes significant image degradation in the pelvis by obscuring the tissue planes of the urinary bladder, female and male genital organs, and rectum. As seen in Figure 1.26, artifact from peristalsis can be diminished by the prescan administration of glucagon (1 mg intramuscularly).[21] However, combined bowel motion and flow artifact can be seen in spite of using compensation techniques as seen in Figure 1.27.

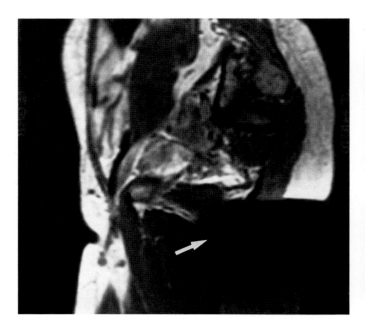

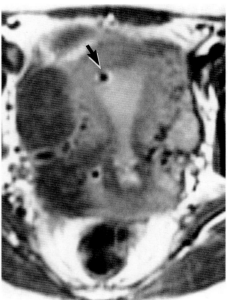

Figure 1.28

Artifact due to safety pin.

Figure 1.29

Metal particle in the uterine cavity (arrow) shed from curette during D & C procedure (1.5 T, TR 2000, TE 20).

Ferromagnetic artifacts

Except for intracranial vascular clips, most ferromagnetic implants can be imaged safely (see also Chapter 3). However, they will cause image artifacts which are usually proportional to the degree of ferromagnetism and to the mass of the object.[22,23] The artifact, shown in Figure 1.28, is typically seen as a round zone of signal void bordered by a circumscribed halo of hyperintensity that fades peripherally. Recognition of the signal aberration as ferromagnetic artifact is usually straightforward. Ferromagnetic particles, shown in Figure 1.29, may be mistaken for calcifications or hemorrhagic residue, and it is important to recognize this appearance as artifact.

Even metal implants without measurable ferromagnetic properties can produce image artifacts. These artifacts are similar to, but less extensive than, those produced by ferromagnetic material of comparable mass as seen in Figure 1.30. They are caused by local eddy currents which are induced by nonferromagnetic conductors in response to changing magnetic fields. In turn, these small currents produce their own electromagnetic fields which can distort the main magnetic field to degrade image quality locally (Figure 1.30).

Instrument-related artifacts

Radiofrequency and gradient coil interference

RF noise (from the patient, the system hardware, or from extrinsic sources) can degrade the MR image. Patient-generated noise is caused by low level eddy currents from the thermal motion of ions in tissue. These currents produce time-varying magnetic fields which represent background noise and limit the resolving power of the MR imager. System hardware which can produce RF interference artifact includes gradient coils, transmitter coils, and amplifiers. Malfunction of system hardware often results in an image artifact with a specific geometric pattern, such as a herring bone pattern. Time-varying magnetic fields such as those produced by the gradient coils can induce currents within the main magnetic field called eddy currents. The types of artifacts that will result from eddy currents are bonded and occur mostly at the periphery of the images. Eddy current artifacts are most commonly observed in GRE sequences. An example of eddy current on GRE sequences is illustrated in Figure 1.31. The use of shielded gradient

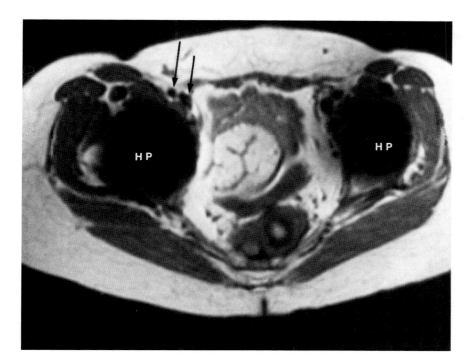

Figure 1.30

Bilateral nonferromagnetic hip prostheses (HP) cause signal voids. There is only minor degradation of image quality resulting in shadowing around the prosthesis. Visualization of adjacent external iliac vessels (arrows) is still possible.

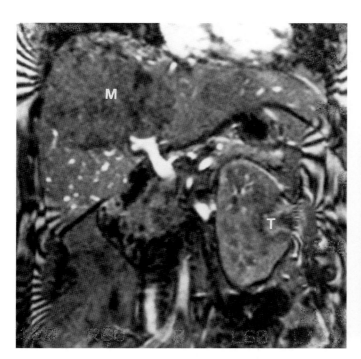

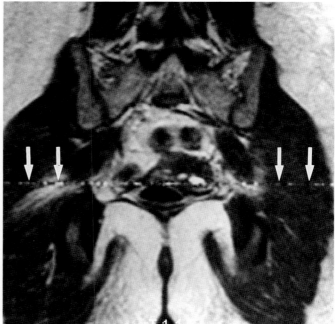

Figure 1.31

Artifact due to eddy currents (1.5 T, GRE TR 33, TE 13) on gradient-recall-echo image. (M)–liver metastasis, (T)–renal tumor.

Figure 1.32

Extrinsic radiofrequency noise causing linear artifact (arrows) along the phase encoding direction.

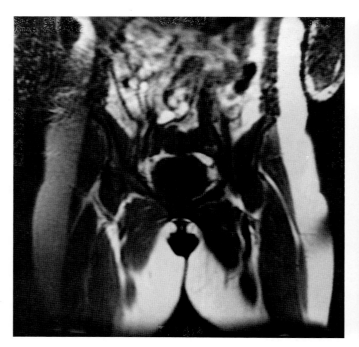

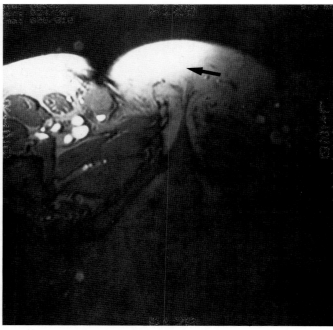

Figure 1.33

Uneven signal intensity
between subcutaneous tissue on
the right and left side caused by
RF coil inhomogeneity.
Shading, also seen at the
bottom of the image.

Figure 1.34

Nonuniformity of surface coil
image. The area near the
conductor of the surface coil
(arrow) produces the highest
signal intensity with a drop in
signal intensity beyond the
diameter of the coil.

coils alleviates this problem to a large extent. Extrinsic
RF noise produces a characteristic, discrete linear
artifact most commonly in a phase encoding direction
as shown in Figure 1.32. Less commonly, the artifact
will be a bend-like projection oriented along the
frequency encoded direction (see Figure 1.33).

Inhomogeneous RF signal reception

Lack of uniformity across the RF coil also produces
image artifact. In superconducting magnets, RF coils
that surround a patient consist of at least two saddle
sections, one above and one below the patient. The coil
is most sensitive to tissue near the four long straight
parts of the saddles, and these areas produce bright
regions on images. The center of the coil is the least
sensitive region, producing areas that are dimmer than
the surrounding ones. **Quadrature coils** produce a
more uniform image because they add at least two
saddles at the right and left of the patient, producing
eight sensitive areas. More complicated coils have even
more conductors and give even better uniformity
across the coil. Since all coils lose sensitivity along
their axes as the end of the coil is approached, sagittal
and coronal images are dimmer at the top and bottom
of the coil as seen in Figure 1.33. **Surface coils** have
the most extreme nonuniformity.[24] Due to their design
they are sensitive near the surface of the patient and
are insensitive to regions deeper than the diameter of
the coil. Areas near the conductor of the surface coil
produce the highest intensity signal as shown in Figure
1.34. A circular coil produces a ring-shaped area of
bright tissue.

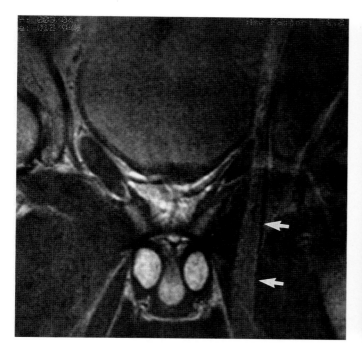

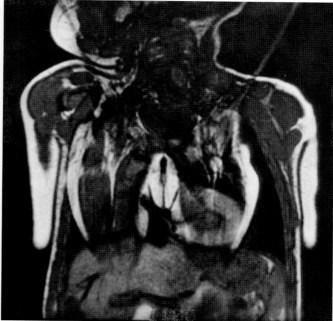

Figure 1.35

Wrap-around artifact in the phase encoding direction (arrows) due to choice of too small a field-of-view. The artifact is unilateral since the patient was postioned asymmetrically within the magnet.

Figure 1.36

Aliasing artifact in the frequency encoding direction in the coronal plane. The patient's pelvis is projected over his chest.

Aliasing

This artifact is seen when the selected field-of-view is smaller than the anatomic area which is excited, and structures that extend peripherally are aliased or 'wrapped around' on the opposite edge of a cross-sectional image.[24] Aliasing can be seen in either the phase (see Figure 1.35) or the frequency encoding direction as shown in Figure 1.36.

Partial volume averaging

Partial volume averaging occurs because cross-sectional imaging is a two-dimensional representation of a three-dimensional section of tissue. As a result, the volume of tissue represented by each pixel has an additional dimension—the slice thickness. The gray scale level of any individual pixel is determined by the average signal intensity of the anatomic components contained within the corresponding voxel. Partial volume averaging is more pronounced when thick section slices are used (see Figure 1.14).

References

1 ABRAGAM A, *The Principles of Nuclear Magnetism*, (Oxford University Press: New York 1961).

2 LAUTERBUR PC, Image formation by induced local interactions: examples employing nuclear magnetic resonance, *Nature* (1973) **242**:190.

3 CROOKS LE, ARAKAWA M, HOENNINGER JC et al, NMR whole body imager operating at 3.5 kGauss, *Radiology* (1982) **143**:169.

4 ERNST RR, BODENHAUSEN G, WOKAUN A, *Principles of Nuclear Magnetic Resonance in One and Two Dimensions*, (Oxford University Press: Oxford 1987).

5 MANSFIELD P, MORRIS PG, *NMR Imaging in Biomedicine*, (Academic Press: New York 1982).

6 MORRIS PG, *Nuclear Magnetic Resonance Imaging in Medicine and Biology*, (Oxford University Press: Oxford 1986).

7 ROSE AA, *Vision: Human and Electronic*, (Plenum Press: New York 1973) Chapter 1.

8 KAUFMAN L, CROOKS LE, Instrumentation. In: Margulis AR, Higgins CB, Kaufman L et al, eds.*Clinical Magnetic Resonance Imaging*, (Radiology Research and Education Foundation: San Francisco 1983) 31–9.

9 KELLER PJ, *Basic Principles of Magnetic Resonance Imaging*, (GE Medical Systems: Milwaukee 1988).

10 CROOKS LE, ORTENDAHL DA, KAUFMAN L et al, Clinical efficiency of nuclear magnetic resonance imaging, *Radiology* (1983) **146**:123–8.

11 KELLER PJ, HUNTER WH, SCHEMALBROCK P, Multisection fat–water imaging with chemical shift selective presaturation, *Radiology* (1987) **164**:539–41.

12 BYDDER GM, YOUNG IR, MR imaging: clinical use of the inversion recovery sequence, *J Comput Assist Tomogr* (1985) **9**:659–75.

13 BRADLEY WG, TSURUDA JS, MR sequence parameter optimization: an algorithmic approach, *AJR* (1987) **149**:815–23.

14 WALUCH V, BRADLEY WG, NMR even echo rephasing in slow laminar flow, *J Comput Assist Tomogr* (1984) **8**:594–8.

15 BRADLEY WG, WALUCH V, Blood flow: magnetic resonance imaging, *Radiology* (1985) **154**:443–50.

16 BABCOCK EE, BRATEMAN L, WEINREB JC et al, Edge artifact in MR images: chemical shift effect, *J Comput Assist Tomogr* (1985) **9**:252–7.

17 HENKELMAN RM, BRONSKILL MJ, Artifacts in magnetic resonance imaging. In: *Reviews of Magnetic Resonance Imaging* (Pergamon: New York 1987) Vol 2, No. 1.

18 WOOD M, HENKELMAN R, MR image artifacts from periodic motion, *Med Phys* (1985) **12**:143–51.

19 FELMLEE JP, EHMAN RL, Spatial presaturation: a method for suppressing flow artifacts and improving depiction of vascular anatomy in MR imaging, *Radiology* (1987) **164**:559–64.

20 HAACKE EM, LENZ GW, Improving MR image quality in the presence of motion by using rephasing gradients, *AJR* (1987) **148**:1251–8.

21 WINKLER ML, HRICAK H, Pelvis imaging with MR: technique for improvement, *Radiology* (1986) **158**:848–9.

22 NEW PFJ, ROSEN BR, BRADY TJ et al, Nuclear magnetic resonance: potential hazards and artifacts of ferromagnetic and nonferromagnetic surgical and dental materials and devices in nuclear magnetic resonance imaging, *Radiology* (1983) **147**:139–48.

23 FINN EJ, DICHIRO G, BROOKS RA et al, Ferromagnetic materials in patients: detection before MR imaging, *Radiology* (1985) **156**:139–41.

24 SCHENCK JF, HART HR JR, FOSTER TH et al, High resolution magnetic resonance imaging using surface coils. In: Kressel HY, ed. *Magnetic Resonance Annual 1986*, (Raven Press: New York 1986).

2

Contrast Agents

Bernadette Carrington

With its excellent soft tissue contrast and multiplanar imaging capability, MRI has improved the diagnostic evaluation of many diseases. Limitations have been recognized, however, especially in relation to accurate tumor detection, estimation of tumor volume and stage, and assessment of relative tumor viability. Some of these difficulties were originally identified in neuroradiology, where problems existed in identifying meningiomas, in differentiating between tumor and edema, and in evaluating the postoperative brain. Similar limitations affect pelvic imaging, especially in the assessment of neoplasms and in the evaluation of lymphadenopathy. In addition, abdominal and pelvic MRI suffer from a lack of gastrointestinal contrast, which may make differentiation between bowel loops and mass lesions difficult. The development of MR contrast media (primarily intravenous contrast agents), which enable improved tissue specificity, and increased sensitivity and diagnostic accuracy, has been instrumental in overcoming some of the limitations of MRI and making the technique more widely acceptable.

Mechanism of action

To be effective, an MR contrast agent, whatever its route of administration, has to alter T1 or T2 tissue relaxation parameters, thereby changing MR signal intensity. Alteration of T1 relaxation with paramagnetic contrast agents results from the interaction of individual proton magnetic moments with the electron magnetic moments of the agent, causing T1-shortening. T2 relaxation is similarly affected, but is also influenced by localized changes in the magnetic field due to induced magnetism (magnetic susceptibility) within the MR contrast agent. The latter adds to local field inhomogeneity, and promotes more rapid proton dephasing—T2-shortening. It is desirable for MR contrast agents to possess unpaired electron spins because their large magnetic moment (650 times greater than a proton)[1] contributes to T1-shortening and also indicates high magnetic susceptibility for T2-shortening.

Potential MR contrast materials may be classified into one of three groups—**ferromagnetic, paramagnetic** or **superparamagnetic**—depending on their atomic structure and susceptibility.[2] (Diamagnetic substances, which include most organic and inorganic compounds, have a negligible effect on adjacent protons because they do not possess unpaired electrons.) Ferromagnetic substances have a high magnetic susceptibility since they contain unpaired electrons in domains, equivalent to solid microscopic volumes within which all the unpaired electron spins are permanently aligned. The domains are randomly arranged in the unmagnetized state but will align in the presence of an external field resulting in the ferromagnetic material becoming magnetized. Moreover, the resultant induced magnetization is permanent, that is, the domains maintain their alignment even after the external field is removed. This property of retained magnetism, which can cause aggregation of particles, makes ferromagnetic materials less suitable as MR contrast agents and, in reality, only paramagnetic or superparamagnetic substances (see below) are feasible contrast agents.

Paramagnetic agents

Paramagnetic agents have independently acting atomic or molecular moments, which tend to align in the presence of an external field. Because the alignment is weak and largely overcome by thermal motion, any net magnetization is lost when the paramagnetic is removed from the field. Paramagnetic agents are generally soluble, allowing administration in an aqueous medium and facilitating flexible magneto-pharmaceutical design.

Although paramagnetic agents have their greatest relaxation on protons in water molecules actually bound to the paramagnetic (limited by the rate of exchange between bound and free water), protons in the immediate vicinity of the paramagnetic also undergo augmented relaxation without necessarily directly binding to it. This effect is less marked, since the strength of any interaction between the paramagnetic and adjacent proton is inversely proportional to the sixth power of the distance between them.[3] The only paramagnetic material in clinical use is the lanthanide, gadolinium.

Gadolinium-DTPA

Gadolinium, with seven unpaired electrons, has the highest magnetic moment of any element. However, free gadolinium is highly toxic in vivo and reported side-effects include hypotension, coagulopathy, fatty liver, and hepatic necrosis.[4,5] To negate these side-effects, gadolinium has been chelated to diethylene-triaminepentaacetic acid (DTPA). The resulting ion gadolinium-DTPA (Gd-DTPA) has a high binding constant (10^{23}) making it extremely stable and safe for administration.[2] Unfortunately chelation reduces the availability of binding sites, leaving only one available for exchange of water molecules.

Pharmacokinetics

Gadolinium-DTPA is administered as the ionic di-N-methylglucamine salt gadopentetate dimeglumine (Magnevist), at a recommended dose of 0.1 mmol/kg (0.2 ml/kg), maximum total dose 20 ml.[6] It is an intravascular, extracellular agent similar to iodinated contrast media and does not pass through normal cell membranes, the placenta, or an intact blood–brain barrier.[7] Less than 0.2 per cent has been identified in breast milk of experimental animals. In healthy male volunteers Gd-DTPA has a mean distribution half life of 12 ±7 min and an elimination half life of 100 min. It is eliminated by renal glomerular filtration, and a small proportion can be identified in feces.[8] Eighty per cent of any intravenous dose of Gd-DTPA is eliminated in the first 6 hours and 90 per cent within the first 24 hours. During clinical trials there has been no evidence of any significant accumulation of Gd-DTPA in the tissues, and no metabolites have been identified in the urine. Vicarious excretion has been seen in the presence of renal impairment, when Gd-DTPA remains stable within the body but may have a prolonged elimination half-life of up to 12 hours.

Effect on MR tissue signal intensity

Unlike iodinated contrast media, with which there is a linear relationship between contrast concentration and radiographic density, the relationship between Gd-DTPA concentration and MR signal intensity is more complex. Both T1 and T2 relaxation times are shortened by Gd-DTPA. At lower concentrations (0.6–6 mmol/l), however, T1-shortening predominates, resulting in an increase in signal intensity of the tissue on T1-weighted sequences.[9] At higher concentrations of gadolinium (25–50 mmol/l), T1-shortening is already maximal and T2-shortening is the dominant effect, resulting in decreased tissue signal intensity on T1-weighted images.[9,10] The dependence of signal intensity on concentration is well illustrated by the effect of Gd-DTPA on the signal intensity of urine within the bladder, as seen in Figure 2.1. At the recommended dose, the T1-shortening effect of Gd-DTPA predominates, resulting in increased tissue signal intensity on T1-weighted images.

Side-effects

The incidence of side-effects encountered in 500 patients at the investigational new drug stage was 25 per cent.[11] However, in only 15 per cent were the adverse reactions judged to be related to gadolinium administration. A larger cohort of 4000 patients has been assessed during routine clinical use of gadolinium, and the incidence of all adverse responses was only 3 per cent.[11] A study of pediatric patients identified side-effects due to gadolinium in only 1.3 per cent.[12] An allergic history increases the risk of adverse reactions by a factor of 3.5, and the incidence of side-effects is also dose-dependent, increasing from 0.5 per cent when the dose is 0.1 mmol/kg to 1.5 per cent for a dose of 0.1–0.2 mmol/kg in the most recent studies.[12]

During the investigational new drug stage, the most common side-effects reported were headache (9.8 per cent), nausea (4.1 per cent), and vomiting (2 per cent). The risk of vomiting was associated with rapid injection of the contrast media and recent food ingestion.[11] Discomfort at or near the injection site

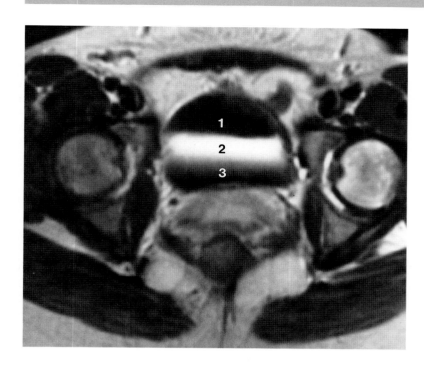

Figure 2.1

Effect of Gd-DTPA concentration on signal intensity. 1.5 T, transaxial T1-weighted image SE 600/20. Three layers can be identified within the bladder: unopacified urine with long T1 and long T2, and low signal intensity (1). Urine with low concentrations of Gd-DTPA (0.6–6 mmol/l) with resulting T1-shortening and high signal intensity (2). Urine containing high concentrations of Gd-DTPA (25–50 mmol/l) where T1-shortening is maximal and T2-shortening effects predominate, resulting in low signal intensity (3).

occurred in less than 2 per cent of patients. Grand mal seizures were reported in 3 of 1068 patients.[13] However, these patients suffered from seizure disorders and no definite association with Gd-DTPA has been identified. Only one death has been recorded; this was due to an acute myocardial infarction occurring a few hours following gadolinium administration.[11] However, Gd-DTPA was not considered responsible for this fatality.

Alterations in certain laboratory parameters have been noted after the administration of Gd-DTPA. A rise in total serum iron levels may be observed two to four hours post-injection in 26 per cent of men and 18 per cent of women.[13] Iron levels may remain above baseline at 24 hours, but they return to baseline values in virtually all patients by 48 hours after administration.[13] Similar changes are seen in total bilirubin, but elevation above baseline occurs in less than 5 per cent of patients.[13]

New developments in paramagnetic agents

New gadolinium chelates are being assessed for clinical use. Gadolinium has been chelated to tetraazacyclododecanetetraacetic acid (DOTA) and the chelate **gadolinium-DOTA** (Gd-DOTA) has a higher binding constant (10^{28}) than Gd-DTPA.[14,15] Whereas Gd-DTPA is divalent, Gd-DOTA is monovalent, and its lower osmolarity[16] may allow administration of higher doses.

Other paramagnetic substances under investigation as possible MR contrast agents include **liposomal derivatives of gadolinium, molecular oxygen,** and **nitroxide spin labels.** Particles of liposomal Gd-DTPA may be incorporated into hepatocytes, or into the phagocytes of the reticuloendothelial system.[17] The effect of high concentrations of oxygen has been assessed, but its paramagnetic effect is weak compared to other contrast agents.[18] In animals, nitroxide spin labels have been administered intravenously and intrathecally but their high chemical reactivity and lower magnetic susceptibility necessitate a high dose. Diradical nitroxide spin labels, with two free radicals, allow more effective enhancement at lower concentrations.[19] Potential long-term concerns include the ability of nitroxide spin labels to promote DNA cross-linkages, and the fact that unstable free radicals are known intermediates in carcinogenesis. However, as demonstrated by the sister chromatid exchange assay, prototype nitroxide spin labels and their metabolites have no mutagenic effects.[20] Clearly, further trials of safety and efficacy are indicated.

Superparamagnetic agents

Superparamagnetic materials are independent single domain particles consisting of aggregates of paramagnetic ions held rigidly in a crystalline lattice.[21] Compared to the component ions, these particles possess a greater magnetic susceptibility, which increases linearly with low field strengths and then plateaus at high field strengths. The particles act by destructive interference of the local magnetic field, caused by the large, abrupt change in the field as it passes through the superparamagnetic material. Small but locally intense magnetic gradients are formed which lead to rapid proton dephasing, promoting T2-shortening.[22] The magnetism within the particles declines to zero after the external field is removed. Superparamagnetic agents are necessarily solid particles, which are usually administered in suspension. One superparamagnetic agent under clinical evaluation is ferrite.

Ferrite

Ferrite is a crystalline iron oxide with a median particle diameter in the region of 50 nm.

Pharmacokinetics

Ferrite is available as a colloidal suspension and is administered by slow intravenous injection at a dose of 10–50 micromol/kg (0.05–0.2 ml/kg body weight).[23] It is highly tissue-specific, and passes into the reticuloendothelial system after intravenous injection. At one hour, 70 per cent of the dose is in the liver, 10 per cent in the spleen, and 10 per cent has accumulated in the lung.[24] At this time, blood levels are less than 0.5 per cent of the injected dose. In early patient studies the half life (T½) of ferrite has been shown to vary markedly, with an early phase T½ of 4.5 to 22 minutes and a late phase T½ between 79 and 309 minutes.[23]

Effect on MR tissue signal intensity

At the recommended dose, ferrite has powerful T2-shortening effects and little effect on T1. The overall result of ferrite administration is a loss of signal intensity in reticuloendothelial organs such as the liver and spleen. However, tumor cells which do not contain any reticuloendothelial component, maintain their T2 values and their conspicuity increases in contrast to the low signal intensity normal tissue. Gradient-echo techniques are twice as sensitive to the effects of ferrite as single spin-echo sequences.[25]

Side-effects

Careful patient monitoring is required during administration of ferrite, since some patients may experience allergic reactions to the iron. These reactions most commonly manifest as rash or hypotension.[23] Serum iron and ferritin levels have been shown to rise during the 24 hours after ferrite has been administered, since iron is released from ferrite and adds 1–2 per cent to total body iron levels.[23]

Although the maximum potential for ferrite is in assessing the liver and spleen for the presence of metastases, it may be of use within the pelvis as a lymphographic agent or as a negative intraluminal bowel contrast agent.

Gastrointestinal contrast agents

Potential bowel contrast agents may be divided into those producing either a positive or a negative signal within the bowel lumen. Positive agents act by T1-shortening effects, and include oils, iron salts and paramagnetic agents such as gadolinium. Ferrites and gas-producing substances produce negative contrast. There are two main disadvantages associated with positive agents: first, their high signal inevitably increases the noise due to bowel motion and, second, their effect varies with both the pulse sequence used and contrast concentration within the bowel.[26] For example, gadolinium is a positive contrast agent at low concentrations, but becomes a negative contrast agent when present in high concentrations. Negative contrast agents which act by T2-shortening do not have these disadvantages. Such agents are generally low in signal intensity, which also simplifies dose considerations. However, high concentrations of negative agents such as ferrite result in image distortion with blurring of adjacent structures. In addition, the required dose of ferrite for adequate bowel opacification in humans approaches 400 mg iron.[26] Since this is a potentially toxic dose, enteral ferrite solution must have low solubility to prevent systemic absorption.

Another consideration in design of reliable bowel contrast agents relates to their miscibility. Miscible substances, such as gadolinium, iron salts, and ferrite are preferred, since they can be administered in small volumes and will mix with the bowel content already present. As with oral contrast agents in computed tomography, if the agents do not mix in every portion of the bowel, then an unopacified dependent loop could be mistaken for a mass lesion. When immiscible agents are used in high volume to replace the bowel contents, problems may occur due to poor palatability and gastrointestinal disturbances.

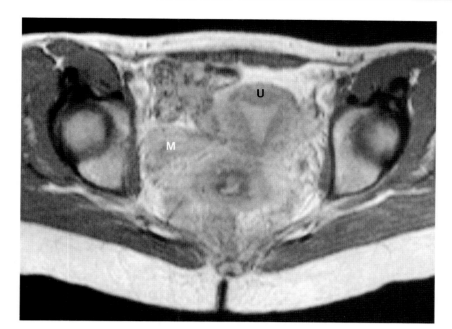

a

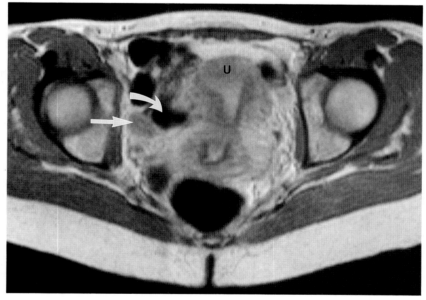

b

Figure 2.2

PFOB as MR gastrointestinal contrast agent. 1.0 T, transaxial SE image 2600/20, (**a**) without oral contrast and (**b**) with PFOB bowel contrast. An apparent adnexal mass (M) represents the right ovary (straight arrow) and bowel loops (curved arrow). (U)– uterus. (Courtesy of Dr JJ Brown.)

Both positive and negative bowel contrast agents are undergoing clinical trials. Gd-DTPA has been administered as an enteral contrast agent, but did cause diarrhea in some patients.[27] Ferrite suspensions are also being evaluated.[26,28] The clay minerals kaolin and bentonite, have been used in aqueous suspension to cause negative bowel opacification. They may operate by diamagnetic effect.[29] Another MR gastrointestinal agent is the perfluorochemical, perfluoroctylbromide (PFOB).[30] PFOB is an organic substance in which all the hydrogen atoms have been replaced by fluorine. On MR images, it appears of low signal intensity within the bowel lumen due to lack of mobile protons (Figure 2.2).

Future developments in contrast media

Intravascular macromolecular agents such as labeled dextran and albumin have already been evaluated in animal models and may prove useful in the assessment of tissue vascularity and capillary integrity.[31,32] Future contrast agent design may also involve the synthesis of tissue specific contrast-labeled antibodies. MR may thus play a role in the assessment of normal physiology and abnormal organ function.

References

1 WESBEY GE, Magnetopharmaceuticals. In: Wehrli FW, Shaw D, Kneeland JB, eds. *Biomedical Magnetic Resonance Imaging: Principles, Methodology and Applications*, (VCH: New York 1988) 157–88.

2 ENGELSTAD BL, WOLF GL, Contrast agents. In: Stark DD, Bradley WG, eds. *Magnetic Resonance Imaging*, (CV Mosby: Washington DC 1988).

3 MCNAMARA MT, Paramagnetic contrast material. In: Higgins CB, Hricak H, eds. *Magnetic Resonance Imaging of the Body*, (Raven Press: New York 1987) 547–59.

4 ARVELA P, Toxicity of rare-earths, *Prog Pharmacol* (1979) **2(3)**:71–114.

5 HALEY TJ, Pharmacology and toxicology of the rare earth elements, *J Pharm Sci* (1965) **54(5)**:663–70.

6 Magnevist (gadopentetate dimeglumine) Prescribing Information. Berlex Laboratories, Inc., Wayne, New Jersey, 07470.

7 KIEFFER SA, Gadopentetate dimeglumine: observations on the clinical research process, *Radiology* (1990) **174**:7–8.

8 WEINMANN HJ, BRASCH RC, PRESS WR et al, Characteristics of gadolinium-DTPA complex: a potential NMR contrast agent, *AJR* (1984) **142**:619–24.

9 KIKINIS R, VON SCHULTHESS GK, JAGER P et al, Normal and hydronephrotic kidney: evaluation of renal function with contrast-enhanced MR imaging, *Radiology* (1987) **165**:837–42.

10 ELSTER AD, SOBOL WT, HINSON WH, Pseudolayering of Gd-DTPA in the urinary bladder, *Radiology* (1990) **174**:379–81.

11 WOLFE GL, Current status of MR imaging contrast agents: special report, *Radiology* (1989) **165**:837–42.

12 NIENDORF HP, Tolerance of Gd-DTPA, clinical experience. International Workshop: Contrast Media in MRI, Berlin. February 1–3, 1990.

13 GOLDSTEIN HA, KASHANIAN FK, BLUMETTI RF et al, Safety assessment of gadopentetate dimeglumine in US clinical trials, *Radiology* (1990) **174**:17–23.

14 BOUSQUET JC, SAINI S, STARK DD et al, Gd-DOTA: characterization of a new paramagnetic complex, *Radiology* (1988) **166**:693–8.

15 RUNGE VM, JACOBSON S, WOOD ML et al, MR imaging of rat brain glioma: Gd-DTPA versus Gd-DOTA, *Radiology* (1988) **166**:835–8.

16 BRASCH RC, BENNETT HF, Considerations in the choice of contrast media for MR imaging, *Radiology* (1988) **166**:897–9.

17 KABALKA G, BUONOCORE E, HUBNER K et al, Gadolinium-labeled liposomes: targeted MR contrast agents for the liver and spleen, *Radiology* (1987) **163**:255–8.

18 RUNGE VM, STEWART RG, CLANTON JA et al, Work in progress: potential oral and intravenous paramagnetic NMR contrast agents, *Radiology* (1983) **147**:789.

19 EHMAN RL, BRASCH RC, MCNAMARA MT et al, Diradical nitroxyl spin label contrast agents for magnetic resonance imaging: a comparison of relaxation effectiveness, *Invest Radiol* (1986) **21**:125–36.

20 AFZAL V, BRASCH RC, NITECKI DE et al, Nitroxyl spin label contrast enhancers for magnetic resonance imaging: studies of acute toxicity and mutagenesis, *Invest Radiol* (1984) **19**:549–52.

21 STARK DD, GROMAN EV, SAINI S et al, Ferrite: a superparamagnetic contrast agent for MR imaging (Abstract), *Magn Reson Med* (1986) **4**:15–16.

22 GIBBY WA, MR contrast agents: an overview, *Radiol Clin North Am* (1988) **26**:1047–58.

23 STARK DD, WEISSLEDER R, GUILLERMO E et al, Superparamagnetic iron oxide: clinical application as a contrast agent for MR imaging of the liver, *Radiology* (1988) **168**:297–301.

24 MAJUMDAR S, ZOGHBI S, POPE CT et al, Quantitation of MR relaxation effects of iron oxide particles in liver and spleen, *Radiology* (1988) **169**:653–5.

25 MAJUMDAR S, ZOGHBI S, GORE JC, The influence of pulse sequence on the relaxation effects of superparamagnetic iron oxide contrast agents, *Magn Reson Med* (1989) **10**:289–301.

26 HAHN PF, STARK DD, SAINI S et al, Ferrite particles for bowel contrast in MR imaging: design issues and feasibility studies, *Radiology* (1987) **164**:34–41.

27 LANIADO M, KORNMESSER W, HAMM B et al, MR imaging of the gastrointestinal tract: value of Gd-DTPA, *AJR* (1988) **150**:817–21.

28 LÖNNEMARK M, HEMMINGSSON A, BACH-GANSMO T et al, Effect of superparamagnetic particles as oral contrast medium at magnetic resonance imaging, *Acta Radiol* (1989) **30**:193–6.

29 LISTINSKY JJ, BRYANT RG, Gastrointestinal contrast agents: a diamagnetic approach, *Magn Reson Med* (1988) **8**:285–92

30 MATTREY RF, HAJEK PC, GYLYS-MORIN VM et al, Perfluorochemicals as gastrointestinal contrast agents for MR imaging: preliminary studies in rats and humans, *AJR* (1987) **148**:1259–63.

31 SCHMIEDL U, OGLAN M, PAAJANEN H et al, Albumin labeled with Gd-DTPA as an intravascular, blood-pool enhancing agent for MR imaging: biodistribution and imaging studies, *Radiology* (1987) **162**:205–21.

32 WANG S, WIKSTRÖM MG, WHITE DL et al, Evaluation of Gd-DTPA-labeled dextran as an intravascular MR contrast agent: imaging characteristics in normal rat tissues, *Radiology* (1990) **175**:483–8.

3
Biosafety

Bernadette Carrington

At the present time, no immediate or delayed deleterious effects of clinical MRI have been identified. This probably reflects the physical limits applied to MR magnetic field strengths, which are significantly below the levels at which alterations in biological systems occur. Consequently, the Food and Drug Administration (FDA) has reclassified MR imagers to Class II (performance standards), the same category as computed tomography scanners.[1] Table 3.1 lists the FDA guidelines for MR systems,[2] as well as the British National Radiological Protection Board (NRPB) guidelines and those of the German Federal Office.[3,4]

Effects of MRI on patients

Effects related to type of field

Any short-term physiological changes detected during MRI are due to the electromagnetic fields used to obtain the image. A patient undergoing an MR examination is subject to three types of magnetic fields: a static field which aligns the body's protons; a time-varying gradient magnetic field which enables spatial localization of these protons; and a pulsed

Table 3.1 Guidelines for clinical MR units: maximum magnetic field strengths and radiofrequency exposure

	Static field (Tesla)	Radiofrequency SAR (Watts/kg)	Time-varying magnetic field
USA	2.0	0.4 (whole body) 2.0 (any gram of tissue)	3 Tesla/second
UK	2.5	0.4 (whole body)	20 Tesla/second (pulses>10 msec) $(\Delta B/\Delta T)^2 t<4$ (pulses<10 msec)
West Germany	2.0	1.0 (whole body) 5.0 (in any kg of tissue, except eyes)	*30 mA/m² or 0.3 V/min (pulses>10 msec) 0.3/t mA/A² or 3/t mV/m (pulses shorter than t= 10 msec)

*Effect measured as induced whole-body current (milliamperes/metre²; mA/m²) or induced electric field strength (volts/metre; V/m).
SAR = specific absorption rate

radiofrequency electromagnetic field to raise the protons to a higher energy state. At clinical field strengths, a small number of temporary biological effects may be recognized due to each of these fields.

Static magnetic field

Two transient effects may be observed at field strengths less than 2 Tesla. The first is **increased T-wave amplitude** on the electrocardiogram, which results from eddy currents produced by electrolytes in blood flowing through a magnetic field. This is called the magnetohydrodynamic effect.[5,6] It occurs at field strengths greater than 0.3 Tesla, and the small electric potentials generated are believed to superimpose on the normally occurring bipotential, causing T-wave augmentation.[7] The T-wave artifact resolves immediately when the patient leaves the magnetic field. Theoretically, similar eddy currents should reduce blood flow by 1 per cent at 1 Tesla, but in an experimental model using monkeys, no blood flow alteration was detected at 1.5 Tesla.[8] Indeed, no other cardiovascular changes have been identified.[9]

The second effect of a static magnetic field is **magnetic anisotropy.** This refers to the molecular realignment which occurs in a strong field to achieve the lowest possible energy state. Its clinical relevance relates to the paramagnetic deoxyhemoglobin in sickled erythrocytes, which will realign in MRI fields to a limited extent.[10] However, no measurable harm has been reported from this temporary realignment.

In all studies performed so far, no significant bioeffects have been detected for static field strengths less than 2 Tesla.[11]

Time-varying magnetic field

For a time-varying magnetic field (TVMF), the induction of eddy currents depends on the change in magnetic field per unit time. Other factors, such as pulse strength and pulse rate, also govern TVMF effects. Clinically, TVMFs are responsible for two phenomena. One is the bone-healing effect of extremely low frequency fields, utilized in orthopedics to promote healing of fractures. The other is of possible relevance in MRI, and relates to the production of magnetophosphenes. These are perceived as flashes of light and are thought to originate from the torque effect of a TVMF inducing electrical stimulation of the retinal cones.[5] They are completely reversible and are not associated with any long-term sequelae. The threshold values needed to obtain magnetophosphenes are usually in excess of those found in clinical MR

units, and therefore, this phenomenon is unlikely to occur in clinical practice. In clinical units, the eddy currents generated by TVMFs do not interfere with either nerve conduction or cardiac function.[8]

Radiofrequency magnetic field

The most important radiofrequency (RF) effect is heat generation. During an MR scan, the amount of energy deposited in the tissues depends on the number and type of RF pulses in a sequence, the pulse width, repetition time and type of coil used. Patient mass and the area imaged are also important, in that the amount of RF energy absorbed increases as body mass decreases, but less RF power is needed in smaller patients to obtain 90° or 180° pulses. Overall, the RF energy per kilogram required is approximately equal in patients of different body habitus.[12]

RF absorption is measured indirectly in terms of tissue heating (the specific absorption rate, SAR and is calculated in watts/kilogram (W/kg). Although such thermal effects are potentially damaging, experiments on both animals and humans have demonstrated no deleterious effects at clinical exposure levels.[9,11] Core body temperature does rise by a mean 0.3°C during a 20-minute scan on a 1.5 Tesla (64 MHz) machine,[13] but this is at an SAR of 4 W/kg, which exceeds the FDA guidelines by a factor of 10. Moreover, in a normal individual, core temperature may demonstrate daily fluctuations of up to 2°C. After RF exposure, skin temperature may show a greater rise, up to 3°C, but this effect has not been documented above 39°C.[11] Skin regions nearer the RF coil show a greater rise in temperature than regions more remote from the coil. For example, in a body coil it is the skin temperature of the chest and abdominal wall that increases most, whereas that of the head increases least.

Particular attention has been paid to estimating RF effects on two vulnerable superficial organs, the eye and the testis. In all experimental models, the maximum temperature increase of the corneal and vitreous humor has been less than 1.5°C, well below the levels needed for cataract formation.[14] Testicular dysfunction has only been identified at SAR levels which greatly exceed those of clinical units.[9,15]

Concern about RF thermal effects has led the FDA to include patients with impaired thermoregulation and decompensated cardiac patients in the warning statement concerning MR scanners.[16] However, an effective air circulation system within the magnet keeps temperature increases to a minimum. Another benefit of effective air circulation is a decrease in claustrophobic episodes, resulting in fewer failed MR examinations.[8]

Potential carcinogenic effect

To date, no increased risk of cancer has been documented at clinical RF exposures. Animal ovarian cells and human lymphocytes have been kept over long periods in moderate or high strength fields without cytogenetic damage.[17] Nonetheless, statistical validation of these results requires confirmation over a longer follow-up period.

MRI in the pregnant patient

It is inappropriate to scan pregnant women routinely, especially in the first trimester, unless a termination of pregnancy is planned. The FDA recommends that the possible risks of the procedure be weighed against the diagnostic benefits and also against the known hazards of ionizing radiation from other imaging modalities.[2] On the few occasions that patients have been inadvertently scanned during the first trimester, the babies have been normal at birth and have not exhibited any developmental or teratogenic abnormality.[8] A substantial number of women have had MR examinations in the second and third trimesters, without any reported abnormalities in their children.[8]

Effects of MRI on operators

Technicians are exposed to the static magnetic field when they assist patients in and out of the magnet bore. In the Soviet Union, some studies of industrial workers involved in the construction of permanent magnets have documented a variety of complaints including headaches, fatigue and dizziness.[18] However, other studies have not confirmed any of these findings. In particular, no evidence exists that intermittent short-term exposures to static magnetic fields carry any risk.[5,19]

General safety of MRI

Ferromagnetic projectiles

The most serious hazard posed by any MR unit is the possibility of injury from metallic projectiles. Small objects, such as hairpins, may reach a terminal velocity of 40 mph when entering the bore of a 1.5 Tesla magnet.[8] Consequently, it is important for all metal objects to be removed from the patient, and for staff to be aware of the risks from any loose metal objects

they may be carrying, for example, keys or loose change in their pockets. Appropriate warning signs should be posted at all entrances to the MR unit. It is also necessary to secure the MR suite during non-operational periods.

Implanted metal objects

Concerns about metallic implants relate to their **electroconductivity, heat conductivity**, and **ferromagnetism**.

Electroconductivity

Both the radiofrequency and time-varying magnetic fields induce currents in implants, which could interfere with electromagnetically operated devices such as cardiac pacemakers or biostimulators. There is also a similar, but temporary, effect from the static magnetic field as the patient is moved in or out of the magnet bore. The FDA has addressed the problem of implanted electromagnetic devices, and contraindications and guidelines in MR imaging of metal implants are discussed below.[16]

Heat conductivity

Induced electric currents, together with absorbed radiofrequency energy, may potentially contribute to heating of the metal with consequent dissipation of heat to the adjacent tissue. However, in vitro experiments have identified no significant heating effects in or near metallic implants at clinical field strengths.[20]

Ferromagnetism

The ferromagnetic properties of a metal determine its force of attraction by a magnetic field, and a turning effect, or **torque**, occurs when a metal object attempts to align its long axis parallel to the static magnetic field. Known ferromagnetic metals include iron, nickel and cobalt. Nonferromagnetic metals include gold, silver, copper and titanium. However, most metals are not implanted in the pure state, but rather as alloys. An alloy is most commonly composed of two or more metals mixed together and fused, usually while in the molten state. Occasionally alloys may be made of an admixture of a metal and non-metal; for example, steel is made of iron and carbon. It is this 'mix', or relative proportion of constituents in the alloy, which governs its degree of ferromagnetism. Other factors to be considered before scanning a ferromagnetic implant include the strength of the time-varying and static magnetic fields, the geometry of the implant, its orientation in situ, and the length of time it has been in place (in order to allow for fixation by fibrous tissue that may occur over time).

Metals also possess weak paramagnetic or diamagnetic effects, which are not significant in the clinical situation and, therefore, are not discussed here. When any doubt exists about the ferromagnetic qualities of a metallic implant, it is advisable to contact the manufacturers.

Guidelines and contraindications in MR scanning of metal implants

The FDA has prepared guidelines and established contraindications to MRI study in the presence of metal implants.[16]

Scanning patients with **intracranial aneurysm clips** is contraindicated, unless it is certain that the clip is made of a nonferromagnetic material such as titanium.[16] In general, other **surgical clips** contain more than 11 per cent nickel and are only weakly ferromagnetic. Another important contraindication to MR scanning is the presence of **intra-ocular metal fragments**. In one patient such fragments migrated, resulting in the loss of sight of one eye.[9] It is recommended that patients be questioned specifically about their occupation and about the possibility of metal fragments in or near the eye.

The presence of a **cardiac pacemaker** is also a specific contraindication to MRI, because the electromagnetic fields produced by the MR unit may interfere with pacemaker function. Although **prosthetic heart valves** do exhibit deflection in a static magnetic field, the forces involved are considerably less than those generated by heart motion. Valves manufactured after 1964 may be safely scanned up to 1.5 Tesla.[21] **Vena cava filters** made of stainless steel are also subject to torque in static magnetic fields up to 1.5 Tesla. However, in a study of properly positioned Greenfield filters, in vitro models have not demonstrated migration or caval wall penetration.[22,23] Since 1988, a nonferromagnetic titanium Greenfield filter has been available for clinical use. All vascular and suture material may be safely examined with MRI.[16]

MRI studies may be performed in the presence of an **intrauterine contraceptive device**, since neither migration nor heating effect has been documented at medium or high field strengths.[24] **Penile prostheses** may also be safely imaged.[25,26] There is no contraindication to scanning patients with **orthopedic implants**, most of which are nonferromagnetic and which have shown no significant heating or motion.[8,20]

In addition to cardiac pacemakers, other electrically, magnetically, or mechanically activated implants are contraindicated, including **biostimulators** and **neurostimulators, drug infusion devices, hearing aids**, and **cochlear implants**.[16] However, recent studies have indicated that some neurostimulators are not affected by MR exposure (Gleason CA, unpublished communication). In particular, patients with the Meditronic single channel SE4 (model 3424) may be safely scanned. In addition, patients with the Avery Model 1 110A, the Meditronic dual channel Model 7560A, and the Meditronic Itrel I may also be scanned, provided the stimulator is at least 40 cm away from zero reference in order to avoid RF interference or heating. However, the Cordis MKII implanted programmable pulse generator is subject to strong linear force and torque effects by the static magnetic field, and it is **not safe** to scan patients with this device.

Bullets pose a potential hazard during MR imaging due to the possibility of migration. Although commercial sporting ammunition is generally not ferromagnetic, police and military bullets are usually made of steel and may experience torque in MR magnetic fields.[27]

References

1 Radiological Health Bulletin 1988; 22(10).

2 *Guidelines for evaluating electromagnetic exposure risks for trials of clinical NMR systems*, US, February 25, 1982, Center for Devices and Radiological Health, Food and Drug Administration.

3 SMITH H, Revised guidance on acceptable limits of exposure during nuclear magnetic resonance clinical imaging, The National Radiological Protection Board ad hoc Advisory Group on Nuclear Magnetic Resonance Clinical Imaging, *Br J Radiol* (1983) **56**:974–7.

4 Recommendations on preventing health risks caused by the magnetic and high frequency electromagnetic fields produced in NMR tomography and in-vivo NMR spectroscopy, *Bundesgesundheitsblatt*, Federal Republic of Germany (1984) **27(3)**:92–6.

5 BUDINGER TF, Nuclear magnetic resonance (NMR) in-vivo studies: known thresholds for health effects, *J Compt Asst Tomogr* (1981) **5(6)**:800–11.

6 BUDINGER TF, CULLANDER C, Health effects of in-vivo nuclear magnetic resonance. In: James TL, Margulis AR, eds. *Biomedical Magnetic Resonance*, (Radiology Research and Education Foundation: San Francisco 1984) 421–41.

7 BEISCHER DE, KNEPTON JC, Influence of strong magnetic fields on the electrocardiogram of squirrel monkeys (Saimiri Scuireus), *Aerospace Med* (1964) **35**:939–44.

8 PAVLICEK W, Safety considerations. In: Stark DD, Bradley WG, eds. *Magnetic Resonance Imaging* (CV Mosby: Washington DC 1988).

9 SHELLOCK FG, Biological effects of MRI: a clean safety record so far, *Diagnostic Imaging*, February 1987, 96–101.

10 TENFORDE TS, Biological effects of high DC magnetic fields, Report No. LBL-12954, Lawrence Berkeley Laboratory, University of California, 1981.

11 SCHAEFER DJ, Safety aspects of magnetic resonance imaging. In: Wehrli FW, Shaw D, Kneeland JB, eds. *Biomedical Magnetic Resonance Imaging: Principles, Methodology, and Applications* (VCH: New York 1988) 553–78.

12 GOTTSCHALK SC, GAUSS RC, RF power deposition measurements at GOM #2 patient size, *Abstracts Soc Mag Reson Med* (1986) **3**:1040–1.

13 SCHAEFER DJ, BARBER BJ, GORDON CJ, Thermal effects of magnetic resonance imaging (MRI) (Abstract) Fourth Annual Meeting of the Society of Magnetic Resonance Imaging, London UK August 1985, 925–6.

14 SHELLOCK FG, CRUES JV, Changes in corneal temperature produced by high-field magnetic resonance imaging: experience in 118 patients, (Abstract) *Magn Reson Imaging* (1986) **4**:95.

15 NCRP Report No 86, Biological effects and exposure criteria for radiofrequency electromagnetic fields, National Council on Radiation Protection and Measurements, Bethesda, 1986.

16 PAVLICEK W, Contraindications in MR, In: Prepared by American College of Radiology Committee on Clinical Applications. *Clinical Applications of Magnetic Resonance Imaging* (1989) 63–4.

17 WOLFF S, JAMES TL, YOUNG GB et al, Magnetic resonance imaging: absence of in vitro cytogenetic damage, *Radiology* (1985) **55**:163–5.

18 VYALOV AM, Magnetic fields as a factor in the industrial environment, *Vestn Akad Med Nauk SSSR* (1967) **8**:72–4.

19 SAUNDERS RD, SMITH H, Safety aspects of NMR clinical imaging, *Brit Med Bull* (1984) **40**:148–52.

20 BUCHLI R, BOESIGER P, MEIER D, Heating effects of metallic implants by MRI examinations, *Mag Reson Med* (1988) **7**:255–61.

21 SOULEN RL, BUDINGER TF, HIGGINS CB, Magnetic resonance imaging of prosthetic heart valves, *Radiology* (1985) **154**:705–7.

22 TEITELBAUM GP, BRADLEY WG, KLEIN BD, MR imaging artifacts, ferromagnetism and magnetic torque of intravascular filters, stents and coils, *Radiology* (1988) **166**:657–64.

23 LIEBMAN CE, MESSERSMITH RN, LEVIN DN et al, MR imaging of inferior vena caval filters: safety and artifacts, *AJR* (1988) **150**:1174–6.

24 MARK AS, HRICAK H, Intrauterine contraceptive devices: MR imaging, *Radiology* (1987) **162**:311–14.

25 HRICAK H, MAROTTI M, GILBERT TJ et al, Normal penile anatomy and abnormal penile conditions: evaluation with MR imaging, *Radiology* (1988) **169**:683–90.

26 SHELLOCK FG, MR imaging of metallic implants and materials: a compilation of the literature, *AJR* (1988) **151**:811–14.

27 WILLIAMS KD, GIESZL BS, KELLER PJ et al, Fired missile projectiles: evaluation of potential ferromagnetic hazards in MR imaging (Abstract), 75th Scientific Assembly and Annual Meeting of the Radiological Society of North America, Chicago, 1989, p 274.

4

Anatomy of the Pelvis

Bernadette Carrington
Hedvig Hricak

The pelvis consists of a bony ring containing the reproductive organs, the lower urinary tract, the small bowel, the colon and rectum, blood vessels, nerves, lymphatics, fat, and supporting musculature. Both the inferior portion of the peritoneal cavity and the anterior and posterior pararenal spaces extend into the pelvis. Detailed descriptions of the normal anatomy of the reproductive organs, the bladder, the urethra and the rectum will be provided at the beginning of the relevant chapters on these organs.

Pelvic compartments

True and false pelvis

By convention, an oblique line passing from the sacral promontory to the superior aspect of the symphysis pubis divides the pelvis into two compartments—the false (greater) pelvis and the true (lesser) pelvis, as shown in Figure 4.1.[1] Laterally, the arcuate and iliopectineal lines of the pelvic brim form the boundary between the true pelvis and the false pelvis (Figure 4.2). The false pelvis communicates with the abdomen anteriorly and superiorly and contains most of the small bowel, the ascending, descending and sigmoid colon, and the common iliac vessels. The true pelvis contains some small bowel, the rectum, the bladder and pelvic ureters, and the reproductive organs. It is separated from the perineum by the levator ani muscles.

Peritoneal recesses

As illustrated in Figure 4.3, the peritoneal reflections divide the pelvis into intraperitoneal and extraperitoneal compartments. This division is of greater clinical

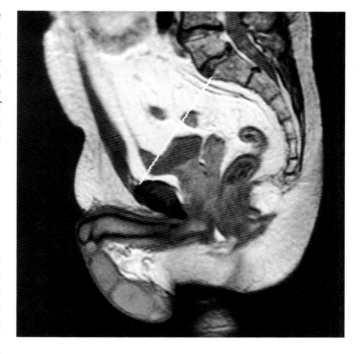

Figure 4.1

Division into true and false pelvis on sagittal proton density image of male pelvis, with computer-generated line from the sacral promontory to the superior border of the symphysis pubis.

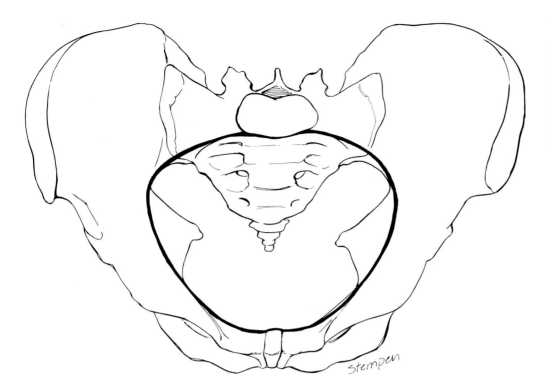

Figure 4.2

Schematic drawing of anteroposterior pelvis illustrating symphysis pubis, pectineal line, arcuate line and sacral promontory, the boundaries between true and false pelvis.

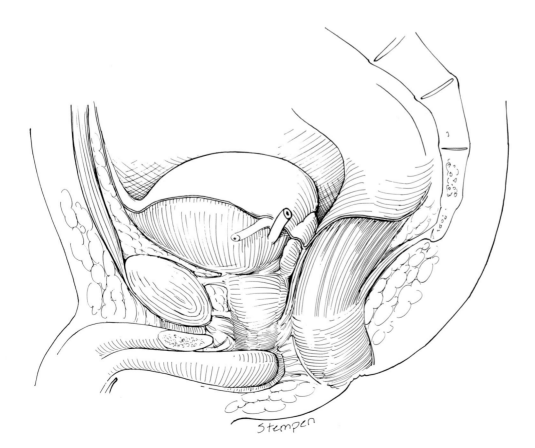

Figure 4.3

Schematic drawing illustrating the peritoneal reflections in the male pelvis.

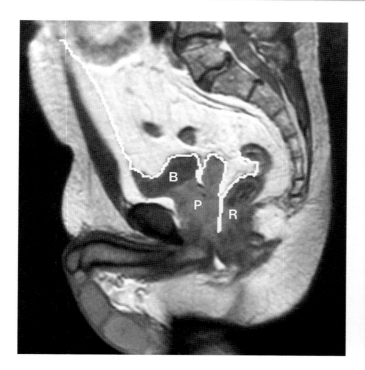

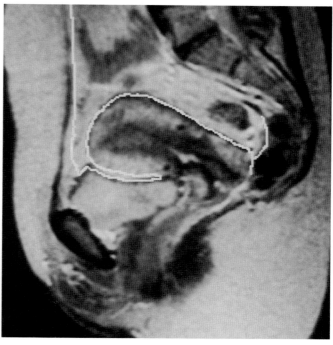

Figure 4.4

Peritoneal reflections in the male pelvis on sagittal MR image with computer tracing. The peritoneum passes inferiorly from the umbilicus investing the median umbilical fold, bladder dome (B) and seminal vesicles. The peritoneum fuses between prostate (P) and rectum (R) forming Denonvilliers' fascia.

Figure 4.5

Sagittal MR image with computer tracing to outline the peritoneal reflections in the female.

significance than that of the true and false pelvis, since it governs the pathways of tumor dissemination. The peritoneal reflections also form several recesses in which abnormal fluid collections and drop metastases may accumulate.

Intraperitoneal recesses

As shown in Figures 4.4 and 4.5, the **rectovesical space**, situated between the rectum and bladder at the level of the second to fourth sacral vertebrae, is the most caudal portion of the peritoneal cavity.[2] In the male, the anterior and posterior peritoneal layers

lining the rectovesical recess fuse inferiorly and extend caudally to form **Denonvilliers' fascia**, which separates the prostate and rectum (Figure 4.4). In the female, the uterus divides the rectovesical space into a smaller vesicouterine recess and a larger rectouterine cul-de-sac (**pouch of Douglas**).[2] Figure 4.5 illustrates the **rectovaginal septum** in the female, which is formed by inferior extension of the fused rectouterine peritoneum.[2] The rectovesical space extends along the lateral margins of the rectum forming the **pararectal fossae**, as demonstrated in Figure 4.6. The left pararectal fossa is often more shallow than the right due to indentation from the sigmoid colon (Figure 4.6). Because it is the most dependent portion of the

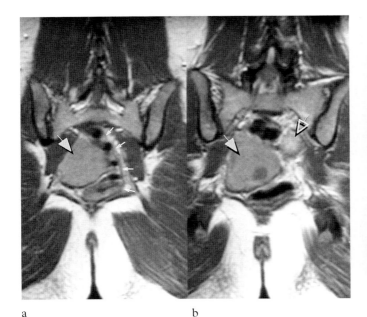

a   b

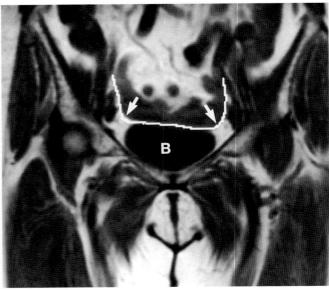

Figure 4.6

Fluid filled pararectal fossae on
two consecutive coronal
sections (**a**) and (**b**). Note the
lower position of the right
pararectal fossa (arrow)
compared to the left pararectal
fossa (open arrow), due to the
location of rectosigmoid (small
white arrows).

Figure 4.7

Coronal section demonstrating
urinary bladder (B) computer
tracing of the paravesical spaces
(arrow).

peritoneal cavity, fluid collections are initially visualized within the rectovesical space. For the same
reason, it is the most frequent site of intraperitoneal
tumor implants.

The intraperitoneal **paravesical spaces** are formed
by indentations of the pelvic peritoneum, and can be
seen on either side of the distended urinary bladder
(Figure 4.7).[3] Each paravesical space is further subdivided by the umbilical folds. Posterior indentations
of the obliterated umbilical arteries are called the
medial umbilical folds, and indentations of the
inferior epigastric vessels are called the **lateral umbilical folds** (Figure 4.8). These intraperitoneal paravesical spaces are usually occupied by bowel, but may
be filled by ascites, abscesses, or peritoneal tumor
implants.

There is also a **supravesicular space** extending
above the bladder between the medial umbilical folds.
It is occupied by small bowel loops or by the fundus
of the distended bladder.

Extraperitoneal recesses

The largest extraperitoneal recess is the **prevesical
space** (Figure 4.9), which is situated between the
transversalis fascia of the anterior abdominal wall
anteriorly and the umbilicovesical fascia posteriorly.
Cranially it extends to the umbilicus, and inferiorly its
extent is delineated by the puboprostatic ligament in
the male and the pubovesical ligament in the female.
Both of these ligaments run from the bladder base to

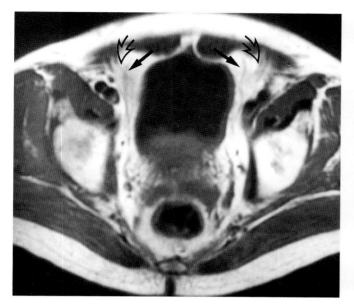

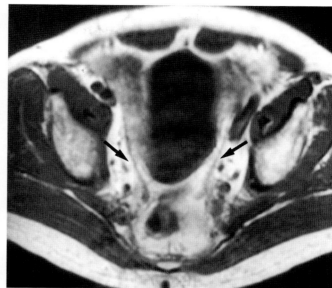

a

b

Figure 4.8

Medial and lateral umbilical folds. (**a**) and (**b**) are consecutive transaxial sections demonstrating the medial umbilical folds (black arrows) anteriorly (**a**) and posteriorly (**b**) as they pass to join the internal iliac vessels. The orientation and position of the medial umbilical folds allow differentiation from the ductus deferens. The lateral umbilical folds are also identified (white arrows).

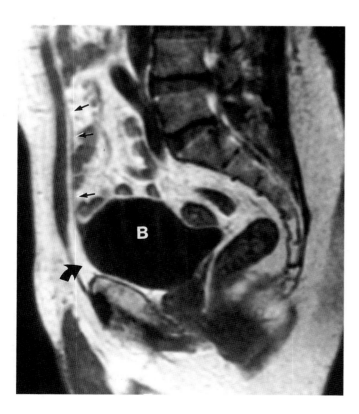

Figure 4.9

Prevesical space. Sagittal section showing prevesical space (curved black arrow) anterior to the bladder (B) and extending superiorly to the umbilicus (small black arrows).

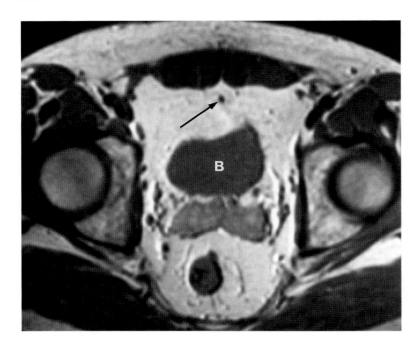

Figure 4.10
The median umbilical fold. Transaxial section showing the midline median umbilical fold (arrow) which contains the obliterated urachus. (B)– bladder.

the symphysis pubis. Laterally the prevesical space merges into the paravesical connective tissue.

The bladder, urachus and obliterated umbilical arteries lie within the perivesical space surrounded by the umbilicovesical fascia. The urachus, as illustrated in Figure 4.10, is contained within the **median umbilical fold**, which runs from the apex of the bladder to the umbilicus.

Normal MR appearance

Blood vessels

On MR scans blood vessels can be visualized in all three orthogonal planes without intravenous contrast.

Patent blood vessels with normal flow velocity are easily distinguished from surrounding fat and pelvic muscles, typically appearing as areas of signal void on spin-echo images. However, the signal intensity from blood depends on flow direction and velocity in addition to imaging parameters (see also Chapter 1). For example, if the MR plane of section cuts a blood vessel obliquely, the vessel may demonstrate medium signal intensity, preventing differentiation from lymph nodes. Gradient-recall-echo imaging sequences should resolve this problem, as illustrated in Figure 4.11.

On pelvic MRI scans the abdominal aorta is depicted as it divides into the common iliac arteries at the level of the third to fourth lumbar vertebrae. The common iliac arteries are situated anterior to the common iliac veins, and course inferiorly, dividing into external and internal iliac branches at the level of

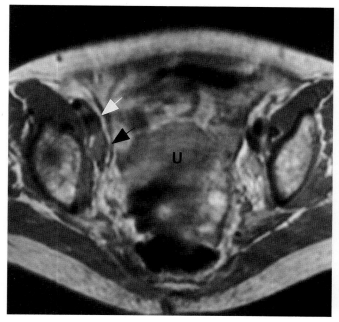

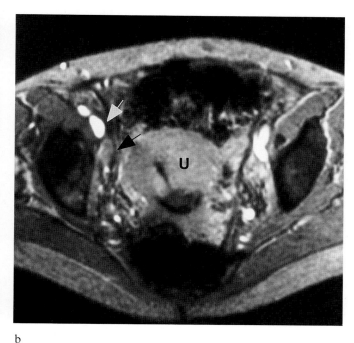

a

b

Figure 4.11

Differentiation between blood vessels and lymph nodes using gradient-recall-echo imaging. (**a**) Spin-echo image; (**b**) gradient-recall-echo image. On the spin-echo image medium signal intensity within the right external iliac vein (white arrow) and the adjacent lymph node (black arrow) is seen. On the gradient-recall-echo image, flowing blood is of high signal intensity and this allows differentiation between the vein (white arrow) and the lymph node (black arrow). (U)–uterus.

the fifth lumbar to first sacral vertebrae, as shown in Figure 4.12a.

External iliac vessels

The external iliac arteries are situated anterolateral to the external iliac veins (Figures 4.12b, c, and d). Two branches may be identified on MRI scans. The inferior epigastric artery arises from the external iliac artery just above the inguinal ligament. It extends in an anterosuperior direction along the medial margin of the internal inguinal ring to the anterior abdominal wall (Figure 4.12c), thereafter coursing cranially behind the rectus abdominis muscle. Figure 4.12d shows the deep circumflex iliac vessels as they ascend anterolaterally from the external iliac vessels, behind

the inguinal ligament and the internal inguinal ring, to the anterosuperior iliac spines.

Internal iliac vessels

The internal iliac arteries pass in a posteroinferior direction to the lower margin of the sacroiliac joints, where they divide into anterior and posterior trunks. The anterior trunk gives rise to obturator, umbilical, vesical, prostatic, rectal and uterine branches before terminating in the inferior gluteal and internal pudendal arteries. The obturator vessels, depicted in Figure 4.12e, are an important anatomical landmark for locating the surgical obturator lymph nodes. The posterior internal iliac trunk divides into the iliolumbar, lateral sacral, and superior gluteal arteries.

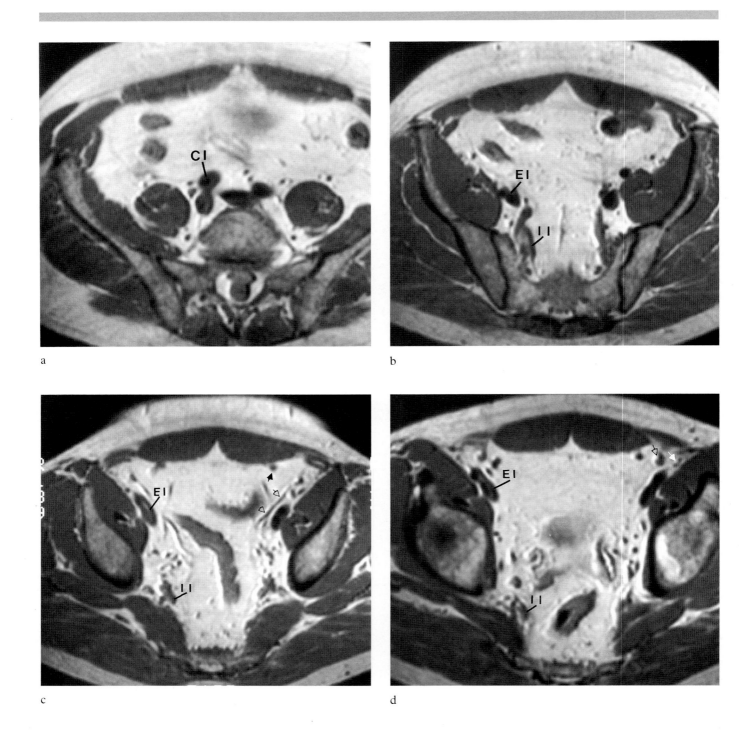

a

b

c

d

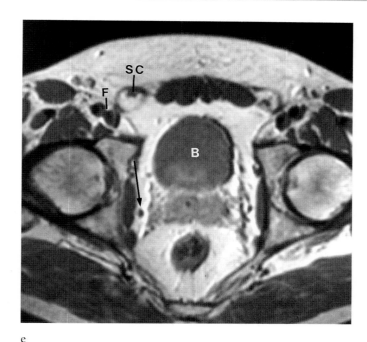

e

Figure 4.12

Branching of pelvic blood vessels. (**a**) Common iliac vessels (CI). (**b**) Division of common iliac vessels into external (EI) and internal (II) vessels. (**c**) and (**d**) External (EI) and internal (II) vessels and inferior epigastric artery (small black solid arrowhead). Deep circumflex iliac artery (small white arrow). Ductus deferens (black open arrowhead). (**e**) At the level of the inguinal ring where the external iliac vessels become the femoral artery and vein (F). The arteries are situated anterior to the veins. Obturator vessel (long black arrow). (SC)– spermatic cord, (B)–bladder.

The oblique course of the vessels is best appreciated on off-axis images (as illustrated in Figure 4.13).

Pelvic lymphatics

The lymphatic vessels, which originate within connective tissue as blind-ending capillaries and merge to form larger vessels (lymphatics), have muscular walls and contain valves. The lymphatics drain into lymph nodes, which are arranged in chains and serve as filters for the lymphatic fluid. Each nodal chain accompanies an artery, and generally receives lymph from viscera supplied by that artery. Nodal groups are usually named after their companion arteries and are subdivided according to their position relative to that artery.

The lymph nodes of abdominal organs are situated at the vascular hilum of each organ, which is relatively immobile. However, the midline urogenital organs in the pelvis do not possess a hilum, and lymph drainage occurs **bilaterally** to pelvic nodal chains and to the retroperitoneum.[4] Figure 4.14 and Table 4.1 sum-

marize pelvic lymphatic anatomy. Appreciation of these diverse lymphatic pathways is important when staging pelvic tumors.

MR appearance of lymph nodes

On T1-weighted MR images lymph nodes are of medium signal intensity. On T2-weighted images the signal intensity varies, although it is always greater than muscle. T1-weighted sequences provide maximum contrast differentiation between medium signal intensity lymph nodes and high signal intensity fat, whereas T2-weighted images allow optimum distinction between higher signal intensity nodes and lower signal intensity muscle. The signal from lymph nodes is enhanced after gadolinium-DTPA injection, sometimes allowing nodes to be differentiated from ovary or bowel. Enhancement is not tissue specific, however, and neither non-neoplastic inflammatory nodal hyperplasia nor tumor deposits in normal size nodes can be identified on MR scans. Normal nodal size varies with site, and in the pelvis, nodes should be less than 1.0 cm in diameter.

Figure 4.13

Off-axis section illustrating the course of the external iliac vessels (black arrows) (**a**) with accompanying schematic drawing (**b**).

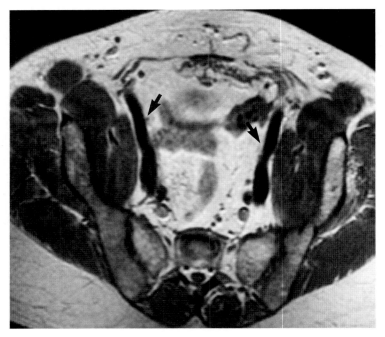

a

Figure 4.14

Schematic drawing of pelvic lymph node chains. Posterior nodal chains are shown in broken lines.

Note that the proximal obturator nodes are the surgical nodes and the distal node at the obturator foramen is the anatomical obturator node.

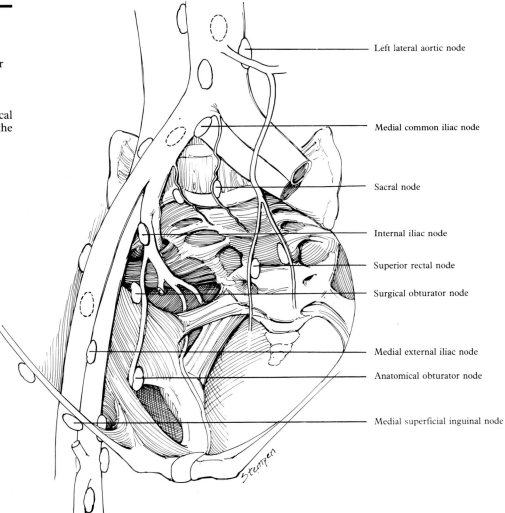

Left lateral aortic node

Medial common iliac node

Sacral node

Internal iliac node

Superior rectal node

Surgical obturator node

Medial external iliac node

Anatomical obturator node

Medial superficial inguinal node

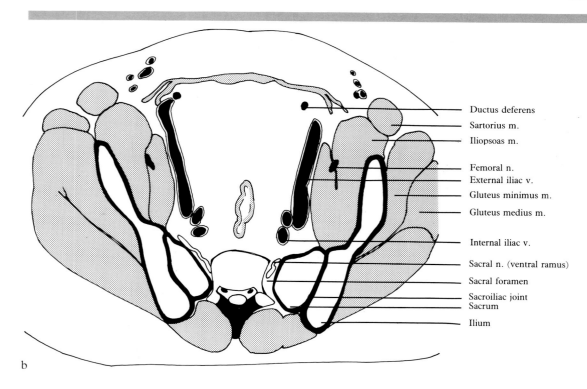

Ductus deferens
Sartorius m.
Iliopsoas m.

Femoral n.
External iliac v.
Gluteus minimus m.
Gluteus medius m.

Internal iliac v.

Sacral n. (ventral ramus)

Sacral foramen

Sacroiliac joint
Sacrum

Ilium

b

Inguinal lymph nodes

The most peripheral nodes draining the pelvis are the inguinal nodes, which are also the terminal nodes for lymphatic drainage of the lower limb. Figure 4.15 illustrates the inguinal lymph nodes, which are subdivided into superficial and deep chains.

Superficial inguinal lymph nodes are situated immediately below the inguinal ligament. Lymph vessels from the anus, the perianal skin, and the round ligament of the uterus drain to the superficial inguinal nodes. The lateral nodes of this group receive lymph from the gluteal region and from the adjoining part of the anterior abdominal wall below the level of the umbilicus. The medial nodes of the group receive superficial lymphatics from the perineal genitalia, including the vagina, below the hymen. A lower group of superficial inguinal nodes, situated vertically along the terminal part of the great saphenous vein, receives all the superficial lymph drainage from the lower limb except for the back and lateral side of the calf. All superficial inguinal nodes send efferents to the external iliac lymph chain.

There are one to three **deep inguinal lymph nodes**, which are situated on the medial side of the femoral vein. They receive efferents from the deep lymph vessels which accompany the femoral vessels, a small

number of efferents from the superficial inguinal nodes, and drainage from the glans penis or clitoris. The deep inguinal nodes also drain to the external iliac lymph nodes.

External iliac lymph nodes

As seen in Figure 4.16, the external iliac lymph nodes accompany the external iliac vessels and are divided into three groups—medial, posterior (intermediate), and lateral. The medial group consists of three to four nodes which receive efferents from the bladder and prostate, the membranous part of the urethra, the cervix, and the upper part of the vagina. The posterior group comprises three nodes which receive lymph from the internal iliac nodes, via the surgical obturator lymph nodes situated adjacent to the obturator nerve and vessels. The lateral group, which also contains three to four nodes, receives lymph from the superficial and deep inguinal nodes, and therefore from the lower limb, the anterior abdominal wall, the perineum, the anal canal, the vagina (lower part), the uterine fundus, the scrotum, and the penis or clitoris. The external iliac vessels drain to the posterior and lateral common iliac nodes.

Table 4.1 Major pelvic lymphatic drainage pathways

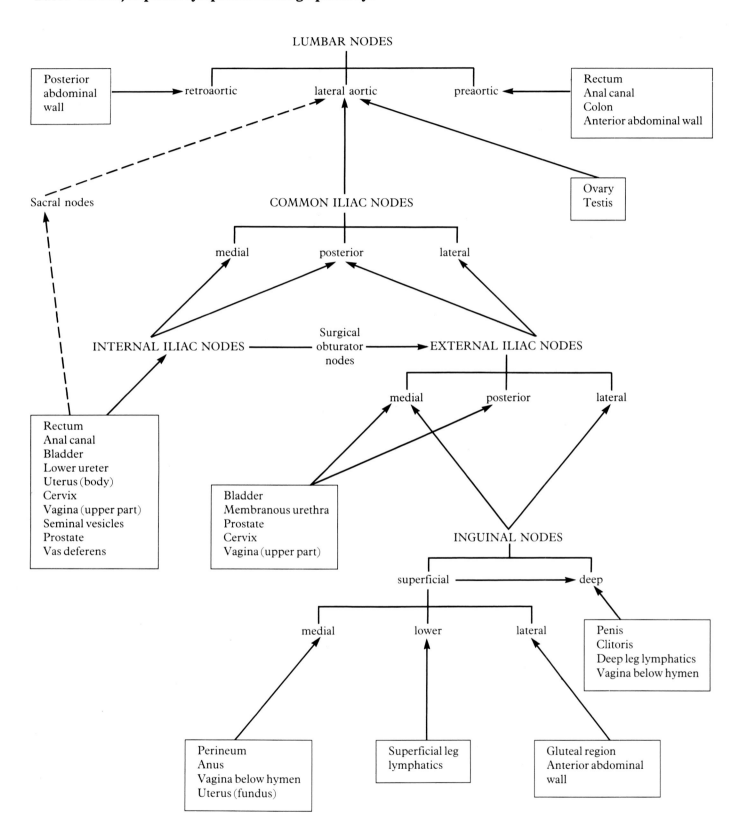

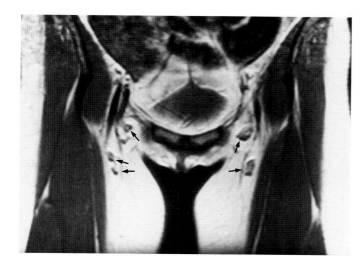

Figure 4.15

Coronal section demonstrating bilateral superficial inguinal nodes (black arrows).

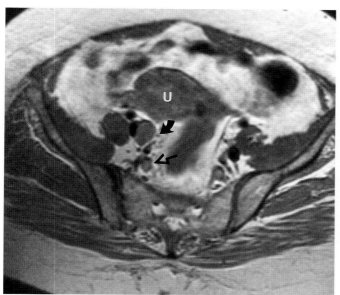

a

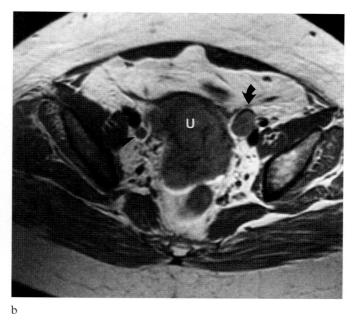

b

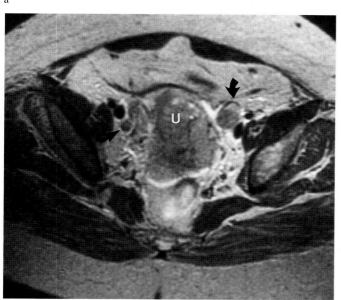

c

Figure 4.16

Lymphadenopathy in patient with carcinoma of the uterus. (**a**) Proton-density image demonstrating medial external (curved black arrow) and internal (open arrow) lymph nodes. (**b**) Proton-density and (**c**) T2-weighted image at the same anatomical level demonstrating medial external (curved black arrow) and posterior external (straight black arrow) lymph nodes, both of which decrease in signal intensity on the T2-weighted image, thereby differentiating them from the ovarian tissue. (U)–uterus.

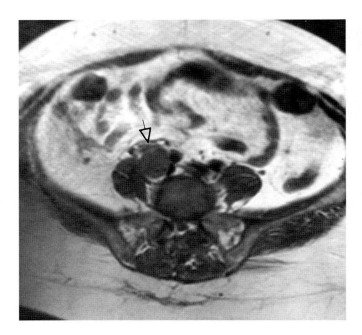

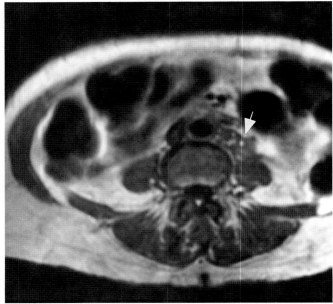

Figure 4.17

Enlarged lateral common iliac
lymph nodes (open arrow).

Figure 4.18

Left paraaortic lymph nodes
(white arrow).

Internal iliac lymph nodes

Figure 4.16 also illustrates the internal iliac nodes
surrounding the internal iliac vessels. They receive
efferents from all the pelvic viscera (the body of the
uterus, the prostate gland, the upper part of the
vagina, the seminal vesicles, the vas deferens, the
lower part of the ureters, and the bladder) as well as
the deeper parts of the perineum, the buttock muscles,
and the posterior aspect of the thigh. Efferents from
the internal iliac lymphatics pass to the common iliac
nodes (medial and posterior group) and to the external
iliac chain via the obturator nodes. The sacral lymph
nodes (situated along the median and lateral sacral
vessels) and the anatomic obturator lymph nodes

(occasionally present in the obturator canal) are
members of the internal iliac group. The sacral nodes
drain directly into the lumbar lymphatics.

Common iliac lymph nodes

Figure 4.17 shows the common iliac lymph nodes.
There are four to six nodes in this chain, which is
further subdivided into lateral, medial and posterior
groups, depending on the relationship to the common
iliac artery. The lateral group usually comprises two
nodes and is the direct continuation of the external
iliac lymph nodes. The posterior group consists of two
to four nodes and receives efferents from the internal

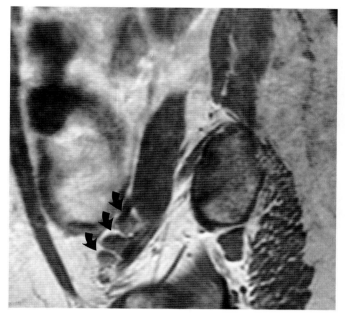

a

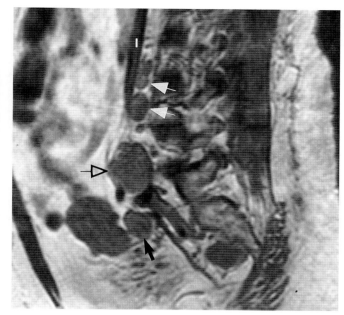

b

Figure 4.19

Pelvic and retroperitoneal lymph nodes as seen on sagittal MR images. (**a**) External iliac lymphadenopathy (curved black arrows). (**b**) Posterior external iliac lymph node (straight black arrow), common iliac lymph node (open black arrow). Right lateral paraaortic nodes (white arrow) seen posterior to the inferior vena cava (I).

and external iliac nodes. The medial common iliac group consists of two nodes and is situated below the aortic bifurcation anterior to the fifth lumbar vertebra or the sacral prominence. It receives lymph from the internal iliac nodes. The common iliac nodes drain into the left and right lateral aortic nodal chains, which are part of the lumbar nodes.

Lumbar lymph nodes

Figure 4.18 depicts the lumbar lymph nodes, which are divided into three groups of terminal nodes—right lateral aortic, left lateral aortic, and preaortic. The right lateral aortic chain includes paracaval and retro-caval nodes, and the preaortic chain incorporates precaval nodes. Both lateral aortic groups drain the viscera and other structures supplied by the lateral and dorsal branches of the aorta, as well as efferent lymphatics from the iliac nodes. Therefore, the lateral aortic nodes constitute the terminal groups for the pelvic viscera (except the gastrointestinal tract), the testes, the ovaries, the ureters, the kidneys, and the posterior abdominal wall. The preaortic lymph nodes drain the viscera supplied by the ventral branches of the aorta, including the abdominal and pelvic bowel. A subsidiary lumbar nodal group of retroaortic lymph nodes does not drain a specific area or viscus; it is considered to represent peripheral nodes from both lateral aortic groups. Lymph nodes are identified on

Figure 4.20

The sciatic nerve (white arrow) seen on off-axis. (**a**) Coronal plane with accompanying schematic drawing (**b**) and (**c**) off-axis transaxial plane with accompanying schematic drawing (**d**).

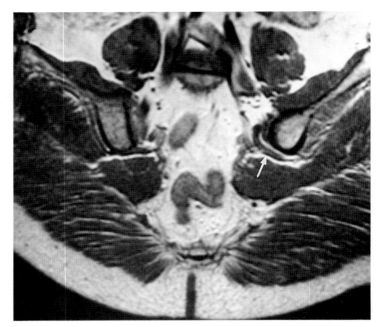

a

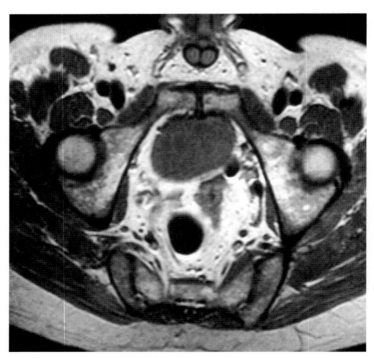

c

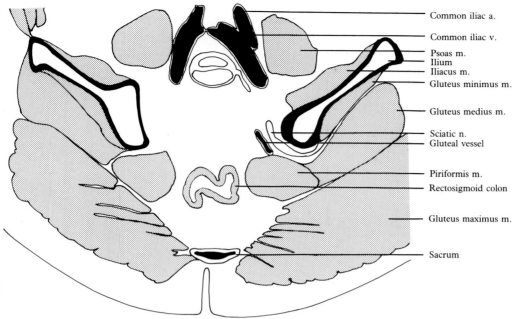

Common iliac a.

Common iliac v.

Psoas m.
Ilium
Iliacus m.
Gluteus minimus m.

Gluteus medius m.

Sciatic n.
Gluteal vessel

Piriformis m.
Rectosigmoid colon

Gluteus maximus m.

Sacrum

b

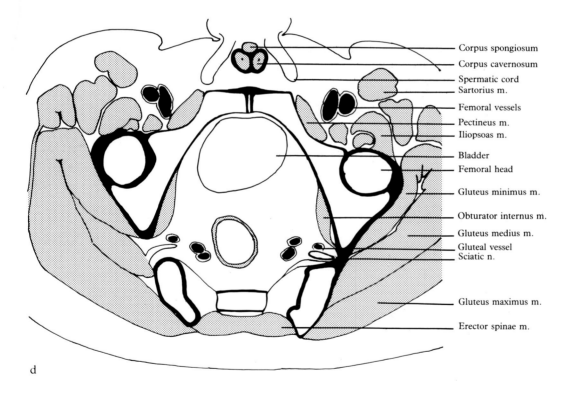

Corpus spongiosum

Corpus cavernosum

Spermatic cord
Sartorius m.

Femoral vessels

Pectineus m.
Iliopsoas m.

Bladder
Femoral head

Gluteus minimus m.

Obturator internus m.

Gluteus medius m.

Gluteal vessel
Sciatic n.

Gluteus maximus m.

Erector spinae m.

d

Figure 4.21

The femoral nerve. Off-axis coronal image (**a**) and accompanying schematic drawing (**b**) demonstrating the groove between the psoas and iliacus muscles (long white arrows), within which the femoral nerve resides.

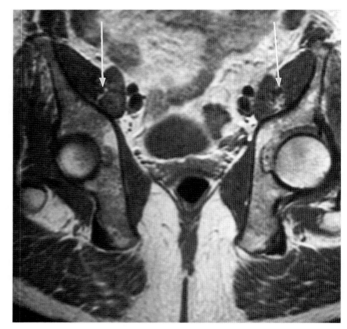

a

Figure 4.22

The obturator sulcus. The obturator nerve, artery and vein are identified within the obturator sulcus (white arrows).

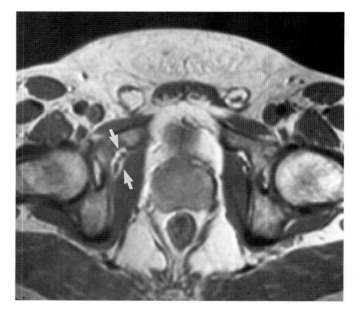

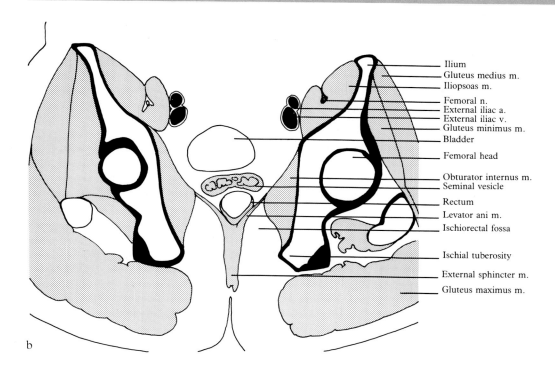

Ilium
Gluteus medius m.
Iliopsoas m.
Femoral n.
External iliac a.
External iliac v.
Gluteus minimus m.
Bladder
Femoral head
Obturator internus m.
Seminal vesicle
Rectum
Levator ani m.
Ischiorectal fossa
Ischial tuberosity
External sphincter m.
Gluteus maximus m.

b

sagittal sections and their relation to vessels can be appreciated (Figure 4.19).

Nerves

Peripheral nerves are of low signal intensity on both T1- and T2-weighted images. After gadolinium-DTPA administration, perineural tissue enhances. The sacral plexus and the sciatic nerves (Figure 4.20) are the only peripheral nerves routinely demonstrated on MR pelvic images. The **sacral plexus**, an oval structure of low signal intensity, may be identified lying on the fascial plane anterior to the piriformis muscle in the superior aspect of the greater sciatic foramen, which is situated immediately beneath the sacro-iliac joint. The **sciatic nerve** may be identified as it leaves the pelvis through the greater sciatic foramen, below the piriformis muscle, and descends into the posterior thigh lateral to the ischial tuberosity.

The femoral and obturator nerves may also be visualized on MR images. In Figure 4.21 the **femoral nerve** can be seen as it passes along the lateral border of the psoas muscle, in the groove between the psoas and iliacus muscles, and leaves the pelvis inferior to

the inguinal ligament. The **obturator nerve** may be seen running from the medial border of the psoas, passing inferior and lateral to the ureter, across the lateral wall of the pelvis, to exit through the obturator foramen with the obturator artery and vein (Figure 4.22).

Fat

As illustrated in Figure 4.22, fat demonstrates homogeneous high signal intensity on T1-weighted images. With increasing repetition and echo times, the high signal intensity of fat is preserved relative to other tissues. Although pathophysiologic studies have identified distinct subtypes of fat cells at different anatomical locations, the MR signal intensity of fat is uniform throughout the body.

Muscle

Striated muscle is of medium signal intensity on T1-weighted images and demonstrates decrease in signal

Figure 4.23

Male perineum. (**a**) MR image, (**b**) schematic drawing at a similar level.

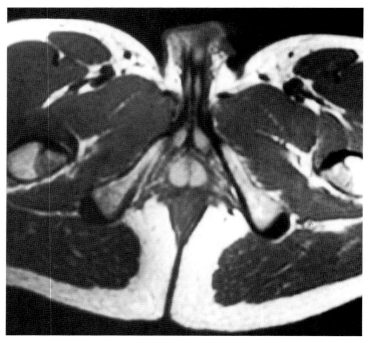

a

Figure 4.24

Female perineum. (**a**) MR image, (**b**) schematic drawing at a similar level.

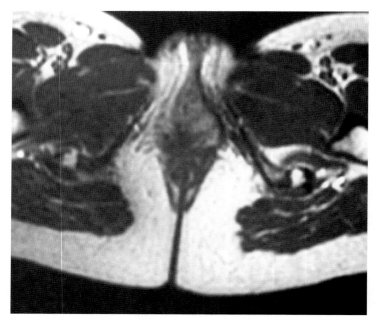

a

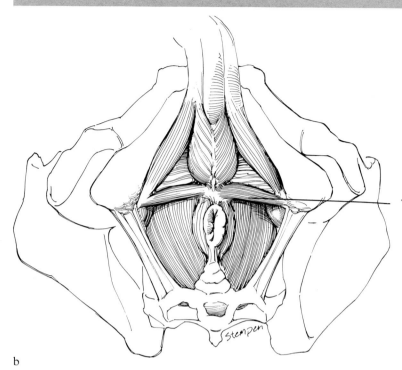

Transversus perinei superficialis m.

b

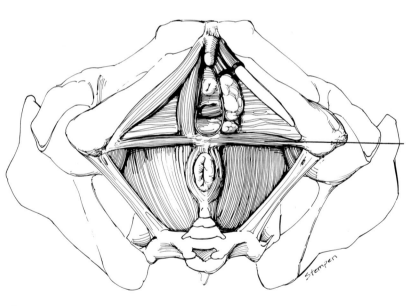

Transversus perinei superficialis m.

b

intensity on T2-weighted images. A detailed demonstration of muscle anatomy is provided in all three orthogonal planes (Figures 4.25 to 4.50).

The **iliopsoas muscles** are the major muscles of the false pelvis. The psoas component originates from the vertebral bodies and transverse processes of the twelfth thoracic to fourth lumbar vertebrae. The iliacus muscle originates from the upper two-thirds of the iliac fossa and sacral ala. Psoas and iliacus unite at the level of first sacral vertebra and pass anteriorly to leave the pelvis beneath the antero-inferior iliac spine and inguinal ligament, inserting on the lesser trochanter of the femur. Between the psoas and iliacus muscle is a small groove containing the iliac fascia and the femoral nerve.

The musculature of the true pelvis consists of the muscles of the pelvic diaphragm plus two lower limb muscles. The major muscles of the pelvic diaphragm are the **levator ani** and **coccygeus**. The levator ani muscle arises from the superior surface of the pubic rami, the fascia of the obturator internus muscle, and the inner surface of the ischium to insert on the last two coccygeal segments and the anococcygeal raphe. It is readily identifiable on all MR sequences, but is best differentiated from adjacent organs (the rectum and prostate in the male and the vagina and urethra in the female) on T2-weighted images. The coccygeus muscle arises from the ischial spine and attaches to the coccyx posterior to the levator ani muscles, in contiguity with the sacrospinous ligament.

The remaining pelvic floor muscles are the deep and superficial transversus perinei muscles, the ischiocavernosus and bulbocavernosus muscles, and the external anal sphincter muscle. The **transversus perinei profundus muscle** originates from and inserts into the pubis, merging posteriorly with the central perineal tendon, which it braces. The urogenital diaphragm passes through the deep transversus perinei muscle. The **transversus perinei superficialis muscle** originates on the dorsal surface of the ischium and inserts on the contralateral muscle and the external anal sphincter. It braces the urogenital diaphragm and is usually absent in females. The **ischiocavernosus muscle** originates from the ramus of the ischium and inserts into the tunica albuginea of the penis or clitoris. It compresses the crus penis and helps erection. The **bulbocavernosus muscle** originates from the central perineal tendon and corpus spongiosum and inserts into the inferior fascia of the urogenital diaphragm. It has multiple functions including emptying the urethra when the bladder neck is closed and assisting in erection and ejaculation.

The **external anal sphincter muscle** is divided into three portions by septae which insert into the longitudinal muscle of the rectum. It is supplemented by the medial portion of the levator ani, called the puborectalis muscle, and acts as part of the anal continence mechanism.

Both obturator internus and piriformis muscles are lower limb muscles originating in the true pelvis and forming part of the pelvic sidewall. The **obturator internus** arises from the anterolateral wall of the true pelvis and the **piriformis muscle** from the lateral aspect of the sacrum. Both muscles insert onto the greater trochanter of the femur.

Bone

The bony pelvis consists of the paired innominate bones together with the sacrum and coccyx. Bony anatomy is illustrated in all three orthogonal planes (Figures 4.25 to 4.50). Cortical bone is of low signal intensity on all MR sequences. The signal intensity of bone marrow varies with magnetic field strength, MR sequence, and age.[5,6,7] On T1-weighted spin-echo sequences, marrow is of intermediate signal intensity at both low and high field strengths, but on T2-weighted spin-echo sequences, the signal intensity of marrow increases at low field strengths and decreases at high field strengths.

Perineum

The perineum, depicted in Figures 4.23 and 4.24, is situated inferior to the pelvic floor muscles. It is a diamond-shaped space bounded anteriorly by the symphysis pubis and arcuate pubic ligament, and laterally by the inferior pubic ramus, the ischial ramus, and the ischial tuberosity. It may be divided into two compartments: the anterior or urogenital triangle, which contains the external urogenital organs; and the posterior or anal triangle, which contains the anus. The two triangles are separated by the superficial transversus perinei muscle. Fat within the ischiorectal fossae occupies the posterolateral perineum.

Cross-sectional atlas

The final section of this chapter is a cross-sectional atlas showing normal pelvic anatomy in the transaxial, sagittal, and coronal planes.

References

1 WILLIAM PL, WARWICK R (eds), *Gray's Anatomy*, (Churchill Livingstone: Edinburgh 1980) 791–800.

2 RUBENSTEIN WA, AUH YH, ZIRINSKY K et al, Posterior peritoneal recesses: assessment using CT, *Radiology* (1985) **156**:461–68.

3 AUH YH, RUBENSTEIN WA, MARKISZ JA et al, Intraperitoneal paravesical spaces: CT delineation with US correlation, *Radiology* (1986) **159**:311–17.

4 LIERSE W, The lymphatic system in the pelvis. In: Lierse W, ed. *Applied Anatomy of the Pelvis*, (Springer Verlag: Berlin 1984) 79–84.

5 DOOMS GC, FISHER MR, HRICAK H et al, Bone marrow imaging: magnetic resonance studies related to age and sex. *Radiology* (1985) **155**:429–32.

6 VOGLER JB III, MURPHY WA, Bone marrow imaging, *Radiology* (1988) **168**:679–93.

7 MOORE SG, DAWSON KL, Red and yellow marrow in the femur: age-related changes in appearance at MR imaging, *Radiology* (1990) **175**:219–23.

SECTION A: MALE PELVIC ANATOMY INCLUDING GENERAL ANATOMY

Transaxial plane

Figures 4.25 to 4.31 are representative transaxial proton-density MR images of male pelvic anatomy with accompanying schematic drawings. (**a**) MR figure, (**b**) schematic drawing.

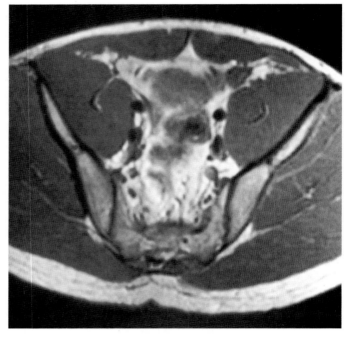

a

Figure 4.25

Figure 4.26

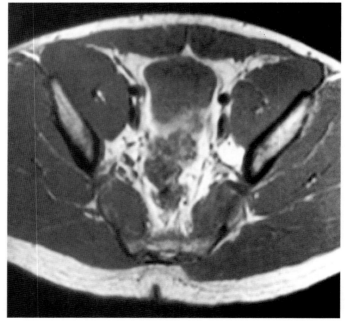

a

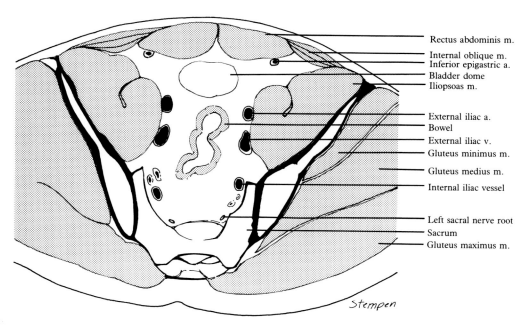

Rectus abdominis m.
Internal oblique m.
Inferior epigastric a.
Bladder dome
Iliopsoas m.

External iliac a.
Bowel
External iliac v.
Gluteus minimus m.

Gluteus medius m.

Internal iliac vessel

Left sacral nerve root
Sacrum
Gluteus maximus m.

Stempen

b

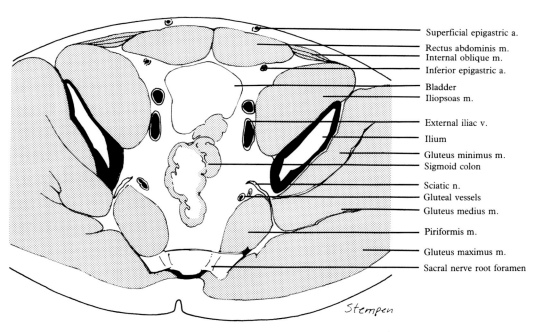

Superficial epigastric a.

Rectus abdominis m.
Internal oblique m.

Inferior epigastric a.

Bladder
Iliopsoas m.

External iliac v.

Ilium

Gluteus minimus m.
Sigmoid colon

Sciatic n.
Gluteal vessels
Gluteus medius m.

Piriformis m.

Gluteus maximus m.
Sacral nerve root foramen

Stempen

b

Figure 4.27

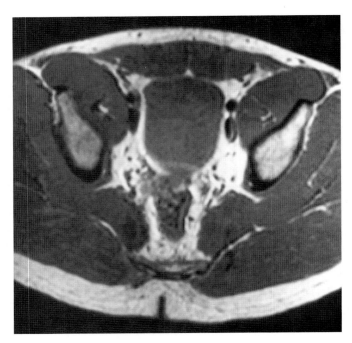

a

Figure 4.28

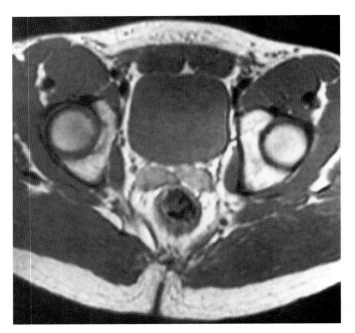

a

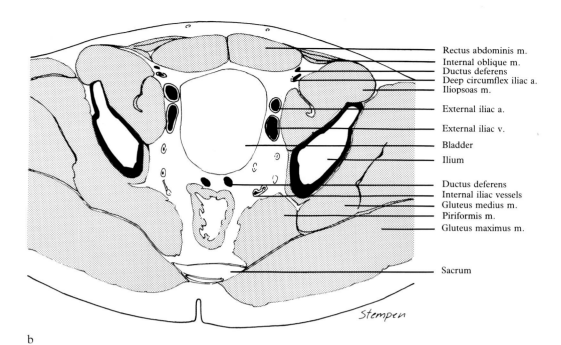

Rectus abdominis m.
Internal oblique m.
Ductus deferens
Deep circumflex iliac a.
Iliopsoas m.

External iliac a.

External iliac v.

Bladder
Ilium

Ductus deferens
Internal iliac vessels
Gluteus medius m.
Piriformis m.
Gluteus maximus m.

Sacrum

Stempen

b

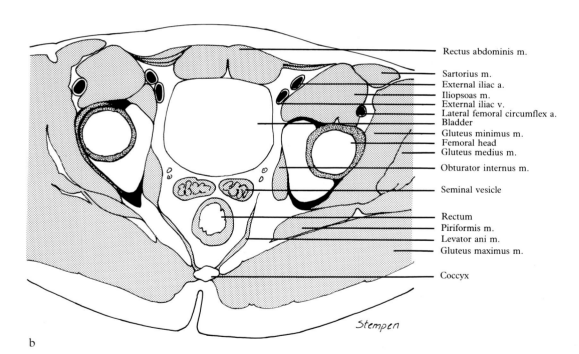

Rectus abdominis m.

Sartorius m.
External iliac a.
Iliopsoas m.
External iliac v.
Lateral femoral circumflex a.
Bladder
Gluteus minimus m.
Femoral head
Gluteus medius m.
Obturator internus m.

Seminal vesicle

Rectum
Piriformis m.
Levator ani m.
Gluteus maximus m.

Coccyx

Stempen

b

Figure 4.29

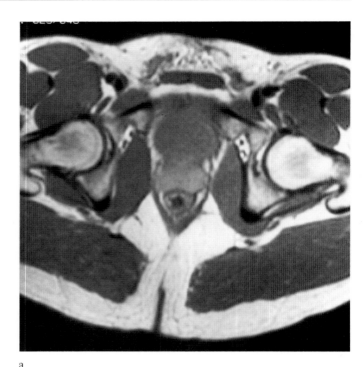

a

Figure 4.30

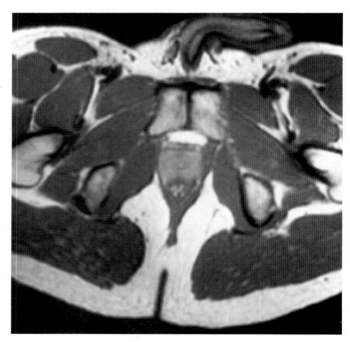

a

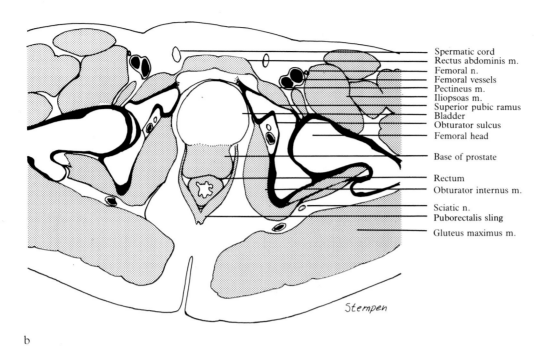

Spermatic cord
Rectus abdominis m.
Femoral n.
Femoral vessels
Pectineus m.
Iliopsoas m.
Superior pubic ramus
Bladder
Obturator sulcus
Femoral head

Base of prostate

Rectum
Obturator internus m.

Sciatic n.
Puborectalis sling

Gluteus maximus m.

Stempen

b

Spermatic cord
Sartorius m.

Femoral vessels

Symphysis pubis
Iliopsoas m.
Pectineus m.

Obturator externus m.

Preprostatic space
Prostate (mid-gland)
Obturator internus m.
Levator ani m.

Anal canal
Ischium
Puborectalis m.
Ischiorectal fossa

Gluteus maximus m.

Stempen

b

Figure 4.31

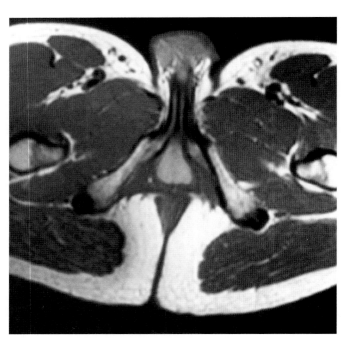

a

Sagittal plane

Figures 4.32 to 4.36 are representative sagittal proton-density images of male pelvic anatomy with accompanying schematic drawings. (**a**) MR figure, (**b**) schematic drawing.

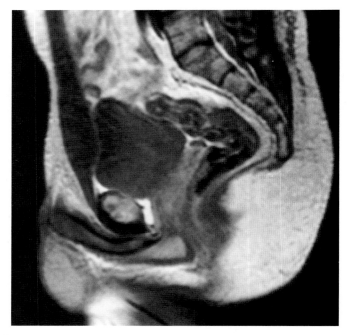

Figure 4.32

a

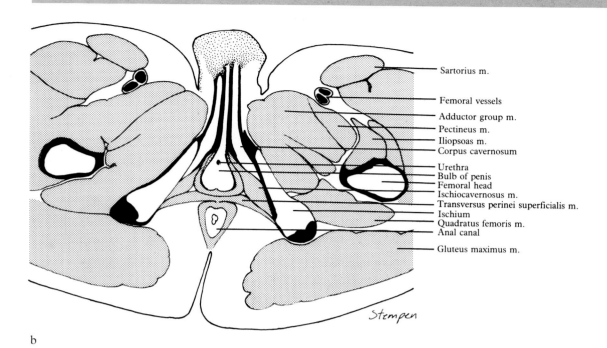

Sartorius m.

Femoral vessels

Adductor group m.

Pectineus m.

Iliopsoas m.

Corpus cavernosum

Urethra
Bulb of penis
Femoral head
Ischiocavernosus m.
Transversus perinei superficialis m.
Ischium
Quadratus femoris m.
Anal canal

Gluteus maximus m.

b

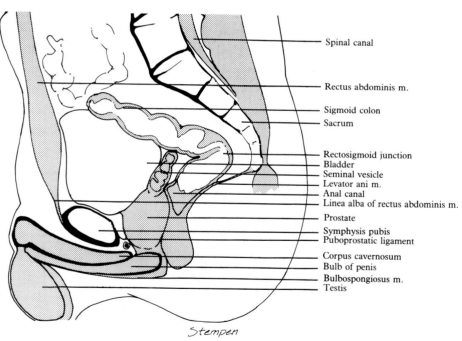

Spinal canal

Rectus abdominis m.

Sigmoid colon
Sacrum

Rectosigmoid junction
Bladder
Seminal vesicle
Levator ani m.
Anal canal
Linea alba of rectus abdominis m.
Prostate
Symphysis pubis
Puboprostatic ligament
Corpus cavernosum
Bulb of penis
Bulbospongiosus m.
Testis

b

Figure 4.33

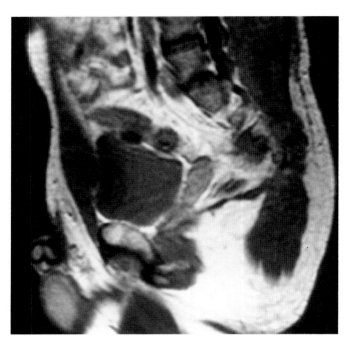

a

Figure 4.34

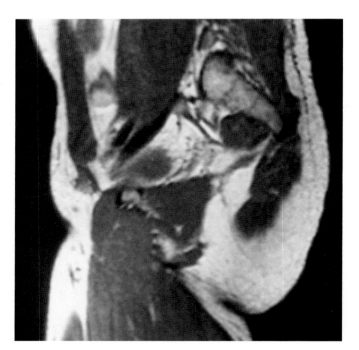

a

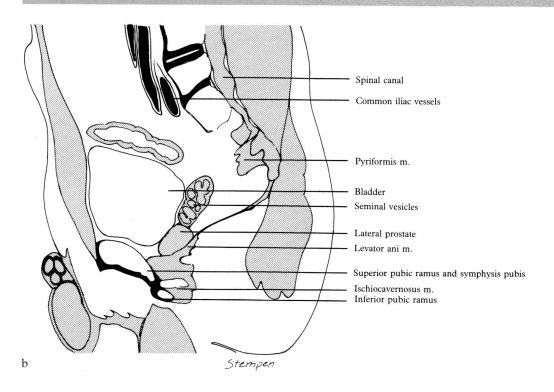

Spinal canal

Common iliac vessels

Pyriformis m.

Bladder
Seminal vesicles

Lateral prostate
Levator ani m.

Superior pubic ramus and symphysis pubis

Ischiocavernosus m.
Inferior pubic ramus

b

Stempen

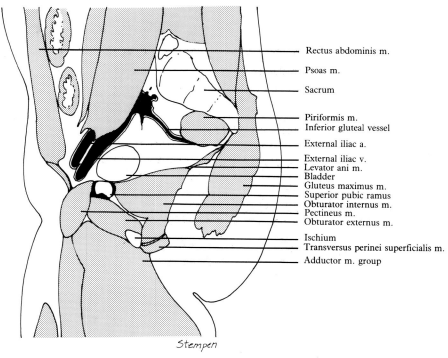

Rectus abdominis m.

Psoas m.

Sacrum

Piriformis m.
Inferior gluteal vessel

External iliac a.

External iliac v.
Levator ani m.
Bladder
Gluteus maximus m.
Superior pubic ramus
Obturator internus m.
Pectineus m.
Obturator externus m.

Ischium
Transversus perinei superficialis m.

Adductor m. group

b

Stempen

Figure 4.35

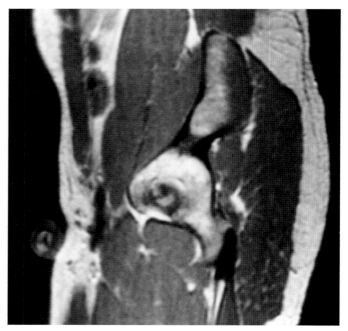

a

Figure 4.36

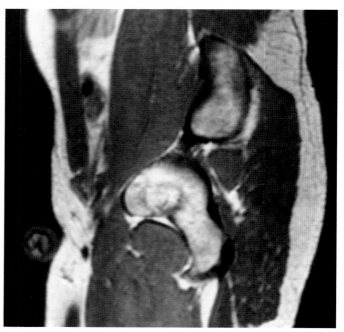

a

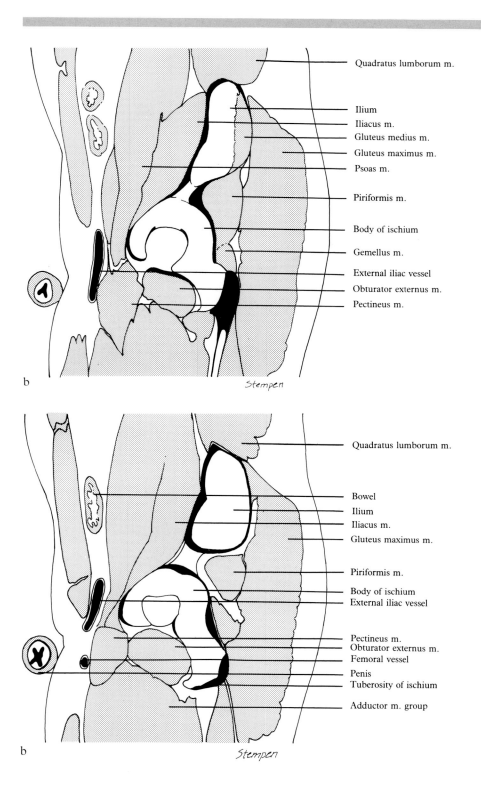

Quadratus lumborum m.

Ilium
Iliacus m.
Gluteus medius m.
Gluteus maximus m.
Psoas m.

Piriformis m.

Body of ischium

Gemellus m.

External iliac vessel
Obturator externus m.
Pectineus m.

b

Stempen

Quadratus lumborum m.

Bowel
Ilium
Iliacus m.
Gluteus maximus m.

Piriformis m.

Body of ischium
External iliac vessel

Pectineus m.
Obturator externus m.
Femoral vessel
Penis
Tuberosity of ischium

Adductor m. group

b

Stempen

Coronal plane

Figures 4.37 to 4.42 are representative coronal proton-density images of male pelvic anatomy with accompanying schematic drawings. (**a**) MR figure, (**b**) schematic drawing.

Figure 4.37

Figure 4.38

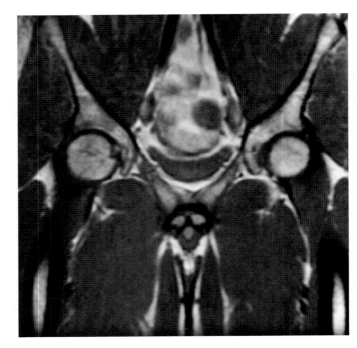

a

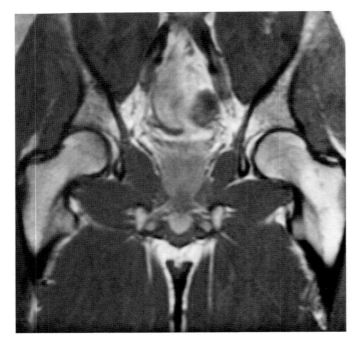

a

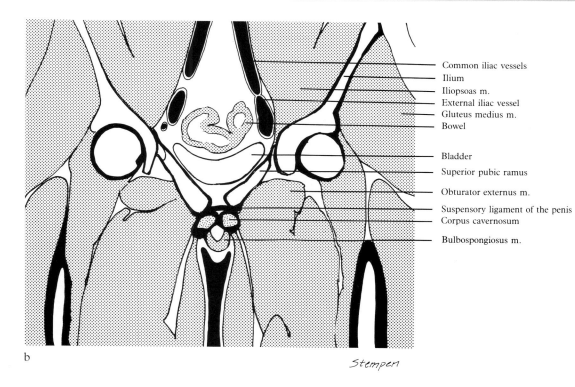

Common iliac vessels
Ilium
Iliopsoas m.
External iliac vessel
Gluteus medius m.
Bowel

Bladder
Superior pubic ramus

Obturator externus m.

Suspensory ligament of the penis
Corpus cavernosum

Bulbospongiosus m.

b

Stempen

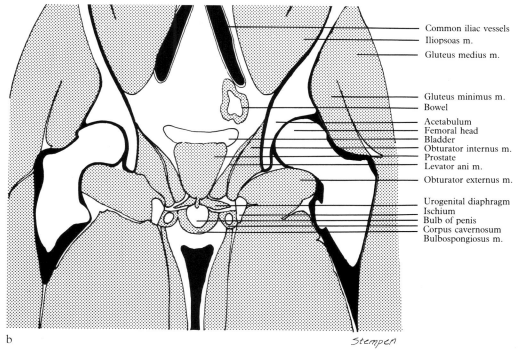

Common iliac vessels
Iliopsoas m.

Gluteus medius m.

Gluteus minimus m.
Bowel

Acetabulum
Femoral head
Bladder
Obturator internus m.
Prostate
Levator ani m.

Obturator externus m.

Urogenital diaphragm
Ischium
Bulb of penis
Corpus cavernosum
Bulbospongiosus m.

b

Stempen

Figure 4.39

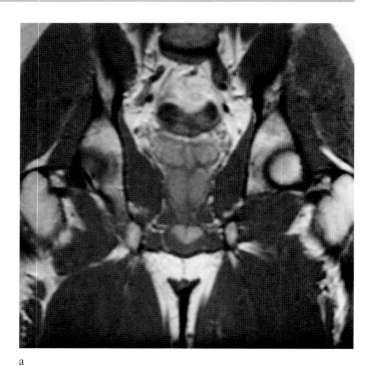

a

Figure 4.40

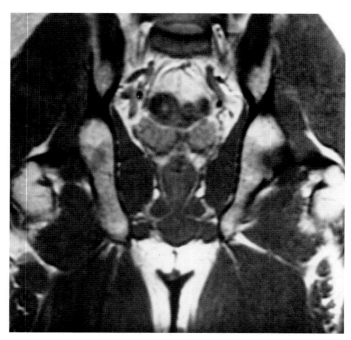

a

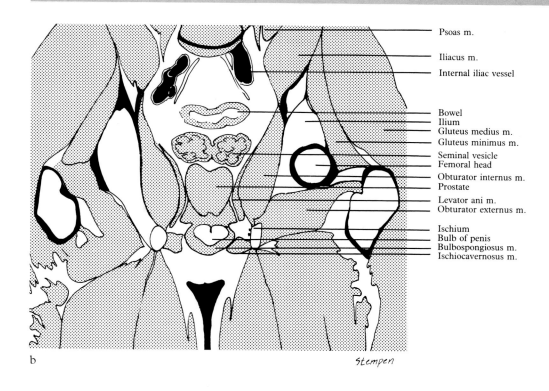

Psoas m.
Iliacus m.
Internal iliac vessel

Bowel
Ilium
Gluteus medius m.
Gluteus minimus m.
Seminal vesicle
Femoral head
Obturator internus m.
Prostate
Levator ani m.
Obturator externus m.

Ischium
Bulb of penis
Bulbospongiosus m.
Ischiocavernosus m.

b   *Stempen*

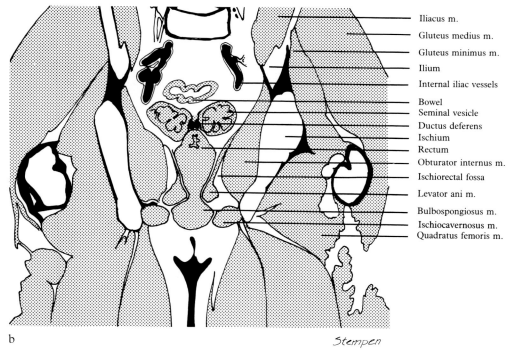

Iliacus m.
Gluteus medius m.
Gluteus minimus m.
Ilium
Internal iliac vessels
Bowel
Seminal vesicle
Ductus deferens
Ischium
Rectum
Obturator internus m.
Ischiorectal fossa
Levator ani m.
Bulbospongiosus m.
Ischiocavernosus m.
Quadratus femoris m.

b   *Stempen*

Figure 4.41

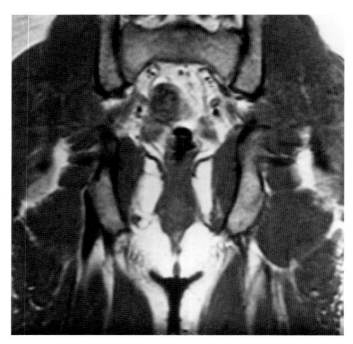

a

Figure 4.42

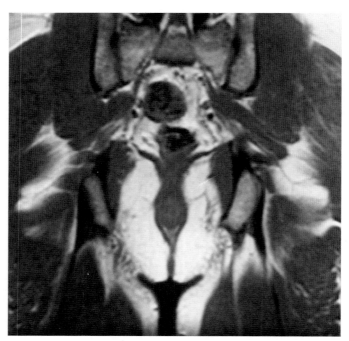

a

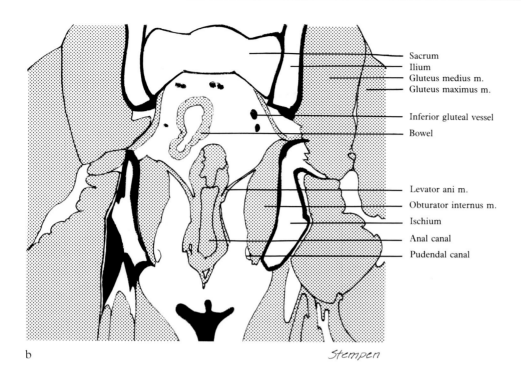

Sacrum
Ilium
Gluteus medius m.
Gluteus maximus m.

Inferior gluteal vessel

Bowel

Levator ani m.
Obturator internus m.
Ischium
Anal canal
Pudendal canal

b

Stempen

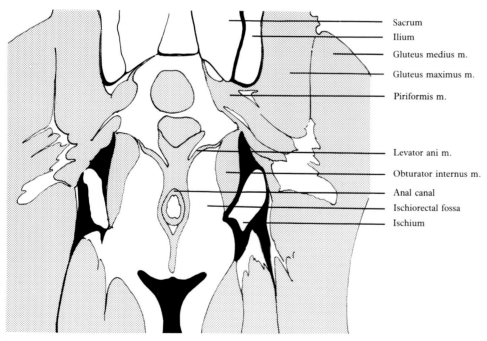

Sacrum
Ilium

Gluteus medius m.

Gluteus maximus m.

Piriformis m.

Levator ani m.

Obturator internus m.

Anal canal
Ischiorectal fossa
Ischium

b

Stempen

SECTION B: FEMALE PELVIC ANATOMY

All images are T2-weighted to enhance zonal anatomy and facilitate organ identification.

Transaxial plane

Figures 4.43 to 4.46 are representative transaxial T2-weighted images of female pelvic anatomy with accompanying schematic drawings. (**a**) MR figure, (**b**) schematic drawing.

Figure 4.43

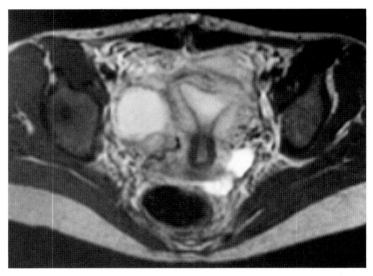

a

Figure 4.44

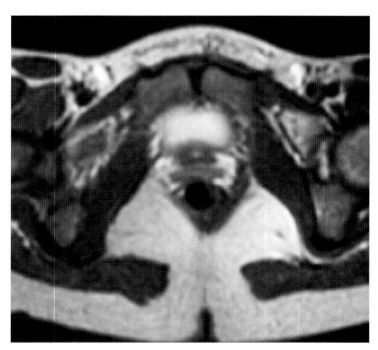

a

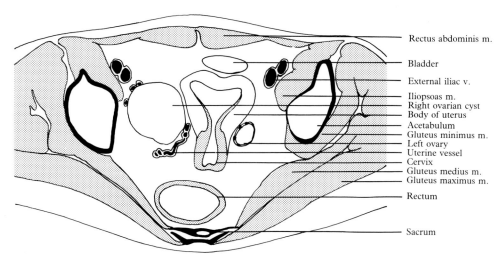

Rectus abdominis m.

Bladder

External iliac v.

Iliopsoas m.
Right ovarian cyst
Body of uterus
Acetabulum
Gluteus minimus m.
Left ovary
Uterine vessel
Cervix
Gluteus medius m.
Gluteus maximus m.

Rectum

Sacrum

b

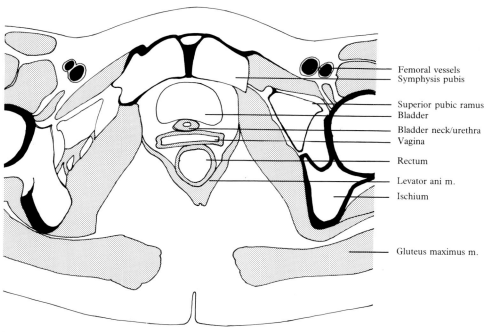

Femoral vessels
Symphysis pubis

Superior pubic ramus
Bladder

Bladder neck/urethra
Vagina

Rectum

Levator ani m.

Ischium

Gluteus maximus m.

b

Figure 4.45

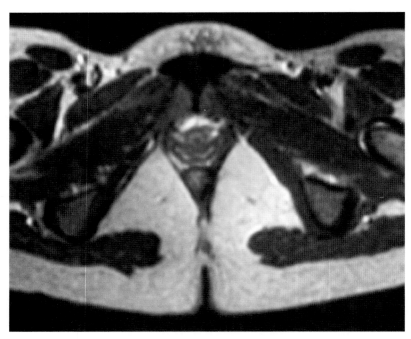

a

Figure 4.46

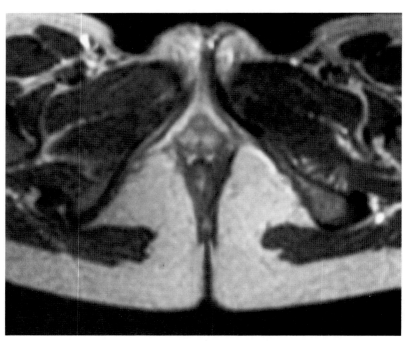

a

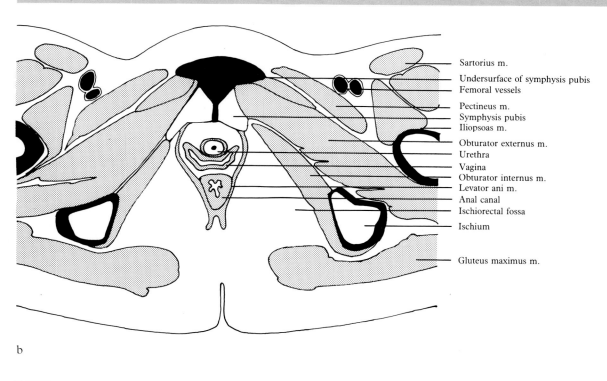

Sartorius m.

Undersurface of symphysis pubis
Femoral vessels

Pectineus m.
Symphysis pubis
Iliopsoas m.

Obturator externus m.
Urethra
Vagina
Obturator internus m.
Levator ani m.
Anal canal
Ischiorectal fossa
Ischium

Gluteus maximus m.

b

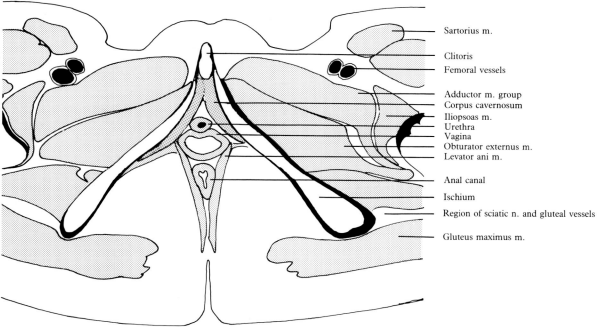

Sartorius m.

Clitoris
Femoral vessels

Adductor m. group
Corpus cavernosum
Iliopsoas m.
Urethra
Vagina
Obturator externus m.
Levator ani m.

Anal canal

Ischium

Region of sciatic n. and gluteal vessels

Gluteus maximus m.

b

Sagittal plane

Figures 4.47 to 4.48 are representative sagittal T2-weighted images of female pelvic anatomy with accompanying schematic drawings. (**a**) MR figure, (**b**) schematic drawing.

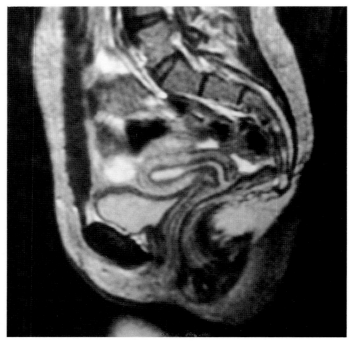

a

Figure 4.47

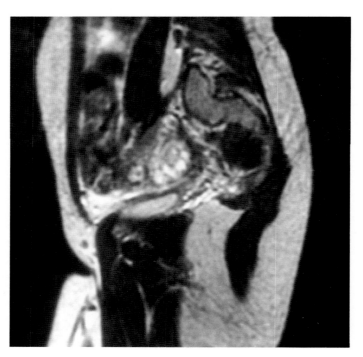

a

Figure 4.48

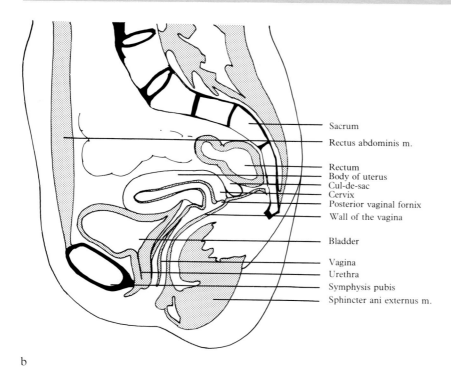

Sacrum
Rectus abdominis m.

Rectum
Body of uterus
Cul-de-sac
Cervix
Posterior vaginal fornix
Wall of the vagina

Bladder

Vagina
Urethra
Symphysis pubis
Sphincter ani externus m.

b

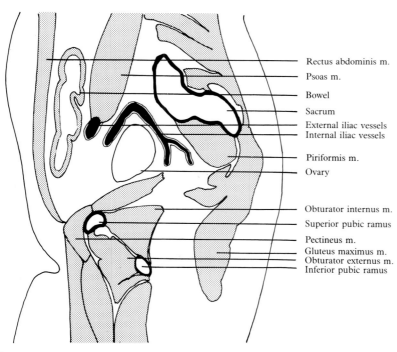

Rectus abdominis m.
Psoas m.

Bowel

Sacrum
External iliac vessels
Internal iliac vessels

Piriformis m.

Ovary

Obturator internus m.
Superior pubic ramus

Pectineus m.
Gluteus maximus m.
Obturator externus m.
Inferior pubic ramus

b

Coronal plane

Figures 4.49 and 4.50 are representative images of female pelvic anatomy with accompanying schematic drawings. (**a**) MR figure, (**b**) schematic drawing.

Figure 4.49

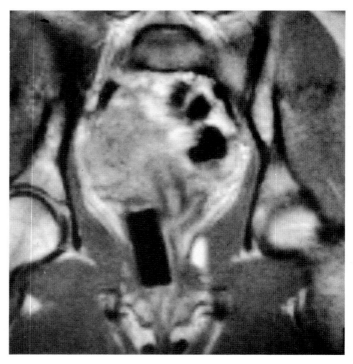

a

Figure 4.50

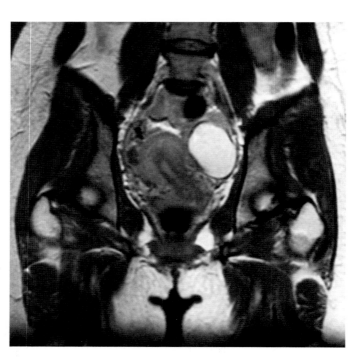

a

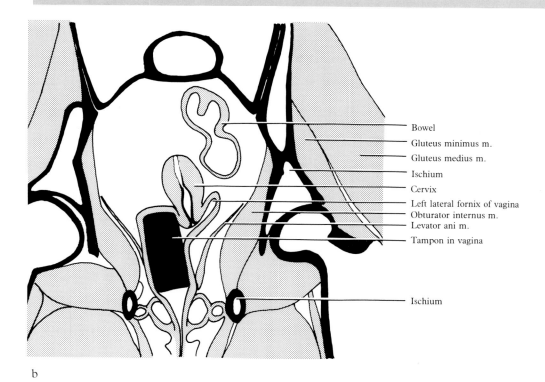

Bowel
Gluteus minimus m.
Gluteus medius m.
Ischium
Cervix
Left lateral fornix of vagina
Obturator internus m.
Levator ani m.
Tampon in vagina

Ischium

b

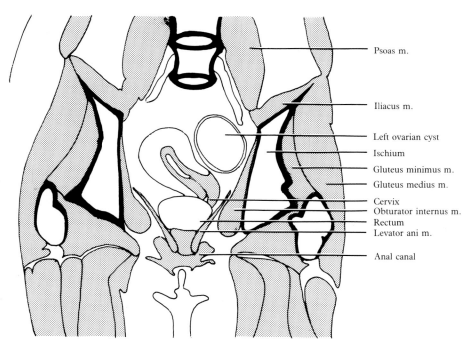

Psoas m.

Iliacus m.

Left ovarian cyst
Ischium
Gluteus minimus m.
Gluteus medius m.
Cervix
Obturator internus m.
Rectum
Levator ani m.

Anal canal

b

5

The Uterus and Vagina

Bernadette Carrington
Hedvig Hricak

Magnetic resonance imaging (MRI) is now recognized as an important modality in the evaluation of the female pelvis. In benign pelvic disease, ultrasonography remains the most appropriate initial investigation, and MRI is reserved for those patients in whom ultrasound is suboptimal or equivocal. In the evaluation of pelvic malignancy, however, MRI is the primary imaging modality. The excellent contrast resolution achieved with MRI and the capability for direct multiplanar imaging are valuable tools in the staging of endometrial, cervical, and vaginal neoplasms.

Normal anatomy of the uterus and vagina

The uterus, cervix, and upper-third of the vagina are formed by fusion of the medial portions of the müllerian ducts which are derived from embryonic mesoderm. The unfused lateral portions of the müllerian ducts form the fallopian tubes.[1] The lower two-thirds of the vagina is derived from the sinovaginal bulb, which arises from the posterior aspect of the urogenital sinus.[2]

Uterus

The uterus is located posterior to the bladder and anterior to the rectum. It is divided into three major portions: (1) the fundus, which is that part of the body (corpus) cephalad to an imaginary line connecting the origin of the two fallopian tubes, (2) the body (corpus), and (3) the cervix.

Fundus and corpus

The anterior (vesical) and posterior (intestinal) surfaces of the uterus are covered by peritoneum, which continues laterally to form the anterior and posterior leaves of the broad ligament. Anteriorly, the peritoneum is reflected off the uterus onto the bladder, forming the **vesicouterine pouch**. Posteriorly it is reflected onto the rectum, forming the **rectouterine pouch (pouch of Douglas, cul-de-sac)**. As illustrated in Figure 5.1, anteriorly the peritoneal reflection is more cephalad and there is a 'bare area' between the uterus and bladder–vesicouterine extraperitoneal space. Posteriorly, the peritoneum extends a greater distance caudally before reflecting onto the rectum. Therefore, the peritoneum invests the entire posterior uterine surface and also covers the posterior vaginal fornix.[1,2]

Cervix

The cervix is narrower and more cylindrical than the corpus and bulges into the vagina. It is divided into supravaginal and infravaginal portions at the attachment of the vaginal fornices. The **external os** (the opening between the cervix and the vagina) is precisely defined and is marked histologically by the **squamocolumnar juction**. The **internal os** (the opening between the cervix and the isthmus—the lower uterine segment) is not as exactly demarcated. It is marked histologically by the change from cervical fibrous stroma and endocervical mucosa to the mixed histology of the isthmus, which is intermediate between uterine and cervical tissue. As shown in Figure 5.2, the internal os is delineated anatomically by waisting of the uterine contour and by the entrance of the uterine vessels.

93

Parametrium

The parametrium is a cellular connective tissue contiguous with the so-called 'bare areas' of the uterus (areas which remain uncovered by the peritoneum).[1,2] Anatomically, the connective tissue adjacent to the myometrium is called the **parametria**, the tissue adjacent to the cervix is called **paracervical** and the tissue adjacent to the vagina is called the **paracolpos**. Clinically, all these tissues are referred to as parametria. As shown in Figures 5.2 and 5.3, the parametrium is found adjacent to the lateral margins of the uterus, where the peritoneum reflects to form the broad ligaments. The 'bare area' is also present anteriorly between the uterus and the bladder (beneath the peritoneal reflection of the vesicouterine pouch).[1] The uterine vessels pass through the lateral parametrium to reach the uterus at the level of the internal os. Parametrial tissue is vascular, and contains many efferent lymphatics. It also contains the ureters, which pass 2 cm lateral to the supravaginal cervix in a posteroanterior direction, and then incline medially to reach the bladder. The floor of the lateral parametrium is formed by the **cardinal ligament** which extends towards the pelvic sidewall and separates the parametrial connective tissue from the paravaginal connective tissue. The lateral margin of the parametrial tissue anteriorly is formed by the **uterovesical ligaments**.

Uterine ligaments

The **broad ligaments**, formed by the anterior and posterior reflections of the peritoneum as it passes over the fallopian tubes, are illustrated in Figure 5.3. In addition to the fallopian tubes, the broad ligaments enclose the round ligaments, the uterine vessels inferiorly, and the ovarian ligament laterally.[1]

The **round ligaments**, which originate at the lateral angles of the uterus close to the interstitial portion of the fallopian tubes, are depicted in Figure 5.3. They pass through the inguinal canal to insert into the labia majora. Some lymphatics travel with the round ligaments and drain the fundus of the uterus to the inguinal nodes.[1]

There are three main **suspensory ligaments** for the uterus—the **vesicouterine, cardinal**, and **uterosacral ligaments**.[1,2] All are localized condensations of the subserous fascia (Figure 5.4). The vesicouterine ligaments pass between the cervix and the bladder base. The cardinal ligaments are situated laterally, and start at the level of the levator ani muscles. They divide into anterior and posterior slips which encircle the cervix and continue to the contralateral pelvic sidewall. The uterosacral ligaments pass posteriorly from the cervix to the sacrum, encircling the rectum and forming the medial border of the lateral ligament of the rectum,

adjacent to the superior extent of the perirectal fascia. The uterosacral ligaments are covered by and indent the peritoneum, forming the **rectouterine folds**, which are the lateral boundaries of the pouch of Douglas.

The uterine suspensory ligaments are clinically significant because they form local pathways for tumor spread, particularly in cervical carcinoma.

Vascular supply

The uterus is supplied by the **uterine artery**, a branch of the internal iliac artery. It passes through the parametrium, above the cardinal ligament, and enters the uterus at the level of the internal os. The uterine artery branches to form arcuate vessels, which supply the myometrium. The **ovarian artery** and **vaginal artery** also supply branches to the uterus. Venous drainage is via intramural veins which anastomose at the lateral borders of the uterus to form the **uterovaginal venous plexus** which drains to the internal iliac vessels.

Lymphatic drainage

The fundus and upper-third of the uterus drain via the round ligament to the **superficial inguinal nodes** and laterally via the mesovarium to the **lumbar paraaortic nodes**. The body of the uterus drains to the **internal and common iliac nodes**.[2]

The cervix drains to **internal iliac, obturator and sacral nodes**.[2]

Vagina

The vagina is a fibromuscular tube lined by stratified epithelium. It extends from the vestibule, the cleft between the labia minora, to the uterus and is located between the bladder and urethra anteriorly and the rectum and anal canal posteriorly as seen in Figure 5.5. The vagina ascends posterosuperiorly at an angle of over 90° to the uterine axis. The angle, however, may vary depending on the contents of the bladder and rectum. The inner surfaces of the vaginal walls are ordinarily in contact, and on cross-section the lumen of the lower part of the vagina forms an 'H' configuration. The anterior wall of the vagina is approximately 7.5 cm in length and the posterior wall is approximately 9 cm. Vaginal width increases superiorly. The upper vagina terminates at its attachment to the uterine cervix near the external os. This attachment is higher on the posterior than on the anterior cervical wall, and the posterior recess, which is called the

posterior vaginal fornix, is therefore deeper than the **anterior vaginal fornix**.[1]

Vascular supply

The vagina is supplied by the **internal iliac artery** via the uterine, middle rectal, inferior vesical, and internal pudendal branches. Venous drainage is via the **uterine** and **vaginal plexuses**.

Lymphatic drainage

The upper-third of the vagina drains to the **internal iliac** and **sacral nodes**. The middle-third drains to the **internal iliac** and **common iliac nodes**. The lower-third of the vagina, beneath the hymen, drains to **deep inguinal** and **ano-rectal nodes**.

MRI appearance of the uterus and vagina

Both the uterus and vagina are clearly visualized on MR images, and their appearance is governed by the age and hormonal status of the patient.[3,4,5]

Uterus

In women of reproductive age, the uterus is normally 6–9 cm in length (the corpus is 4–6 cm long and the cervix is 2.5–3.2 cm).[3–6] Uterine volume varies with the menstrual cycle and is greatest during the secretory phase. As illustrated in Figure 5.5, on T1-weighted scans the uterus images with medium to low signal intensity. On T2-weighted images, three distinct uterine layers can be differentiated—the **endometrium**, **junctional zone**, and **myometrium**.[7,8]

The endometrium, which images with high signal intensity on T2-weighted scans, occupies the central portion of the uterus. Endometrial thickness varies with the menstrual cycle (Figure 5.6). At its thinnest, immediately after menstruation and in the beginning of the proliferative phase, the endometrium measures between 1 and 3 mm. At its thickest, during the mid-secretory phase, it measures between 3 and 7 mm.[4,5]

The myometrium images with medium signal intensity on T2-weighted scans, and it increases in signal intensity in the mid-secretory phase. As shown in Figure 5.6, myometrial arcuate vessels are also most prominent in the mid-secretory phase.

The myometrium is separated from the endometrium by a low signal intensity region called the **junctional zone**. There is no histological equivalent to the junctional zone, but in vitro measurements of endometrial and myometrial width indicate that it represents inner myometrium.[3,8] The junctional zone has been shown to have a lower water content (79 per cent) than the outer myometrium (81 per cent),[8] and this may account for the disparity in MR signal intensity between the two zones. The combined width of the outer myometrium and the junctional zone is between 14 and 21 mm.[3,8] Although three uterine zones can also be identified on sonograms, they differ in width from the zones depicted on MR scans and are not directly comparable.[9]

Figure 5.7 illustrates uterine zonal anatomy as identified in the neonate, due to the influence of maternal estrogens. In the child the cervix is longer than the body of the uterus, and continues to account for greater than half the uterine length until approximately the thirteenth year.[10] In premenarchal females, the uterus is approximately 4 cm in length.[10] On T2-weighted images the endometrium is either minimal or absent, and the junctional zone is indistinct. The myometrium has a lower signal intensity than in postmenarchal females (Figure 5.8).

Figure 5.9 illustrates the uterus in postmenopausal women. The zonal anatomy is indistinct, the endometrium is less than 3 mm thick and the myometrium is of lower signal intensity as compared to the uteri of premenopausal females.[4]

Exogenous hormone therapy. In addition to age and reproductive status, exogenous hormones affect the MRI appearance of the uterus. As depicted in Figure 5.10, the myometrium in women taking **oral contraceptives** images with higher than normal signal intensity on T1-weighted images, and increases in signal intensity on T2-weighted images.[4] With prolonged use of oral contraceptives the corpus may decrease in size.[11]

Administration of **gonadotropin-releasing hormone analogs** causes a hypoestrogenic state and results in involution of the uterus (Figure 5.11). The MRI appearance of the uterus is similar to that in a postmenopausal woman.[12]

As shown in Figure 5.12, the MRI appearance of the uterus in a postmenopausal woman taking **exogenous hormones** is similar to that of the uterus in a woman of reproductive age.[4]

Cervix

On T2-weighted images the cervix demonstrates an inner area of high signal intensity with a surrounding predominantly low signal intensity stroma (Figure 5.13). The inner, central zone is believed to represent epithelium and mucus.[3,4] The stroma of the cervix, which has a high concentration of elastic fibrous tissue within its inner portion, demonstrates low signal intensity on T2-weighted images. Smooth muscle strands predominate towards the periphery of the cervix, resulting in an area of medium signal intensity similar to that of myometrium[13] as illustrated in Figures 5.14, 5.15, and 5.16. The relative proportions of fibrous stroma and smooth muscle varies among normal females.

Parametrium

The parametrium demonstrates medium signal intensity on T1-weighted images and shows varying increases in signal intensity on T2-weighted images (Figures 5.14 and 5.15).

Vagina

The vagina is conventionally divided into thirds with the upper-third encompassing the vaginal fornices (Figures 5.17a and b), the middle-third at the level of the bladder base (Figure 5.17c), and the lower-third adjacent to the urethra (Figures 5.17d and e). On T1-weighted scans the vagina images with medium signal intensity, similar to the urethra anteriorly and the rectum posteriorly. However, on T2-weighted images (Figure 5.17) vaginal anatomy can be appreciated and the vagina can be separated from adjacent organs. The vascular paracolpos images with higher signal intensity, as illustrated in Figures 5.17b and 5.17c.

The placement of a vaginal tampon is not only unnecessary for identification of the vagina, but the presence of the tampon will obliterate the anatomical details of the wall of the vagina as seen in Figure 5.18. Figure 5.19 illustrates the variations in the appearance of the vagina with the menstrual cycle in women of reproductive age.[14] In the early proliferative phase (Figure 5.19), there is excellent contrast between the low signal intensity vaginal wall and the high signal intensity central mucosa. However, as illustrated in Figure 5.19, there is less contrast between the vaginal wall and central mucus or adjacent fat in the mid-secretory phase.

In pregnancy, especially during the third trimester, the vaginal wall, the central mucus, and the surrounding tissue all image with homogeneous medium to high signal intensity on T2-weighted images. Figure 5.20 illustrates the poor distinction among these structures.

In premenarchal females and postmenopausal women the vaginal wall is of low signal intensity on T2-weighted images, and there is only a thin, attenuated high signal intensity central mucosa (Figure 5.21).

Contrast enhancement

After administration of intravenous gadolinium-DTPA (Gd-DTPA) (0.1 mmol/kg), the zonal anatomy of the uterus is displayed on T1-weighted images. As depicted in Figure 5.22, the endometrium and myometrium are enhanced, but the junctional zone remains of lower signal intensity, most likely because of its more compact structure and decreased extracellular space.[15]

The effects of Gd-DTPA administration in the cervix are shown in Figure 5.23. Both the paracervical tissue and inner mucosal epithelium are enhanced, whereas the compact cervical stroma remains of lower signal intensity.[15]

Both the wall of the vagina and the submucosa are enhanced after Gd-DTPA administration (Figure 5.23). In some patients a low signal intensity central line may be observed, the nature of which is uncertain. It may represent inner epithelium or the vaginal lumen.[15]

Intrauterine contraceptive devices

Intrauterine contraceptive devices (IUDs) are safely imaged with MR. All IUDs demonstrate a signal void on T1- and T2-weighted images (Figures 5.24 and 5.25 respectively) and their appearance varies according to the type of the device (Figures 5.24 and 5.26).

Suggested imaging sequences

Both T1- and T2-weighted images are necessary to evaluate the uterus and vagina. T1-weighted images provide excellent organ outline and help in tissue characterization and in the evaluation of the nature of any fluid collections. T2-weighted images are necessary to identify uterine and vaginal zonal anatomy and to depict intrauterine pathology.

Gadolinium-DTPA enhanced images allow visualization of zonal anatomy on T1-weighted images. The use of T1-weighted sequences results in a shorter imaging time (less motion artifact) and therefore Gd-DTPA enhanced MR imaging may be used for patients who are seriously ill, uncooperative, or claustrophobic, and in whom T2-weighted imaging will result in inferior results. Gd-DTPA is routinely recommended for endometrial carcinoma staging.

MRI offers three orthogonal planes of imaging, each of which has specific advantages in the assessment of the female pelvis. In the transverse plane the uterus and cervix are well demonstrated as is the region of the uterosacral ligaments and the presacral space. Vaginal anatomy is best displayed in this plane, using a T2-weighted spin-echo image. The transverse plane is optimal for evaluation of the parametrium.

In the sagittal plane, the uterus is seen along its long axis allowing appreciation of its zonal anatomy. The uterovesical ligament is visualized and the relationship of the uterus and vagina to the bladder and rectum can be assessed. The sagittal plane is also invaluable in confirming the presence of presacral disease.

The coronal plane is a complementary plane in the evaluation of the female pelvis. It can be used as an adjunct in the assessment of the uterus, parametrium, vagina, and exocervix, and it offers an opportunity to identify lymphadenopathy.

Off-axis imaging may be of value in assessment of the uterine corpus and cervix, when precise measurements are required or contour abnormalities need to be evaluated.[16]

Pathology of the uterus and vagina

Congenital anomalies

Müllerian duct anomalies

Müllerian duct anomalies (MDAs) result from non-development or partial or complete nonfusion of the müllerian ducts. They occur in 1–15 per cent of women.[17] MDAs are clinically relevant because they are associated with an increased incidence of impaired fertility and menstrual disorders.[18] In particular, women with MDAs have a significant risk of obstetric complications, such as spontaneous abortion, still-birth, and preterm delivery.[19,20] MDAs may be associated with renal anomalies, particularly renal agenesis or ectopia which occurs in 50 per cent of patients with vaginal agenesis, and may be seen in obstructed duplications.[21,22] Table 5.1 summarizes a clinical classification of MDAs proposed by Buttram and Gibbons.[23]

Uterine agenesis or hypoplasia. Uterine agenesis or hypoplasia is due to nondevelopment or rudimentary development of the müllerian ducts. It may occur as one feature of a congenital syndrome or as a consequence of chromosomal defects. It is sometimes found in isolation in patients with primary amenorrhoea.

MRI appearance. In uterine agenesis there is no identifiable uterine tissue. Patients with uterine hypoplasia have a small endometrial cavity with a reduced intercornual diameter (less than 2 cm) as seen in Figure 5.27. When the uterus is hypoplastic due to hormonal dysfunction (infantile uterus), not only is the uterus small but on T2-weighted images it demonstrates abnormally low signal intensity with poorly differentiated zonal anatomy (Figure 5.28).

Unicornuate uterus. The unicornuate anomaly results from nondevelopment or incomplete development of one müllerian duct. With incomplete development of one müllerian duct, three separate subtypes of unicornuate anomaly are recognized: a unicornuate uterus with a rudimentary horn that does not contain endometrium; a unicornuate uterus with a rudimentary horn which does contain endometrium but does not communicate with the main uterine cavity; and a unicornuate uterus which has a rudimentary horn which contains endometrium and does communicate with the main uterine cavity.

MRI appearance. Figure 5.29 illustrates the 'banana'-shaped uterine cavity which results when there is nondevelopment of one müllerian duct. Endometrial and myometrial width are normal. When there is incomplete development of one müllerian duct, the unicornuate uterus has a rudimentary horn which either does or does not contain endometrium, as shown in Figure 5.30.

Table 5.1 Classification of MDAs[23]

Class I: Segmental Agenesis or Hypoplasia
    A Vaginal
    B Cervical
    C Fundal
    D Tubal
    E Combined

Class II: Unicornuate
    A1 Rudimentary horn contains endometrium. Horn may (a) or may not (b) communicate with main uterine cavity.
    A2 Rudimentary horn without endometrium
    B No rudimentary horn

Class III: Uterus Didelphys

Class IV: Bicornuate
    A Complete – division down to internal os
    B Partial
    C Arcuate

Class V: Septate
    A Complete down to internal/external os
    B Incomplete

Didelphys uterus. The didelphys anomaly results from nonfusion of the müllerian ducts, with the development of two separate normal sized uteri and cervices with an upper longitudinal vaginal septum (Figure 5.31).

MRI appearance. Two uteri, cervices and a septate upper vagina are seen. The two uterine horns are widely separated as seen in Figures 5.31a and b. The endometrial and myometrial width are preserved.

Bicornuate uterus. A bicornuate uterus results from partial failure of müllerian duct fusion. The resulting septum is composed of myometrium and surgery is required for correction. The septum may extend to the external os (**bicornuate bicollis uterus**) as seen in Figure 5.32 or to the internal os (**bicornuate unicollis uterus**) as seen in Figure 5.33. An **arcuate uterus** represents a mild form of the bicornuate anomaly in which there is a partial septum composed of myometrium (Figure 5.34).

MRI appearance. On MRI scans the intercornual distance can be seen to be increased, and there is an outward fundal concavity compared with the normal convexity. Endometrial and myometrial width and ratio are normal. In arcuate uteri the fundal surface is flattened or slightly concave.

Septate uterus. Failure of resorption of the final fibrous septum between the müllerian duct components results in a septate uterus (Figure 5.35).

MRI appearance. As illustrated in Figure 5.35 the septum in septate uteri demonstrates low signal intensity on both T1- and T2-weighted images. If the septum reaches to the internal os it is complete. If it terminates above the internal os it is partial. The fundal contour is normal, with an outward fundal convexity.

Complications associated with MDAs. In addition to impaired fertility and obstetric complications (as seen in Figure 5.36), MDAs are associated with an increased incidence of endometriosis. Obstructed uterine drainage may occur in two types of MDAs. One type is a unicornuate uterus with a rudimentary horn which contains endometrium that does not communicate with the main uterine cavity (Figure 5.37). The

other is uterus didelphys, when one of the duplicated vaginas has an obstructing transverse septum in its upper-third (Figure 5.38). Both types of patients present with hematometra, but only the patients with obstructed didelphys also have hematocolpos. The hematocolpos associated with uterus didelphys can be differentiated from hematocolpos due to an imperforate hymen, by demonstration of the level of the obstruction. In uterus didelphys the obstruction is in the upper-third of the vagina (Figure 5.38) while the imperforate hymen causes obstruction at the lower-third of the vagina (Figure 5.39). Differentiation between a unicornuate and didelphys uterus as a cause of obstruction depends on the identification of a compressed unicornuate uterine cavity rather than a separate normal uterus. The unicornuate anomaly has a single cervix and vagina, whereas the didelphys anomaly has a double cervix and duplicated upper vagina.

MRI in relation to other imaging modalities. Hysterosalpingography (HSG) and laparoscopy or surgery have until now been the mainstays for diagnosis of MDAs. Ultrasound has also been used, particularly in the pregnant patient.[24] All of these modalities have inherent limitations, however, particularly in the differentiation between septate and bicornuate uteri.[25] MRI has been shown to be an accurate and noninvasive method for the evaluation of MDAs.[26,27] Because of the capability for tissue characterization (as seen in Figure 5.40), MRI is particularly useful in patients in whom surgical unification is anticipated. A bicornuate uterus requires open surgical repair while in biseptate uteri, the septate can be corrected hysteroscopically. MRI is also helpful in elucidating the etiology of obstructed MDAs.[28]

Ambiguous genitalia

Intersex problems occur in 1 in 1000 live births, and may be subdivided into those with or without ambiguous genitalia. The role of radiology lies in the assessment of patients with ambiguous genitalia when evaluation of the internal genital anatomy is vital to patient management. Disorders of ambiguous genitalia are divided into four categories: male and female pseudohermaphroditism; mixed gonadal dysgenesis; and true hermaphroditism.[29]

Female pseudohermaphroditism. Female pseudohermaphrodites are genetic females with normal female internal genitalia, as seen in Figure 5.41. Virilization is caused by androgen excess, due to congenital adrenal hyperplasia, maternal ingestion of androgens, or a maternal virilizing tumor.

Male pseudohermaphroditism. Male pseudohermaphrodites are genetic males with testicular tissue, but with decreased androgen synthesis or end-organ androgen insensitivity. The testicular feminization syndrome is common in these patients, and they often present with undescended testes (see Chapter 10).

Mixed gonadal dysgenesis. Patients with mixed gonadal dysgenesis have chromosomal abnormalities, most commonly the XO/XY karyotype. Usually there is a streak gonad or absent gonad on one side, and a testis on the other. The side with the streak or absent gonad usually has a fallopian tube, and the side with the testis has a vas deferens.

True hermaphroditism. True hermaphrodites have both ovarian and testicular tisue. The most common combination, seen in Figure 5.42, is an ovotestis on one side with an ovary or testis on the other side. The internal genitalia are variable.

MRI appearance. MRI is particularly well suited to the noninvasive determination of the presence or absence of a uterus, vagina, gonads, and phallus. The position of undescended testes may be identified preoperatively, and the presence of corpora cavernosa and spongiosum, or the identification of partial vaginal agenesis, is helpful in selecting appropriate treatment and determining the correct surgical approach.[30,31]

MRI in relation to other imaging modalities. Ultrasound is often used initially in the assessment of ambiguous genitalia, but the examination may be limited by a poorly distended bladder in the neonate. MRI is of value in the evaluation of internal genital anatomy, particularly where multiple complex congenital anomalies are present.

Congenital vaginal agenesis

Vaginal agenesis may be partial or complete, and is often associated with müllerian duct anomalies. It is also associated with unilateral renal agenesis or ectopia in up to 50 per cent of patients.[21] Management of vaginal agenesis depends on whether the vagina is completely or partially absent, on the length of the atretic segment, and on the presence or absence of a uterus.

MRI appearance. As seen in Figure 5.43, T2-weighted axial images are optimal for confirming the absence of the vagina or assessing the length of the atretic segment.[14,32] T2-weighted sagittal images, however, are preferable for determining whether the patient has a uterus.

MRI in relation to other imaging modalities. Ultrasound is the primary modality in evaluation of vaginal atresia. The length of the atretic vagina can be accurately measured with transperineal sonography,[33] and the presence of a uterus can be determined by transabdominal sonography. MRI is reserved for those cases in which sonography is equivocal or other pelvic anomalies are suspected.

Uterine tumors

Leiomyoma

Leiomyomata are the most common uterine neoplasms, found in up to 40 per cent of women of reproductive age.[10] They are well circumscribed benign tumors, made up of smooth muscle with a variable amount of fibrous tissue. They are surrounded by a pseudocapsule of areolar tissue and supplied by one or two large vessels. Leiomyomata may be solitary or multiple, and over 90 per cent arise from the uterine corpus. Five percent are known to occur in the cervix, and a small number are found in the broad ligament.

Depending on their position in relation to the uterine wall, leiomyomata are classified as **submucosal**, **intramural**, or **subserosal**. Five to 10 percent of leiomyomata are submucosal and project into the uterine cavity. They most often come to clinical attention because of infertility, recurrent abortion, or hypermenorrhoea with anemia. Intramural leiomyomata are also associated with infertility. Depending on their size and location, submucosal and intramural leiomyomata may obstruct labor. Subserosal leiomyomata, which project into the abdomen or pelvis, may undergo torsion causing the patient to present with acute abdominal pain.

Treatment of leiomyomata depends on their size and location. Small submucosal lesions may be treated by hysteroscopic removal. Intramural lesions are treated by myomectomy, particularly in those women desiring uterine preservation or pregnancy. A pregnancy rate of 40–50 per cent has been reported after myomectomy. Treatment with gonadotropin-releasing hormone analogs causes a hypoestrogenic state and promotes atrophy of the leiomyomata.[12,34]

MRI appearance. The characteristic appearance of nondegenerative leiomyomata is illustrated in Figure 5.44. On T1-weighted scans they appear as well circumscribed, rounded lesions which image with a medium intensity signal, often indistinguishable from adjacent myometrium. On T2-weighted scans they usually image with a homogeneous low intensity signal.[35–37]

Occasionally, calcification causes leiomyomata to image with low signal intensity on both T1- and T2-weighted scans (Figure 5.45). Sometimes only the periphery of a leiomyoma is calcified as depicted in Figure 5.46.

Degenerative leiomyomata have various and nonspecific MRI appearances. On T1-weighted scans they image with medium or high signal intensity and on T2-weighted scans (Figure 5.47) they demonstrate heterogeneous predominantly high signal intensity. Degeneration can be hyaline, myxomatous, fatty, or carneous. The latter is caused by muscle infarction during periods of rapid tumor growth, such as in pregnancy (so-called red degeneration), and may present a more uniform high signal intensity appearance on T2-weighted images.[37]

There is no improvement in the detection or characterization of leiomyomata after intravenous administration of gadolinium-DTPA.[15] As depicted in in Figure 5.48, nondegenerative leiomyomata demonstrate no signal enhancement. Degenerative lesions demonstrate variable enhancement, as illustrated in Figure 5.49.

Classification of leiomyomata by location can be accurately assessed with MRI. **Submucosal leiomyomata** can be identified protruding into the endometrial cavity, as shown in Figure 5.50. **Intramural leiomyomata** are recognized by their epicenter, located within the myometrium (Figures 5.48 to 5.50). In Figure 5.51 the epicenter of **subserosal leiomyomata** can be seen to be outside the myometrium. In addition, the position of leiomyomata in relation to the uterus can be evaluated with MRI. Leiomyomata may be fundal, as shown in Figures 5.45 and 5.47, located within the corpus (Figures 5.48 and 5.49), or they may extend into the lower uterine segment (Figure 5.52).

MRI in relation to other imaging modalities. Most leiomyomata are detected clinically or by ultrasound. However, sonograms have resulted in false negative diagnoses in up to 20 per cent of patients,[38] and leiomyomata may be mistaken for adnexal masses,

particularly where other anomalies (such as a retroverted uterus, duplicated uterus, or other pelvic disease) are present.[39] Small lesions, less than 2 cm, may be missed, and extremely large leiomyomata, as shown in Figure 5.53, may be impossible to assess.

MRI, which has been shown to have a sensitivity of 92 per cent for the diagnosis of leiomyomata as small as 0.5 cm,[3,5] is indicated when ultrasound results are inconclusive or limited.[40] It is especially useful in the search for submucosal leiomyomata in infertile patients. It is possible to differentiate between leiomyoma and adenomyosis with MRI,[37] and it may also be used prior to myomectomy, when the location and size of leiomyomata need to be known. It can also facilitate assessment of response to hormone analog treatment as depicted in Figure 5.54.[34]

Adenomyosis

Typically adenomyosis is a disease of females in the fifth decade and has been identified in 15–27 per cent of hysterectomy specimens.[10,41] Its incidence is increased in multiparous women. It is defined as the presence of endometrial glands and stroma within the myometrium, at least 2.5 mm from the endometrial basalis layer.[10] The endometrial glands and stroma become interdigitated within the myometrium and are surrounded by hypertrophied smooth muscle. Since the trapped endometrium is of basalis origin and is resistant to hormonal stimuli, typical cyclical endometrial changes are not seen.

The clinical manifestations of adenomyosis are variable. Most frequently patients present with hypermenorrhea and anemia, secondary dysmenorrhea, perimenstrual pelvic pain, and an enlarged uterus. Hysterectomy is the only treatment, and, until recently, the diagnosis could only be confirmed at surgery since it is not possible to distinguish adenomyosis from leiomyomata clinically or by ultrasound.

MRI appearance. There are two forms of adenomyosis, a diffuse and a focal type. In **diffuse adenomyosis**, the uterine body and fundus are diffusely enlarged. The low signal intensity junctional zone is increased in thickness (widened), and segmentally (Figure 5.55) or diffusely (Figure 5.56) extends peripherally through the myometrium.[36] In some patients high signal intensity foci can be detected within the adenomyosis. When these foci occur on both T1- and T2-weighted images, they are thought to represent hemorrhage. When they are seen only on T2-weighted images, however, it is postulated that they represent endometrial tissue.[42] Figure 5.57 illustrates distortion of the endometrium which may occur if the adenomyosis is extensive.[37]

Focal adenomyosis (also called an **adenomyoma**) is seen as a mass of low signal intensity which appears similar to a leiomyoma. Differentiation between an adenomyoma and a leiomyoma depends on the configuration, margin, and site of the lesion.[36,37] As depicted in Figure 5.57, an adenomyoma is oval in contour compared to the rounded leiomyoma. In adenomyoma the margin of the lesion is ill-defined at its interface with the myometrium, whereas the leiomyoma margin is sharply demarcated.

MRI in relation to other imaging modalities. MRI is the investigation of choice in the preoperative evaluation of suspected adenomyosis. In patients with a smoothly enlarged uterus, other imaging modalities like US and CT offer little information. MRI is also recommended when patient counselling concerning surgical treatment options (ie, hysterectomy versus myomectomy) is required. While the diagnosis of diffuse adenomyosis is accurately achieved with MRI, the differentiation between an adenomyoma and a leiomyoma may sometimes be difficult. As illustrated in Figure 5.58a, degenerative leiomyoma may exhibit heterogeneous signal intensity with indistinct margins toward the myometrium, making the differentiation from an adenomyoma difficult.

Endometrial polyps

Endometrial polyps are sessile or pedunculated endometrial projections composed of hyperplastic endometrium. They arise in the fundus or cornua of the uterus, and 80 per cent occur in females between 30 and 60 years of age. Although they are found in 10–30 per cent of patients with endometrial carcinoma, carcinomatous change is only rarely identified within them.[43] Patients typically present with abnormal intermenstrual or postmenopausal bleeding.

MRI appearance. On T1-weighted scans endometrial polyps image with a medium signal intensity similar to normal endometrium. On T2-weighted scans polyps may image with a signal intensity similar to or slightly lower than the endometrium, and they may be seen to cause widening of the endometrial cavity as illustrated in Figure 5.59. Endometrial polyps enhance after intravenous gadolinium-DTPA (Figure 5.59). Figure 5.60 illustrates a polyp which has undergone degeneration and, as a result, becomes more heterogeneous in appearance on T1- and T2-weighted images. Occasionally polyps may prolapse through the cervix.

Endometrial carcinoma

Endometrial carcinoma is the fourth most common female cancer with 34 000 new cases per year in the USA and 4000 deaths.[44] Most patients are postmenopausal, but between 2 and 5 per cent of tumors occur in patients under 40 years of age. The disease occurs twice as often in white women as in blacks, and there is an association between endometrial carcinoma and endocrine or metabolic disorders, particularly obesity, diabetes mellitus, and Stein-Levanthal syndrome. Nulliparous women are also at greater risk. The development of endometrial carcinoma is promoted by unopposed estrogen stimulation of the uterus. This was recognized in the early 1970's, when postmenopausal estrogen replacement without any concomitant progesterone caused an increase in endometrial carcinoma.

Tumors may be localized or diffuse. Localized endometrial cancers are polypoid or exophytic in nature, with only superficial attachment to the endometrium. Diffuse tumors demonstrate extensive invasion of the entire endometrium. Initial tumor spread through the myometrium, involving both corpus and cervix, is followed by extension outside the uterus, and then involvement of adjacent organs. Lymphatic spread is to the pelvic, paraaortic, and inguinal nodes. Distant metastases occur most often in the peritoneum, lung, liver, and supraclavicular lymph nodes.

Patients most frequently present with postmenopausal bleeding. If the tumor secondarily obstructs the endocervical canal, pyometra or hematometra may occur. Rarely, patients present with pain due to metastatic disease.

More than 15 prognostic variables—including clinical, histologic (grade of tumor), morphologic (depth of myometrial invasion), and the presence of nodal metastases—have been ascribed to endometrial carcinoma. It is the depth of myometrial invasion, however, which governs the incidence of lymph node metastases.[45] With superficial myometrial invasion the incidence of lymph node metastases is only 3 per cent, whereas with deep myometrial invasion lymph node metastases occur in 40 per cent of patients.[46] Clinical staging, according to the system of the International Federation of Gynecology and Obstetrics (FIGO), is known to understage the disease in 15–20 per cent of cases.[46,47] Understaging results primarily from the inability to evaluate the depth of myometrial invasion, intraperitoneal implants, nodal metastases, and adnexal metastases. Therefore a surgical FIGO staging system has been proposed (Table 5.2).[48]

Hysterectomy, with or without radiotherapy, is the primary form of treatment for early stage I disease. Radiotherapy, sometimes followed by hysterectomy, is recommended for more advanced disease. Stage IV endometrial carcinoma is treated by local radiation to

Table 5.2 Surgical FIGO staging and TNM classification of endometrial carcinoma

TNM categories	FIGO surgical stages[48]	Criteria
TX		Primary tumor cannot be assessed
T0		No evidence of primary tumor
Tis	0	Carcinoma in situ
T1	I	Tumor confined to corpus
T1a	Ia	Tumor limited to endometrium
T1b	Ib	Invasion of less than half of the myometrium
	Ic	Invasion of more than half of the myometrium
T2	II	Tumor invades cervix but does not extend beyond uterus
T3	III	Tumor extends beyond the uterus, adnexa but not outside the true pelvis
T4	IVa	Tumor invades mucosa of bladder or rectum and/or extends beyond the true pelvis
M1	IVb	Distant metastasis

TNM = Tumor, node, metastasis
FIGO = International Federation of Gynecology and Obstetrics

control bleeding and hormonal therapy or chemotherapy.

MRI appearance. As illustrated in Figure 5.61, on nonenhanced MR images, the signal intensity of small endometrial cancers is similar to that of normal endometrium, limiting accurate tumor delineation.[49] Indirect signs of the presence of endometrial cancer include increased thickness or lobularity of the uterine cavity.[49,50] Larger tumors cause widening of the endometrial cavity. A low signal intensity focal mass may be identified on T2-weighted images as seen in Figure 5.62.[49] These changes are not diagnostic, however, and similar changes may be seen in a submucosal degenerating leiomyoma, adenomatous hyperplasia, and blood clots.[49]

After gadolinium-DTPA administration, endometrial carcinoma demonstrates enhancement as illustrated in Figure 5.63. The contrast between tumor and normal endometrium is accentuated, and it becomes possible to identify small tumors confined to the endometrium. On contrast-enhanced images, it is also possible to differentiate tumor from necrosis, allowing accurate assessment of tumor volume and leading to an overall improvement in staging accuracy.[15,51] Furthermore, while a nonenhanced scan often cannot differentiate between retained fluid (eg hematometra, pyometra) and tumor as a cause for the enlarged uterus, this distinction is possible after Gd-DTPA administration. The use of Gd-DTPA in the differentiation between fluid and tumor expansion of the endometrial cavity is shown in Figures 5.64 and 5.65.

MRI staging. The MRI staging classification for endometrial carcinoma follows the surgical FIGO staging system, taking into account the depth of myometrial invasion and lymph node involvement.[49]

Stage I endometrial carcinoma is carcinoma confined to the uterine corpus. Stage I tumors are further subdivided depending on the degree of myometrial invasion. The MRI/surgical FIGO subdivisions of stage I tumors are: (1) stage Ia—tumor confined to the endometrium; (2) stage Ib—invasion confined to the inner half of the myometrium; and (3) stage Ic—invasion of the outer half of the myometrium. Tumors are considered to be confined to the endometrium (stage Ia) when the junctional zone is preserved, as seen in Figure 5.62, or there is a sharp tumor–myometrium interface (Figure 5.64). Stage Ib endometrial carcinoma is indicated by disruption of the junctional zone with an irregular myometrial/endometrial interface and/or by increased signal intensity tumor in the inner-half of the myometrium, with preservation of the outer myometrium, as depicted in Figures 5.63 and 5.65. The most reliable MRI criterion for myometrial invasion (stage Ib) is disruption of the junctional zone, although this zone is not always visualized in postmenopausal women. Deep myometrial invasion (stage Ic) is suggested by high signal intensity tumor in the outer half of the myometrium, with an intact, although thinned, outer stripe of normal myometrium (Figure 5.66).[49] In addition to myometrial invasion, MRI can be used to measure the size of the uterus and the length of the endometrial cavity. In clinical FIGO staging an endometrial cavity length of less than 8 cm was considered stage Ia, while a length of greater than 8 cm was considered stage Ib. MRI can accurately follow these guidelines but as it was realized that uterine size does not correlate with patient prognosis, this finding is no longer used for staging.

Stage II endometrial cancer indicates involvement of the cervix. Invasion of the cervix is easily assessed on multiplanar MR images.

MR may also be used to evaluate extrauterine tumor spread (stages III and IV), as shown in Figures 5.67 and 5.68. The bladder or rectum are considered to be invaded when their wall demonstrates focal loss of normal low signal intensity on T2-weighted images. The accuracy in detection of pelvic lymph node involvement by MRI is similar to that of CT. Both techniques rely on increased nodal size for tumor detection and neither MRI nor CT can distinguish between malignant and hyperplastic nodes (Figure 5.69).

MRI in relation to other imaging modalities. Transabdominal ultrasound is not a reliable staging modality for endometrial carcinoma.[52] The value of endovaginal ultrasound in the detection and staging of endometrial carcinoma needs to be defined. CT is of use in the later stages of disease, but differentiation between stages I and II is difficult, as is assessment of the depth of myometrial invasion.[53,54]

MRI is accurate in the staging of endometrial carcinoma, with a reported overall accuracy rate of between 83 per cent and 92 per cent.[49,55] The primary advantage of MRI is in the assessment of the depth of myometrial invasion, with a reported accuracy of approximately 80 per cent.[49,55] The usefulness of MRI in staging the endometrial cancer, including the assessment of the depth of myometrial invasion, detection of extrauterine tumor spread, and involvement of the cervix has been ascertained.[49,51,55,56] Indications for staging by MRI include patients in whom physical examination is limited due to obesity, patients who are unsuited for surgical FIGO staging, patients in whom the extent of tumor may alter the surgical approach, or patients in whom a concomitant lesion makes assessment difficult. MRI is also useful in monitoring response before and after radiotherapy.

Recurrent endometrial carcinoma

70 per cent of treatment failures for endometrial carcinoma occur within the first three years. The pattern of disease recurrence depends on the primary treatment. In those patients who received whole pelvis radiation therapy, recurrence is more likely to be due to extrapelvic metastases in the abdomen, liver, lung or bony skeleton.[46] In nonirradiated patients, recurrent disease is often seen on the pelvic sidewall, in retained parametrium or at the vaginal apex.[46] When recurrence is isolated and occurs at the vaginal apex, there is a 25–50 per cent cure rate after surgery.[57]

Treatment is by surgical resection of the recurrent disease. Exenteration may be performed for large lesions and for those patients who have undergone prior radiotherapy.

MR appearance. Recurrent intrapelvic endometrial carcinoma is visualized as a mass lesion of medium signal intensity on T1-weighted images and high signal intensity on T2-weighted images. Tumor recurrence at the vaginal cuff is seen as a lobulated mass of medium signal intensity on T1-weighted images and increased signal intensity on T2-weighted images. Involvement of pelvic sidewall muscles is depicted by the evidence of loss of fat planes and the identification of direct extension of irregular high signal intensity tumor within the muscle (Figure 5.70). Tumor recurrence invading the bladder, or lymph node invasion, can also be detected (Figure 5.71).

Recurrent endometrial tumor may be distinguished from long-standing radiation fibrosis, which is typically of low signal intensity on both T1- and T2-weighted images. However, the appearances of recurrent disease may be indistinguishable from inflammatory or early radiation changes and therefore histologic confirmation remains essential.

MRI in relation to other imaging modalities. The role of radiology in recurrent endometrial carcinoma is to define the extent of the recurrence and thereby help in management decisions. The multiplanar imaging capability of MR, together with its superior contrast resolution, currently offer the best radiological assessment of intrapelvic disease. Both MRI and CT may be used to identify enlarged lymph nodes.

Malignant mixed müllerian tumors

Malignant mixed müllerian tumors, sarcomas derived from pluripotential stromal cells, have both carcinomatous and sarcomatous elements. Like endometrial carcinoma, they occur in postmenopausal women and have similar risk factors, including obesity, hypertension, and diabetes mellitus.[46] In up to 30 per cent of patients there is a history of prior pelvic radiation treatment.[58] These tumors are typically massive and aggressive, with early myometrial invasion. One-third of apparent stage I lesions have extrauterine disease at laparotomy, and peritoneal involvement is seen in over 50 per cent of cases which extend beyond the uterus.[10]

Patients usually present with nonspecific clinical symptoms including postmenopausal bleeding, pelvic pain, and discharge. Occasionally, fragments of malignant tissue may be passed into the vagina and, on physical examination, tumor may be seen projecting through the cervical os.[10] Treatment is by hysterectomy and whole pelvis radiotherapy, but the overall survival rate is only 25–30 per cent at five years.

MRI appearance. The uterus is usually enlarged at presentation due to the aggressive nature of the lesion. The endometrial cavity is expanded and often there is evidence of deep myometrial invasion, as shown in Figure 5.72. The lesion may be of homogeneous low signal intensity on T1-weighted images, or areas of hemorrhage may cause focal regions of high signal intensity, as seen in Figure 5.73. On T2-weighted scans the tumor images with heterogeneous, medium to high signal intensity.[50,59]

Müllerian sarcomas cannot be differentiated from large endometrial carcinomas on MRI scans. Findings suggestive of a sarcoma include a large tumor with extensive myometrial and serosal extension and the presence of ovarian or intraperitoneal metastases.

Metastatic involvement of the uterus

The uterus may be involved by metastatic spread from other gynecologic malignancies, particularly ovarian or cervical carcinoma. When extragenital tumors metastasize to the uterus, it is usually in the context of known metastatic disease elsewhere. The most common extragenital metastases to involve the uterus are those from breast carcinomas (47 per cent).[60] Gastrointestinal carcinoma originating in the stomach, colon, or pancreas has given rise to uterine metastases, as have renal cell carcinoma and melanoma.[60]

Metastases may involve the endometrium or myometrium and patients commonly present with abnormal bleeding. Diagnosis is by dilatation and curettage.

MRI appearance. Endometrial metastatic disease cannot be differentiated from primary endometrial tumors. Myometrial deposits have a variable appearance, which may resemble degenerative uterine leiomyomata, with medium or high signal intensity on T1-weighted images and heterogeneous medium or high signal intensity on T2-weighted images as illustrated in Figure 5.74. Therefore, the findings for both endometrial and myometrial tissue metastases are nonspecific.

MRI in relation to other imaging modalities. All imaging modalities are nonspecific in the diagnosis of uterine metastases and histologic diagnosis is required.

Diseases of the cervix

Cervical stenosis

Cervical stenosis, most commonly involving the external os, usually occurs as a sequel to infection or as a result of interventions such as cauterization, conization, cryosurgery, and radiotherapy. Senile atrophy may also cause stenosis. Mechanical stenosis may be caused by tumor growth blocking the endocervical canal, as may occur in endometrial and cervical cancers.

MRI appearance. Cervical stenosis can be identified on MRI scans, and the location of the stenosis can be determined. When stenosis is secondary to tumor obstruction, the uterus is seen to be distended and expanded, usually the result of retained secretions, pyometra, or hematometra. The signal intensity of the uterine cavity varies, depending on the nature of its contents (protein and blood content). On T1-weighted images, the MRI appearance may be homogeneous or heterogeneous and signal intensities may be low, medium, or high. On T2-weighted images the uterine cavity is usually of high signal intensity, as shown in Figure 5.75.

Cervical incompetence

Sixteen percent of second and third trimester abortions are caused by cervical incompetence. Incompetence may be congenital, associated with uterine malformations or diethylstilbestrol (DES) exposure, or it may be caused by a low collagen content within the cervix. Acquired incompetence is usually secondary to obstetric or gynecologic trauma, multiple gestations, or increased prostaglandin production.[61]

MRI appearance. Four MR characteristics, which may occur alone or in combination, are suggestive of cervical incompetence.[62] Features that should be assessed include the length of the cervical canal (normal is greater than 3 cm), the width of the internal os (normal is less than 3.5 mm), the appearance of the endocervical canal (normally symmetrical), and the signal intensity characteristics of the cervical tissue.

In patients with cervical incompetence unrelated to DES exposure, the cervix is often of normal length, but shortening (to less than 3 cm) of the endocervical canal can be seen. The most common feature is asymmetrical widening of the endocervical canal (most probably post-traumatic) which may be associated with normal (Figure 5.76) or abnormally thin (Figure 5.77) underlying stroma. The MRI finding of localized or diffuse thinning (Figure 5.78) or absence of low signal intensity stroma is very suggestive of cervical incompetence. An additional finding is widening of the internal os. The width of the internal os (identified by the entrance of the uterine vessels and waisting of the uterine contour) is increased to over 4 mm.

When the uterine anomalies are due to DES exposure, as shown in Figure 5.79, the length of the cervical canal is reduced, usually measuring less than 2.5 cm.[62] The internal os is of normal width or narrower, as is the width of the endocervical stroma. The signal intensity of the stroma is unremarkable, although relatively thin. The uterus of DES offspring may, however, have normal measurements, as seen in Figure 5.80.

MRI in relation to other imaging modalities. Hysterosalpingography (HSG) has been used in the past to identify widening of the internal os and isthmus. However, in today's practice HSG is not performed in the mid-secretory phase, when the changes due to cervical incompetence are most pronounced, and furthermore HSG cannot provide information concerning the tissue composition of the cervix. Therefore, HSG is no longer recommended for the evaluation of cervical incompetence. Ultrasound is the method of choice for the diagnosis of cervical incompetence during pregnancy. Sonographic findings of an internal os measuring more than 15 mm during the first trimester and 20 mm during the second trimester indicate cervical incompetence.[63] However, no information is available on the diagnosis of cervical incompetence in the nonpregnant female. With MRI, cervical length and the diameter of the internal os can be accurately measured. In addition, the shape of the endocervical canal and the characteristics of the cervical stroma can be assessed.[62] While further studies are needed to explore the potential of MRI in the evaluation of cervical incompetence, the unique potential of MRI is undisputable.

DES exposure

Diethylstilbestrol (DES) is a synthetic estrogen that at one time was used in pregnant women to prevent miscarriage. The female offspring of these patients, exposed in utero to DES, have an increased risk of congenital abnormalities of the uterine cavity, such as hypoplasia, T-shaped deformity, and constrictions. These occur in up to two-thirds of patients. One in three patients with DES exposure has vaginal adenosis, and there is also an estimated increased risk of developing clear cell adenocarcinoma of the vagina in the order of 1 in 100 to 1 in 4000.[64]

MRI appearance. Uterine changes consistent with DES exposure can be identified on MRI studies. Hypoplasia of the uterine cavity has been identified with a length less than 3.3 cm.[65] Uterine constrictions can also be identified, due to increased width of the junctional zone in the region of the constriction.[65] However these changes are not present in all cases of DES exposure. The cervix is shown to be shortened (usually less than 2.5 cm) mainly due to loss of the infravaginal portion.[66] On T2-weighted images, as depicted in Figure 5.80, adenosis in DES exposed patients can be identified as multiple foci of high signal intensity.

Nabothian cysts

Nabothian cysts are small, 1–3 mm, nodules on the surface of the cervix caused by mucus distention of endocervical glands or clefts. When small they are rarely symptomatic, and require no treatment. Occasionally nabothian cysts grow to 2–4 cm in diameter and have been reported to simulate a cystic adnexal mass.[67]

MRI appearance. A nabothian cyst appears as a small focus of medium to high signal intensity on T1-weighted images, and increases in signal intensity on T2-weighted images, as demonstrated in Figure 5.81. Their small size and well defined margin differentiate nabothian cysts from most cervical neoplasms. However, postbiopsy changes or tiny foci of endometriosis may not be readily differentiated.

Cervical carcinoma

Overall, cervical carcinoma is the third most common gynecologic malignancy, with 16 000 new cases per year in the USA and 7400 deaths.[44] However, it is the **most** common malignancy in women under 50 years of age. Carcinoma starts at the squamocolumnar junction which marks the junction of ecto- and endocervix, and in young females it occurs on the lips of the cervix. In older women, however, the squamocolumnar junction shifts to a higher location in the endocervical canal, and tumors are more likely to involve the supravaginal portion of the cervix. Overall 20 per cent of tumors occur inside the endocervical canal.[10]

There are two main histological types of cervical carcinoma: squamous cell carcinoma and adenocarcinoma. Squamous cell carcinoma accounts for 80–90 per cent of cases, and known risk factors include lower socioeconomic status, promiscuity, smoking, and a variety of genital infections including herpes simplex, human papilloma virus, and genital warts.[68] Adenocarcinoma occurs in approximately 10 per cent of cases, and carries a worse prognosis than squamous cell cervical carcinoma.

Table 5.3 TNM classification and clinical FIGO staging of cervical cancer

TNM	FIGO	System description
TX	0	Primary tumor cannot be assessed
T0		No evidence of primary tumor
Tis		Carcinoma in situ
T1	I	Cervical carcinoma confined to uterus (extension to corpus should be disregarded)
T1a	Ia	Preclinical invasive carcinoma, diagnosed by microscopy only
T1a1	Ia1	Minimal microscopic stromal invasion
T1a2	Ia2	Tumor with invasive component 5 mm or less in depth, taken from the base of the epithelium, and 7 mm or less in horizontal spread
T1b	Ib	Tumor larger than T1a2
T2	II	Cervical carcinoma invades beyond uterus but not to pelvic wall or to lower third of the vagina
T2a	IIa	Without parametrial invasion
T2b	IIb	With parametrial invasion
T3	III	Cervical carcinoma extends to pelvic wall and/or involves the lower third of the vagina and/or causes hydronephrosis or nonfunctioning kidney
T3a	IIIa	Tumor involves lower third of the vagina, no extension to pelvic wall
T3b	IIIb	Tumor extends to pelvic wall and/or causes hydronephrosis or nonfunctioning kidney
T4	IVa	Tumor invades mucosa of bladder or rectum and/or extends beyond true pelvis. Note: The presence of bullous edema is not sufficient evidence to classify a tumor T4
M1	IVb	Distant metastasis
NX		Regional lymph nodes cannot be assessed
N0		No regional node metastasis
N1		Regional lymph node metastasis

TNM = Tumor, node, metastasis
FIGO = International Federation of Gynecology and Obstetrics

Patients usually present with vaginal bleeding or discharge and are clinically categorized according to the International Federation of Gynecologic Oncology (FIGO) system (Table 5.3). Prognosis depends on the histologic grade of the tumor, its size (transverse diameter), its location within the cervix (exocervix versus endocervix), the depth of stromal invasion, adjacent tissue extension, and the presence of lymph node metastases. Clinical FIGO staging is inaccurate because of limitations in the assessment of parametrial and pelvic sidewall tumor extension. In addition, the depth of stromal invasion and presence of lymphadenopathy cannot be assessed by physical examination.

Hysterectomy is the treatment of choice for patients with stage Ib and small IIa disease. Stages IIb–IV are primarily treated by pelvic radiation. Adenocarcinoma of the cervix is usually treated by both surgery and radiotherapy.

MRI appearance. On T2-weighted images cervical carcinoma is identified as an abnormal area of high signal intensity, distinct from the normal low signal intensity of the cervical stroma, as shown in Figure 5.82.[50,69] Tumor location is accurately demonstrated on MRI. Tumors in the exocervix are located in the anterior (Figure 5.82) or posterior (Figure 5.83) cervical lip, or are circumferential (Figure 5.84). Similarly, as depicted in Figure 5.85, tumors originating in the endocervix (the most difficult tumor location for adequate physical examination) are well displayed on MRI. As illustrated in Figure 5.86, small lesions, less than 0.5 cm, are difficult to depict. Administration of intravenous gadolinium-DTPA causes variable enhancement of the tumor, and may render it isodense with surrounding cervical tissue (Figure 5.87). Although contrast enhancement allows distinction between viable tumor and areas of necrosis (Figure 5.88), it has not been shown to increase diagnostic accuracy in tumor depiction.[15]

MRI staging. Stage Ib tumors are confined to the cervix. On MRI, in addition to staging the tumor size, the depth of stromal invasion can be assessed. In partial stromal invasion, the uninvolved stroma is demonstrated on T2-weighted images as a peripheral low signal intensity stripe (Figure 5.89). In full thickness stromal involvement, tumor signal intensity is seen extending through the stroma, although the configuration and symmetry of the parametrial tissue is preserved, as shown in Figure 5.85. In stage IIa disease, tumor extends into the upper-third of the vagina. On T2-weighted images, in addition to the tumor presence the low signal intensity of the vaginal wall is no longer seen, as illustrated in Figure 5.90. Parametrial invasion classifies the tumor as stage IIb cervical carcinoma. Parametrial invasion occurs by direct tumor spread from the endocervix and is often present when the tumor with full thickness stromal invasion is located in or extending into the upper endocervical canal, or when the tumor involves the lower uterine segment. The MRI appearance of parametrial invasion is characterized by asymmetry of the parametrium, or direct visualization of an abnormal tumor tissue extending into the parametrial region, often encasing the parametrial vessels (Figures 5.91, 5.92, and 5.93).[70,71]

On T2-weighted images anterior tumor extension is seen as high signal intensity involving the anterior parametrium and uterovesical ligament, as illustrated in Figure 5.94. When the bladder is involved, as shown in Figure 5.95, tumor replaces the normal low signal intensity bladder wall, resulting in thickening and abnormally high signal intensity on T2-weighted images. Rectal involvement can occur by direct invasion from a large volume tumor, or by tumor spread along the uterosacral ligaments (Figure 5.96). The presacral space may also be invaded due to tumor infiltration along the uterosacral ligaments (Figure 5.97). Tumor extension to the pelvic sidewall is indicated on T2-weighted images by abnormal signal intensity in the piriformis, obturator internus, or levator ani muscles, as depicted in Figure 5.98. The use of Gd-DTPA-enhanced imaging is helpful in the evaluation of advanced disease, particularly when invasion of the bladder or rectum is suspected (Figure 5.99). The presence of lymph node metastasis is a proven prognostic factor. Cervical carcinoma spreads to endometrial nodes (Figure 5.92), followed by obturator nodes (Figures 5.96 and 5.97) and then internal and external iliac chains (Figure 5.100).

MRI in relation to other imaging modalities. CT may be used in staging cervical carcinoma, but its primary usefulness is in the assessment of lymph node metastases. CT is quite limited in the identification of vaginal and parametrial involvement (stages II and III), and it may also be difficult to determine bladder or rectal invasion with CT.

MRI has been shown to be superior to CT in the staging of cervical carcinoma.[72] MRI is more accurate in assessing tumor size (70–100 per cent accuracy), in determining parametrial and vaginal involvement (85–100 per cent accuracy), and in detecting the presence of nodal disease.[70,73] The most important staging factor which influences treatment is the presence of invasive disease, and in this regard the accuracy of MRI staging has been shown to be greater than 95 per cent.[71] Overall staging accuracy ranges between 80 and 90 per cent.[70,71]

MRI is indicated in patients with cervical carcinoma when the transverse diameter of the tumor is greater than 2 cm on clinical examination. Primary endocervical lesions and predominantly infiltrative tumors should also be evaluated by MRI, since the extent of disease cannot be accurately assessed clinically. In patients who are pregnant or who have concomitant uterine lesions, staging by MRI may also be superior to clinical assessment.

Recurrent cervical carcinoma

Recurrent or persistent cervical carcinoma occurs in 50 per cent of treated patients. The risk factors for the recurrence of cervical carcinoma include the grade and histologic tumor type, the tumor size, the presence and the depth of stromal invasion and the presence of involved lymph nodes at the time of presentation. Those patients in whom disease recurs after primary surgical treatment are usually managed by pelvic radiation therapy. Re-irradiation for recurrent pelvic disease is not performed except in very select cases because of the associated high morbidity and limited efficacy. Pelvic disease, involving the cervix, vagina, bladder, rectum or parametrium is theoretically curable by pelvic exenteration, and this is also the treatment choice in patients who have had prior radiation.

Intranodal recurrence or pelvic sidewall disease is treated with resection, radiation, chemotherapy, or the most appropriate therapeutic combination. In this setting, treatment is only rarely curative.

MR appearance. Recurrent cervical carcinoma is found at the vaginal vault in 20 per cent of cases.[74] The combination of sagittal and transaxial planes of MR imaging is helpful in tumor detection (a localized mass is seen in Figure 5.101) while the combination of T1- and T2-weighted images allows tissue characterization. Recurrent tumor is illustrated in Figure 5.102 and demonstrates increased, often heterogeneous, high signal intensity. Following Gd-DTPA injection, recurrent tumor shows various degrees of enhancement as seen in Figure 5.103. While lesions larger than 1 cm are accurately depicted, smaller lesions are more difficult to assess as their characterization may suffer from partial volume averaging. Tumor extension into the bladder (Figures 5.103 and 5.104) and rectum (Figure 5.105) causes abnormal high signal intensity of their walls on T2-weighted images. The use of Gd-DTPA is helpful in the assessment of bladder and rectal invasion. The presence of pelvic sidewall invasion (Figure 5.106) makes the patient ineligible for curative exenteration. The presence of enlarged lymph nodes can also be assessed.

MRI in relation to other imaging modalities. MRI is the most appropriate investigation for the evaluation of suspected cervical carcinoma recurrence. The extent of intrapelvic disease can be evaluated and this helps in the assessment of patient suitability for exenteration. Two findings are essential in deciding on the feasibility of surgery: pelvic wall invasion, and presence of malignant lymph nodes. MRI is accurate in the assessment of pelvic wall invasion but in the identification of lymphadenopathy both MR and CT rely on nodal enlargement as the sole indicator of tumor involvement.

MR may be used in patients with a palpable mass in the vaginal vault or cul-de-sac, which could represent tumor or fibrosis. Long-standing post-operative or postradiation fibrosis is characteristically of low signal intensity on both T1- and T2-weighted images.

Disorders of the vagina

Bartholin's cysts

Bartholin's cysts, caused by retained secretions within the vulvovaginal glands, usually occur secondary to chronic inflammatory reactions or trauma. Most patients are asymptomatic, although sometimes the cysts become infected and require drainage.

MRI appearance.   A Bartholin's cyst can be identified as an area of abnormal signal intensity located in the posterolateral aspect of the lower third of the vagina, as shown in Figure 5.107. Depending on its fluid composition, the cyst is usually of medium to high signal intensity on T1-weighted images, and increases in intensity on T2-weighted images because of its proteinaceous content. Bartholin's cysts are usually an incidental finding noted during the course of an MRI examination.

Vaginal carcinoma

Primary vaginal carcinomas account for less than 2 per cent of gynecologic neoplasms. Vaginal tumors are usually adenocarcinomas, and there is an increased risk of clear cell adenocarcinoma in patients with a history of DES exposure.[64] Patients present with bleeding, discharge, or pain.

Treatment is by radiation therapy or surgery for early stage disease. Late stage disease or local failure may be treated by pelvic exenteration.

MRI appearance.   On T1-weighted scans vaginal neoplasms image with medium signal intensity, and their presence can be appreciated only when they are large enough to alter the vaginal contour.[75] However, on T2-weighted images a medium to high signal intensity mass can be appreciated, and its location and extent can be accurately assessed, as seen in Figure

Table 5.4 TNM classification of and clinical FIGO staging of vaginal cancer

TNM	FIGO	System description
TX		Primary tumor cannot be assessed
T0		No evidence of primary tumor
Tis		Carcinoma in situ
T1	I	Tumor confined to vagina
T2	II	Tumor invades paravaginal tissues but does not extend to pelvic wall
T3	III	Tumor extends to pelvic wall
T4	IVa	Tumor invades mucosa of bladder or rectum and/or extends beyond the true pelvis
M1	IVb	Distant metastasis
NX		Regional lymph nodes cannot be assessed
N0		No regional node metastasis
N1		Upper two-thirds of vagina Regional lymph node metastasis
N1 N2		Lower-thirds of vagina Regional lymph node metastasis Bilateral inguinal lymph node metastasis

5.108. The MRI appearance of vaginal tumors, how-ever, is not specific, and sometimes, when vaginal carcinoma involves the cervix it may be difficult to decide whether the carcinoma is primarily vaginal or cervical in origin. As illustrated in Figure 5.109, if the bulk of the tumor is in the vagina, then a vaginal origin is favored. Inflammatory changes or congestion of the vagina may mimic the changes found in vaginal carcinoma.

MRI staging.   MRI staging of vaginal neoplasms can be correlated with the FIGO clinical staging system (Table 5.4). FIGO stage I tumors correspond to the MRI appearance of superficial vaginal tumors. The normal low signal intensity vaginal wall may be preserved on T2-weighted images, or there may be areas of abnormal medium signal intensity which extend through the vaginal wall. In the latter case the surrounding fat remains of high signal intensity and continues to be distinct from the vagina. In stage II there is extension into the paravaginal tissue, and the interface between fat and tumor is indistinct. Tumor invasion of the urinary bladder with formation of a vesicovaginal fistula can also be demonstrated on MRI. The diagnosis of vesicovaginal fistula is re-inforced with use of Gd-DTPA, as seen in Figure

5.110. In stage III disease the tumor has reached the pelvic sidewall, and involves the levator ani, the obturator internus, or the piriformis muscles.[75]

MRI in relation to other imaging modalities. The diagnosis of vaginal carcinoma is primarily a clinical one, obtained by physical examination and biopsy. Because of their inferior soft tissue contrast resolution, other imaging modalities such as CT and US are limited in assessing the extent of early disease. The utility of MRI lies in identifying the extent and stage of disease, thereby facilitating treatment planning.

Metastatic disease of the vagina

Vaginal metastases are more common than primary vaginal carcinoma. Metastatic spread of tumor to the vagina is often the result of direct tumor extension from a cervical or vulvar primary. For example, recurrent cervical carcinoma involves the vagina in 20 per cent of cases.[74] Endometrial carcinoma also has a predilection for metastasizing to the vagina.

MRI appearance. The MRI appearance of vaginal metastases is similar to that of primary vaginal neoplasms. The metastasis can be a sessile or polypoid mass of medium signal intensity on T1-weighted images and high signal intensity on T2-weighted images, as seen in Figure 5.111. The sessile type of metastasis is difficult to differentiate from an inflammatory process.

MRI in relation to other imaging modalities. Metastatic vaginal tumors are usually diagnosed clinically, although the accuracy of MRI in assessment of tumor spread to the vagina has been reported to be 92 per cent. However, MRI plays an important role in differentiating radiation fibrosis from recurrent tumor in patients who have undergone radiotherapy and in whom there is a mass. In contrast to metastatic disease, most commonly fibrosis images with low signal itensity on T1-and T2-weighted images.[75,76]

Vulvar carcinoma

Vulvar carcinoma accounts for 3–5 per cent of all female genital malignances and there is a recognized association with carcinoma of the cervix or vagina. Patients are typically aged 60–65 years at presentation, although vulvar carcinoma does occur in younger women who have chronic granulomatous diseases such as lymphogranuloma venereum or vulvar dystrophy.[77] Vulvar neoplasms typically involve the labia and are almost invariably squamous cell carcinoma, of which 80 per cent are mature, well differentiated lesions.

The predominant clinical symptom is pruritus. Patients may also complain of vulvar bleeding or a mass. Lesions are graded according to the TNM system recorded in Table 5.5. The most important prognostic variable is the presence of lymphadenopathy.[78] Vulvar carcinoma spreads to the ipsilateral superficial inguinal nodes, then to deep inguinal nodes, contralateral inguinal nodes, and iliac nodes. Five year survival rates are 80–95 per cent when the inguinal nodes are not involved but only 30–40 per cent when inguinal nodes are positive. Other prognostic indicators are lesion size and depth of penetration, lesion type (exophytic or infiltrative), histological grade and the presence of clitoral involvement.

Treatment is primarily surgical, and traditionally entailed a vulvectomy with bilateral superficial inguinal, deep inguinal and femoral node dissection. However, current practice is to modify this approach by performing an ipsilateral superficial lymph node dissection and only progress to deep inguinal and contralateral nodal dissection if the ipsilateral nodes are positive.[79]

Table 5.5 TNM classification of vulvar cancer

TNM	System description
TX	Primary tumor cannot be assessed
T0	No evidence of primary tumor
Tis	Carcinoma in situ
T1	Tumor confined to vulva, 2 cm or less in greatest dimension
T2	Tumor confined to vulva, more than 2 cm in greatest dimension
T3	Tumor invades any of the following: urethra, vagina, perineum, anus
T4	Tumor invades any of the following: bladder mucosa, upper part of urethral mucosa, rectal mucosa, or tumor fixed to the bone
Nx	Regional lymph nodes cannot be assessed
N0	No nodes palpable
N1	Nodes palpable in either groin, not enlarged, mobile (not clinically suspicious of neoplasm)
N2	Nodes palpable in either groin, enlarged, firm and mobile (clinically suspicious of neoplasm)
N3	Fixed or ulcerated nodes

MRI appearance.   On MRI, vulvar carcinoma is seen as an abnormal focus of medium signal intensity on T1-weighted images increasing in signal intensity on T2-weighted images, as demonstrated in Figure 5.112. The extent of the primary lesion and extension into adjacent structures such as the vagina or the clitoris (Figure 5.113) can be evaluated. The presence of inguinal node metastases is readily appreciated on MRI, as seen in Figure 5.114.

MRI in relation to other imaging modalities.   The diagnosis of vulvar carcinoma and superficial inguinal node involvement remains clinical. Cross-sectional imaging modalities such as CT and MRI are of use in the detection of deep inguinal and pelvic lymph node enlargement. The superior soft tissue contrast resolution offered by MRI may be of value in the assessment of involvement of adjacent structures.

References

1 WILLIAM PL, WARWICK R, eds. *Gray's Anatomy*, (Churchill Livingstone: Edinburgh 1980) 791–800.

2 LIERSE W, *Applied Anatomy of the Pelvis*, (Springer Verlag: Berlin 1984) 272–83.

3 LEE JKT, GERSELL DJ, BALFE DM et al, The uterus: in vitro MR-anatomic correlation of normal and abnormal specimens, *Radiology* (1985) **157**:175–9.

4 DEMAS BE, HRICAK H, JAFFE RB, Uterine MR imaging: effects of hormonal stimulation, *Radiology* (1986) **159**:123–6.

5 MCCARTHY JS, TAUBER C, GORE J, Female pelvic anatomy: MR assessment of variations during the menstrual cycle and with use of oral contraceptives, *Radiology* (1986) **160**:119–23.

6 LANGLOIS LP, The size of the normal uterus, *J Reprod Med* (1970) **4(6)**:31–9.

7 HRICAK H, ALPERS C, CROOKS LE et al, Magnetic resonance imaging of the female pelvis: initial experience, *AJR* (1983) **141**:1119–28.

8 MCCARTHY S, SCOTT G, MAJUMDAR S et al, Uterine junctional zone: MR study of water content and relaxation properties, *Radiology* (1989) **171**:241–3.

9 MITCHELL DG, SCHONHOLZ L, HILPERT PH et al, Zones of the uterus: discrepancy between US and MR images, *Radiology* (1990) **174**:827–31.

10 HENDRICKSON MR, KEMPSON RL, *Surgical Pathology of the Uterine Corpus*, (WB Saunders: Philadelphia 1980) 452.

11 MOGHISSI K, Effects of steroidal contraceptives on the reproductive system. In: Hafez E, ed. *Human Reproduction*, (Harper & Row: Hungerstown 1980) 529–37.

12 ANDREYKO JL, BLUMENFELD Z, MARSHALL LA et al, Use of an agonistic analog of GnRH (NAFARELIN) to treat leiomyomata: assessment by magnetic resonance imaging, *Am J Obstet Gynecol* (1988) **158**:903–10.

13 DANFORTH DN, The distribution and functional activity of the cervical musculature, *Am J Obstet Gynecol* (1954) **68**:1261–71.

14 HRICAK H, CHANG YCF, THURNHER S et al, Evaluation of the vagina by magnetic resonance imaging: Part I Normal anatomy and congenital anomalies, *Radiology* (1988) **169**:169–74.

15 HRICAK H, HAMM B, WOLF K-J, Use of Gd-DTPA in MR imaging of the female pelvis, Proceedings of Contrast Media in MRI, Berlin 1990.

16 BAUMGARTNER BR, BERNARDINO ME, MR imaging of the cervix: off-axis scan to improve visualization of zonal anatomy, *AJR* (1989) **153**:1001–2.

17 SORENSON SS, Estimated prevalence of Müllerian anomalies, *Acta Obstet Gynecol Scand* (1988) **67**:441–5.

18 SORENSON SS, Hysteroscopic evaluation and endocrinological aspects of women with Müllerian anomalies and oligomenorrhoea, *Int J Fertil* (1987) **32(6)**:445–52.

19 PENNES DR, BOWERMAN RA, SILVER TM et al, Failed first trimester pregnancy termination: uterine anomaly as etiologic factor, *J Clin Ultrasound* (1987) **15**:165–70.

20 FEDELE L, ZAMBERLETTI D, VERCELLINI P et al, Reproductive performance of women with unicornuate uterus, *Fertil Steril* (1987) **47(3)**:416–19.

21 FORE SR, HAMMOND CB, PARKER RT et al, Urologic and genital anomalies in patients with congenital absence of the vagina, *Obstet Gynecol* (1975) **46(4)**:410–15.

22 BERMAN L, STRINGER DA, STONGE O et al, Unilateral hematocolpos in uterine duplication associated with renal agenesis, *Clin Radiol* (1987) **38**:545–7.

23 BUTTRAM VC, GIBBONS WE, Müllerian anomalies: a proposed classification (an analysis of 144 cases), *Fertil Steril* (1979) **32(1)**:40–6.

24 MALINI S, VALDES C, MALINAK R, Sonographic diagnosis and classification of anomalies of the female genital tract, *J Ultrasound Med* (1984) **3**:397–404.

25 REUTER KL, DALY DC, COHEN SM, Septate versus bicornuate uteri: errors in imaging diagnosis, *Radiology* (1989) **172**:749–52.

26 MINTZ MC, THICKMAN DI, GUSSMAN D et al, MR evaluation of uterine anomalies, *AJR* (1987) **148**:287–90.

27 FEDELE L, DORTA M, BRIOSCHI D et al, Magnetic resonance evaluation of double uteri, *Obstet Gynecol* (1989) **74(6)**:844–7.

28 CARRINGTON BM, HRICAK H, NURUDDIN RR MRI evaluation of Müllerian duct anomalies, (Accepted by *Radiology*).

29 FRIEDLAND GW, Miscellaneous congenital anomalies of the genitourinary tract. In: Pollack HM, ed. *Clinical Urography*, (WB Saunders: Philadelphia 1990) 771–86.

30 KOGAN BA, HRICAK H, TANAGHO EA, Magnetic resonance imaging in genital anomlies, *J Urol* (1987) **138**:1028–30.

31 SECAF E, NURUDDIN R, HRICAK H et al, Evaluation of ambiguous genitalia with MRI (work in progress). Radiologic Society of North America, Supplement to *Radiology* (1989):371.

32 TOGASHI K, NISHIMURA K, ITOH K et al, Vaginal agenesis: classification by MR imaging, *Radiology* (1987) **162**:675–7.

33 SCANLAN KA, POZNIAK MA, FAGERHOLM M et al, Value of transperineal sonography in the assessment of vaginal atresia, *AJR* (1990) **154**:545–8.

34 ZAWIN M, MCCARTHY S, SCOUTT L et al, Monitoring therapy with a gonadotropin-releasing hormone analog: utility of MR imaging, *Radiology* (1990) **175**:503–6.

35 HRICAK H, TSCHOLAKOFF D, HEINRICHS L et al, Uterine leiomyomas: correlation of MR, histopathologic findings and symptoms, *Radiology* (1986) **158**:385–91.

36 MARK AS, HRICAK H, HEINRICHS LW et al, Adenomyosis and leiomyoma: differential diagnosis with MR imaging, *Radiology* (1987) **163**:527–9.

37 TOGASHI K, OZASA H, KONISHI I et al, Enlarged uterus: differentiation between adenomyosis and leiomyoma with MRI, *Radiology* (1989) **171**:531–4.

38 GROSS BH, SILVER TM, JAFFE MH, Sonographic features of uterine leiomyomas, *J Ultrasound Med* (1983) **2**:401–6.

39 BALTAROWICH OH, KURTZ AB, PENNELL R et al, Pitfalls in the sonographic diagnosis of uterine fibroids, *AJR* (1988) **151(4)**:725–8.

40 WEINREB JC, BARKOFF ND, MEGIBOW A et al, The value of MR imaging in distinguishing leiomyomas from other solid pelvic masses when sonography is indeterminate, *AJR* (1990) **154**:295–9.

41 KILKKU P, ERKKOLA R, GRONROOS M, Nonspecificity of symptoms related to adenomyosis: a prospective comparative survey, *Acta Obstet Gynecol Scand* (1984) **63**:229–31.

42 TOGASHI K, NISHIMURA K, ITOH K et al, Adenomyosis: diagnosis with MR imaging, *Radiology* (1988) **166**:111–14.

43 SCULLY RE, Definition of endometrial carcinoma precursors, *Clin Obstet Gynecol* (1982) **25**:39–48.

44 SILVERBERG E, LUBERA J, Cancer statistics, *A Cancer Journal for Clinicians* (1987) **36**:9–25.

45 CHEN SS, LEE L, Retroperitoneal lymph node metastases in stage I carcinoma of endometrium: correlation with risk factors, *Gynecol Oncol* (1983) **16**:319–25.

46 MORROW PC, TOWNSEND DE, Tumors of the endometrium. In: Morrow PC, Townsend DE, eds. *Synopsis of Gynecologic Oncology*, 3rd edn, (Churchill Livingstone: New York 1987) 159–205.

47 COWLES TA, MAGRINA JF, MASTERSON BJ et al, Comparison of clinical and surgical staging in patients with endometrial carcinoma, *Obstet Gynecol* (1985) **66**:413–6.

48 Announcements: FIGO stages, 1988 revision, *Gynecol Oncol* (1989) **35**:125–7.

49 HRICAK H, STERN JL, FISHER MR et al, Endometrial carcinoma staging by MR imaging *Radiology* (1987) **162**:297–305.

50 WORTHINGTON JL, BALFE DM, LEE JKT et al, Uterine neoplasms: MR imaging, *Radiology* (1986) **159**:725–30.

51 HRICAK H, Use of gadolinium in MR imaging of the pelvis. In: Gooding CA, ed. *Diagnostic Radiology 1990*, (Radiology Research and Education Foundation: UCSF 1990) 97–102.

52 KERR-WILSON RH, SHINGLETON HM, ORR JW et al, The use of ultrasound and computed tomography scanning in the management of gynecologic cancer patients, *Gynecol Oncol* (1984) **18**:54–61.

53 WALSH JW, GOPLERUD DR, Computed tomography of primary, persistent and recurrent endometrial malignancy, *AJR* (1982) **139**:1149–54.

54 BALFE DM, VAN DYKE J, LEE KT et al, Computed tomography in malignant endometrial neoplasms, *J Comput Assist Tomogr* (1982) **7**:677–83.

55 HRICAK H, RUBINSTEIN LV, GHERMAN GM et al, MRI in the evaluation of endometrial carcinoma: results of an NCI cooperative study, *Radiology* (submitted).

56 CHEN SS, RUMANCIK WM, SPIEGEL G, Magnetic resonance imaging in stage I endometrial carcinoma, *Obstet Gynecol* (1990) **75**:274–7.

57 PHILIPS GL, PREM KA, ADCOCK LL et al, Vaginal recurrence of adenocarcinoma of the endometrium, *Gynecol Oncol* (1982) **13**:323–8.

58 WILLIAMSON EO, CHRISTOPHERSON WM, Malignant mixed Müllerian tumors of the uterus, *Cancer* (1972) **29**:585–92.

59 SHAPEERO LH, HRICAK H, Mixed Müllerian sarcoma of the uterus: MR imaging findings, *AJR* (1989) **153**:317–19.

60 KUMAR NB, HART WB, Metastases to the uterine corpus from extragenital cancer: a clinicopathologic study of 63 cases, *Cancer* (1982) **50**:2163–9.

61 ANSARI AH, REYNOLDS RA, Cervical incompetence: a review, *J Reprod Med* (1987) **32**:161–71.

62 HRICAK H, CHANG YCF, CANN CE et al, Cervical incompetence: preliminary evaluation with MR imaging, *Radiology* (1990) **174**:821–6.

63 MAHRAN M, The role of ultrasound in the diagnosis and management of the incompetent cervix. In: Kurjak A, ed. *Recent Advances in Ultrasound Diagnosis* (Volume 2). International Congress series no. 498, (Elsevier: Amsterdam 1980) 505–14.

64 MORROW PC, TOWNSEND DE, Vaginal adenosis, adenocarcinoma and diethylstilbestral. In: Morrow PC, Townsend DE, eds. *Synopsis of Gynecologic Oncology*, 3rd edn. (Churchill Livingstone: New York 1987) 45–55.

65 VAN GILS APG, THAM RTOTA, FALKE THM et al, Abnormalities of the uterus and cervix after diethylstilbestrol exposure: correlation of findings on MR and hysterosalpingography, *AJR* (1989) **153**:1235–8.

66 HANEY AF, HAMMOND CB, SOULES MR et al, Diethylstilbestrol-induced upper genital tract abnormalities, *Fertil Steril* (1979) **31**:142–6.

67 TOGASHI K, NOMA S, OZASA H, CT and MR demonstration of Nabothian cysts mimicking a cystic adnexal mass, *J Comput Assist Tomogr* (1987) **11**:1091–2.

68 MORROW PC, TOWNSEND DE, Tumors of the cervix. In: Morrow PC, Townsend DE, eds. *Synopsis of Gynecologic Oncology*, 3rd edn. (Churchill Livingstone: New York 1987) 103–58.

69 TOGASHI K, NISHIMURA K, ITOH K et al, Uterine cervical cancer: assessment with high-field MR imaging, *Radiology* (1986) **160**:431–5.

70 HRICAK H, LACEY CG, SANDLES LG et al, Invasive cervical carcinoma: comparison of MR imaging and surgical findings, *Radiology* (1988) **166**:623–31.

71 TOGASHI K, NISHIMURA J, SAGO T et al, Carcinoma of the cervix: staging with MR imaging, *Radiology* (1989) **171**:245–51.

72 KIM SH, CHOI BI, LEE HP et al, Uterine cervical carcinoma: comparison of CT and MR findings, *Radiology* (1990) **175**:45–51.

73 GRECO A, MASON P, LEUNG AWL et al, Staging of carcinoma of the uterine cervix: MRI-surgical correlation, *Clinical Radiology* (1989) **40**:401–5.

74 CHEN NJ, Vaginal invasion by cervical carcinoma, *Acta Med Okayama* (1984) **38**:305–13.

75 CHANG YCF, HRICAK H, THURNHER S et al, Evaluation of the vagina by magnetic resonance imaging: Part II Neoplasm, *Radiology* (1988) **169**:569–71.

76 EBNER F, KRESSEL HY, MINTZ MC et al, Tumor recurrence versus fibrosis in the female pelvis: differentiation with MR at 1.5T, *Radiology* (1988) **166**:333–40.

77 WILKINSON EJ, FRIEDRICH EG, Diseases of the vulva. In: Kurman RJ, ed. *Blaustein's Pathology of the Female Genital Tract*, (Springer-Verlag: New York 1987) 36–140.

78 MORROW PC, TOWNSEND DE, Tumors of the vulva. In: Morrow PC, Townsend DE, eds. *Synopsis of Gynecologic Oncology*, 3rd edn, (Churchill Livingstone: New York 1987) 57–89.

79 EDWARDS CL, STRINGER CA, Management of early stage carcinoma of the vulva. In: Rutledge FN, Freedman RS, Gershenson DM, eds. *Gynecologic cancer: Diagnosis and Treatment Strategies*, (University of Texas Press: Austin 1987) 285–90.

Figure 5.1

Drawing in sagittal plane illustrating the anterior and the posterior peritoneal reflections between the uterus, bladder and rectum.

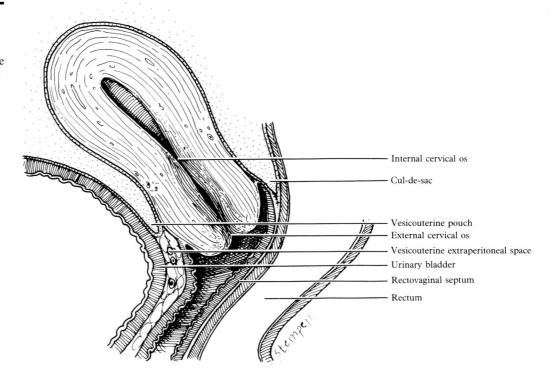

- Internal cervical os
- Cul-de-sac
- Vesicouterine pouch
- External cervical os
- Vesicouterine extraperitoneal space
- Urinary bladder
- Rectovaginal septum
- Rectum

Figure 5.2

Drawing in coronal plane demonstrating landmarks of the internal and external cervical os as well as the lateral extension of the parametria.

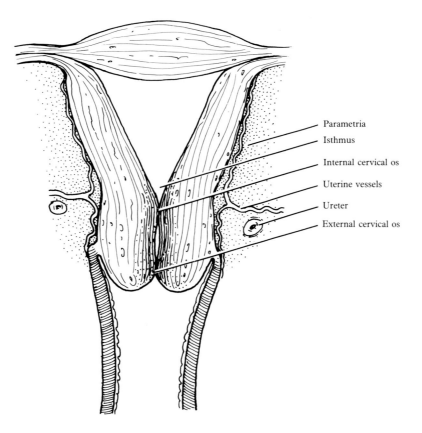

- Parametria
- Isthmus
- Internal cervical os
- Uterine vessels
- Ureter
- External cervical os

Figure 5.3

Three-dimensional drawing in
an oblique plane demonstrating
the peritoneal reflections,
parametria, the broad and
round ligaments. (**a**) Drawing
with major pelvic organs
present. (**b**) The bladder is
removed in order to better
illustrate anterior peritoneal
reflections.

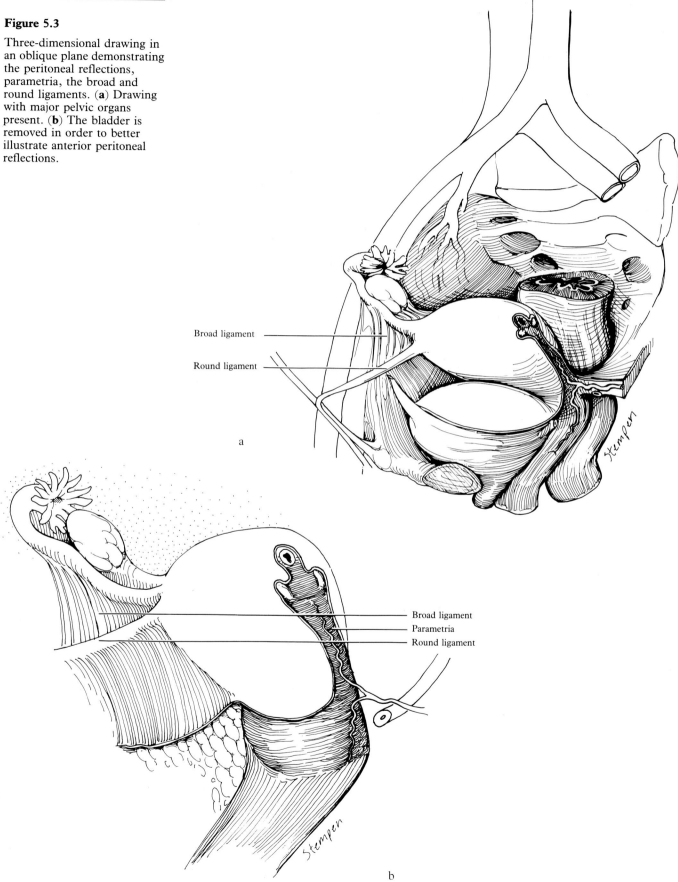

Broad ligament

Round ligament

a

Broad ligament
Parametria
Round ligament

b

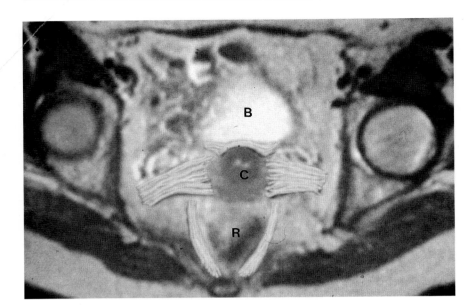

Figure 5.4

The uterine ligaments. T2-weighted transaxial image with computer drawings of the anterior uterovesical ligaments, the posterior uterosacral ligaments and the region of the lateral parametria, of which the cardinal ligaments form the base. (C)–cervix; (B)–urinary bladder; (R)–rectum.

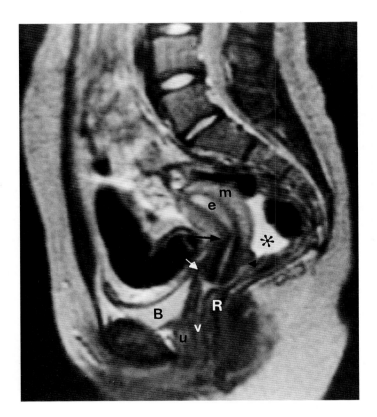

Figure 5.5

Anatomy of the uterus and the vagina as seen on T2-weighted sagittal image. Within the corpus uterus, the myometrium (m) and the endometrium (e) are separated by the low signal intensity junctional zone. The cervix extends from the level of the internal os (black arrow) to the external os which protrudes into the vagina (v) located between the bladder (B) and the urethra (u) anteriorly and the rectum (R) posteriorly. Both the anterior (white arrowhead) and the posterior (black arrowhead) vaginal fornices are seen. Fluid in the cul-de-sac (asterisk).

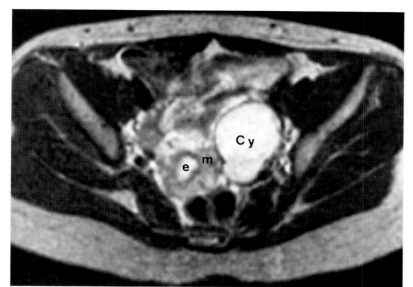

a

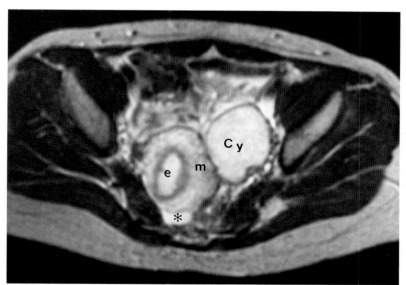

b

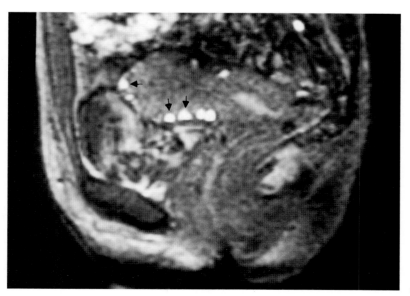

c

Figure 5.6

Appearance of the uterus during menstrual cycle. T2-weighted image (**a**) proliferative phase, (**b**) secretory phase, and (**c**) sagittal GRE image (TR 33 TE 13, angle 30°). The uterus is large in the secretory phase with increased thickness of the endometrium (e) and increased width and signal intensity of the myometrium (m). Arcuate vessels (arrows) demonstrate high signal intensity. (Cy)–left ovarian cyst; (asterisk)–fluid in the cul-de-sac.

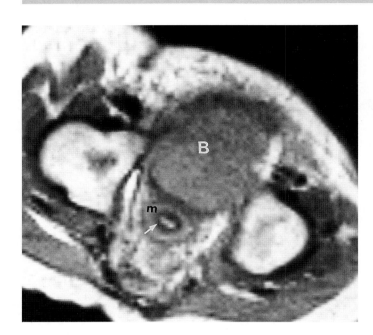

Figure 5.7

Effect of maternal estrogens on neonatal uterus. Transaxial T2-weighted image demonstrating zonal anatomy of the uterus with differentiation between medium signal intensity myometrium (m), high signal endometrium and low signal intensity junctional zone (small white arrow). (B)–urinary bladder. (0.35T.)

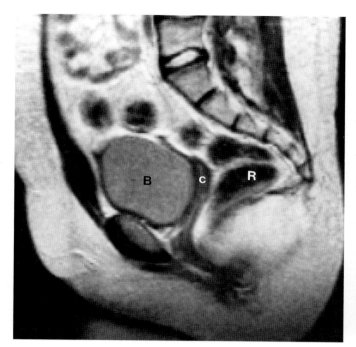

a

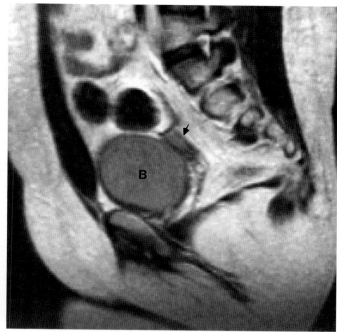

b

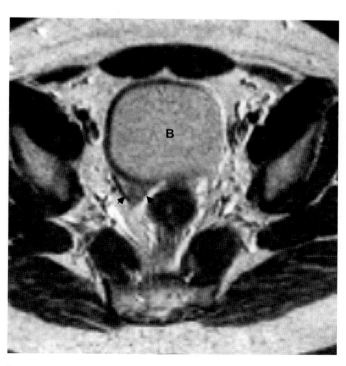

c

Figure 5.8

Premenarchal female. (**a**) and
(**b**) are two consecutive sagittal
T2-weighted images and (**c**) is
in the transaxial plane. A small
corpus uterus (arrows) with no
identifiable endometrium and a
low signal intensity
myometrium is seen. (B)–
bladder; (R)–rectum; (C)–
cervix.

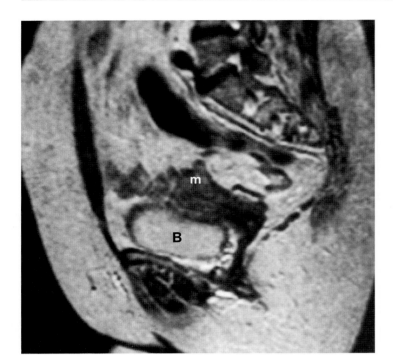

Figure 5.9

Postmenopausal uterus. T2-weighted image shows low signal intensity uterus with indistinct zonal anatomy and low signal intensity myometrium (m). (B)-urinary bladder.

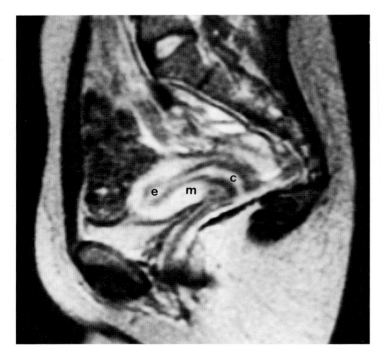

Figure 5.10

Patient taking oral contraceptive pill, sagittal T2-weighted image. The myometrium (m) is of abnormally high signal intensity. The endometrium (e) is atrophic; (c)-cervix.

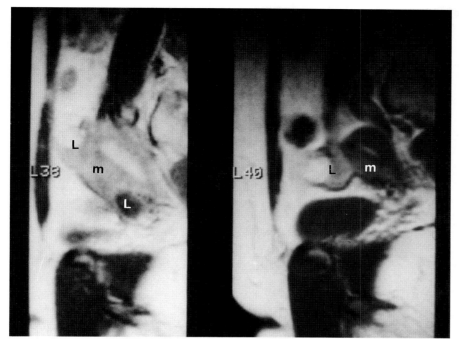

a

b

Figure 5.11

Effect of gonadotropin releasing hormone analogs on the MRI appearance of the uterus, T2-weighted sagittal image (**a**) before and (**b**) after six months therapy. Following therapy the uterus is smaller in size and the myometrium (m) shows interval decrease in signal intensity. (L)-leiomyoma. (0.35T.)

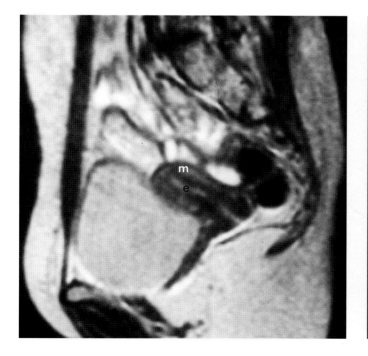

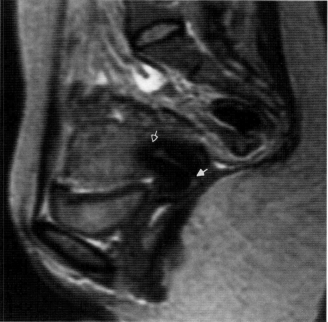

Figure 5.12

Postmenopausal woman (age 73 years) on estrogen/progesterone supplement therapy, T2-weighted sagittal image demonstrating uterus with differentiation of zonal anatomy. (m)-myometrium; (e)-endometrium.

Figure 5.13

Normal cervix; T2-weighted image, sagittal plane. The low signal intensity cervical stroma surrounding the higher signal intensity endocervical canal is seen extending from the internal os (open arrowhead) to the external os (solid arrowhead).

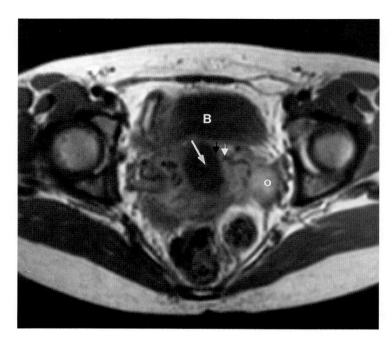

a

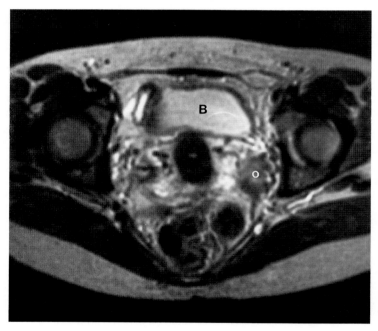

b

Figure 5.14

Normal thick cervical stroma (**a**) proton density (**b**) T2-weighted transaxial images. The compact low signal intensity fibrous cervical stroma is seen surrounding the high signal intensity center (long white arrow). The outer cervical stroma (containing mostly smooth muscle fibers) is of higher signal intensity and is seen extending from the entrance of the uterine vessels (white arrow) to the margin of the fibrous stroma (black arrow). The parametria (tissue surrounding the uterine vessels) show enhancement on T2-weighted images. (O)-hemorrhagic cyst; (B)-urinary bladder.

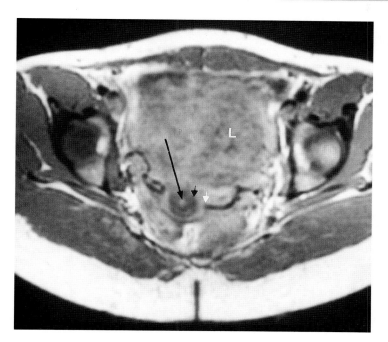

a

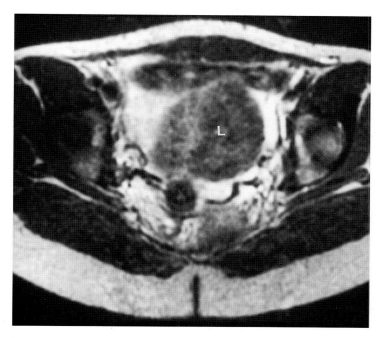

b

Figure 5.15

(**a**) Anatomy of the cervix with differentiation between the high signal intensity center (long black arrow) and the cervical stroma which can be further divided into a low signal intensity inner (fibrous) part and an outer medium signal intensity (predominantly muscular) portion. The latter is extending from the lower intensity stroma (small black arrow) to the entrance of the uterine vessels (white arrow). On the T2-weighted image (**b**), the parametrial region shows marked increase in signal. (L)-large leiomyoma.

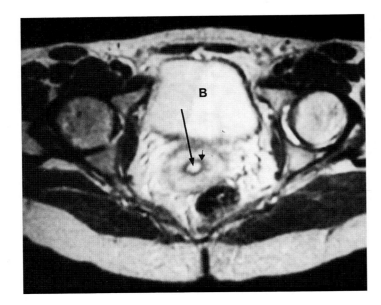

Figure 5.16

Thin fibrous cervical stroma (small solid black arrow) is seen surrounding a high signal intensity central area (long black arrow). The wide peripheral zone is due to a large portion of muscle tissue. T2-weighted image. (B)-urinary bladder.

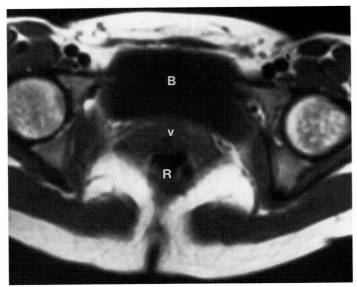

a

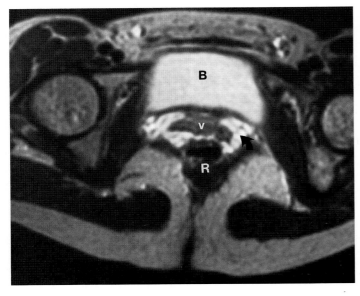

b

Figure 5.17

Normal MR appearance of the vagina at three anatomical levels – upper, middle and lower-third. (**a**) T1- and (**b**) T2-weighted images at the level of the upper third of the vagina (vaginal fornices), (**c**) T2-weighted image at the level of the mid-vagina (bladder base) and (**d**) T1- and (**e**) T2-weighted images at the level of the lower-third of the vagina. On T1-weighted images, the vagina (V) demonstrates medium signal intensity undistinguishable from the adjacent urethra (open arrows) or rectum (R). On T2-weighted images the zonal anatomy of the vagina is well demonstrated (a lower signal wall and higher signal intensity central portion) and the differentiation between vagina and the adjacent bladder (B), urethra or rectum (R) is clear. The paracolpos (black curved arrows) increases in signal intensity on T2-weighted images. (V)-vagina; (B)-urinary bladder and bladder base; urethra-open arrows.

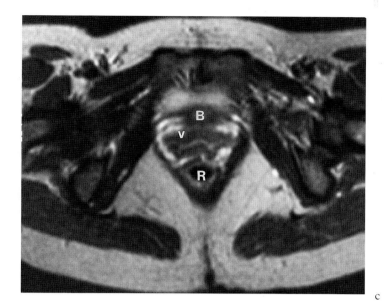

c

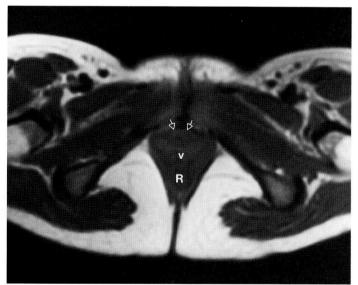

d

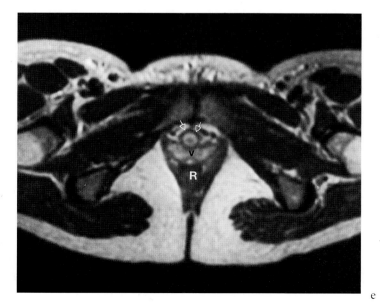

e

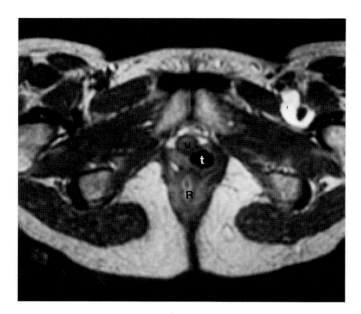

Figure 5.18

Placement of a tampon (t) in the vagina (T2-weighted image) is not only unnecessary for the identification of the vagina [clearly identified between the anterior urethra (u) and posterior placed rectum (R)] but it will distort the normal anatomical relations and tissue detail.

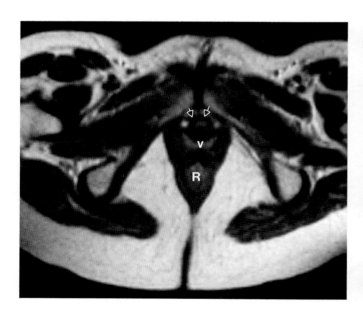

a

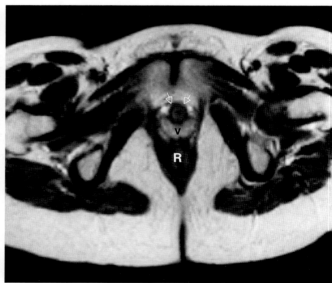

b

Figure 5.19

Appearance of the vagina on T2-weighted images (**a**) in the proliferative phase and (**b**) in the secretory phase of the menstrual cycle. As compared to the proliferative phase, in the secretory phase the wall of the vagina (V) is thin with reduced contrast between the wall and central mucus. Urethra-open arrows; (R)-rectum. (0.35T.)

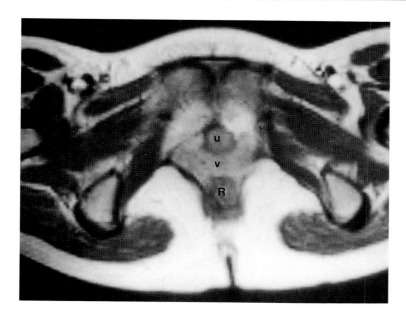

Figure 5.20

Appearance of the vagina in the third trimester of pregnancy on a T2-weighted image. The vagina (v) is engorged and differentiation between the wall and submucosa cannot be made. (U)-urethra; (R)-rectum. (0.35T.)

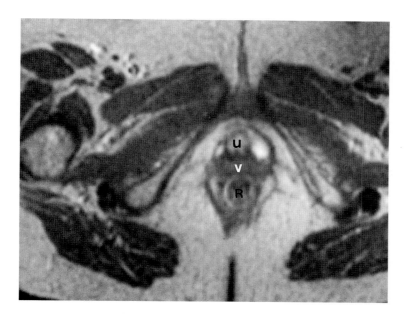

Figure 5.21

Vagina in a postmenstrual patient on a T2-weighted image. The vagina (v) is small and of uniform low signal intensity. (U)-urethra; (R)-rectum.

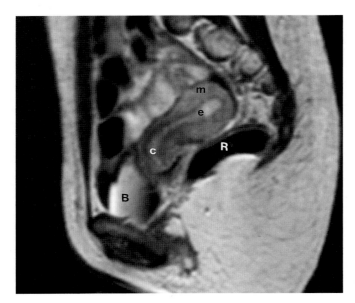

a

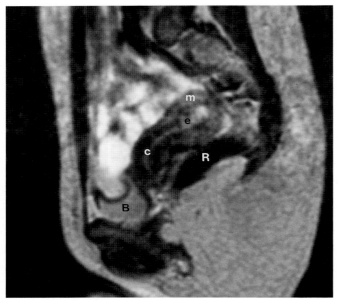

b

Figure 5.22

Gadolinium-DTPA enhancement of the uterus, sagittal (**a**) T1-weighted Gd-DTPA-enhanced image and (**b**) T2-weighted image. Uterine zonal anatomy which is routinely seen on T2-weighted images is also identified on the Gd-DTPA-enhanced T1-weighted image. (e)-endometrium; (m)-myometrium); (c)-cervix; (B)-urinary bladder; (R)-rectum.

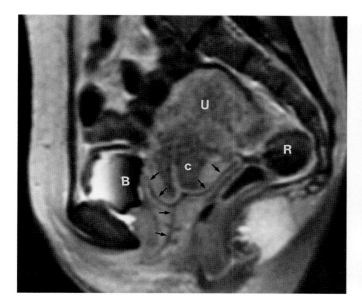

a

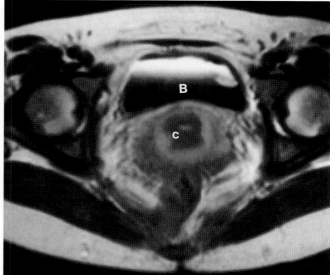

b

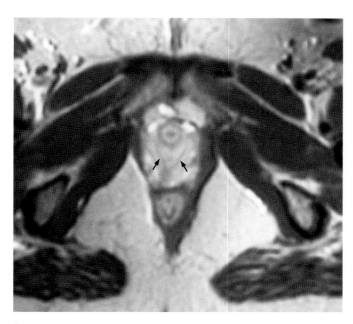

c

Figure 5.23

Gadolinium-DTPA enhancement of the cervix and vagina on T1-weighted images (**a**) sagittal, (**b**) and (**c**) transaxial plane. The compact cervical stroma (c) does not enhance while the central epithelial and peripheral paracervical tissue does. The wall of the vagina enhances but the inner surface does not, allowing demonstration of the vaginal lumen and fornices (small black arrows). (B)-urinary bladder; (R)-rectum; (U)-uterus.

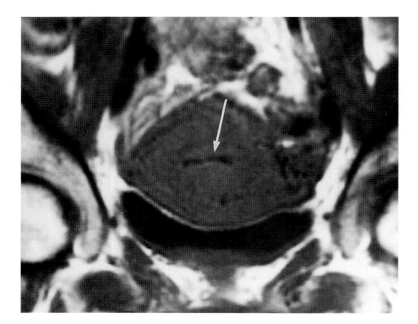

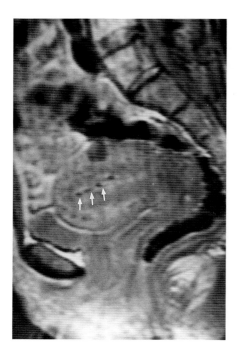

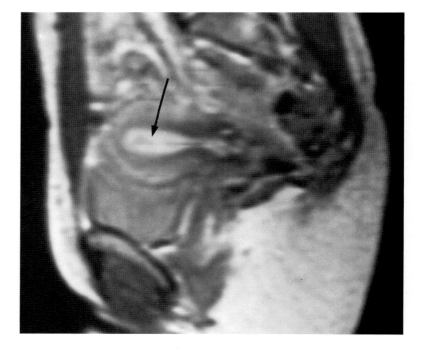

Figure 5.24

Lippes Loop intrauterine contraceptive device (arrow) demonstrating a signal void on a T1-weighted image.

Figure 5.25

Lippes Loop intrauterine contraceptive device (arrows) demonstrating a signal void on a T2-weighted image.

Figure 5.26

Copper-7 intrauterine contraceptive device (arrow). T2-weighted image.

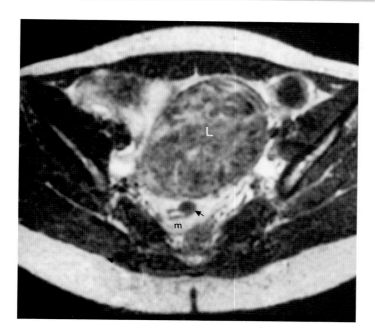

Figure 5.27

Uterine hypoplasia, T2-weighted image. The uterus is small but with good zonal differentiation between myometrium (m) and higher signal intensity endometrium. Small leiomyoma (arrow) and large degenerative subserosal leiomyoma (L).

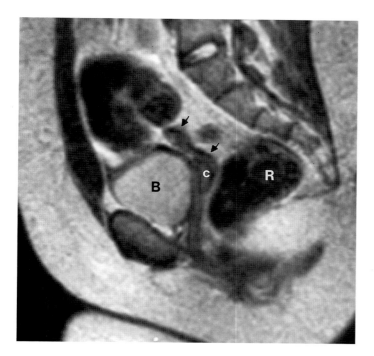

Figure 5.28

Infantile uterus in 25-year-old female with Turner's syndrome. Sagittal T2-weighted image. The uterus (arrows) is small and the zonal anatomy is indistinct. The myometrium is of low signal intensity. (c)-cervix; (B)-urinary bladder; (R)-rectum.

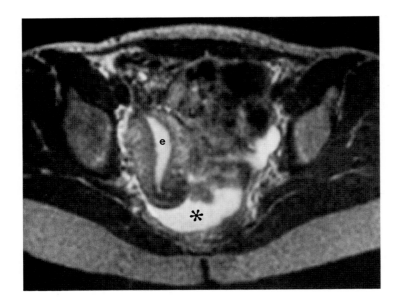

a

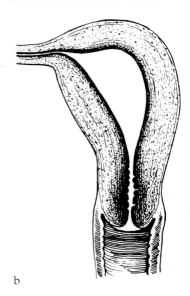

UNICORNUATE UTERUS

b

Figure 5.29

Unicornuate uterus. (**a**) T2-weighted transaxial MR image. (**b**) Schematic drawing. The uterus is 'banana-shaped'. Endometrial (e) and myometrial width are normal. Fluid in the cul-de-sac (asterisk).

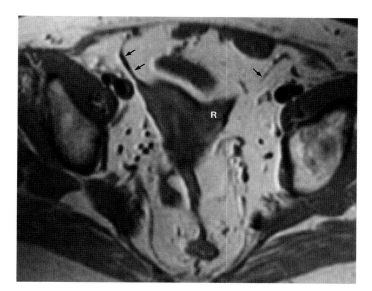

a

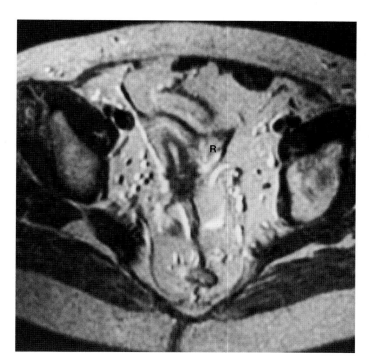

b

Figure 5.30

Unicornuate uterus with non-communicating rudimentary horn. (**a**) Proton density and (**b**) T2-weighted transaxial MR images. (**c**) Schematic drawing. The rudimentary horn (R) is due to incomplete development of one müllerian duct. Round ligaments (small arrows).

UNICORNUATE
(noncommunicating rudimentary horn)

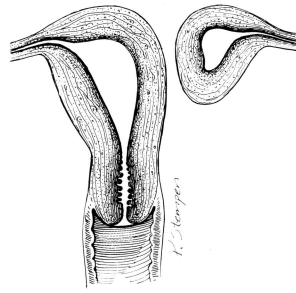

c

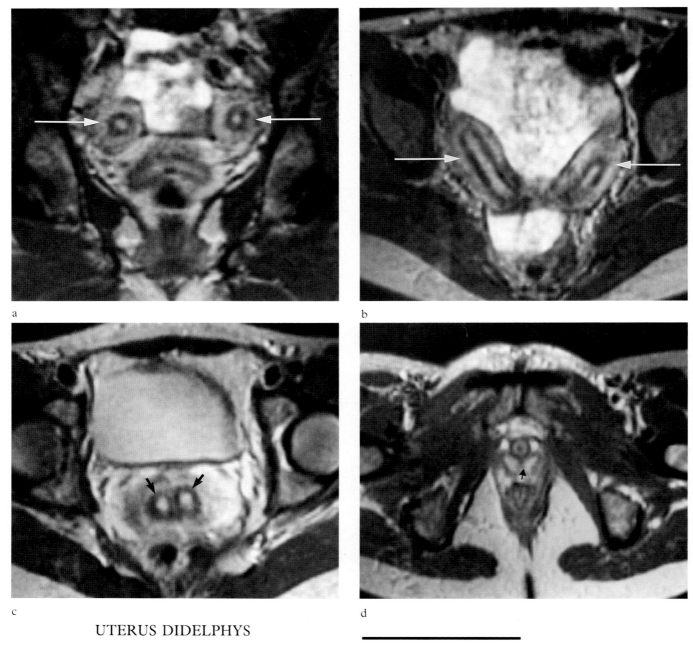

a

b

c

d

UTERUS DIDELPHYS

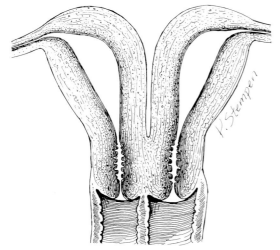

e

Figure 5.31

Didelphys uterus. T2-weighted images (**a**) coronal, and (**b**), (**c**) and (**d**) transaxial planes. (**e**) Schematic drawing. Two separate uterine horns (long white arrows), two cervices (black arrows) and a septum in the upper-third of the vagina (small black arrowhead) are identified.

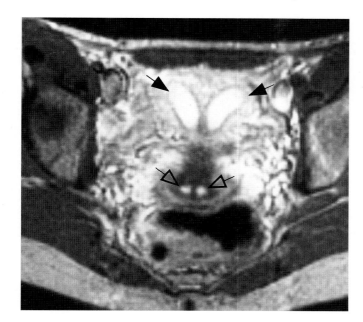

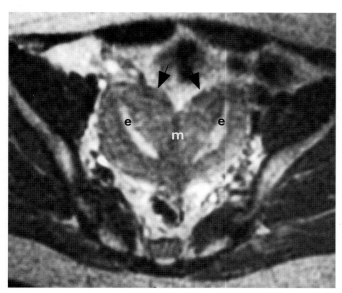

a

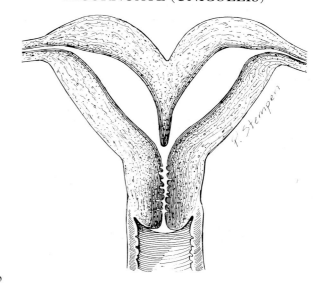

BICORNUATE (UNICOLLIS)

b

Figure 5.32

Uterus bicornuate bicollis. T2-weighted image in the transaxial plane. Two uterine cornua (closed black arrows) and two cervices (open arrowheads) are seen.

Figure 5.33

Uterus bicornuate unicollis. (**a**) Transaxial T2-weighted image. (**b**) Schematic drawing. There are two uterine cornua (black arrowheads) and two endometrial cavities (e) separated by tissue composed of myometrium (m). The outer fundal contour is concave, 'v' configuration.

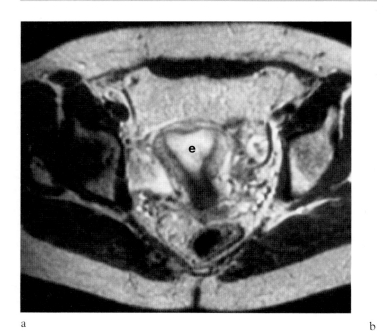

a

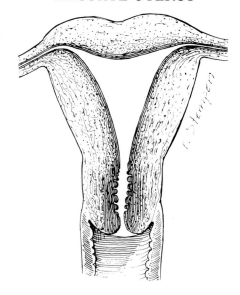

ARCUATE UTERUS

b

Figure 5.34

Arcuate uterus. (**a**) T2-weighted transaxial MR image. (**b**) Schematic drawing. The outer fundal contour is only slightly concave but there is 'heart-shaped' endometrium (e) characteristic of this anomaly.

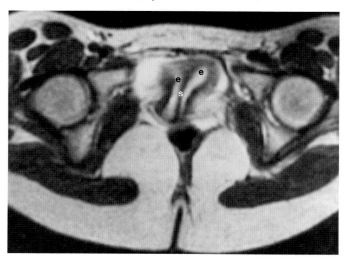

a

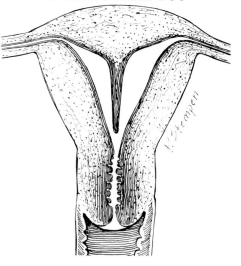

UTERUS BISEPTUS

b

Figure 5.35

Septate uterus. (**a**) Transaxial T2-weighted MR image of uterus biseptus, bicollis. (**b**) Schematic drawing of uterus biseptus unicollis. The complete septum (S) between the two endometrial cavities (e) is of low signal intensity on the T2-weighted image.

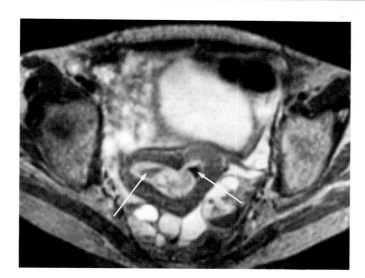

Figure 5.36

Arcuate uterus with bleeding
following first trimester
miscarriage, T2-weighted
transaxial image. The outer
fundal contour is slightly
concave and there is a partial
septum composed of
myometrium. Heterogeneous
signal intensity within the
uterine cavity respresents
bleeding with low signal blood
clots secondary to a recent
miscarriage (arrows).

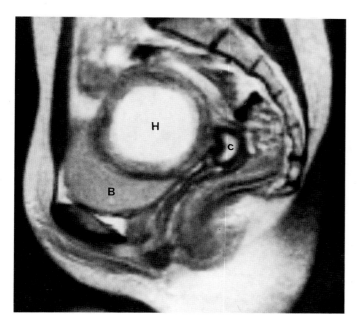

Figure 5.37

Unicornuate uterus with
obstructed rudimentary horn.
T2-weighted images (**a**) in the
sagittal plane, (**b**) and (**c**) in the
transaxial plane. A large
hematometra (H) is seen within
the noncommunicating
rudimentary horn. It indents
the unicornuate uterine cavity
(u). There is a normal, single
cervix (c). (B)-urinary bladder.
(0.35T.)

a

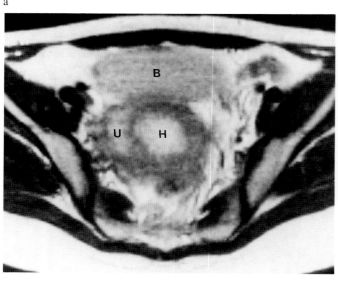

b

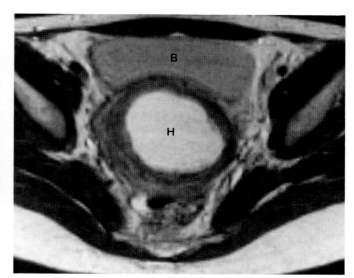

c

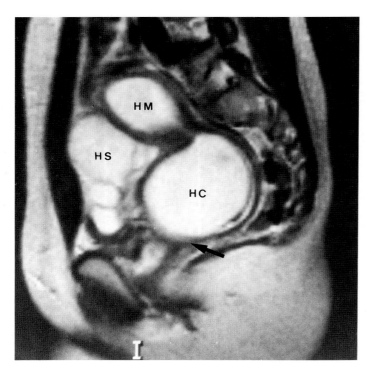

a

Figure 5.38

Uterus didelphys with unilateral obstruction. T2-weighted images (**a**) in the sagittal plane and (**b**) in the transaxial plane. There is hematosalpinx (HS), hematometra (HM) and hematocolpos (HC) due to an obstructing transverse septum in the upper third of the vagina (arrow). The nonobstructed second uterus (U) is identified separately.

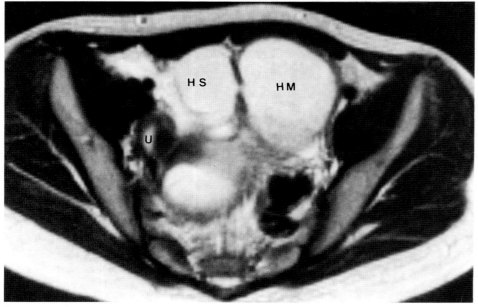

b

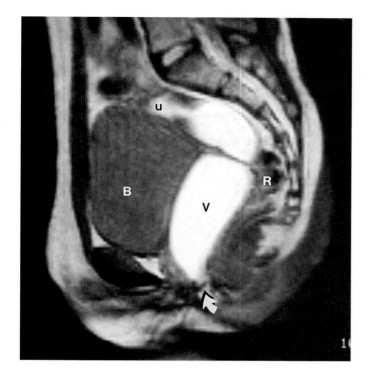

Figure 5.39

Hematocolpos due to imperforate hymen. Proton density sagittal image demonstrating a distended blood-filled vagina (v) and uterus (u) due to an imperforate hymen (curved arrow) which is located at the level of the perineum. (B)-urinary bladder; (R)-rectum.

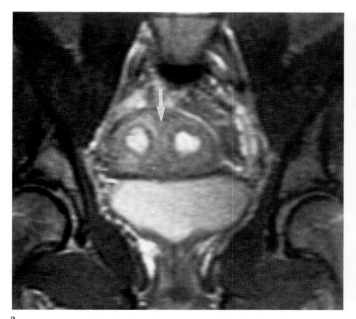

a

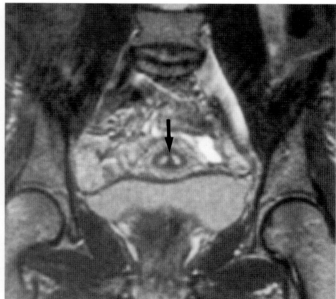

b

Figure 5.40

Septal composition as determined on T2-weighted images. (**a**) Bicornuate and (**b**) biseptate uterus. The septum in the bicornuate anomaly is composed of medium to high signal intensity myometrium (white arrow) while in the septate uterus, the septum demonstrates low signal intensity indicating collagen tissue (black arrow).

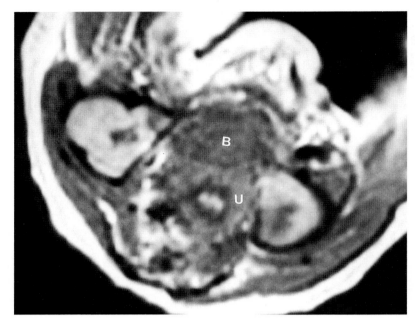

a

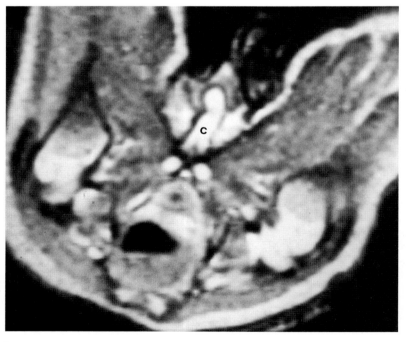

b

Figure 5.41
Newborn with ambiguous genitalia. (**a**) and (**b**) are transaxial transverse T2-weighted images demonstrating the uterus (u) with excellent zonal differentiation and a prominent clitoris (c). (B)-urinary bladder. (0.35T.)

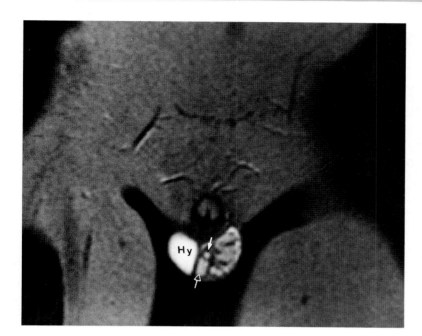

Figure 5.42

True hermaphrodite. T2-weighted image demonstrating the presence of a left ovotestis. Both ovary (solid white arrow) and testis (open white arrow) are seen in the left scrotal sac. The right testis was undescended and the right scrotal sac contains a hydrocele (Hy).

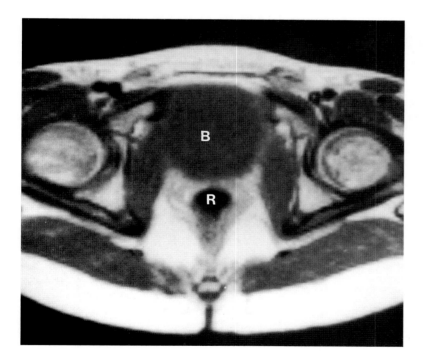

Figure 5.43

Vaginal agenesis. Transaxial proton density image demonstrating no identifiable vaginal tissue between the bladder (B) and the rectum (R).

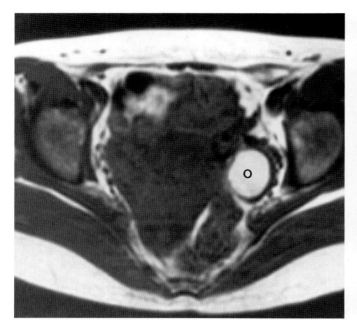

a

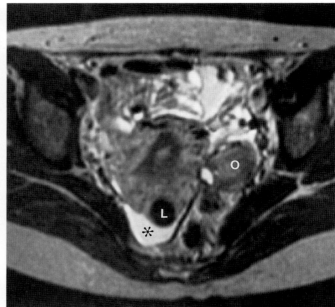

b

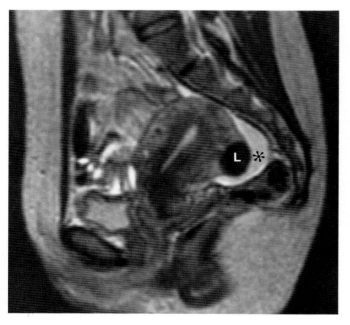

c

Figure 5.44

Nondegenerative leiomyoma on transaxial (**a**) T1- and (**b**) T2-weighted images. (**c**) Sagittal T2-weighted image. On the T1-weighted image a posterior contour abnormality is appreciated. On the T2-weighted images the contrast between the low signal intensity nondegenerative leiomyoma (L) and higher signal intensity myometrium is seen. Fluid in cul-de-sac (asterisk). (O)-hemorrhagic ovarian cyst.

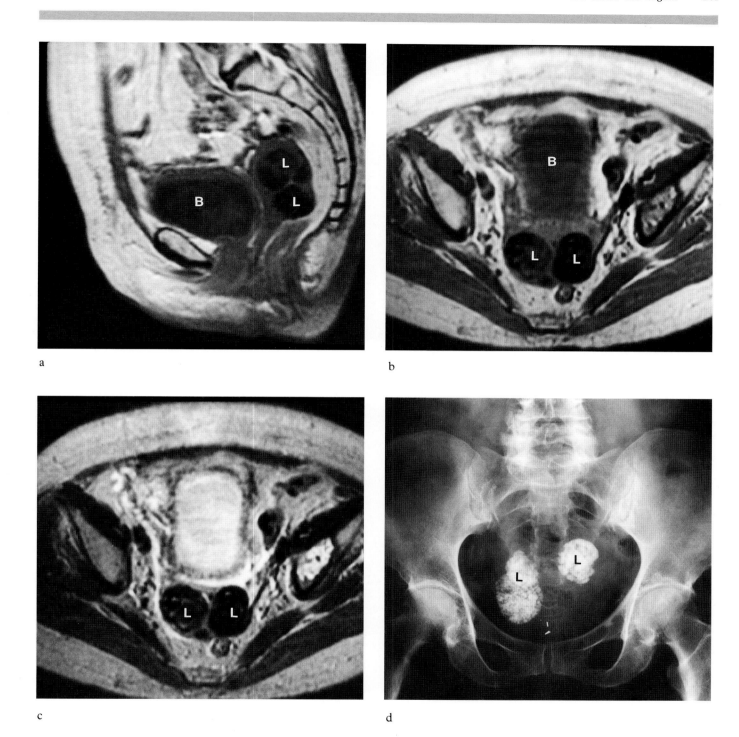

a

b

c

d

Figure 5.45

Calcified leiomyomata in a postmenopausal patient. (**a**) Sagittal T1-weighted image, (**b**) transaxial T1-weighted, (**c**) transaxial T2-weighted images and (**d**) AP radiograph of the pelvis. The uterus has involuted but calcified leiomyomata (L) demonstrate low signal intensity on both T1- and T2-weighted images. The accompanying AP pelvis radiograph shows the typical popcorn calcifications of leiomyomata. (B)-urinary bladder.

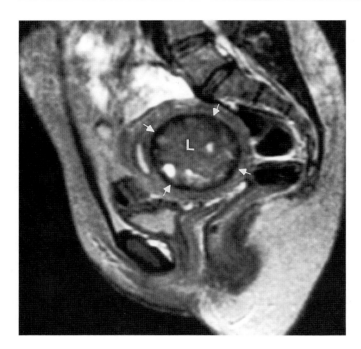

Figure 5.46

Intramural leiomyoma (L) with peripheral thick low signal intensity margin (small arrows) due to calcification. Sagittal T2-weighted image.

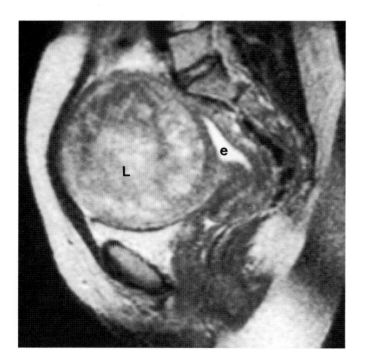

Figure 5.47

Degenerative leiomyoma. There is a fundal intramural heterogeneous high signal intensity leiomyoma (L), with myometrial tissue between the leiomyoma and the endometrial cavity (e).

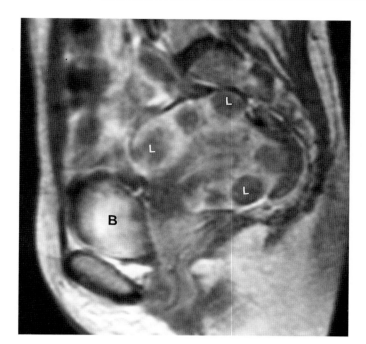

a

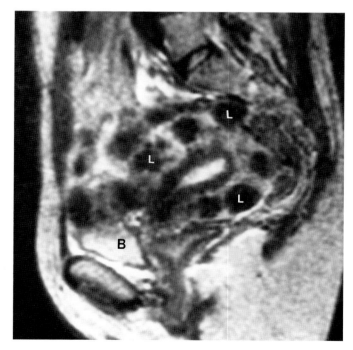

b

Figure 5.48

Nondegenerative intramural leiomyoma (L). (**a**) T1-weighted image following Gd-DTPA injection. (**b**) Nonenhanced T2-weighted image. Following injection of Gd-DTPA, the leiomyomata are of low signal intensity. (B)-urinary bladder.

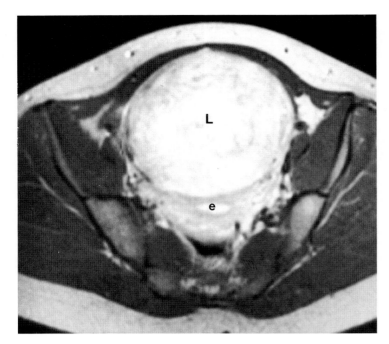

a

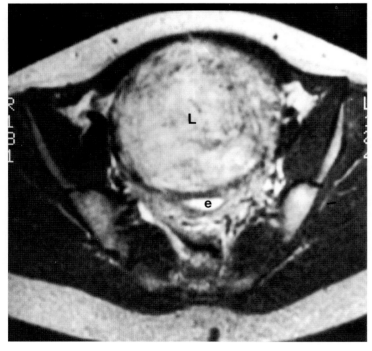

b

Figure 5.49

Degenerative intramural leiomyoma (**a**) post Gd-DTPA-enhanced T1-weighted image and (**b**) T2-weighted image. There is marked enhancement of the leiomyoma (L) after Gd-DTPA injection. The leiomyoma is of heterogeneous high signal intensity on the T2-weighted image. Uterus with enhancement of the endometrium (e).

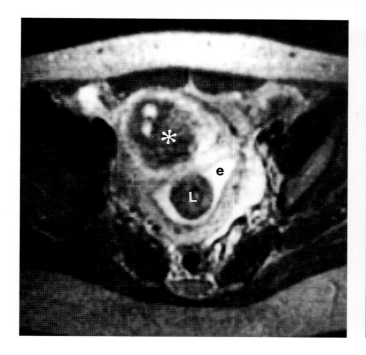

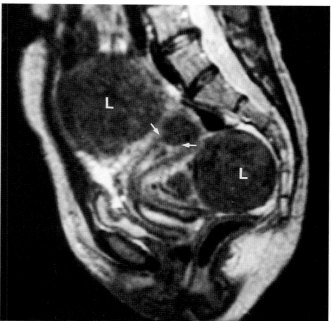

Figure 5.50

Submucosal (L) and intramural (asterisk) leiomyoma on a T2-weighted image. The submucosal leiomyoma protrudes into the endometrial cavity (e).

Figure 5.51

Subserosal (L) and small fundal submucosal (small arrows) nondegenerative leiomyomata demonstrated on this sagittal T2-weighted image.

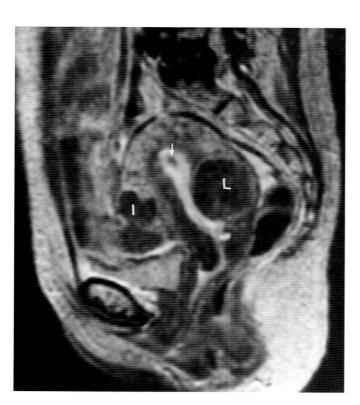

Figure 5.52

Leiomyoma (L) located in the lower uterine segment. Small submucosal leiomyoma (arrow); intramural leiomyoma (l), T2-weighted image.

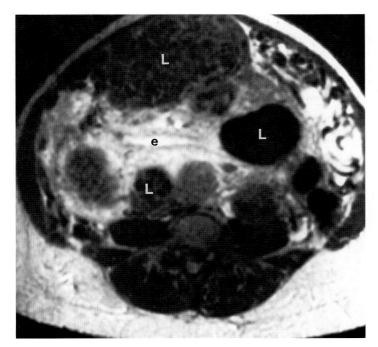

a

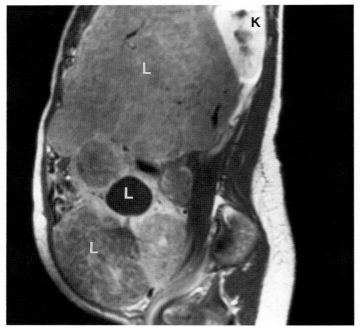

b

Figure 5.53
Multiple large leiomyomata presenting as mass extending from the pelvis to the diaphragm. Neither clinical examination nor ultrasound could assign the organ of origin. (**a**) Transaxial T2-weighted image demonstrating that the multiple low signal intensity masses—leiomyomata (L)—are within the myometrium. (e)-endometrium. (**b**) Gadolinium-enhanced T1-weighted sagittal image demonstrating the extent of the large leiomyomata (L). (K)-kidney.

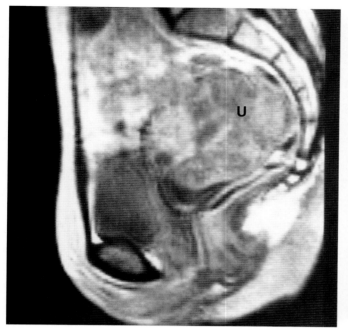

a

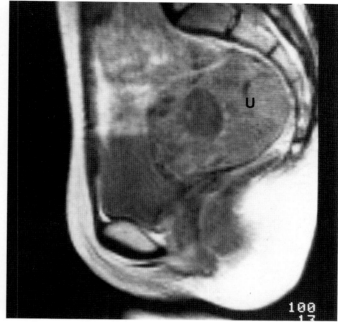

b

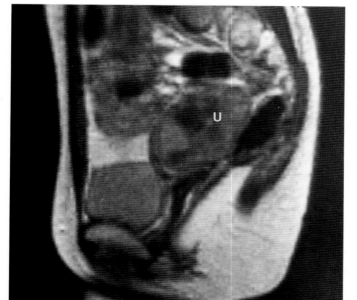

c

Figure 5.54

Response of leiomyomata to hormone analog treatment. Sagittal T2-weighted images (**a**) pretreatment, (**b**) after two months of treatment and (**c**) after six months of treatment. There is a progressive decrease in size and signal intensity of the leiomyomata and the uterus (U).

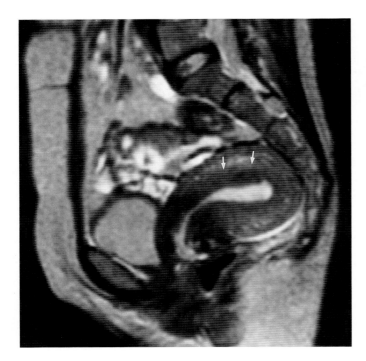

Figure 5.55

Mild form of diffuse adenomyosis (arrows), the findings confirmed at surgery. T2-weighted sagittal image.

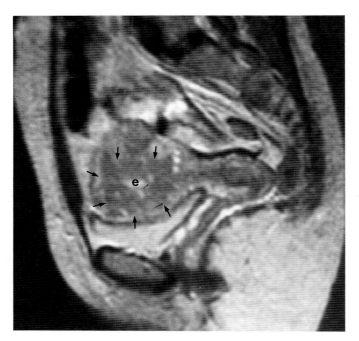

Figure 5.56

Extensive diffuse adenomyosis showing marked widening of the low signal intensity junctional zone (arrows). (e)-endometrium. T2-weighted sagittal image.

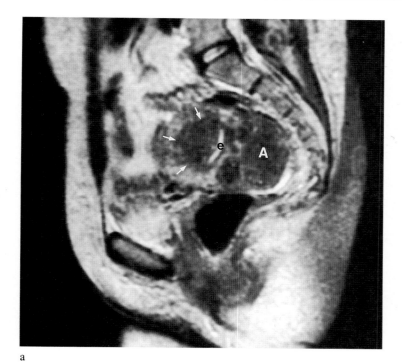

a

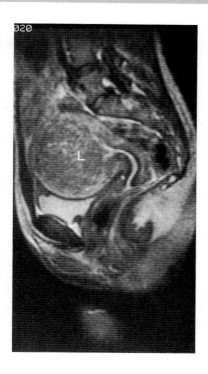

Figure 5.58

Degenerative leiomyoma. T2-weighted sagittal image demonstrating heterogeneous signal intensity of a fundal submucosal leiomyoma (L). The leiomyoma has indistinct margins, and is difficult to differentiate from an adenomyoma.

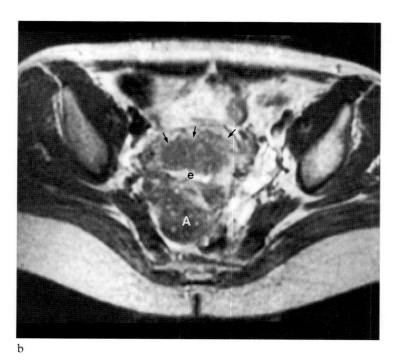

b

Figure 5.57

Adenomyoma and diffuse adenomyosis. T2-weighted (**a**) sagittal and (**b**) transaxial images. The adenomyoma (A) is elliptical in configuration, has indistinct margins and contains multiple high signal intensity foci. Diffuse adenomyosis (arrows) shows an indistinct margin, and segmental widening of the junctional zone.

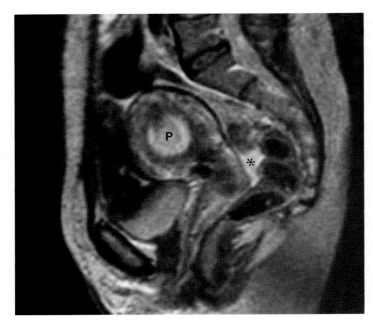

a

Figure 5.59

Endometrial polyp. Sagittal (**a**) T2-weighted and (**b**) Gd-DTPA-enhanced T1-weighted images. The endometrial polyp (P) is seen to expand the endometrial cavity and demonstrates a slightly lower signal intensity than the endometrium. After Gd-DTPA, the endometrial polyp enhances allowing identification of fluid within the endometrial cavity (arrow). (V)-vagina. Fluid in the cul-de-sac (asterisk).

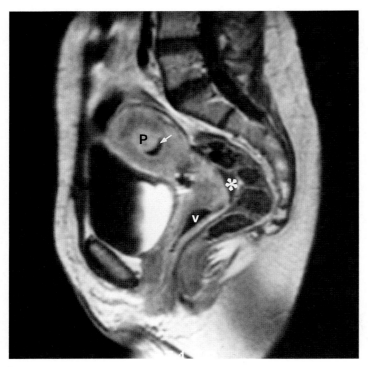

b

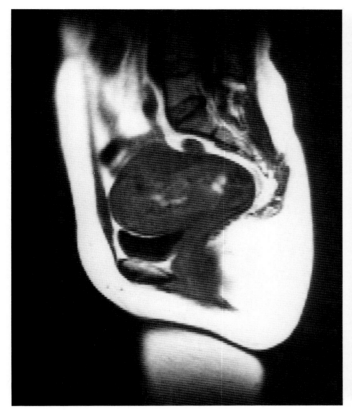

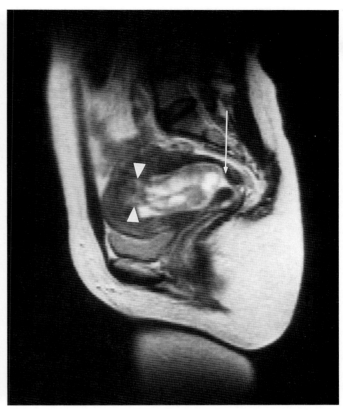

a

b

Figure 5.60

Degeneration in an endometrial polyp. Sagittal (**a**) T1- and (**b**) T2-weighted images. The endometrial cavity is expanded by a heterogeneous mass arising from the fundus (arrowhead) and extending to the internal os (long arrow). High signal intensity on T1- and T2-weighted images indicates hemorrhage. At histology, the diagnosis of degenerative endometrial polyp was made. (0.35T.)

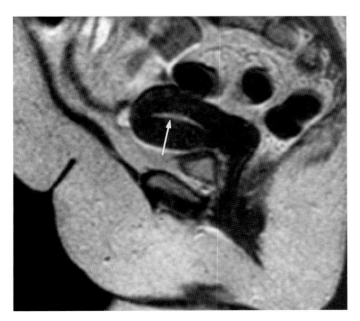

Figure 5.61

Endometrial carcinoma stage Ia – tumor confined to the endometrium. T2-weighted image showing endometrium of normal width and signal intensity (arrow).

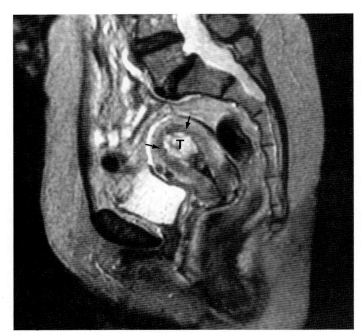

a

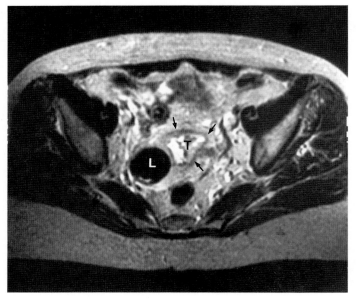

b

Figure 5.62

Endometrial carcinoma stage Ia – tumor confined to corpus without myometrial invasion. Sagittal (**a**) and transaxial (**b**) T2-weighted images showing localized widening of the endometrial cavity due to polypoid endometrial carcinoma (T). The junctional zone (small arrows) remains intact indicating that the tumor is confined to the myometrium. Retained blood within the lower uterine cavity demonstrates low signal intensity. (L)-leiomyoma.

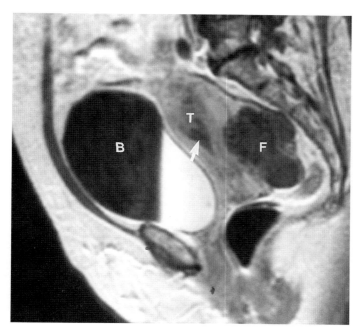

a

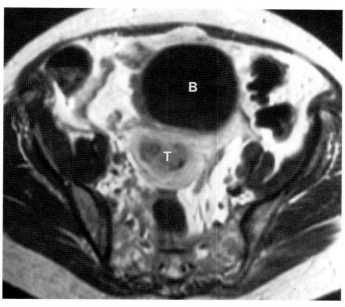

b

Figure 5.63

Endometrial carcinoma stage Ib – tumor confined to corpus. Gd-DTPA-enhanced T1-weighted image with invasion of the inner-half of the myometrium. (**a**) Sagittal and (**b**) transaxial plane. Following Gd-DTPA injection, there is enhancement of the tumor (T) while residual secretions (arrow) do not enhance. (B)-urinary bladder; (F)-ovarian fibroma, which shows no signal enhancement.

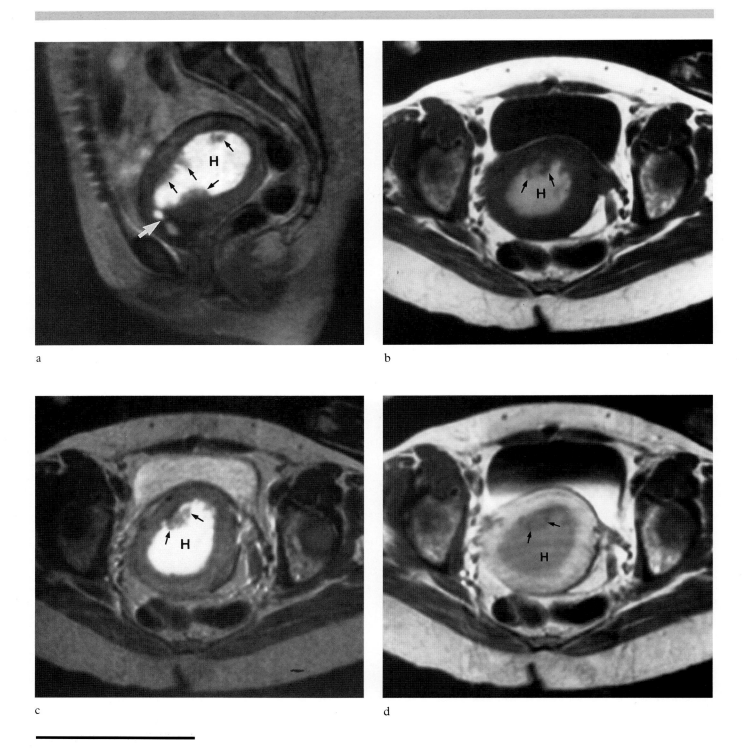

a

b

c

d

Figure 5.64

Endometrial carcinoma stage Ia – tumor confined to endometrium. (**a**) T2-weighted sagittal image and (**b**) T1-weighted , (**c**) T2-weighted and (**d**) Gd-DTPA-enhanced T1-weighted transaxial images. Multiple polypoid tumors (small arrows) which enhance following Gd-DTPA injection are identified. The uterus is enlarged and the endometrial cavity expanded by high signal intensity material which does not enhance after gadolinium injection. Because of its signal characteristics on nonenhanced T1- and T2-weighted images and lack of enhancement after Gd-DTPA, the fluid most likely represents hemorrhage (H). The retained hemorrhage was due to senile cervical stenosis (white arrow).

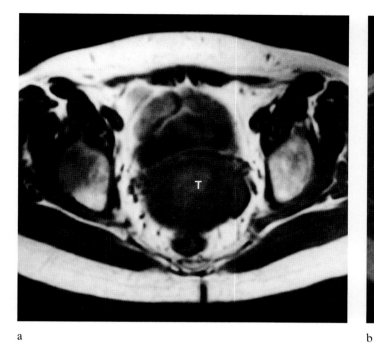

a

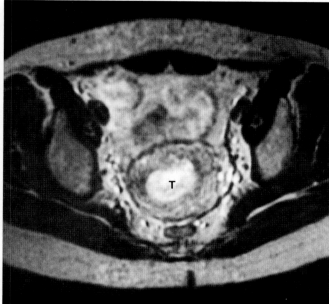

b

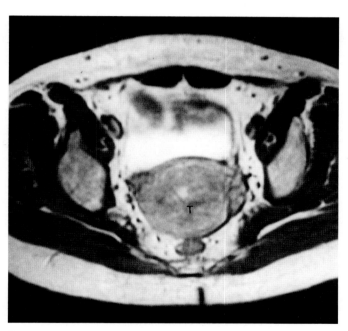

c

Figure 5.65

Endometrial carcinoma stage Ib – large tumor with superficial myometrial invasion. Transaxial (**a**) T1-weighted image, (**b**) T2-weighted image, and (**c**) gadolinium-enhanced T1-weighted images. The uterus is enlarged and its center (T) is of higher signal intensity on the T1-weighted image. The central area (T) further increases in signal intensity on T2-weighted images. However, after gadolinium injection the central area enhances indicating that it represents a large solid endometrial tumor (T).

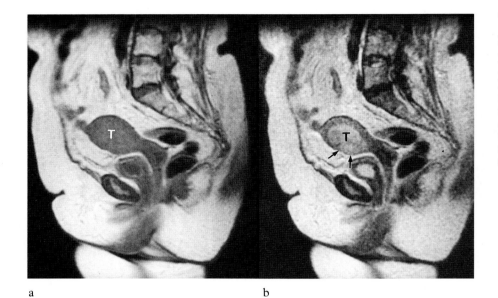

a   b

Figure 5.66

Endometrial carcinoma stage Ic – tumor infiltrating the outer half of the myometrium. Sagittal (**a**) proton density and (**b**) T2-weighted images, demonstrating the endometrial tumor (T) with deep myometrial invasion (arrows) anteriorly.

Figure 5.67

Endometrial carcinoma stage III – vaginal involvement. Sagittal (**a**) T2-weighted image, (**b**) gadolinium-enhanced T1-weighted image. A large tumor (T) is seen extending into the cervix and vagina (V). The bladder wall (black arrows) and rectal wall (white arrows) remain intact and of low signal intensity. Following gadolinium injection, heterogeneous tumor enhancement is seen within the uterus and vagina while the bladder and rectal wall remain normal. (B)-urinary bladder.

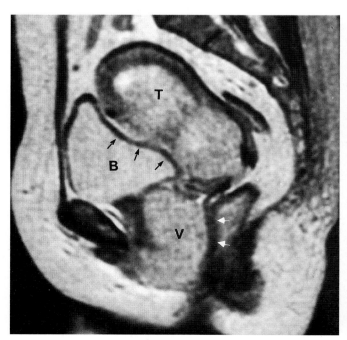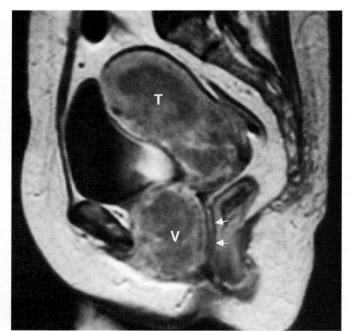

a   b

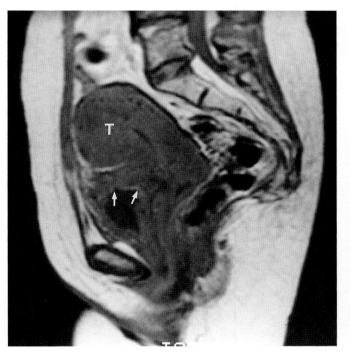

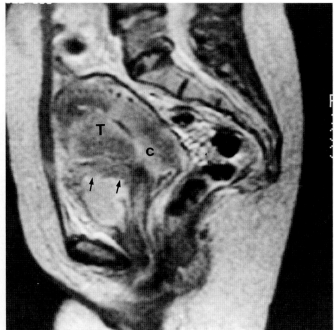

a

b

Figure 5.68

Endometrial carcinoma stage IV – bladder invasion. Sagittal (**a**) proton density and (**b**) T2-weighted images. A large endometrial tumor (T) demonstrates direct invasion into the cervix (c) and posterior bladder wall (small arrows).

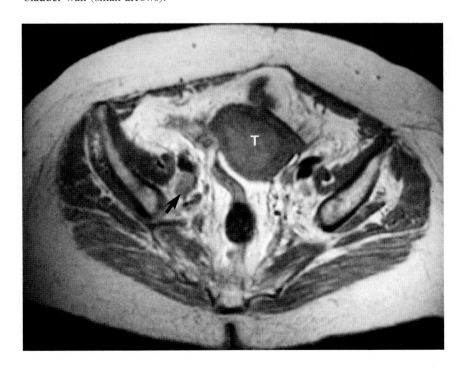

Figure 5.69

Endometrial carcinoma with lymph node metastases to the posterior external iliac nodes (arrow). Proton density image. (T)-endometrial tumor.

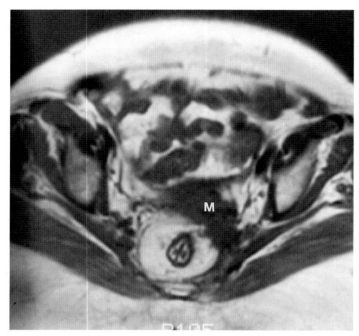

a

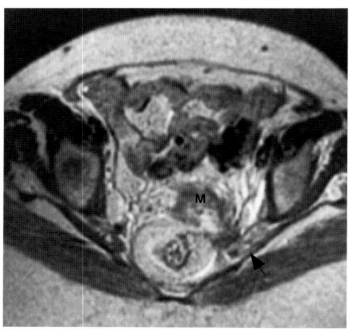

b

Figure 5.70

Recurrent endometrial carcinoma involving the pelvic sidewall. Transaxial (**a**) T1- and (**b**) T2-weighted images demonstrating a mass (M), which is of medium signal intensity on the T1-weighted image and of increased, heterogeneous, signal intensity on the T2-weighted image. The high signal intensity tumor tissue is extending to the pelvic sidewall muscle (black arrow). The rectum demonstrates high signal intensity of its submucosa on the T1-weighted image most probably due to radiation proctitis with bleeding.

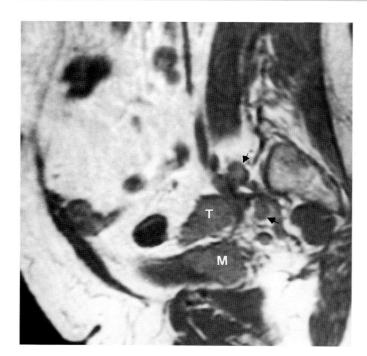

Figure 5.71

Recurrent endometrial carcinoma with invasion of the urinary bladder and metastatic lymphadenopathy. Sagittal proton density image demonstrating multiple enlarged internal iliac lymph nodes (arrows). There is also a lobulated tumor mass (M) invading the posterior aspect of the bladder. A second tumor mass (T) is seen in the region of the posterior external nodal chain.

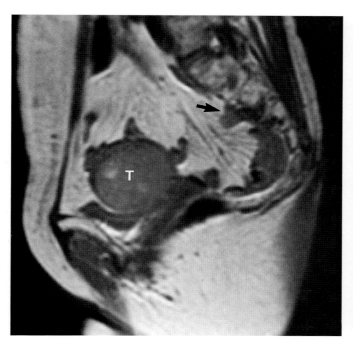

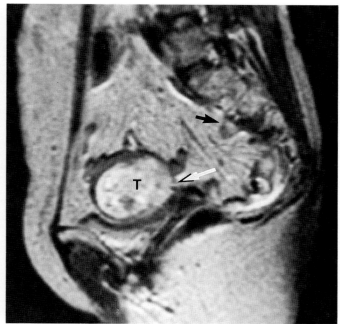

a   b

Figure 5.72

Malignant mixed müllerian tumor sagittal (**a**) T1-weighted and (**b**) T2-weighted images. The tumor (T) demonstrates medium signal intensity on the T1-weighted image and increases in signal intensity on the T2-weighted image. Deep myometrial invasion (white arrow) and tumor metastasis into the presacral region (black arrow) are demonstrated.

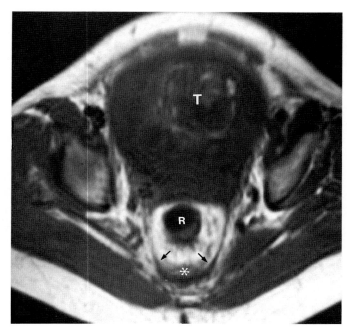

a

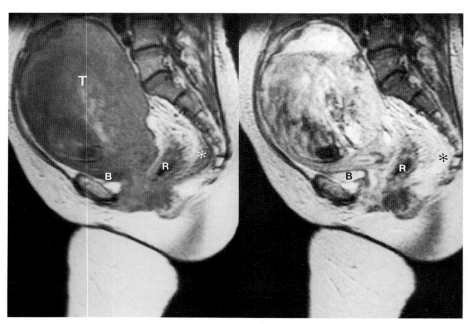

b   c

Figure 5.73

Malignant mixed müllerian tumor. (**a**) T1-weighted transaxial, (**b**) proton density and (**c**) T2-weighted sagittal images. The uterus is markedly enlarged by hemorrhagic heterogeneous signal intensity tumor (T) which demonstrates deep myometrial invasion, tumor extension into the cervix and vagina and extension along the uterosacral ligaments (small arrows) into the presacral space (asterisk). The rectum (R) is displaced anteriorly. The bladder (B) is not invaded.

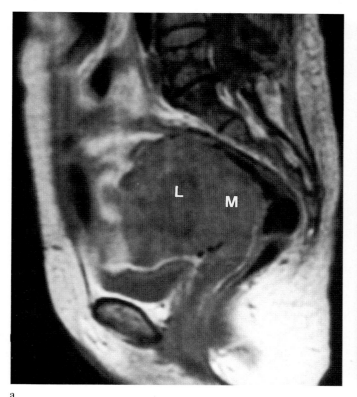

a

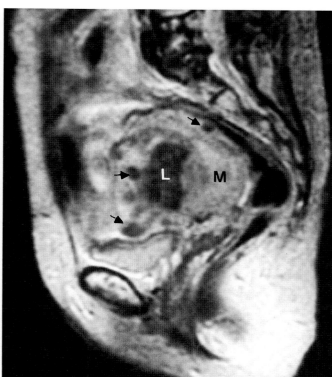

b

Figure 5.74

Uterine metastases from breast carcinoma. Sagittal plane (**a**) proton density and (**b**) T2-weighted images demonstrating low signal intensity leiomyomata (L–large leiomyoma, arrows–small intramural leiomyoma) and posteriorly a medium signal intensity mass (M) due to a metastasis from carcinoma of the breast. Based on MRI signal characteristics, the metastatic tumor (M) cannot be differentiated from a degenerative leiomyoma.

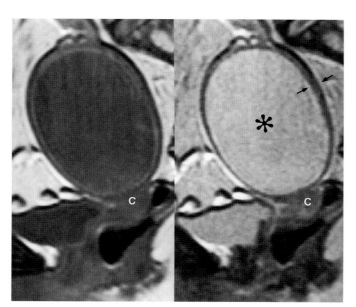

a   b

Figure 5.75

Cervical stenosis with pyometra secondary to radiation therapy. Sagittal (**a**) proton density and (**b**) T2-weighted images demonstrating an expanded uterine cavity with myometrial thinning (arrows) and pyometra (asterisk). (c)-cervix.

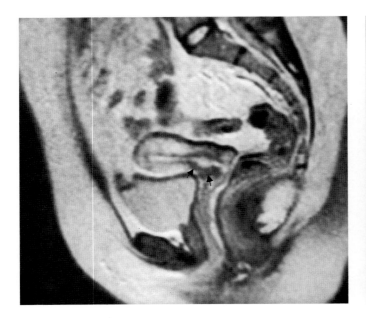

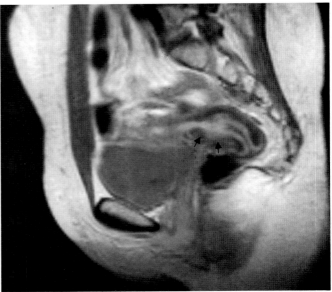

Figure 5.76

Cervical incompetence; T2-weighted sagittal image. There is an asymmetrical widening (black arrows) of the endocervical canal with normal low signal intensity of the underlying stroma. The endocervical canal is 3.3 cm long.

Figure 5.77

Cervical incompetence with decreased thickness of the irregular cervical stroma (black arrows); T2-weighted sagittal image. The length of the endocervical canal is 4.8 cm.

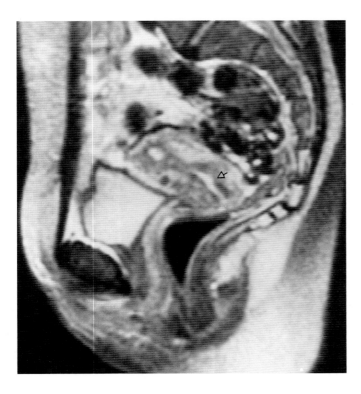

Figure 5.78

Cervical incompetence with minor asymmetrical widening and thin cervical stroma (open arrow) T2-weighted image.

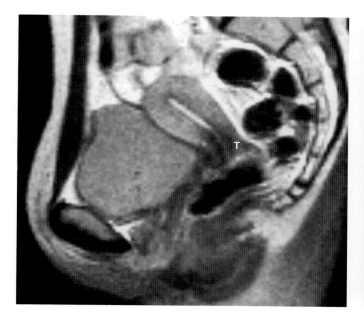

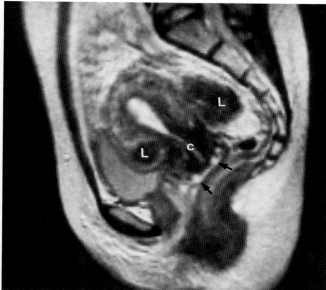

Figure 5.79

Cervical incompetence due to DES exposure. Sagittal T2-weighted image demonstrating a shortened endocervical canal measuring less than 2 cm. There is a cervical carcinoma (T) arising from the posterior cervical lip.

Figure 5.80

Vaginal adenosis due to DES exposure. T2-weighted sagittal image showing multiple foci of high signal intensity (arrows) within the walls of the vagina due to the vaginal adenosis.

Multiple leiomyomata (L) are seen. The uterus is of normal size and configuration. The endocervical canal (c) measures 4 cm in length.

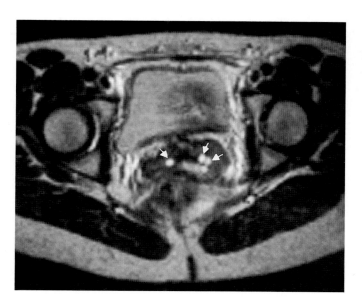

Figure 5.81

Nabothian cysts. Transaxial T2-weighted image demonstrating multiple high signal intensity nabothian cysts (arrows).

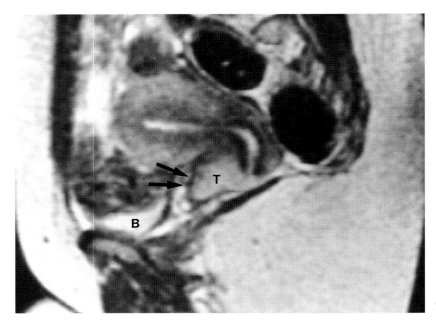

a

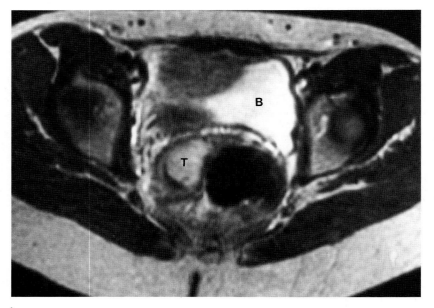

b

Figure 5.82

Carcinoma of the cervix stage I, T2-weighted image, (**a**) sagittal and (**b**) transaxial plane. The cervical tumor (T) is located in the anterior cervical lip. While the carcinoma protrudes into vagina, it does not invade the wall of the vagina. The anterior fornix (arrows) remains of normal low signal intensity. (B)-urinary bladder.

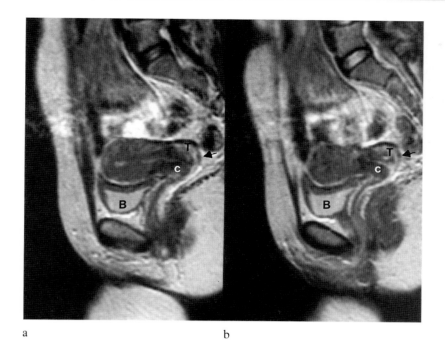

a   b

Figure 5.83

Carcinoma of the cervix stage I, T2-weighted sagittal images. (**a**) and (**b**) are two consecutive sections. A small tumor (T) is seen in the posterior cervical lip elevating the posterior fornix of the vagina (small arrows). The anterior cervical lip (c) is intact. (B)-urinary bladder.

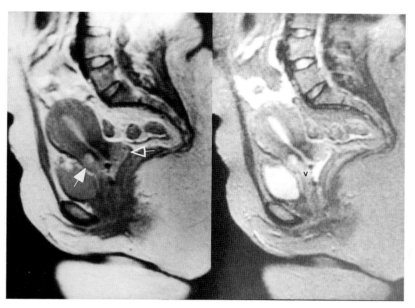

a   b

Figure 5.84

Carcinoma of the cervix stage II, sagittal (**a**) proton density and (**b**) T2-weighted images. The tumor is seen invading the anterior (open arrow) and posterior (closed arrow) lip of the exocervix. The anterior fornix of the vagina (v) is invaded classifying the patient as stage II disease.

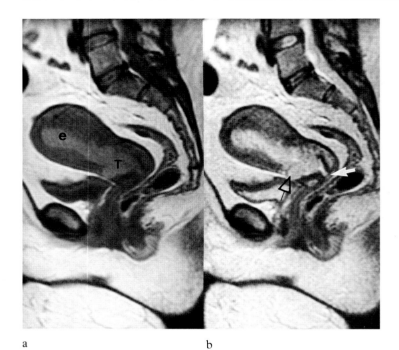

a   b

Figure 5.85

Carcinoma of the cervix stage I, sagittal (**a**) proton density and (**b**) T2-weighted image. The large tumor (T) is in the endocervical canal and is extending into the endometrial cavity (e). The external cervical os (white arrow) is free of tumor and is normal. The tumor demonstrates full thickness stromal invasion anteriorly (open black arrow).

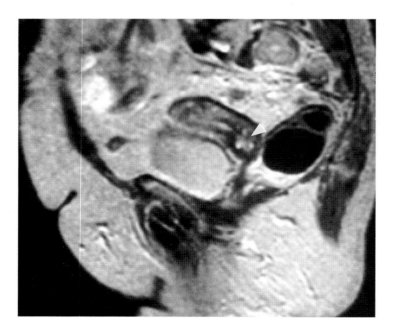

Figure 5.86

Carcinoma of the cervix stage I, sagittal T2-weighted image. In this postmenopausal patient, there is a small tumor mass (arrow) seen within the endocervix.

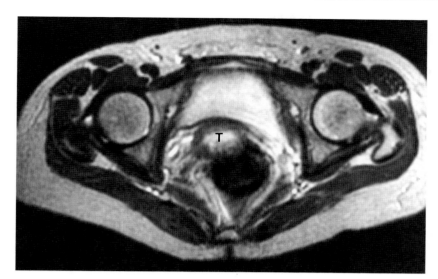

a

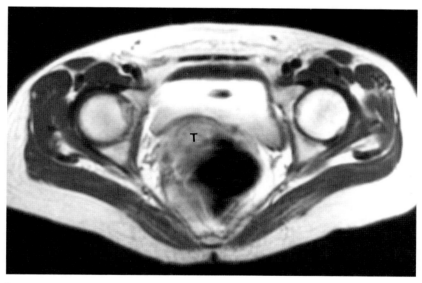

b

Figure 5.87

Carcinoma of the cervix stage I, (**a**) T2-weighted image, (**b**) gadolinium-enhanced T1-weighted image sagittal projection. Following Gd-DTPA injection, there is enhancement of the tumor (T) but tumor margins and depth of stromal invasion are better seen on the T2-weighted nonenhanced scan.

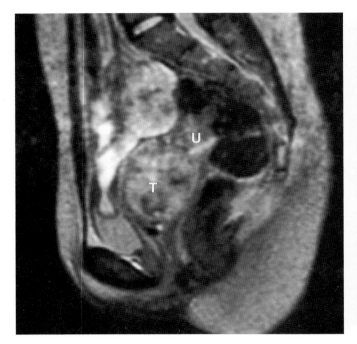

a

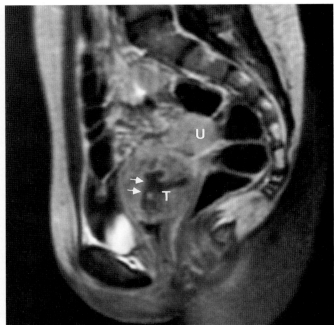

b

Figure 5.88

Carcinoma of the cervix stage IIa. Sagittal plane (**a**) T2-weighted image and (**b**) gadolinium-DTPA-enhanced T1-weighted image. A large cervical tumor (T) is of heterogeneous signal intensity on the T2-weighted image. Following Gd-DTPA injection, a large area of necrosis (arrows) is identified within the cervical tumor (T). (U)-corpus uterus.

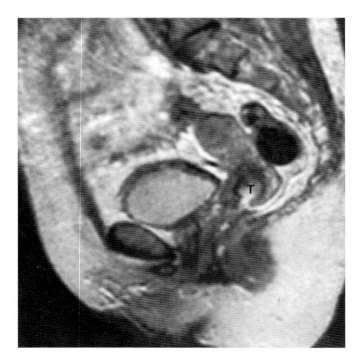

Figure 5.89

Carcinoma of the cervix stage I with partial invasion of the cervical stroma, T2-weighted image. The cervical tumor (T) is imaged with high signal intensity. The residual cervical stroma is seen as a low signal intensity stripe.

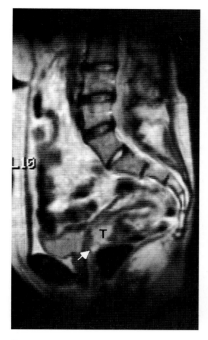

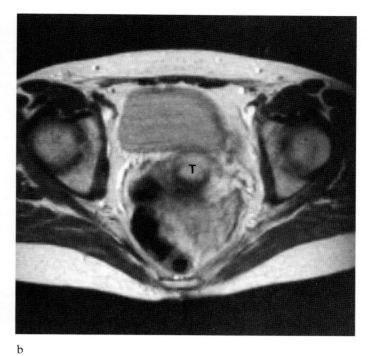

a   b

Figure 5.90

Carcinoma of the cervix stage
IIa invasion of the upper-third
of the vagina. T2-weighted (**a**)
sagittal and (**b**) transaxial
images demonstrating high
signal intensity tumor (T)
invading the anterior vaginal
fornix (arrow). (0.35T.)

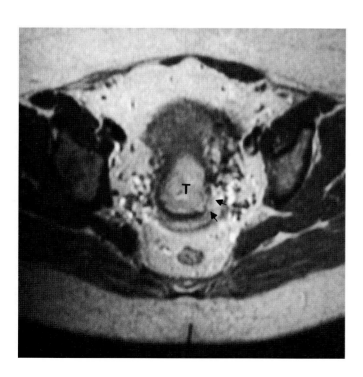

Figure 5.91

Carcinoma of the cervix stage
IIb transaxial T2-weighted
image. A large cervical tumor
(T) shows full thickness stromal
invasion along the left lateral
margin (arrows) with localized
parametrial extension.

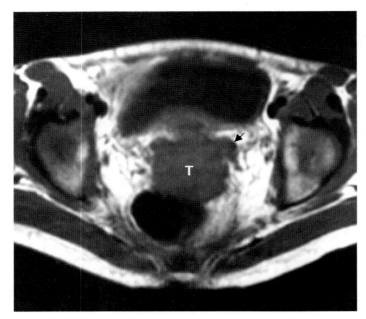

a

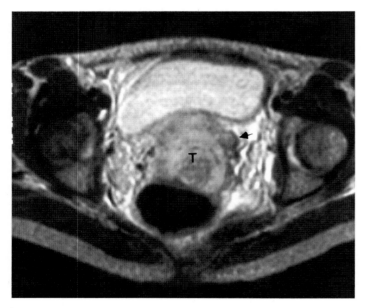

b

Figure 5.92

Carcinoma of the cervix stage IIb transaxial (**a**) T1-weighted and (**b**) T2-weighted images. A large cervical tumor (T) has diffuse and complete full stromal invasion as well as bilateral parametrial extension as seen by the enlargement and irregular margin of the parametria. In addition, there is a left parametrial node (arrow).

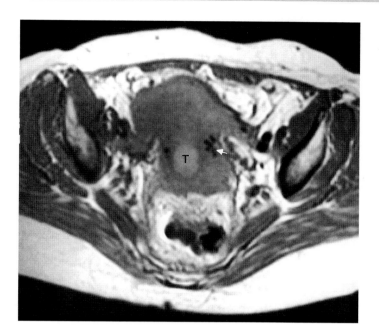

Figure 5.93

Carcinoma of the cervix stage IIb; transaxial proton density image. Parametrial extension is diagnosed by the tumor encasement of uterine vessels (arrow). (T)-cervical tumor.

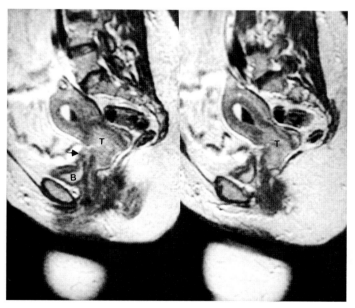

a   b

Figure 5.94

Carcinoma of the cervix stage IIb extension into the anterior uterovesical space. (a) and (b) are two consecutive sagittal T2-weighted images. The cervical tumor (T) is obstructing the internal os causing hematometra within the endometrial cavity. The tumor is extending into the anterior uterovesical space (anterior parametria) (arrow) but the wall of the urinary bladder (B) remains of low signal intensity indicating that it is not invaded.

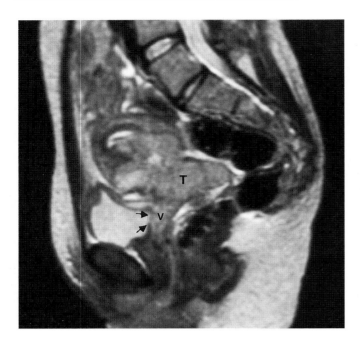

Figure 5.95

Carcinoma of the cervix stage IVa sagittal T2-weighted image. Large cervical tumor (T) is seen extending into the anterior uterovesical space and invading the wall of the urinary bladder (arrows). Bladder invasion is diagnosed by a localized interruption of the normal low signal intensity bladder wall (arrows). The tumor is also invading the vagina (v).

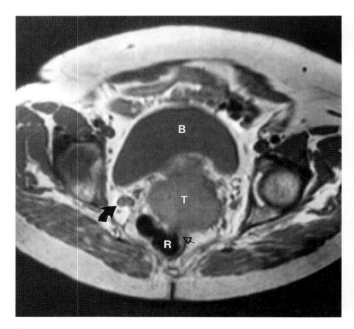

a

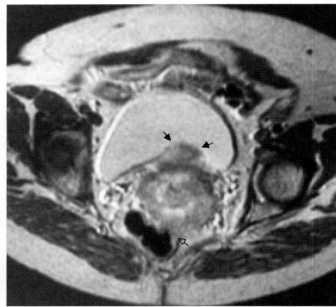

b

Figure 5.96

Carcinoma of the cervix stage IVa with invasion of the rectum, transaxial (**a**) T1- and (**b**) T2-weighted images. The large cervical tumor (T) demonstrates direct extension (open arrow) to the rectum (R). The urinary bladder (B) is also invaded (arrows). Also seen are enlarged obturator nodes (curved arrow).

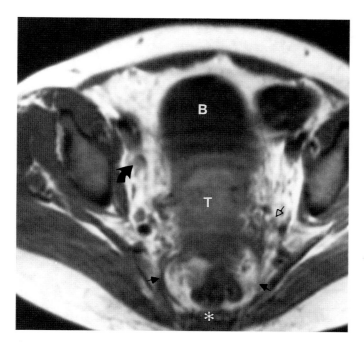

a

Figure 5.97

Carcinoma of the cervix stage IVb with invasion of the uterosacral ligament and tumor extension into the presacral region, (**a**) T1- and (**b**) T2-weighted images. Large tumor (T) shows full thickness stromal invasion and invasion of the parametria. Tumor encasement of the uterine vessels (arrow) is seen. Tumor is extending along the uterosacral ligaments (solid arrows) to the presacral region (asterisk). There is posterior external (curved arrow) and parametrial (open arrow) lymphadenopathy. (B)-urinary bladder. The air within the bladder is due to recent cystoscopy.

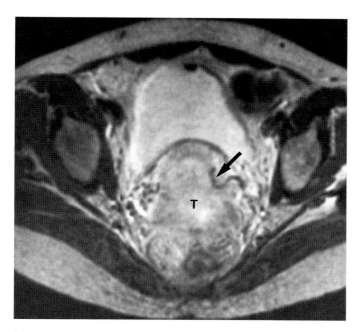

b

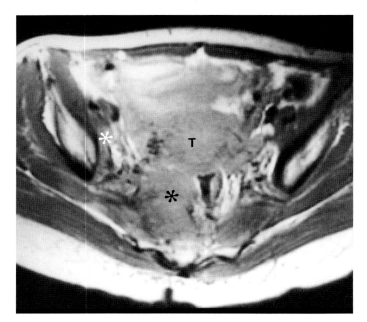

a

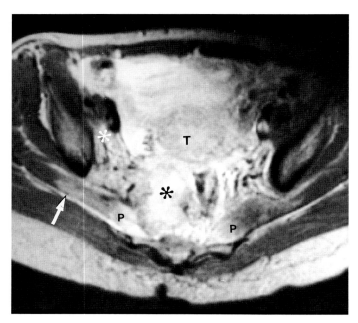

b

Figure 5.98

Carcinoma of the cervix stage IVb with invasion of the pelvic sidewall, transaxial (**a**) proton density and (**b**) T2-weighted images. The cervical tumor (T) shows direct extension to the pelvic sidewall (black asterisk). The tumor is invading both right and left piriformis muscles (p) as well as the right gluteus medius muscle on the right (arrow). There is also invasion of the lateral pelvic sidewall (white asterisks).

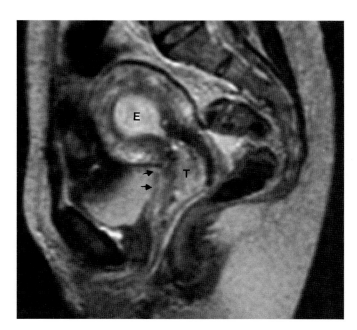

a

Figure 5.99

Carcinoma of the cervix stage IVa with invasion of the urinary bladder, sagittal plane (**a**) T2-weighted and (**b**) Gd-DTPA-enhanced T1-weighted image. Cervical tumor (T) with anterior invasion extending to the bladder wall (arrows). Following Gd-DTPA injection, the region of the tumor invasion (arrows) shows enhancement. An incidental finding is endometrial polyp (E). On Gd-DTPA-enhanced study, retained secretions within the vaginal fornices do not enhance (remain of low signal intensity) contrasting with the enhancing exocervix (open arrows) protruding into the vagina.

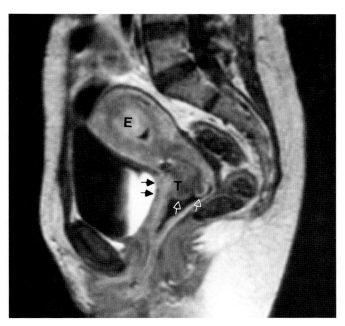

b

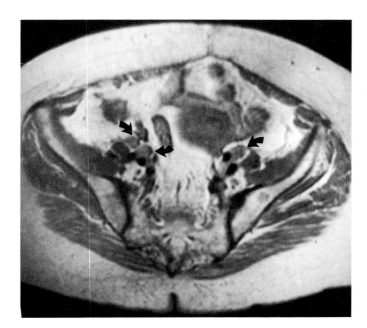

Figure 5.100

Lymphadenopathy in a patient with carcinoma of the cervix, transaxial proton density image. Bilateral enlarged lymph nodes are identified along the external iliac chain (curved arrows).

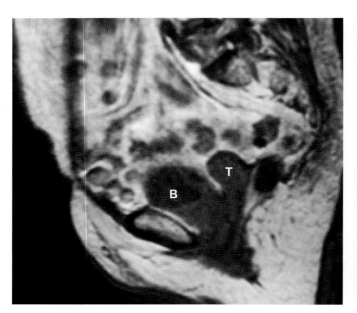

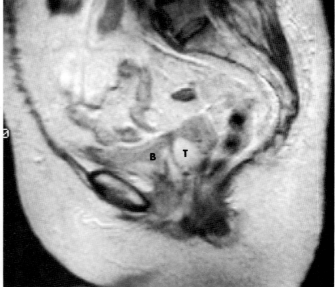

Figure 5.101

Recurrent cervical carcinoma in the vaginal cuff sagittal T1-weighted image. There is enlargement of and a bulbous appearance to the vaginal cuff indicating the presence of tumor (T). However, on the T1-weighted image, a definite diagnosis of tumor recurrence is not possible. (B)-urinary bladder.

Figure 5.102

Recurrence of cervical carcinoma in the vaginal cuff sagittal T2-weighted image. The enlargement of the vaginal cuff exhibits heterogeneous, mostly high signal intensity indicating tumor recurrence (T). Changes within the urinary bladder (B) are due to previous radiation therapy.

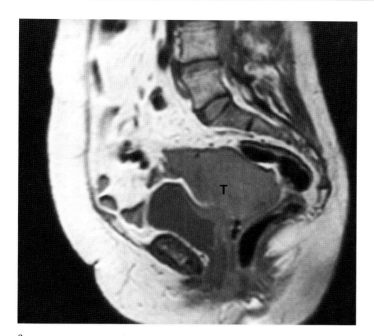

a

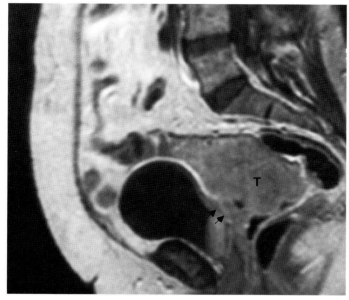

b

Figure 5.103

Recurrence of cervical carcinoma in the region of the vaginal cuff (**a**) T1-weighted image and (**b**) Gd-DTPA-enhanced T1-weighted image. There is large tumor recurrence (T) showing enhancement following gadolinium injection. The tumor recurrence involved the urinary bladder (arrows).

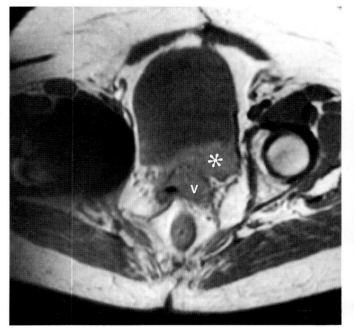

a

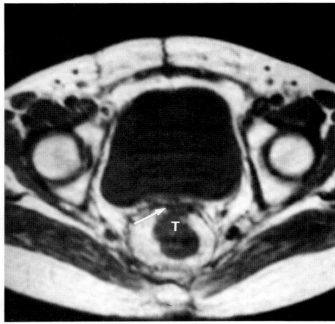

a

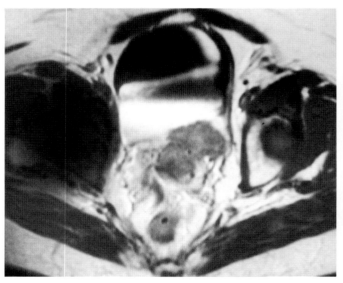

b

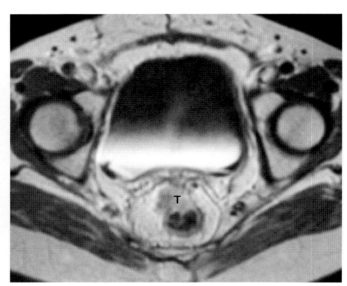

b

Figure 5.104

Recurrence of carcinoma of the cervix in the vagina with extension into the urinary bladder. Transaxial (**a**) T1-weighted and (**b**) Gd-DTPA-enhanced T1-weighted image. The vagina (v) is enlarged and there is tumor mass (asterisk) extending into the urinary bladder. Following gadolinium injection, there is heterogeneous enhancement of the recurrent tumor.

Figure 5.105

Cervical carcinoma tumor recurrence with tumor extension into the rectum. Transaxial (**a**) T1- and (**b**) Gd-DTPA-enhanced T1-weighted image. A small amount of abnormal tissue is seen in the vagina (arrow) and the largest part of the tumor recurrence (T) is invading the rectum. There is tumor enhancement following gadolinium injection.

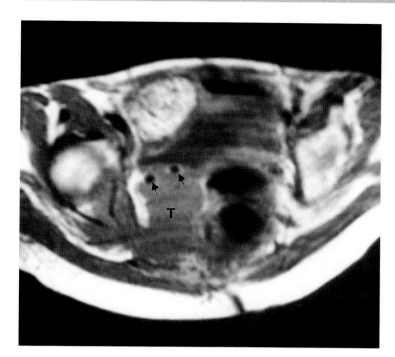

Figure 5.106

Tumor recurrence from carcinoma of the cervix is seen around surgical clips (arrows). The tumor recurrence (T) is extending towards the right lateral pelvic sidewall. Proton density transaxial image.

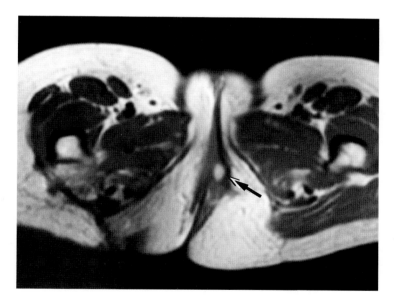

Figure 5.107

Bartholin's cyst transaxial T1-weighted image. A small cyst (arrow) is seen at the posterolateral aspect of the vagina. The diagnosis is made by the characteristic location of the cyst.

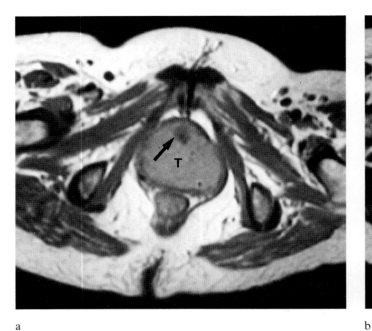

a

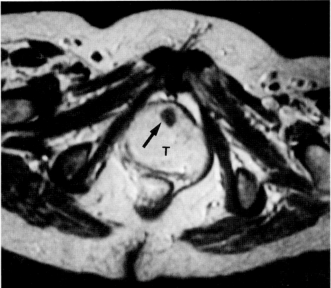

b

Figure 5.108

Carcinoma of the vagina (**a**) proton density and (**b**) T2-weighted transaxial images. The large vaginal tumor (T) is expanding the vagina, altering its contour and invading the urethra (arrow).

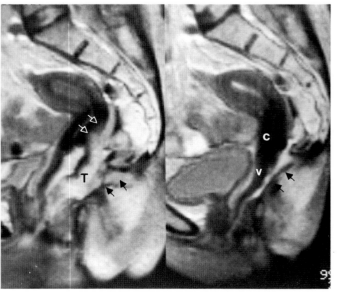

a   b

Figure 5.109

Carcinoma of the vagina sagittal T2-weighted image (**a**) at the time of diagnosis and (**b**) six months after radiation therapy. A large tumor (T) is seen expanding the vagina and invading the levator ani muscles (black arrows). The posterior cervical lip (white arrowhead) is also invaded. There is an excellent tumor response to radiation therapy, as six months following radiation therapy, the cervix, (c) vagina (v) and levator ani muscle are normal. (0.35T.)

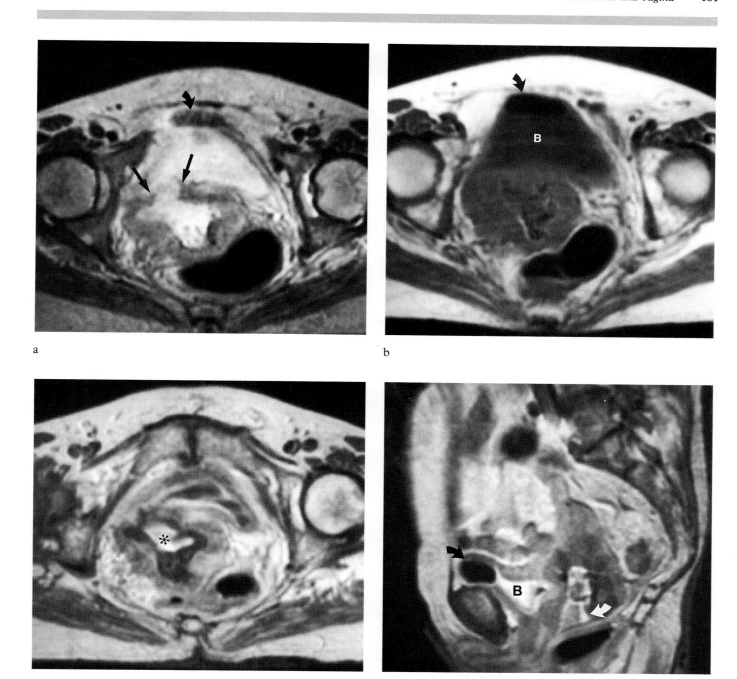

a

b

c

d

Figure 5.110

Carcinoma of the vagina with extension into the urinary bladder causing vesicovaginal fistula. Transaxial (**a**) T2-weighted image, (**b**) T1-weighted image, (**c**) gadolinium-enhanced T1-weighted image and (**d**) sagittal gadolinium-enhanced T1-weighted image. The necrotic tumor is extending into the urinary bladder causing a large vesicovaginal fistula (long arrows). The air (curved arrow) within the bladder (B) is a result of the fistula. On the T2-weighted image, the defect in the vagina and bladder wall can be seen. On the T1-weighted image, the large vaginal tumor is of heterogeneous low signal intensity. It is the gadolinium-enhanced image that confirms the diagnosis of the vesicovaginal fistula as the high signal intensity gadolinium-enhanced urine is seen extending from the urinary bladder to the vagina (asterisks) and can be seen on the sagittal film (white curved arrow).

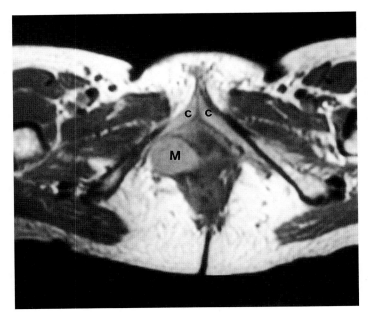

a

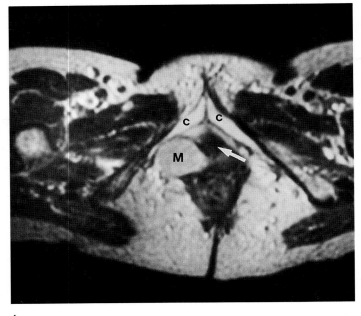

b

Figure 5.111

Endometrial carcinoma metastatic to the vagina, transaxial (**a**) proton density and (**b**) T2-weighted image. The large mass (M) is seen within the right lateral wall of the vagina. The urethra (arrow) is not invaded. (cc)-corpora cavernosa of the female.

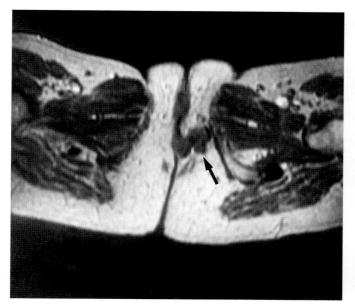

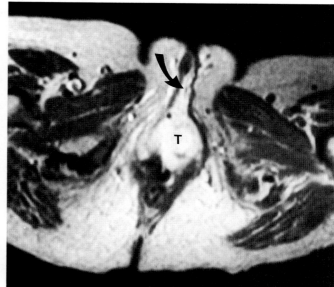

a

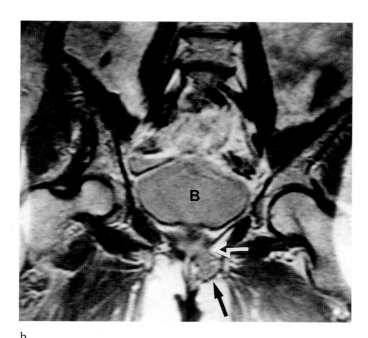

b

Figure 5.113

Carcinoma of the vulva with invasion of the clitoris, transaxial T2-weighted image. A large vulval tumor (T) is extending into the clitoris (curved arrow).

Figure 5.112

Carcinoma of the vulva (**a**) transaxial T1-weighted image and (**b**) coronal T2-weighted image. The tumor (black arrow) has an irregular margin and as depicted on the coronal T2-weighted image, invades the inferior part of the levator ani muscle (open white arrow). (B)-urinary bladder.

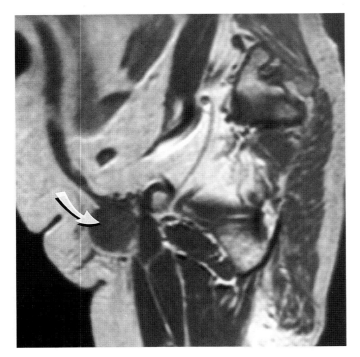

a

Figure 5.114
Left inguinal adenopathy
secondary to vulval carcinoma.
(**a**) sagittal proton density
image, (**b**) transaxial T1- and
(**c**) transaxial T2-weighted
image. A large left inguinal
node (curved arrow) on a T2-
weighted image shows marked
enhancement indicating
necrosis.

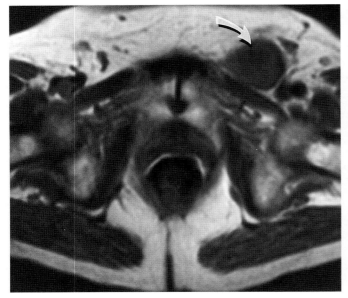

b

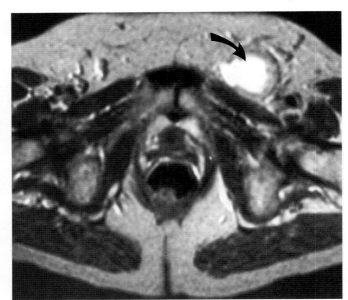

c

6

The Adnexae

Bernadette Carrington

The adnexae may be evaluated by any of the cross-sectional imaging modalities—ultrasound (US), computed tomography (CT) or magnetic resonance imaging (MRI). US is preferred for initial investigations, and CT and MRI are used in cases requiring further assessment. The large field-of-view, superior contrast resolution, and multiplanar facility offered by MRI are advantageous in the evaluation of adnexal lesions.

Normal anatomy of the adnexae

The ovaries develop from the gonadal primordia and migrate caudally from the thoracolumbar region to the pelvis by the end of the first year of life.[1] In the adult the ovaries lie in the **ovarian fossae**, which are lateral pelvic sidewall recesses situated between the obliterated umbilical artery anteriorly and the internal iliac artery and ureter posteriorly.[2] In nulliparous women the long axis of each ovary is vertical. In parous women, however, the position of the ovaries varies due to displacement during the first pregnancy. Ovarian position is also influenced by the filling of adjacent organs such as bladder and bowel.

The anatomy of the ovary is illustrated in Figure 6.1. Each ovary has tubal (superior) and uterine (inferior) extremities as well as lateral and medial surfaces and mesovarian and free borders.[2] The tubal extremity is enveloped by the fimbriae of the fallopian tube and the ovarian suspensory ligament is attached at this point. The uterine extremity is the site of attachment of the tubo-ovarian ligament. The lateral surface of the ovary is contiguous with the parietal peritoneum, which separates it from the obturator vessels and nerve. The medial surface is related to the fallopian tube. The mesovarian border faces anteriorly, towards the broad ligament, and the ovary is attached by a short fold of peritoneum called the **mesovarium.** The free border of the ovary is directed posteriorly, towards the ureter.

The appearance and physiology of the ovary vary with age. At birth the gland measures $1.5 \times 0.5 \times 0.3$ cm, weighs 0.3 gm, and is situated within the false pelvis. In the adolescent the ovary enlarges to reach adult proportions and attains its final position in the true pelvis. In the adult, each ovary is almond-shaped (amygdaloid), measures approximately $3 \times 1.5 \times 1$ cm, and weighs between 2 and 8 gm. After the menopause, the ovary becomes atrophic, measures less than 2 cm in diameter and weighs only 1–2 gm.

The neonatal ovary contains up to 750 000 primary ovarian follicles. No new follicles are made during life and many degenerate during childhood and after puberty. The adult ovary contains 70 000 follicles, and a few develop each month to become **graafian follicles.** One of the graafian follicles matures and releases an ovum at the time of ovulation. The outer cortex of the adult ovary therefore contains immature ovarian follicles, graafian follicles, and postovulatory corpora lutea which mark the site of prior graafian follicles. The adult ovary also has a highly vascular central medulla. After the menopause the ovary contains relatively few follicles and has increased amounts of fibrous tissue.

Ovarian ligaments

As illustrated in Figure 6.1, the **ovarian suspensory ligament** extends from the lateral pelvic wall to the tubal extremity of the ovary and contains the ovarian artery and vein. The **tubo-ovarian ligament** extends from the lateral uterine angle in a postero-inferior direction to the fallopian tube and attaches to the uterine extremity of the ovary.

Vascular supply

The ovary is supplied by the **ovarian artery**, which arises directly from the aorta, and by a small ovarian branch of the **uterine artery**. Each ovary has a venous **pampiniform plexus**, which drains to the ipsilateral **ovarian vein.** The ovarian veins drain to the inferior vena cava on the right side and to the left renal vein on the left side.

Lymphatic drainage

The lymphatic drainage of the ovary is via the **lateral aortic** and **preaortic lymph nodes.**

MRI appearance

On MRI scans normal ovaries can be identified in 85 per cent of women of reproductive age, and measurements ranging from 1.5 to 3 cm have been reported.[3] As shown in Figure 6.2, the ovaries are seen as low or medium signal intensity structures on T1-weighted images, and they increase in signal intensity on T2-weighted images.[3] Occasionally a low signal intensity rim, which may correspond to the fibrous cortical stroma, is seen on T2-weighted images. Although the small vessels around the ovaries help to identify them, distinction from uterus or bowel may be difficult on T1-weighted images, and distinction from fat may be difficult on T2-weighted images. The use of oral MR gastrointestinal contrast agents facilitates visualization of the ovaries, and, as seen in Figure 6.2c, gadolinium-DTPA administration causes enhancement of ovarian tissue and permits recognition of small follicular cysts which do not enhance.[4]

Recommended imaging sequences

It is necessary to use both T1- and T2-weighted spin-echo sequences to identify and evaluate the ovaries. The transverse plane of imaging permits demonstration of the ovaries, particularly if contiguous sections are used. Both the transverse and coronal planes are considered optimal for identification of the ovaries and

for confirmation that a mass originates in the adnexa rather than the uterus.[3,5] The ovaries may also be well visualized on more lateral sagittal sections (Figure 6.3).

The identification of an adnexal mass necessitates evaluation of the upper urinary tract for evidence of renal obstruction. This may be achieved by including the renal area on one imaging sequence or arranging for a separate renal evaluation by sonography.

Adnexal pathology

Tubo-ovarian abscess

A tubo-ovarian abscess is a potential complication of pelvic inflammatory disease (PID). Acute PID occurs in approximately 500 000 women per year in the United States. Use of an intrauterine contraceptive device is a recognized risk factor.[6] In up to 50 per cent of cases the organisms responsible are sexually transmitted **Neisseria gonorrhoeae** or **Chlamydia trachomatis.** Cervicovaginal bacteria such as **Bacteroides fragilis** and anaerobic gram-positive cocci may also cause PID.[7]

Patients present with a history of abdominal pain and tenderness. Recent onset of vaginal discharge or abnormal menstrual bleeding may occur. Pelvic examination discloses bilateral adnexal tenderness which is exacerbated by cervical motion. A palpable fluctuant adnexal mass suggests a tubo-ovarian abscess, which is treated by surgical drainage and antibiotic therapy. PID patients are at greater risk of tubal blockage and hydrosalpinx (see below), and resultant infertility.

MRI appearance

On MRI scans a tubo-ovarian abscess is identified as an adnexal fluid collection with a thickened, irregular wall which incorporates the inflamed ovarian tissue. The signal characteristics of the fluid depend on its protein content and on the presence or absence of hemorrhage. As depicted in Figure 6.4, an abscess uncomplicated by bleeding typically demonstrates low or medium signal intensity on T1-weighted images and high signal intensity on T2-weighted images. Edema and inflammatory infiltration often give the adjacent fat a heterogeneous appearance. If the abscess remains untreated, or is resistent to antibiotic therapy, chronic inflammation may induce a hypervascular state which manifests as an increase in the number of visualized pelvic blood vessels (Figure 6.4). After intravenous gadolinium-DTPA administration the wall of a tubo-ovarian abscess enhances (Figure 6.4d).

MRI in relation to other imaging modalities

The diagnosis of PID is based on history and examination with appropriate bacteriological confirmation. When a complication such as tubo-ovarian abscess is suspected, sonography is the imaging modality of choice. MRI is reserved for those situations where ultrasound diagnosis is difficult due to patient size or the presence of co-existing pathology. MRI may also be used to determine the size and relations of any residual abscess collection in patients who do not respond to initial treatment. This information is helpful in deciding whether further surgical intervention is necessary.

Endometriosis

Endometriosis is defined as the presence of heterotopic secretory endometrium in ectopic locations. It is found in up to 15 per cent of women undergoing laparotomy, and in infertile women its incidence increases to 30–45 per cent. There is also an increased incidence in patients with müllerian duct anomalies, particularly when there is obstructed uterine drainage. The most common sites for endometriosis are the ovaries, which are involved in two-thirds of patients, usually bilaterally.[8] Internal hemorrhage within an area of endometriosis produces ovarian endometrial cysts (**endometriomas**) which predispose to endometrial malignancy, either clear cell carcinoma, endometrioid carcinoma, or mixed müllerian sarcoma. Other sites for endometriotic deposits are the peritoneum, cul-de-sac, vesicouterine pouch, and rectosigmoid colon.[8] The regional lymph nodes are involved in up to 30 per cent of patients and the uterine ligaments may also be involved.

Endometriosis is staged laparoscopically according to a point system based on the presence, size, and location of ovarian endometrial implants; the presence and severity of ovarian and tubal adhesions; and whether or not the cul-de-sac has been obliterated.[9]

Patients usually present with dysmenorrhea and other symptoms are related to the involvement of a particular pelvic organ. Severity of symptoms does not correlate with the extent of disease. Some patients with extensive disease are asymptomatic, and others, with relatively small endometriotic deposits, suffer disabling pelvic pain. Medical treatment of endometriosis includes the use of androgen-like drugs such as danazol. In cases of intractable pain, surgery may be necessary.

MRI appearance

On MRI scans endometriosis produces three distinct lesions: ovarian endometriomas, endometrial implants, or adhesions.

Endometriomas Endometriomas have a characteristic MR appearance (Figure 6.5). They are typically multiloculated and thin-walled, with an indistinct interface with adjacent organs due to adhesions (see below). They also demonstrate variable signal intensity on spin-echo sequences. On T1-weighted scans they may be of homogeneous high signal intensity or they may be more heterogeneous in appearance, but at least one loculus usually demonstrates some high signal intensity on a short TR/TE sequence.[10] On T2-weighted scans they are more likely to be heterogeneous in appearance, with low signal intensity (shading) within loculi, as seen in Figure 6.6. When loculi contain hemorrhagic fluid they image with high signal intensity on both T1- and T2-weighted images.[10,11] A hematocrit effect, which occurs when high signal intensity layering is seen in the dependent portion of the endometrioma, has also been described on T1-weighted images.[12]

After intravenous gadolinium-DTPA administration the wall of an endometrioma may demonstrate rim enhancement (Figure 6.7). Enhancing areas of nodularity or papillary excrescences within the wall may indicate neoplastic change within the endometrioma, as shown in Figure 6.8.

Endometrial implants Endometrial implants may be extra- or intraperitoneal in location. **Extraperitoneal implants** may occur on the ovary, bladder (Figure 6.9), or rectum. Implants may also be found in the vagina (Figures 6.10 and 6.11). They are typically small round lesions which image with medium signal intensity on T1-weighted images and high signal intensity on T2-weighted images, similar to normal endometrium.[11] However, the signal characteristics of the implants are altered by hormonal therapy which may induce hemorrhage. As illustrated in Figure 6.11, lesions may then demonstrate high signal intensity on both T1- and T2-weighted scans.

The signal characteristics of **intraperitoneal endometrial implants** are similar to those of extraperitoneal implants, although, in general, intraperitoneal disease is more difficult to detect on MRI than extraperitoneal deposits or endometriomas.[11] Intraperitoneal implants are most readily identified on the uterine serosal surface, or in the cul-de-sac (Figure 6.11c–e).

Adhesions Adhesions are identified on MRI when a clear interface cannot be demonstrated between an endometrioma and adjacent organs.[10,11] Examples of adhesions are shown in Figures 6.5 and 6.12. Angulation and fixation of bowel loops (Figure 6.12) may also indicate adhesions. Occasionally adherent fluid-filled bowel loops can mimic endometriosis, as seen in Figure 6.13.

MRI in relation to other imaging modalities

Although it is possible to identify endometriomas with US and CT, these modalities have very poor sensitivity in detecting more diffuse forms of endometriosis.[13,14] MRI is the most sensitive (65–70 per cent) imaging modality for the diagnosis of endometriosis, with a specificity ranging from 60 to 80 per cent.[11,15] It is possible to identify endometriomas, ovarian adhesions, and some extraperitoneal endometrial implants on MRI scans, but extraovarian adhesions and intraperitoneal implants cannot be demonstrated reliably.[11] This precludes the use of MRI as a primary staging modality for endometriosis, and laparoscopy remains the procedure of choice. MRI is valuable for assessing areas which are inaccessible to laparoscopy, either due to the presence of multiple adhesions or the extraperitoneal location of disease.[11,15]

Ovarian cysts

Differentiation between benign and malignant ovarian cysts

The characterization of ovarian cystic lesions is a recurrent clinical and radiologic problem. There are surgical and pathologic criteria to differentiate between benign and malignant cysts and to identify borderline malignant lesions.[16] Sonographic and CT criteria have also been developed, which can be used to distinguish simple benign cysts from more complex lesions. These include a well-defined, smooth outline to the cyst, a thin wall; anechoic cyst contents on US or cyst contents of uniform low density on CT; and few or no loculations within the cyst.[17–21]

Similar guidelines may be applied to the MR interpretation of cystic ovarian masses. Table 6.1 summarizes the typical features of benign and malignant ovarian cysts. It has been demonstrated that the most important MR criteria for differentiating a benign from a malignant cyst are: (1) whether the lesion is entirely cystic or has solid components; (2) the thickness of its wall; (3) the presence of vegetations or nodularity arising from the wall; and (4) the identification of necrosis or hemorrhage within the cyst.[22] Secondary criteria which may further aid in differentiation include: (1) the presence of ascites; (2)

Table 6.1   Guidelines for the MR interpretation of ovarian lesions[22,23]

Characteristic	Benign	Malignant
Size	Usually less than 4 cm	Often greater than 4 cm
Definition	Well defined	Indistinct margin
Nature	Cystic	Solid or mixed solid/cystic
Wall thickness	Less than 3 mm	Greater than 3 mm
Vegetations or nodularity	Usually absent	Present
Septations	Absent or few	Multiple
Necrosis	Absent	May be present
Ascites	Absent	May be present
Lymphadenopathy	Absent	May be present
Involvement of other pelvic organs or sidewall	Absent	May be present

lymphadenopathy; (3) peritoneal, mesenteric, or omental disease; and (4) evidence of involvement of pelvic organs or the pelvic sidewall.[22] Using the primary criteria it is possible to characterize approximately 80 per cent of lesions as benign or malignant. When all criteria are included in the analysis the accuracy rate increases to 95 per cent.[22] Other factors to be considered are lesion size and definition, and the presence of internal septations.[23]

Benign ovarian cystic disease

Benign ovarian cysts are typically well defined with a thin wall. Their content depends on their etiology and varies from serous to highly proteinaceous fluid or blood. Benign cystic ovarian disease includes follicular cysts, simple cysts, cystadenomas, dermoids, polycystic ovarian disease, and endometriomas (discussed above).

Follicular cysts   Follicular cysts are the result of failure of ovulation with continued growth of the follicle. They may be multiple and bilateral. Although they are usually asymptomatic, follicular cysts may undergo spontaneous rupture and, rarely, torsion, with subsequent infarction.

MRI appearance   As demonstrated in Figure 6.14, follicular cysts are smooth-walled lesions, usually less than 3 cm. Typically they image with low signal intensity on T1-weighted scans and high signal intensity on T2-weighted scans. Since the protein content of the cysts is hormone dependent, however, the relative signal intensity varies as a result of hormonal changes during the menstrual cycle.

After intravenous Gd-DTPA administration the ovary is enhanced, increasing the contrast between solid ovarian tissue and the fluid content of the follicular cysts. Therefore, the number of cysts visualized may increase after Gd-DTPA enhancement.

Simple cysts A simple ovarian cyst, probably derived from follicular cells, has no identifiable lining. In practice, the category of simple cysts often includes any unilocular cyst filled with serous fluid, including functional cysts and cystadenomas.

MRI appearance Simple cysts are well circumscribed, thin-walled lesions which are unilocular and less than 5 cm in diameter. As shown in Figure 6.15, they image with homogeneous signal intensity which is low on T1-weighted images and rises on T2-weighted images. The fluid content is usually isointense or slightly hyperintense relative to urine.[5] Occasionally, simple cysts undergo hemorrhage, in which case the contents show variable signal intensity on T1- and T2-weighted images, depending on the age of the hemorrhage. A common finding is high signal intensity on both T1- and T2-weighted sequences. Figure 6.16 illustrates the hematocrit layering effect, which occurs when high signal intensity blood products collect in the dependent portion of the cyst. The appearance of a hemorrhagic simple cyst may therefore mimic an endometrioma.

Cystadenomas Cystadenomas, which can be divided into serous and mucinous subtypes, account for 25 per cent of all benign ovarian neoplasms and are seen primarily in women of reproductive age.[24] They are bilateral in 15 per cent of patients. Mucinous cystadenomas comprise 15 per cent of all benign ovarian tumors and 5 per cent of these are bilateral. They are often found in association with dermoid cysts.[24] Both serous and mucinous cystadenomas may develop papillary excrescences.

MRI appearance Cystadenomas are multiloculated, thin-walled lesions with a smooth outer surface. Their fluid content is of variable signal intensity on T1- and T2-weighted images, depending on whether it consists of serous fluid or mucin, and whether secondary hemorrhage has occurred. Layering may be observed within the cyst (Figure 6.17). Occasionally, papillary growth is identified as a localized thickening of the cyst wall which enhances after Gd-DTPA administration.

Dermoids (benign cystic teratomas) Dermoids account for 10–25 per cent of all ovarian neoplasms. Fifty per cent of dermoids are diagnosed in women between the third and fifth decades but there is a wide age distribution and they may be found at any age. In fact dermoids are the most common ovarian neoplasms of childhood.[24]

Dermoid cysts are lined partially or completely by squamous epithelium. A **Rokitansky nodule** or **dermoid plug** arises from the tumor wall and contains mature, well differentiated tissue such as teeth, hair, and fat.[25]

In 25 per cent of cases, patients are asymptomatic and the dermoid is discovered on routine pelvic examination. Some patients experience abdominal discomfort or notice abdominal fullness. Torsion occurs in 10 per cent of cases, causing abdominal pain. Occasionally the dermoid ruptures, leading to granulomatous peritonitis. A small percentage (1–2 per cent) of dermoids become malignant. The risk of malignancy is increased when a dermoid is greater than 10 cm in size and occurs in a postmenopausal patient. The treatment of choice for an uncomplicated dermoid is oophorectomy. However, in younger patients it may be feasible to excise the tumor with preservation of the residual normal ovarian tissue.

MRI appearance Figure 6.18 illustrates the MRI appearance of bilateral dermoid tumors. Dermoids are well defined lesions with a heterogeneous appearance, reflecting their varying contents. The majority of dermoids contain components which are isointense with fat.[3,5,26] Fluid/fluid levels may be seen due to layering of hemorrhagic fluid, or there may be a fat/fluid level which is confirmed by the presence of a chemical shift artifact at the interface between the two layers (Figure 6.19).

Rokitansky nodules are usually oval or round with a regular border and may be identified within the dermoid. The signal intensity of Rokitansky nodules varies depending on their tissue content. Where there is fibrous tissue, calcification, or bone the nodule is of low signal intensity on both T1- and T2-weighted images. Fat within nodules images as high signal intensity on both T1- and T2-weighted sequences. Rokitansky nodules are depicted in Figures 6.18 and 6.20.

Polycystic disease Polycystic ovaries are a component of the **Stein–Leventhal syndrome**, which is also associated with infertility, oligomenorrhea or amenorrhea, and hirsutism. The etiology of the condition is complex, but involves failure of the normal cyclical changes in follicle-stimulating hormone (FSH) and luteinizing hormone (LH) with a persistently elevated LH/FSH level. This results in chronically stimulated but unruptured follicles, which are found in the subcapsular region of the ovaries.[27] There is also an increase in the ovarian fibrous stroma and hypertrophy of the capsule.[28]

MRI appearance Polycystic ovaries are always bilateral and each ovary measures between 3 and 5 cm and demonstrates multiple peripheral cysts. The cysts are of low signal intensity on T1-weighted images and high signal intensity on T2-weighted images.[29] The central ovarian tissue is of low signal intensity on both T1- and T2-weighted images (Figure 6.21), which corresponds to the histological change of an increase in the medullary cellular stroma.[29] In addition, the uterus is often hypoplastic, although normal zonal anatomy is preserved on T2-weighted images.

MRI in relation to other imaging modalities

Ultrasound remains the procedure of choice for assessing cystic adnexal masses and has been shown to have a high sensitivity (84 per cent) for their detection. CT may be performed when the ultrasound examination is degraded due to bowel gas or obesity, and it may be diagnostic in certain cases, for example dermoid cysts.[30] However, the contrast resolution of both US and CT is limited and they may not be able to identify the etiology or tissue characteristics of such masses. As demonstrated in Figure 6.22, MRI can be utilized to identify the origin of an indeterminant mass, to differentiate between cysts and other adnexal lesions, and to determine the relationship of adnexal lesions to the adjacent organs. The ability of MRI to provide information about the nature of the fluid content of ovarian cysts may be valuable in some cases. MRI has also been demonstrated to be superior to ultrasound in the demonstration of polycystic ovarian disease.[29] MRI is thus recommended as a problem-solving modality in the evaluation of cystic ovarian lesions.

Benign solid ovarian disease (fibroma-thecoma tumors)

Ovarian fibroma-thecoma tumors develop from ovarian stromal cells and have a spectrum of histological findings ranging from a purely fibroblastic appearance to a lipid-rich thecal tumor. Fibromas are hormonally inert tumors composed of fibroblasts interspersed with collagen fibres.[24] They are typically unilateral and benign. Fibromas account for 1–5 per cent of all ovarian tumors and occur in postmenopausal women. In one-third of patients fibromas are found in association with ascites. They may occur in conjunction with a right hydrothorax (**Meigs' syndrome**), but this is rare and is seen in less than 1 per cent of cases.[24]

MRI appearance

Ovarian fibromas are well defined, solid adnexal masses which demonstrate medium to low signal intensity on T1-weighted images and low signal intensity on T2-weighted images. They resemble nondegenerative leiomyomata (see Chapter 5), and differentiation between the two may be difficult if a fibroma is situated immediately adjacent to the uterus. Fibromas show no evidence of enhancement after Gd-DTPA administration, as seen in Figures 6.17 and 5.63.

MRI in relation to other imaging modalities

Although ovarian fibromas can be identified on both US and CT, neither modality has the ability to characterize the lesion. With MRI it is possible to confirm that an adnexal lesion represents a fibroma.

Malignant ovarian tumors

Ovarian carcinoma

There are 19 000 new cases of ovarian carcinoma per year in the United States. It is most likely to occur in women in their fifth to seventh decades, and is the most frequent fatal gynecological malignancy, accounting for 11 600 deaths per year.[31] Several predisposing factors are recognized including: lower parity; delayed onset of child-bearing; infertility; and a family history of malignancy. It is also more likely to occur in Caucasian women of both European and North American origin. Women taking oral contraceptives are at lower risk of developing ovarian carcinoma, and this is thought to relate to the reduced frequency of ovulation.

Tumors may originate from the surface coelomic epithelium, germ cells, or stroma; and they are classified according to the cell of origin with the ovary. Of these tumors, 85–90 per cent are of epithelial origin and are either (1) **serous cystadenocarcinoma** (42 per cent); (2) **mucinous cystadenocarcinoma** (12 per cent); (3) **endometrioid carcinoma** (15 per cent); (4)

undifferentiated carcinoma (17 per cent); or (5) **clear cell carcinoma** (6 per cent).[32] Germ-cell tumors are predominantly **dysgerminomas, endodermal sinus tumors**, or **embryonal carcinoma**. Of the stromal tumors, only **granulosa cell tumors** are encountered with any significant frequency.[31]

Epithelial ovarian tumors spread by surface shedding of malignant cells, lymphatic dissemination, and, rarely, by hematogenous spread. Involvement of the contralateral ovary and uterus occurs in a significant number of patients with otherwise early stage disease.

As the tumor grows, it may directly infiltrate the pelvic peritoneum. Intraperitoneal dissemination of malignant cells leads to the formation of metastatic peritoneal implants. Tumor cells circulating in the peritoneal fluid then drain into lymphatic channels located in the diaphragm. Because of respiration, there is preferential flow of peritoneal fluid along the paracolic gutters to the right hemidiaphragm, and 80 per cent of all peritoneal fluid drains to the right hemidiaphragmatic lymphatic capillaries.[32] Subdiaphragmatic tumor deposits are, therefore, more commonly identified on the right side. Eventually, malignant obstruction of the diaphragmatic lymphatics occurs, and exfoliated malignant cells implant on the omentum and serosal peritoneum.

Lymphatic dissemination of ovarian tumors is primarily to the lateral aortic and preaortic lymph nodes. Secondary dissemination to the external and internal iliac nodes may occur via an infiltrated broad ligament, and the external iliac and inguinal nodes may be affected if the round ligament of the uterus is involved.[31] Distant metastases are found most frequently in the liver, lung, or pleura.

Clinical staging of ovarian carcinoma is accomplished at laparotomy, using the FIGO staging system summarized in Table 6.2. At the staging laparotomy, the surgeon performs a bilateral salpingo-oophorectomy, a hysterectomy, and an omentectomy. The peritoneal cavity is then carefully explored for peritoneal implants, with particular attention paid to the undersurfaces of the hemidiaphragms. In addition, multiple peritoneal and lymph node biopsies are performed.

Ovarian carcinoma is noted for its lack of clinical symptoms until the disease is relatively advanced. The most common complaints are abdominal discomfort or pain, an increase in abdominal girth, and vaginal bleeding. Patients may present with a pelvic mass or ascites. As mentioned above, the initial treatment for ovarian carcinoma is surgical, a total abdominal hysterectomy, and bilateral salpingo-oophorectomy and omentectomy performed at the staging laparotomy. If complete surgical removal of the tumor is not possible, then tumor debulking (cytoreduction) is undertaken. The aim of cytoreduction is to reduce the size of residual tumor deposits to less than 2 cm in

Table 6.2 Clinical FIGO staging and TNM classification of ovarian cancer

FIGO	TNM	System description *T-primary tumor*
	TX	Primary tumor cannot be assessed
	T0	No evidence of primary tumor
	Tis	Carcinoma in situ
I	T1	Tumor limited to ovaries
Ia	T1a	Tumor limited to one ovary; capsule intact, no tumor on ovarian surface
Ib	T1b	Tumor limited to both ovaries; capsules intact, no tumor on ovarian surface
Ic	T1c	Tumor limited to one or both ovaries with any of the following: capsule ruptured, tumor on ovarian surface, malignant cells in ascites or peritoneal washings
II	T2	Tumor involves one or both ovaries with pelvic extension
IIa	T2a	Extension and/or implants on uterus and/or tube(s)
IIb	T2b	Extension to other pelvic tissues
IIc	T2c	Pelvic extension (2a or 2b) with malignant cells in ascites or peritoneal washings
III	T3 and or N1	Tumor involves one or both ovaries with microscopically confirmed peritoneal metastasis outside the pelvis and/or regional lymph node metastasis
IIIa	T3b	Microscopic peritoneal metastasis beyond pelvis
IIIb	T3b	Macroscopic peritoneal metastasis beyond pelvis, 2 cm or less in greatest dimension
IIIc	T3c and or N1	Peritoneal metastasis beyond pelvis more than 2 cm in greatest dimension and/or regional lymph node metastasis
IV	M1	Distant metastasis (excludes peritoneal metastasis)

TNM = Tumor, node, metastasis
FIGO = International Federation of Gynecology and Obstetrics

diameter, thereby maximizing the effect of chemotherapy or radiotherapy. In patients who are clinically and radiologically disease-free following chemotherapy and/or radiotherapy, a second look laparotomy is performed to identify clinically unsuspected residual disease and to remove it where possible. Patients with residual tumor are considered for further chemotherapy.

Prognostic indicators in ovarian cancer include: (1) the presence of residual tumor deposits after the initial surgery; (2) tumor grade (degree of cellular differentiation); (3) FIGO stage; (4) patient age; and (5) histologic tumor subtype.[31] The most important of these are residual disease and tumor grade. Overall survival of patients with microscopic or no residual disease and early stage tumors is approximately 80 per cent. Patients with high-grade, high-stage tumors and bulky residual disease have a 5-year survival rate of approximately 10 per cent.

MRI appearance   On MRI images ovarian carcinoma is visualized as a solid or mixed solid and cystic lesion. As depicted in Figures 6.23 and 6.24, tumors are of medium signal intensity on T1-weighted images and of heterogeneous high signal intensity on T2-weighted images. Enhancement of ovarian cancers after Gd-DTPA administration facilitates appreciation of tumor necrosis and identification of the solid or cystic components within the lesion (Figure 6.25). Hemorrhage or multiple loculations within lesions can be identified on MRI scans, and an accurate estimation of the thickness of the tumor capsule can be made.

MRI staging   MRI facilitates assessment of spread of ovarian tumors to the uterus (Figures 6.23 and 6.25), bladder, rectum, and pelvic sidewall. An **omental cake**, demonstrated in Figures 6.26 and 6.27, can also be readily identified on MRI scans. Omental disease shows significant enhancement after Gd-DTPA administration. In some cases, as shown in Figure 6.27, peritoneal implants may be appreciated on MRI images. Although implants are enhanced after the administration of Gd-DTPA, somewhat improving detection rates, interference from peristaltic artifacts and the lack of available oral gastrointestinal contrast agents limit the usefulness of MRI for peritoneal implant identification.

Ascites (Figures 6.25, 6.26, and 6.27) and pelvic and retroperitoneal lymphadenopathy can also be identified on MRI scans.[33] However, MRI does rely on nodal enlargement as the sole criterion for malignant involvement of lymph nodes.

MRI in relation to other imaging modalities   The role of radiology in the staging of ovarian cancer is controversial, and staging laparotomy with identification of histologic type and pathologic grade remains the standard method. Imaging techniques have proved to be of value in assessing patients in whom staging information is suboptimal because of inadequate initial surgical exploration. Imaging may also be required for staging in patients considered unfit for surgery.

In patients with residual disease, radiologic evaluation can provide a baseline for evaluating the efficacy of chemotherapy, without the need for second-look laparotomy. Imaging may also help identify those patients with residual disease after chemotherapy whose tumor is amenable to curative resection.

Currently CT remains the imaging technique of choice in the assessment of ovarian carcinoma because of its proven ability to detect peritoneal and bowel implants.[34] CT is of particular value in identifying intrahepatic metastases which may not be detected by palpation at laparotomy.[35] Ascites is also identifiable on CT scans, as is lymphadenopathy.

Ultrasound cannot reliably identify peritoneal disease, and its inferior contrast resolution precludes reliable evaluation of the extent of tumor spread within the pelvis.

The role of MRI in ovarian cancer remains to be evaluated. MRI has some advantage in the assessment of tumor involvement of pelvic organs because of its superior contrast resolution and multiplanar imaging capability. The detection rates of MR and CT are approximately equal in the identification of pelvic and retroperitoneal lymphadenopathy.[33] The MRI detection of peritoneal implants is limited at present, but the use of gastrointestinal contrast agents and intravenous Gd-DTPA may prove useful in this regard. However, the accurate delineation of intra-abdominal tumor extent necessitates imaging the liver and diaphragmatic regions and this adds considerably to the total examination time required.

Granulosa cell tumors

Granulosa cell tumors (neoplasms of the ovarian stromal cell line) account for approximately 2 per cent of all ovarian tumors. Half are found in postmenopausal women, and 5 per cent occur in prepubertal girls. Granulosa cell neoplasms may produce estrogen, causing clinical symptoms of sexual precocity in children, menorrhagia or irregular bleeding in women of reproductive age, and the resumption of menses in postmenopausal women. Over half of the patients with granulosa cell tumors develop endometrial hyperplasia or polyps due to increased levels of estrogen. There is also a recognized association between granulosa cell tumors and endometrial carcinoma, which occurs in 5–15 per cent of patients in the postmenopausal age group. In 1–3 per cent of cases granulosa cell tumors produce androgens, sometimes causing patients to develop clinical features of virilization. Granulosa cell tumors are liable to rupture, particularly in pregnancy or labor, and may be responsible for severe intra-abdominal bleeding in up to 15 per cent of patients.[36]

Staging for granulosa cell tumors is the same as that for epithelial ovarian cancers. In unilateral stage Ia disease, treatment is by unilateral salpingo-oophorectomy. More advanced disease confined to the ovaries is treated by bilateral salpingo-oophorectomy. In disseminated intra-abdominal disease treatment involves tumor debulking with postoperative adjuvant radiotherapy.[36] Hysterectomy is usually performed in older patients because of the risk of endometrial carcinoma.[36]

Granulosa cell tumors have a propensity to recur locally as late as ten years after removal. Since they are not chemosensitive, treatment is by radiotherapy with or without further tumor debulking.

MRI appearance Granulosa cell tumors are solid lobulated adnexal lesions (Figures 6.28 and 6.29). They are of medium signal intensity on T1-weighted images and heterogeneous high signal intensity on T2-weighted images. Granulosa cell tumors enhance after administration of intravenous Gd-DTPA, as shown in Figure 6.29, and small foci of necrosis are readily identified within the tumor. As with epithelial ovarian cancers, dissemination occurs by intraperitoneal seeding, and there may be adherence to and involvement of adjacent bowel loops (Figure 6.28). Ascites is often associated with more advanced disease.

Granulosa cell tumors are locally invasive and can involve any pelvic organ. Large tumors can directly erode into the sacrum (Figure 6.29d and e) producing symptoms due to sacral nerve root compression or infiltration.

MRI in relation to other imaging modalities As with most ovarian masses, the imaging appearance of granulosa cell tumors is not specific and a tissue diagnosis is required. Clinical and pathologic staging is performed at surgery, and this obviates the need for radiologic staging. However, in patients with large primary tumors or tumor recurrence, radiologic assessment may be valuable in determining the local extent of disease, particularly any involvement of the bony pelvis. CT or MRI can be utilized, but the multiplanar imaging offered by MRI may be advantageous in assessing sacral disease.

Krukenberg tumors

Approximately 6 per cent of ovarian tumors found during exploration for another pelvic or abdominal mass are metastatic.[24] The primary cancers usually arise in the gastrointestinal tract, breast, or thyroid. The term 'Krukenberg tumor' is used for ovarian metastases that contain significant numbers of signet ring cells, and a cellular stroma derived from the ovarian stroma. Almost all Krukenberg tumors represent metastases from the stomach, but some originate in the breast, intestine, or other organs containing mucous glands. Tumor is thought to spread from the stomach to the ovary by retrograde dissemination via the aortic lymphatics, or by hematogeneous or transperitoneal spread. Metastatic spread to the ovary is disproportionately common in premenopausal women, presumably because of the vascularity of the functioning ovary.

Krukenberg tumors are usually solid, kidney-shaped and bilateral. Patients present with abdominal distension or palpable pelvic masses. In the vast majority, the primary malignancy is already known but occasionally initial presentation is with Krukenberg tumors. Prognosis is poor, with a mortality rate of approximately 90 per cent one year after the ovarian masses are discovered.[38]

MRI appearance Figure 6.30 illustrates the typical MRI appearance of Krukenberg tumors. They are bilateral, solid ovarian masses which image with medium signal intensity on T1-weighted sequences and increased signal intensity on T2-weighted sequences. Enhancement is seen after Gd-DTPA administration.

MRI in relation to other imaging modalities The appearance of Krukenberg tumors is non-specific, although the diagnosis may be suspected from the clinical history and the presence of bilateral tumors. Biopsy provides confirmation, and the lesions can be delineated by any of the cross-sectional imaging modalities. In patients without a known history of malignancy, investigation of the gastrointestinal tract may be warranted with special emphasis on the stomach (Figure 6.30).

Lymphoma

Occasionally, lymphoma may present as a gynecological problem, and in rare instances non-Hodgkin's lymphoma is localized to the genital tract. Since the ovary is ordinarily devoid of lymphocytes, however, there is dispute as to whether lymphoma can originate in the ovary.[24] Nonetheless, a small number of well documented cases of primary extranodal ovarian lymphoma have been reported.[37] In these patients, disease is confined to the ovary and its regional lymph nodes. Histologically, ovarian lymphoma is usually lymphoblastic or histiocytic, and it may be of the large-cleaved or non-cleaved type. There is a wide age incidence and patients present with abdominal pain or increased abdominal girth. Although disease may appear to be confined to the ovary at laparotomy, in most patients more generalized disease becomes manifest subsequently. Therefore, treatment is by excision of the ovarian mass followed by radiotherapy and/or chemotherapy.

Disseminated lymphoma, most often poorly differentiated non-Hodgkin's lymphoma, is occasionally discovered when a patient presents with a lymphomatous ovarian mass.[37] Most women are in the reproductive age group, and have generalized symptoms of malaise and weight loss.

MRI appearance Figure 6.31 illustrates the MRI appearance of disseminated lymphoma involving the ovary. Lymphoma is a solid mass, of medium signal intensity on T1-weighted images and high signal intensity on T2-weighted images. Local infiltration and involvement of adjacent organs may be identified. The use of Gd-DTPA produces enhancement of viable tumor tissue and delineates tumor extent. The regional lymph nodes of the ovary (preaortic and lateral aortic chains) may be enlarged due to tumor involvement.

MRI in relation to other imaging modalities There is no pathognomonic feature for ovarian lymphoma, and the diagnosis rests on histologic biopsy. Radiologic staging of the chest and abdomen is then required, and CT remains the modality of choice in these cases. MRI may be useful in the initial evaluation of the pelvic lesion, when its etiology is unknown.

Fallopian tube disorders

Hydrosalpinx

Hydrosalpinx is distension of the fallopian tube and is caused by closure of the fimbriated end of the tube with secondary accumulation of serous fluid or hemorrhagic secretions. The etiology of hydrosalpinx is diverse, but it most commonly occurs after salpingitis.[7] Other causes include adhesions from prior surgery, endometriosis, and obstruction secondary to uterine or fallopian tube tumors.

MRI appearance On transaxial scans, a hydrosalpinx appears as an aggregation of fluid-containing thin-walled cavities in the adnexa which demonstrate low to medium signal intensity on T1-weighted images and high signal intensity on T2-weighted images (Figure 6.32). After Gd-DTPA administration there may be slight enhancement of the tubal wall. On sagittal sections (Figure 6.32d and e) it can be appreciated that the apparent cystic spaces are actually continuous.

MRI in relation to other imaging modalities Hydrosalpinx is usually diagnosed by hysterosalpingography or by laparoscopy. With both US and CT it is difficult to distinguish hydrosalpinx from other types of cystic adnexal masses. On MRI, hydrosalpinx may be more easily recognized when viewed in two planes. Hydrosalpinx is usually identified coincidental to other pathology.

Fallopian tube carcinoma

Primary carcinoma of the fallopian tube accounts for only 0.1–0.5 per cent of all gynecologic malignancies. It has a predilection for women of low parity, is bilateral in 10–15 per cent of cases, and the average age of diagnosis is 55 years.[7] Fallopian tube malignancies are usually adenocarcinomas, histologically similar to ovarian serous carcinoma. Fallopian tube carcinomas also behave like ovarian serous carcinoma, with an initial endophytic growth which expands the lumen of the fallopian tube. Local extension involves the ovary, uterus, sigmoid colon, and other pelvic structures. Intraperitoneal metastatic spread occurs via the tubal lumen, and there is a high incidence of lymphatic metastasis to the aortic and iliac lymph nodes.

Patients commonly present with vaginal bleeding or discharge, a pelvic mass, or pain.[39] Fallopian tube carcinomas are staged surgically, with the FIGO system used for ovarian carcinoma (Table 6.2).

Treatment is primarily by surgical removal, but additional postoperative therapy, such as abdominal radiation or chemotherapy, is usually necessary.[40] Second-look operations may be performed after chemotherapy to assess response. Survival rate depends on the stage of the tumor. Patients with stage I disease have a 60 per cent five-year survival rate and those with stage IV disease have a 19 per cent five-year survival rate.[40]

MRI appearance As illustrated in Figure 6.33, fallopian tube carcinoma presents as a solid adnexal mass which cannot be readily differentiated from ovarian malignancy. On T1-weighted images the tumor exhibits medium signal intensity, and the signal intensity increases on T2-weighted images. Differential enhancement after Gd-DTPA distinguishes viable tumor from necrotic elements. When the mass occludes the fallopian tube, there may be an associated hydrosalpinx (Figure 6.33c–e).

MRI in relation to other imaging modalities Fallopian tube carcinoma is a rare tumor and cannot be differentiated from an ovarian neoplasm by any imaging study. The same indications and limitations that apply to cross-sectional imaging modalities in the evaluation of epithelial and stromal ovarian malignancies apply to the assessment of fallopian tube tumors.

References

1 LIERSE W, *Applied Anatomy of the Pelvis*, (Springer-Verlag: New York 1984), 272–83.

2 WILLIAMS PL, WARWICK R, eds. *Gray's Anatomy*, (Churchill Livingstone: New York 1989) 1435–9.

3 DOOMS GC, HRICAK H, TSCHOLAKOFF D, Adnexal structures: MR imaging, *Radiology* (1986) **158**:639–46.

4 HRICAK H, HAMM B, WOLF K-J, Use of Gd-DTPA in MR imaging of the female pelvis, Contrast Media in MRI (1990), Berlin.

5 MITCHELL DG, MINTZ MC, SPRITZER CE et al, Adnexal masses: MR imaging observations at 1.5 T with US and CT correlation, *Radiology* (1987) **162**:319–24.

6 WESTROM L, BENGTSSON LP, MARDH PA, The risk of pelvic inflammatory disease in women using intrauterine contraceptive devices compared to non-users, *Lancet* (1976) **2**:221–4.

7 WHEELER JE, Pathology of the follopian tube. In: Blaustein A ed. *Pathology of the Female Genital Tract*, (Springer-Verlag: New York 1982) 393–413.

8 WILLIAMS TJ, Endometriosis. In: Mattingly RF, Thompson JD eds. *TeLinde's Operative Gynecology*, (Lippincott: Philadelphia 1985) 257–86.

9 THE AMERICAN FERTILITY SOCIETY: revised American Fertility Society classification of endometriosis: 1985, *Fertil and Steril* (1985) **43**:351–2.

10 NISHIMURA K, TOGASHI K, ITOH K et al, Endometrial cysts of the ovary MR imaging, *Radiology* (1987) **162**:315–18.

11 ARRIVÉ L, HRICAK H, MARTIN MC, Pelvic endometriosis: MR imaging, *Radiology* (1989) **171**:687–92.

12 NYBERG DA, PORTER BA, OLDS MO et al, Imaging of hemorrhagic adnexal masses, *J Comput Assist Tomogr* (1987) **11**:664–9.

13 FRIEDMAN H, VOGELZANG RL, MENDELSON EB et al, Endometriosis detection by US with laparoscopic correlation, *Radiology* (1985) **157**:217–20.

14 FISHMAN EK, SCATARIGE JC, SAKSOUK FA et al, Computer tomography of endometriosis, *J Comput Assist Tomogr* (1983) **7**:257–64.

15 ZAWIN M, MCCARTHY S, SCOUTT L et al, Endometriosis: appearance and detection of MR imaging, *Radiology* (1989) **171**:693–6.

16 MORROW PC, TOWNSEND DE, Tumors of the ovary: general considerations; classification; the adnexal mass. In: Morrow PC, Townsend DE, eds. *Synopsis of Gynecologic Oncology*, 3rd edn. (Churchill Livingstone: New York 1987) 231–56.

17 MEIRE HB, FARRANT P, GUHA T, Distinction of benign from malignant cysts by ultrasound, *Br J Obstet Gynaecol* (1978) **85**:893–9.

18 WALSH JW, TAYLOR KJW, WASSON JFM et al, Gray-scale ultrasound in 204 proved gynecologic masses: accuracy and specific diagnostic criteria, *Radiology* (1979) **130**:391–7.

19 MOYLE JW, ROCHESTER D, SILDER L et al, Sonography of ovarian tumors: predictability of tumor type, *AJR* (1983) 141:985–91.

20 SAWYER RW, VICK CW, WALSH JW et al, Computed tomography of benign ovarian masses, *J Comput Assist Tomogr* (1985) **9**:784–9.

21 FAKUDA T, IKEUCHI M, HASHIMOTO H et al, Computed tomography of ovarian masses, *J Comput Assist Tomogr* (1986) **10**:990–6.

22 STEVENS S, HRICAK H, CARRINGTON BM et al, Detection and characterization of ovarian lesions at 1.5 T using gadolinium-DTPA. Submitted to *Radiology*.

23 MAWHINNEY RR, POWELL MC, WORTHINGTON BS et al: Magnetic resonance imaging of benign ovarian masses, *Br J Radiology* (1988) **61(723)**:179–86.

24 MORROW PC, TOWNSEND DE, Tumors of the ovary: soft tissue and secondary (metastatic) tumors; tumor-like conditions. In: Morrow PC, Townend DE, eds. *Synopsis of Gynecologic Oncology*, 3rd edn. (Churchill Livingstone: New York 1987) 335–44.

25 TALERMAN A, Germ cell tumors of the ovary. In: Kurman RJ, ed. *Blaustein's Pathology of the Female Genital Tract*, (Springer-Verlag: New York 1987) 686–96.

26 TOGASHI K, NISHIMURA K, ITOH K et al, Ovarian cystic teratomas: MR imaging, *Radiology* (1987) **162**:669–73.

27 GOLDZIEHER JW, Polycystic ovarian disease, *Fertil Steril* (1981) **35**:371–94.

28 FUTTERWEIT W, The pathologic anatomy of polycystic ovarian disease. In: Futterweit W, ed. *Polycystic Ovarian Disease* (Springer-Verlag: New York 1984) 41–6.

29 MITCHELL DG, GEFTER WB, SPRITZER CE et al, Polycystic ovaries: MR imaging, *Radiology* (1986) **160**:425–9.

30 BUY J-N, GHOSSAIN MA, MOSS A et al, Cystic teratoma of the ovary: CT detection, *Radiology* (1989) **171**:697–701.

31 YOUNG RC, FUKS Z, HOSKINS W, Cancer of the ovary. *In*: DeVita VT, Hellman S, Rosenberg SA, eds. *Cancer Principles and Practice of Oncology*, (Lippincott:Philadelphia 1989) 1162–96.

32 MEYERS MA, The spread and localization of acute intraperitoneal effusions, *Radiology* (1970) **95**:547–54.

33 DOOMES GC, HRICAK H, CROOKS LE et al, Magnetic Resonance Imaging of lymph nodes: comparisons with CT, *Radiology* (1984) **153**:719–28.

34 BUY J-N, MOSS AA, GHOSSAIN MA et al, Peritoneal implants from ovarian tumors: CT findings, *Radiology* (1988) **169**:691–4.

35 JOHNSON RJ, BLACKLEDGE G, EDDLESTON B et al, Abdominopelvic computed tomography in the management of ovarian carcinoma, *Radiology* (1983) **146:**447–52.

36 GRIFFITHS CT, PARKER L, Cancer of the ovary. In: Knapp RC, Berkowitz RS eds. *Gynecologic Oncology*, (Macmillan: New York 1986) 313–75.

37 TALERMAN A, Mesenchymal tumors and malignant lymphoma of the ovary. In: Blaustein A, ed. *Pathology of the female genital tract*, (Springer-Verlag: New York 1982) 561–80.

38 BLAUSTEIN A, Metastatic carcinoma in the ovary. In: Blaustein A, ed. *Pathology of the Female Genital Tract*, (Springer-Verlag: New York 1982) 705–15.

39 MUNTZ HG, TARRAZA HM, GRANAI CO et al, Primary adenocarcinoma of the fallopian tube, *Eur J Gynaecol Oncol* (1989) **10**:239–49.

40 HOSKINS WJ, PEREZ C, YOUNG RC, Gynecologic tumors. In: DeVita VT, Hellman S, Rosenberg SA, eds. *Cancer Principles and Practice of Oncology*, (Lippincott: Philadelphia 1989) 1099–151.

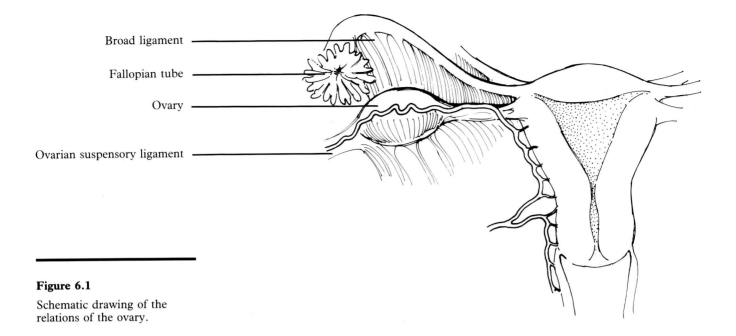

Broad ligament

Fallopian tube

Ovary

Ovarian suspensory ligament

Figure 6.1

Schematic drawing of the
relations of the ovary.

Figure 6.2

Normal MR appearance of the
ovaries. Transaxial (**a**) T1-
weighted, (**b**) T2-weighted, and
(**c**) T1-weighted gadolinium-
enhanced images. The ovaries
(arrows) are of medium signal
intensity on the T1-weighted
image and of high signal
intensity on the T2-weighted
sequence. Follicular cysts
demonstrate markedly high
signal intensity on the T2-
weighted image. On the
gadolinium-enhanced image
there is enhancement of ovarian
tissue but not of the follicular
cysts. (B)-urinary bladder; (U)-
uterus.

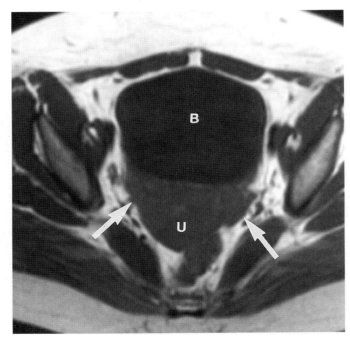

a

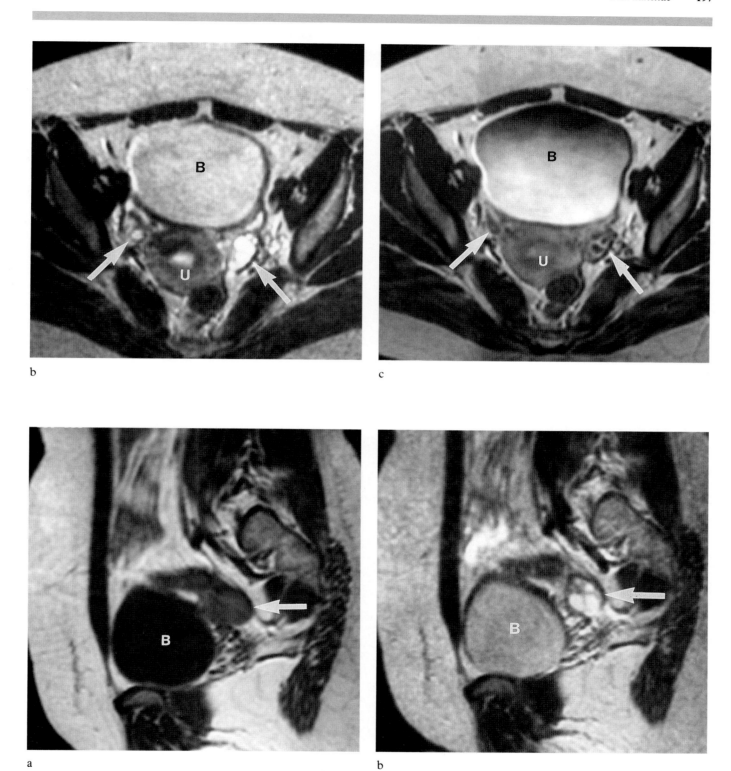

Figure 6.3

Visualization of the ovary in the sagittal plane. (**a**) T1-weighted and (**b**) T2-weighted sagittal images illustrating that the ovary (arrows) may be identified on lateral sagittal sections (B)-urinary bladder.

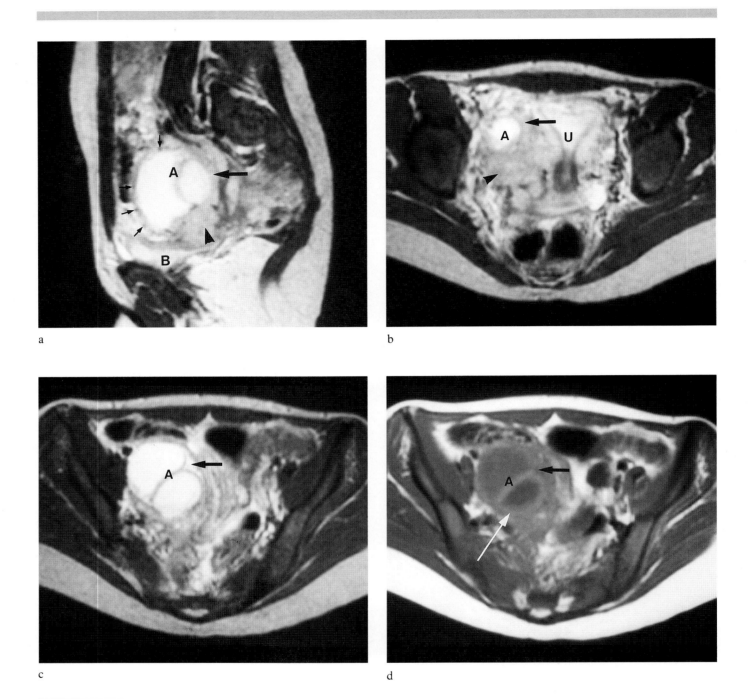

a

b

c

d

Figure 6.4

Tubo-ovarian abscess. (**a**) Sagittal, (**b**) and (**c**) transaxial T2-weighted images and (**d**) gadolinium-enhanced T1-weighted image. The abscess (A) is multiloculated and of high signal intensity with a thickened wall (black arrows). It demonstrates peripheral enhancement after gadolinium (white arrow). An inflammatory mass of tissue (arrowheads) is seen inferior to the loculated fluid. Hypervascularity is identified by the presence of multiple small blood vessels around the abscess (small black arrows). (B)-urinary bladder; (U)-uterus.

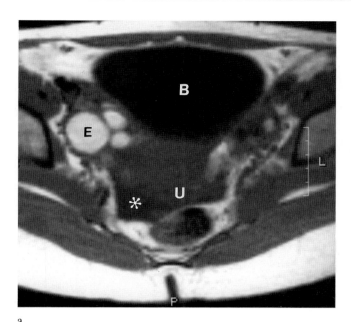

a

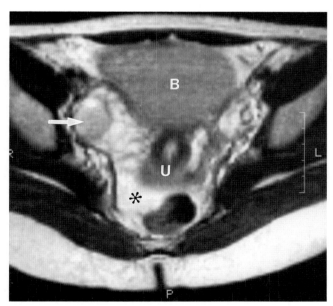

b

Figure 6.5

MR appearance of an endometrioma. (**a**) T1-weighted and (**b**) T2-weighted transaxial images showing a right ovarian endometrioma (E) which is multiloculated, thin-walled, and of high signal intensity on the T1-weighted image. The largest locule demonstrates layering with medium signal intensity occupying the most dependent portion (arrow). The margin between the endometrioma and the uterus is indistinct due to adhesions. (B)-urinary bladder; (U)-uterus; (asterisk)-fluid in the cul-de-sac.

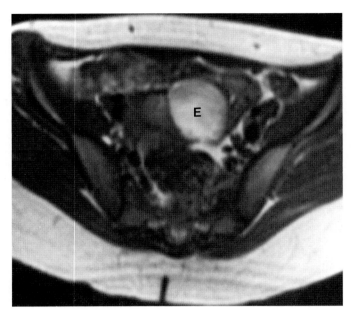

a

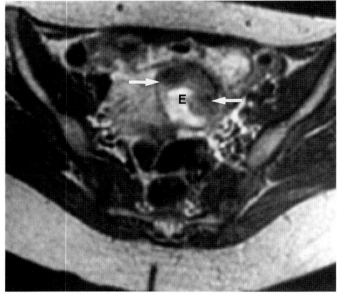

b

Figure 6.6

Endometrioma with shading. Transaxial (**a**) T1-weighted and (**b**) T2-weighted images. The endometrioma (E) is of high signal intensity on the T1-weighted image. On the T2-weighted image it demonstrates heterogeneous intensity with low signal intensity shading (arrows) in a predominantly peripheral distribution.

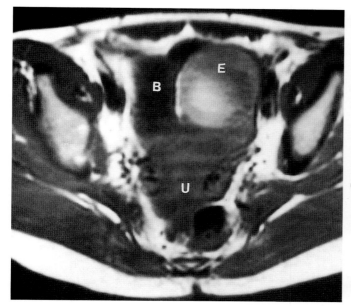

a

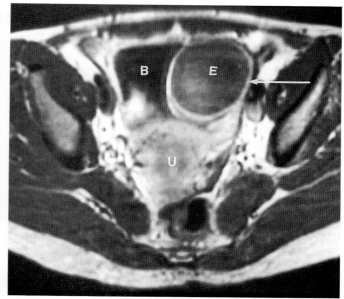

b

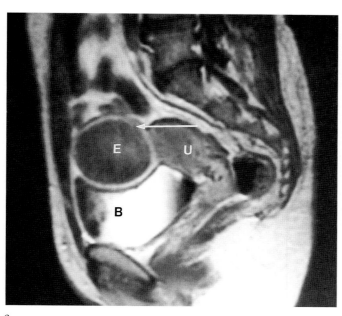

c

Figure 6.7

Gadolinium enhancement of the wall of an endometrioma. Transaxial (**a**) T1-weighted and (**b**) Gd-DTPA-enhanced T1-weighted images, and (**c**) sagittal Gd-DTPA enhanced image. The large endometrioma (E) shows peripheral enhancement of its wall (arrows) after gadolinium administration. The endometrioma is adherent to the fundus of the uterus (U). (B)-urinary bladder.

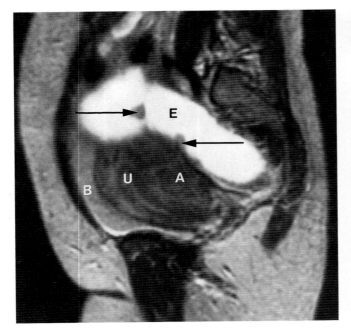

a

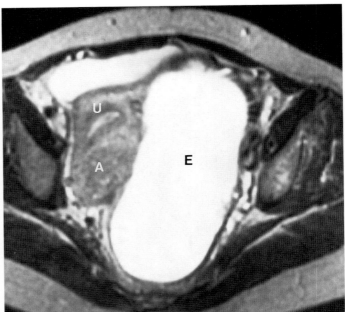

b

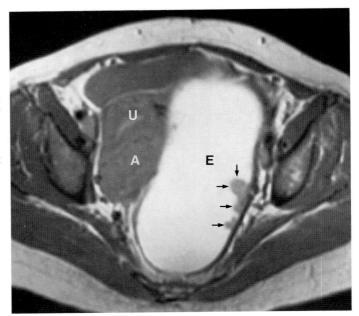

c

Figure 6.8

Endometrioma containing a focus of clear cell carcinoma. (**a**) Sagittal T2-weighted image and transaxial (**b**) T2-weighted and (**c**) Gd-DTPA-enhanced T1-weighted images. A very large endometrioma (E) demonstrates high signal intensity on both the T2-weighted and gadolinium-enhanced images. Areas of nodularity (long black arrows) are seen on the sagittal T2-weighted section. One papillary excrescence (small black arrows) on the left lateral wall of the endometrioma demonstrates enhancement after injection of Gd-DTPA and was a pathologically proven site of clear cell carcinoma. This lesion is not identified on the T2-weighted images since its signal intensity is similar to that of the hemorrhagic fluid content of the endometrioma. An adenomyoma (A) is seen within the uterus (U). (B)-urinary bladder.

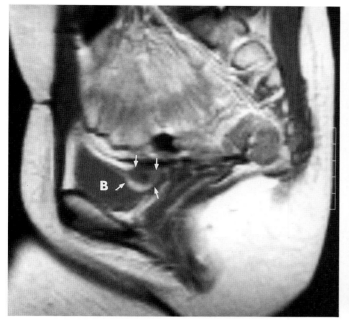

a

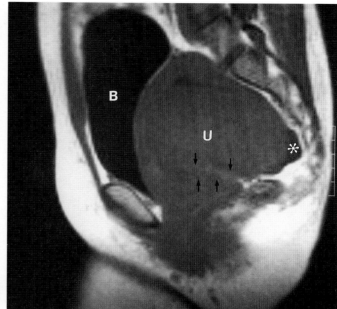

a

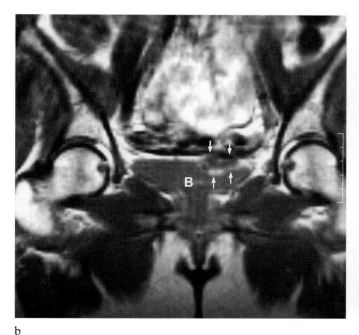

b

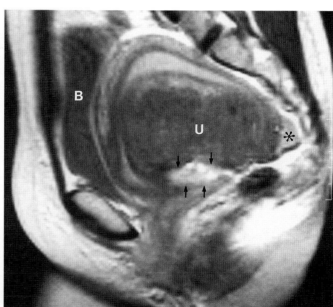

b

Figure 6.9

Bladder endometrial implant.
Proton density (**a**) sagittal and
(**b**) coronal images showing a
medium signal intensity
endometrial implant (arrows) in
the wall of the bladder (B).
Peripheral high signal intensity
within the implant was due to
hemorrhage. (0.35T.)

Figure 6.10

Vaginal endometrial implant.
Sagittal (**a**) T1-weighted and (**b**)
T2-weighted images illustrating
that the implant (arrows) is
indistinct on the T1-weighted
image and of high signal
intensity on the T2-weighted
image. There is a leiomyoma
within the uterus (U) and fluid
(asterisk) within the cul-de-sac.
(B)-urinary bladder. (0.35T.)

Figure 6.11

Intraperitoneal and extraperitoneal endometrial implants. Transaxial (**a**) proton density and (**b**) T2-weighted images at the same anatomical level. (**c**) Proton density and (**d**) T2-weighted images at the same anatomical level and (**e**) sagittal T2-weighted image. There are high signal intensity extraperitoneal endometrial implants in the left vaginal fornix (long white arrows) and in the perirectal tissues (curved white arrows). Intraperitoneal implants are seen in the cul-de-sac (small white arrows) and lateral margin of the vesicouterine pouch (white arrowhead). (B)-urinary bladder; (U)-uterus.

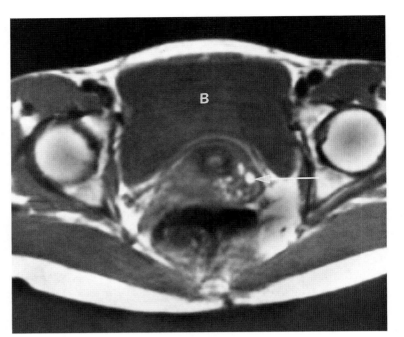

a

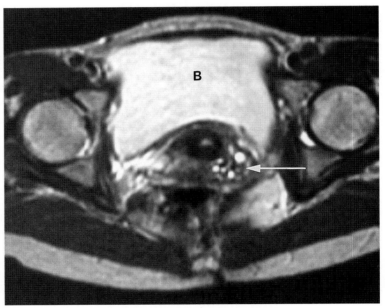

b

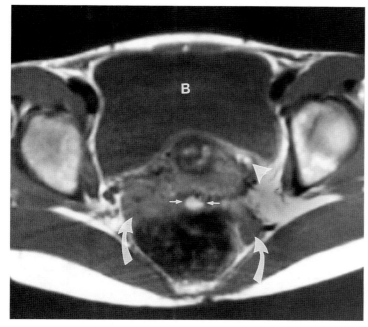

c

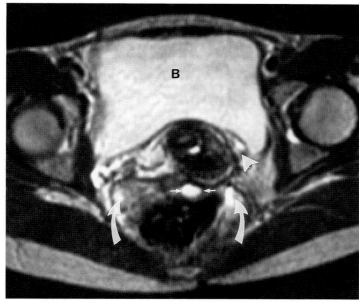

d

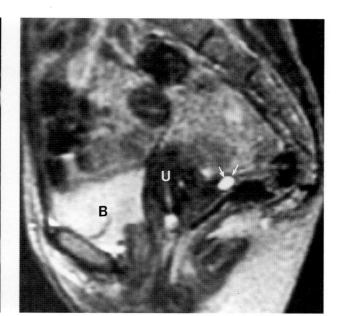

e

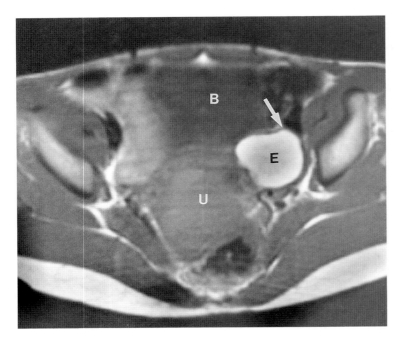

a

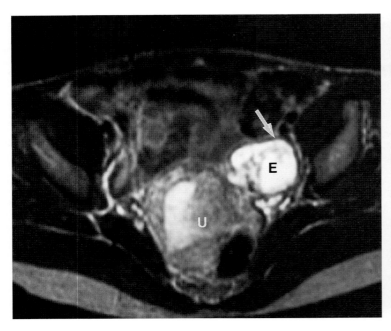

b

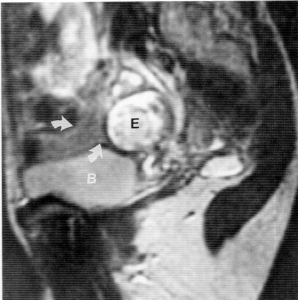

c

Figure 6.12

Adhesions due to endometriosis. Transaxial (**a**) proton density and (**b**) T2-weighted images and (**c**) sagittal T2-weighted image showing a left ovarian endometrioma (E) whose margin with the uterus (U) is indistinct, consistent with adhesions. The endometriomal outline is distorted anterolaterally (arrows) indicating adherence to the pelvic sidewall. An adjacent bowel loop is angulated (curved arrows) most likely due to adhesions. (B)-urinary bladder.

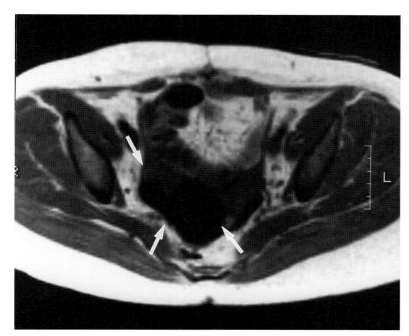

a

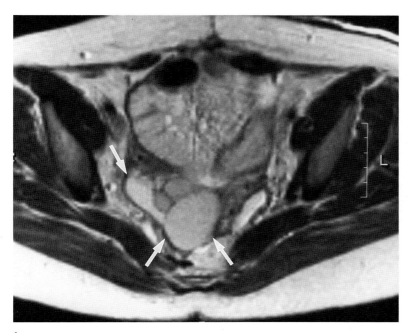

b

Figure 6.13

Adherent fluid-filled bowel loops mimicking endometriosis. Transaxial (**a**) T1-weighted and (**b**) T2-weighted sections demonstrating bowel loops (arrows) of varied size and signal intensity encased by adhesions due to inflammatory bowel disease. These findings may be mistaken for an ovarian endometrioma.

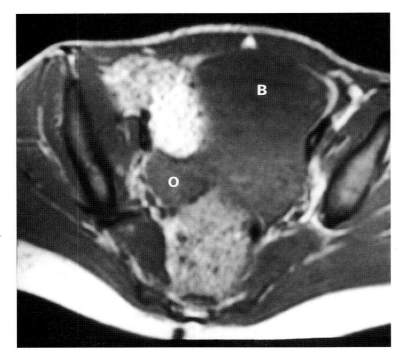

a

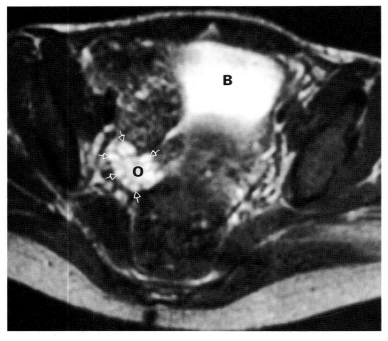

b

Figure 6.14

Follicular ovarian cysts. Transaxial (**a**) T1- and (**b**) T2- weighted images demonstrating the right ovary (O) with multiple, peripheral high signal intensity cysts (arrows) visualised on the T2-weighted image. (B)-urinary bladder.

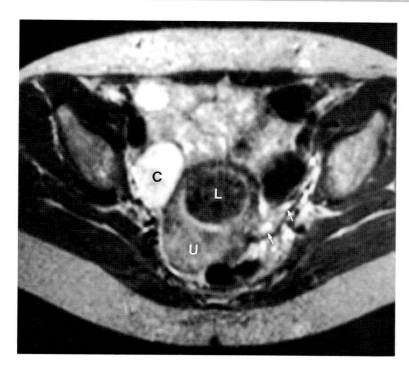

a

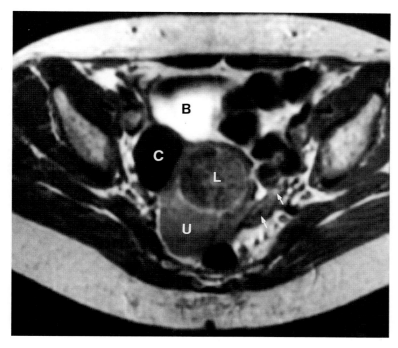

b

Figure 6.15

Simple cyst of the ovary. Transaxial (**a**) T2-weighted and (**b**) Gd-DTPA-enhanced T1-weighted images demonstrating a right sided, unilocular well circumscribed cyst (C) which is of uniform high signal intensity on the T2-weighted image and of uniform low signal intensity on the gadolinium-enhanced image. There is no enhancement of the cyst wall. The left ovary contains small follicular cysts (arrows). The uterus (U) contains a leiomyoma (L). (B)-urinary bladder.

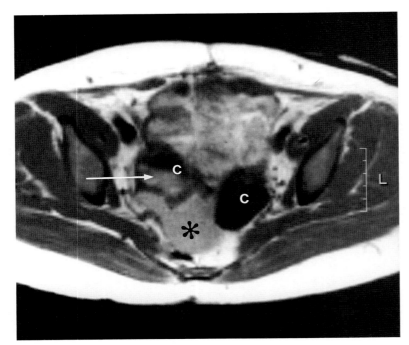

a

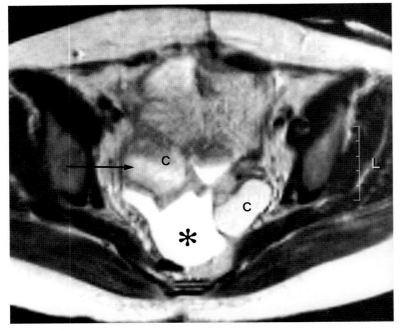

b

Figure 6.16

Hemorrhage within bilateral simple ovarian cysts. Transaxial (**a**) T1-weighted and (**b**) T2-weighted images showing bilateral ovarian cysts (C) with high signal intensity layering in one cyst (arrows) on both T1- and T2-weighted images. This represents the accumulation of blood products within the dependent portion of the cyst. High signal intensity hemorrhagic fluid (asterisk) is also seen in the cul-de-sac.

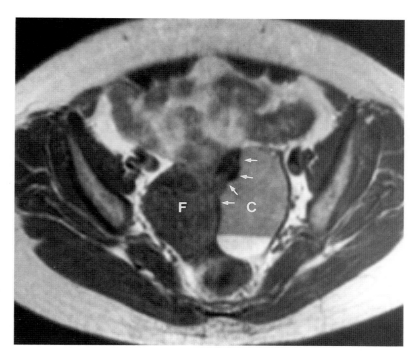

a

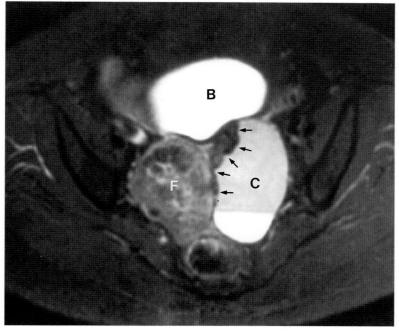

b

Figure 6.17

Ovarian cystadenoma and ovarian fibroma. Gadolinium-enhanced transaxial (**a**) T1-weighted and (**b**) fat saturation T1-weighted images showing a well demarcated cystadenoma (C) in the left ovary. A fluid/fluid level can be identified, as can a localized papillary excrescence (arrows) of the wall, which shows some focal enhancement. The patient also has a solid ovarian fibroma (F) in the right ovary. It demonstrates low signal intensity and shows no enhancement after gadolinium. (B)-urinary bladder.

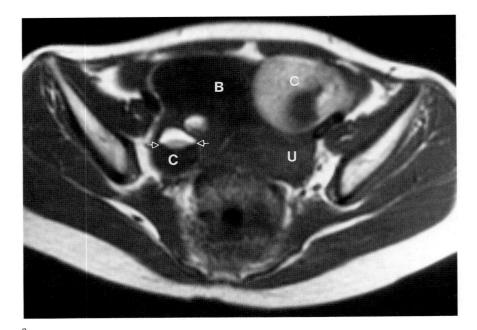

a

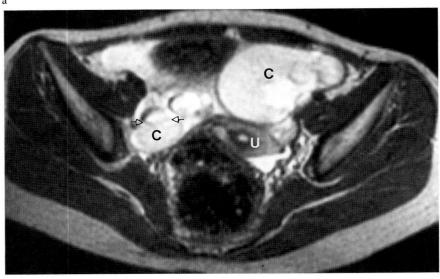

b

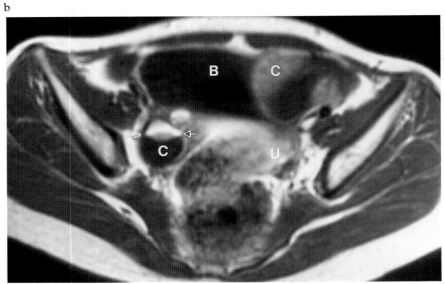

c

Figure 6.18

Bilateral dermoid cysts. Transaxial (**a**) T1-weighted, (**b**) T2-weighted, and (**c**) Gd-DTPA-enhanced T1-weighted images, with (**d**) a contrast-enhanced CT scan at the same level. (**e**) T1-weighted and (**f**) T2-weighted transaxial sections demonstrate the Rokitansky protuberance. The dermoid cysts (C) have a heterogeneous appearance with high signal intensity fat (arrows) forming fat/fluid levels. There is a small amount of free fluid around the uterus (U). On the companion CT scan the presence of fat/fluid levels can be identified, but the size of the left dermoid and the position of the uterus are difficult to appreciate. The Rokitansky protuberance (curved arrows) is clearly seen arising from the left dermoid wall and projecting into the cyst cavity. Its heterogeneous nature is also evident. (B)-urinary bladder.

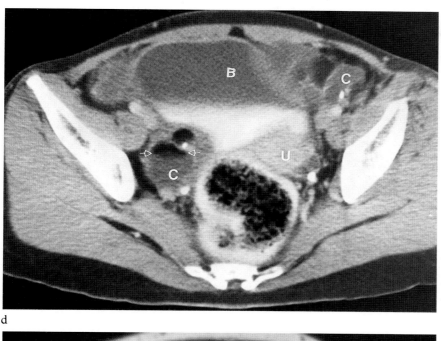

d

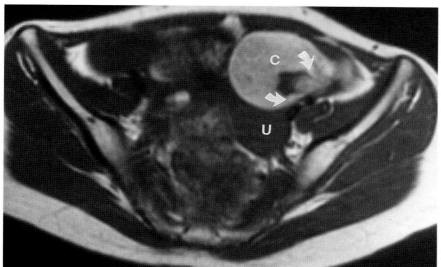

e

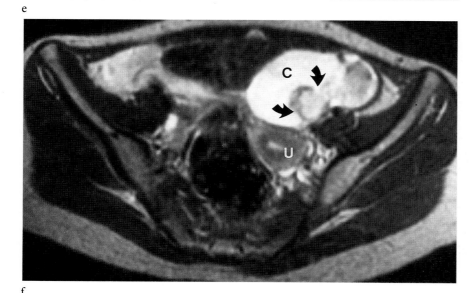

f

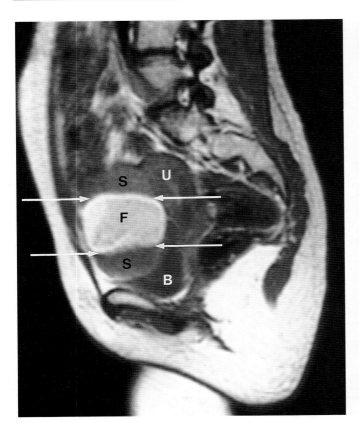

a

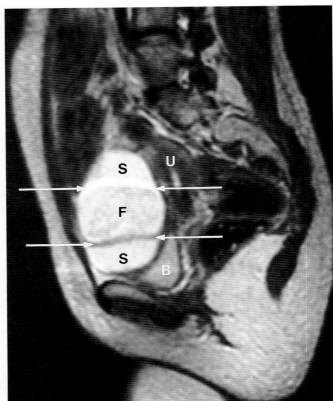

b

Figure 6.19

Chemical-shift artifact at the fat/fluid interface within a dermoid cyst. Sagittal (**a**) proton density and (**b**) T2-weighted images demonstrating a chemical-shift artifact (arrows) at the interface between the fat (F) within the Rokitansky protuberance and serous fluid (S) within the dermoid cyst cavity proper. (B)-urinary bladder; (U)-uterus.

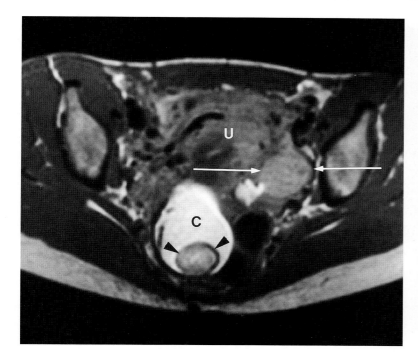

a

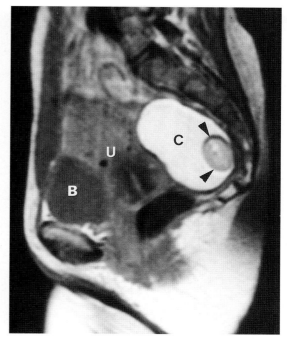

c

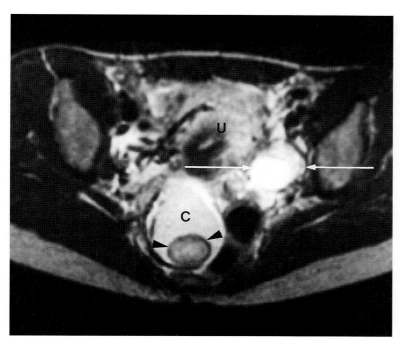

b

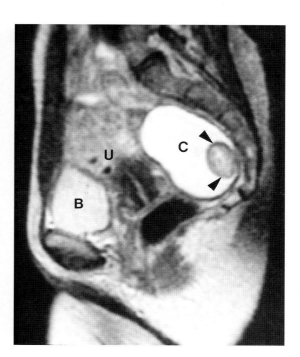

d

Figure 6.20

Rokitansky protuberance within dermoid cyst. Transaxial (**a**) proton density and (**b**) T2-weighted images. Sagittal (**c**) proton density and (**d**) T2-weighted images. The dermoid cyst (C) is of high signal intensity on all sequences and contains a medium signal intensity oval-shaped Rokitansky protuberance (arrowheads). There is also a left ovarian cyst (arrows). (B)-urinary bladder; (U)-uterus.

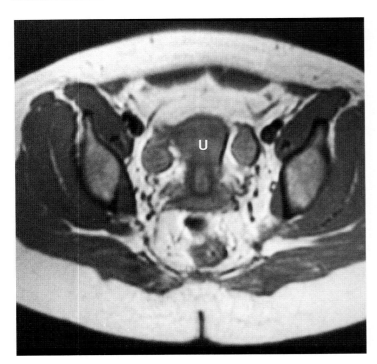

a

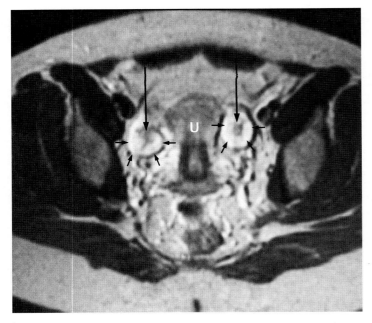

b

Figure 6.21

Polycystic ovaries. Transaxial (**a**) proton density and (**b**) T2-weighted images showing normal sized ovaries with a rim of high signal intensity due to multiple peripheral cysts (short arrows). Medullary low signal intensity (long arrows), due to increased amounts of fibrous tissue, can be identified on the T2-weighted image. The uterus (U) is small, but the zonal anatomy is preserved.

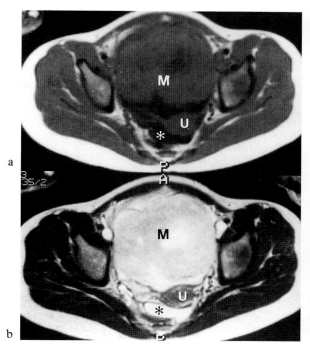

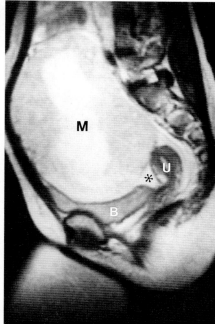

Figure 6.22

Large ovarian tumor. Transaxial (**a**) T1-weighted and (**b**) T2-weighted images and (**c**) sagittal T2-weighted image. This large ovarian mass (M) was originally thought to be a degenerative leiomyoma on ultrasound and CT. On MRI it is obviously entirely separate from the uterus (U) and represents an ovarian tumor. Ascites (asterisk) is present in the pelvis. (B)-urinary bladder. (0.35T.)

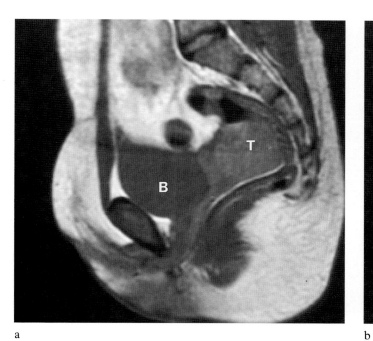

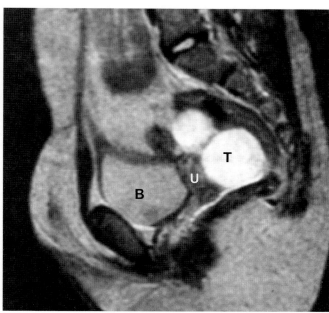

Figure 6.23

Ovarian carcinoma. Sagittal (**a**) proton density and (**b**) T2-weighted images showing a lobulated ovarian tumor (T) in the region of the cul-de-sac. It demonstrates medium signal intensity on the proton density image and high signal intensity on the T2-weighted image. The tumor is contiguous with the uterus (U), which is small and images with low signal intensity due to prior intracavitary radiation therapy for cervical carcinoma. (B)-urinary bladder.

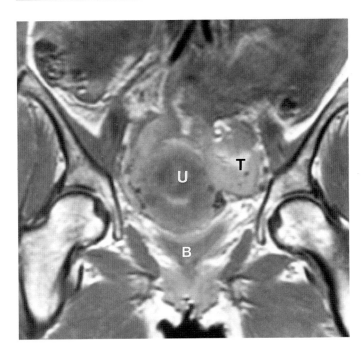

a

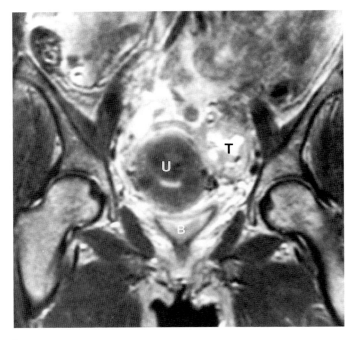

b

Figure 6.24

Ovarian carcinoma. Coronal (**a**) proton density and (**b**) T2-weighted images depicting a heterogeneous left adnexal ovarian carcinoma (T) with a high signal intensity central portion due to necrosis. Intramural leiomyomata are present in the uterus (U). (B)-urinary bladder.

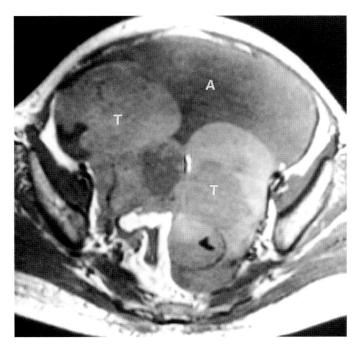

a

Figure 6.25

Bilateral endometrioid carcinoma. Transaxial (**a**) proton density, (**b**) T2-weighted, and (**c**) Gd-DTPA-enhanced T1-weighted images showing large bilateral ovarian tumors (T) and ascites (A). On the unenhanced scans it is unclear which portions are solid and which are cystic. After injection of gadolinium, the cystic (c) and solid (s) components can be identified, and a papillary tumor (arrows) is well visualized. The fundus of the uterus (U) is seen to be enveloped by the tumor.

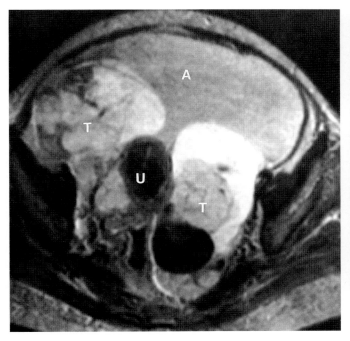

b

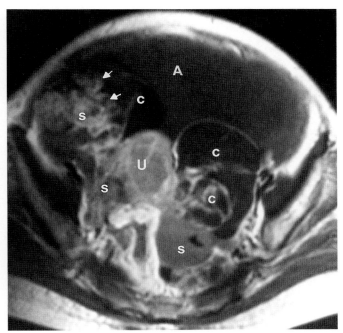

c

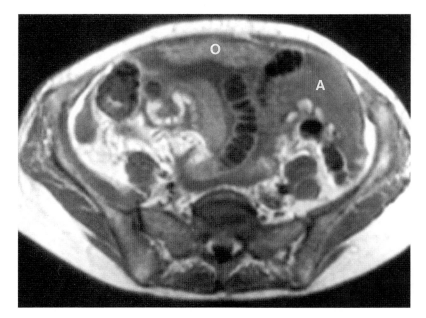

a

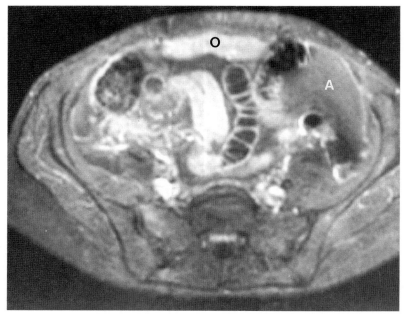

b

Figure 6.26

Omental cake due to ovarian carcinoma. Transaxial (**a**) Gd-DTPA-enhanced and (**b**) fat saturation Gd-DTPA-enhanced T1-weighted images demonstrating ascites (A) and an omental cake (O).

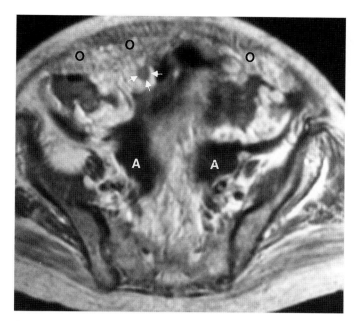

a

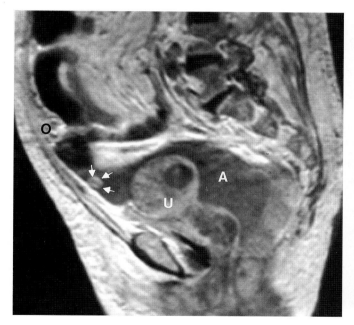

b

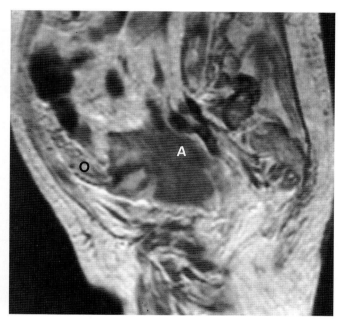

c

Figure 6.27

Peritoneal implants and omental cake due to ovarian carcinoma. Gd-DTPA-enhanced T1-weighted (**a**) transaxial and (**b**) and (**c**) sagittal images showing heterogeneous medium and high signal intensity of the infiltrated omentum (O) and small rounded medium to high signal intensity peritoneal implants (arrows). A large volume of ascites (A) is present. There is an intramural leiomyoma in the uterus (U).

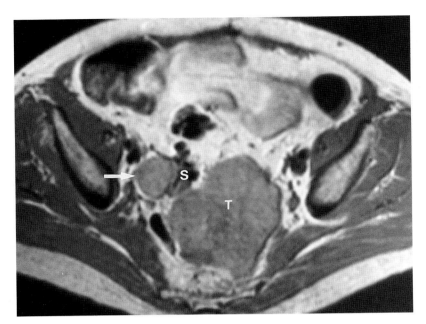

a

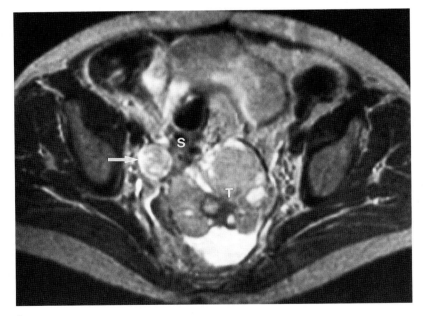

b

Figure 6.28

Granulosa cell tumor. Transaxial (**a**) proton density and (**b**) T2-weighted images illustrating a solid tumor mass (T) which contains foci of high signal intensity on the T2-weighted image due to areas of necrosis. The tumor is adherent to the sigmoid colon (S) and there is a serosal tumor deposit (arrows).

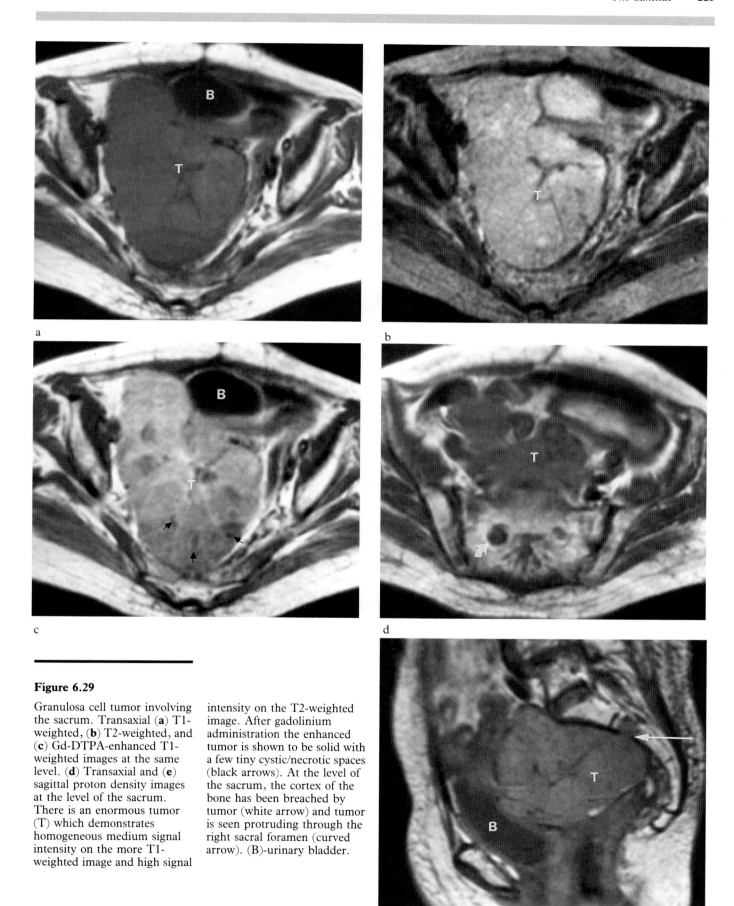

Figure 6.29

Granulosa cell tumor involving the sacrum. Transaxial (**a**) T1-weighted, (**b**) T2-weighted, and (**c**) Gd-DTPA-enhanced T1-weighted images at the same level. (**d**) Transaxial and (**e**) sagittal proton density images at the level of the sacrum. There is an enormous tumor (T) which demonstrates homogeneous medium signal intensity on the more T1-weighted image and high signal intensity on the T2-weighted image. After gadolinium administration the enhanced tumor is shown to be solid with a few tiny cystic/necrotic spaces (black arrows). At the level of the sacrum, the cortex of the bone has been breached by tumor (white arrow) and tumor is seen protruding through the right sacral foramen (curved arrow). (B)-urinary bladder.

Figure 6.30

Krukenberg tumor due to metastases from a stomach primary. Transaxial (**a**) T1-weighted, (**b**) T2-weighted, and (**c**) Gd-DTPA-enhanced T1-weighted images. (**d**) Coronal Gd-DTPA-enhanced image, (**e**) contrast enhanced CT scan through the renal hila, and (**f**) and (**g**) films from upper GI study of the stomach. A large solid tumor (T) is seen extending to both sides of the midline and enhances after gadolinium injection. A coronal section reveals a right perirenal urine collection (PF) due to ureteric compression by the pelvic mass. CT confirms the presence of right hydronephrosis (H) and perinephric fluid. The stomach wall (S) is thickened (arrows), and a barium study reveals thickened gastric folds (f) with an irregular margin to the greater curve (arrows) due to the presence of a diffusely infiltrating carcinoma. (U)-uterus.

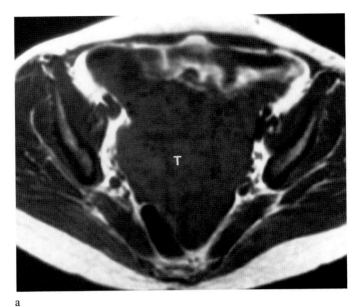

a

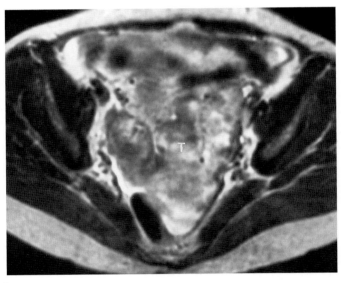

b

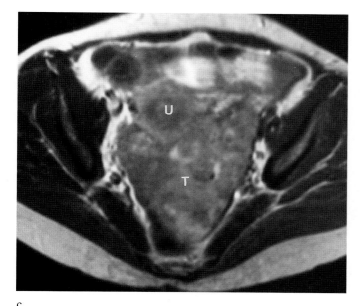

c

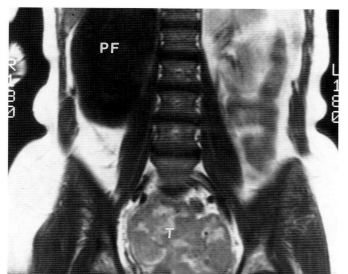

d

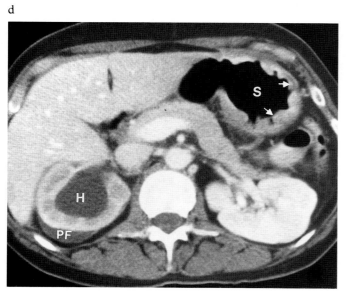

e

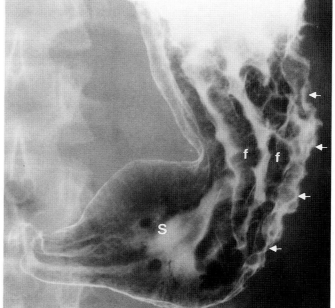

f

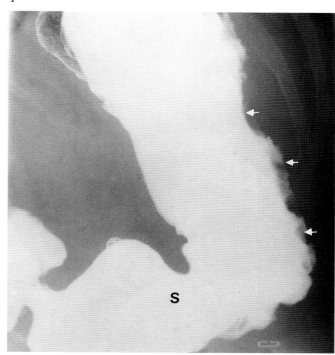

g

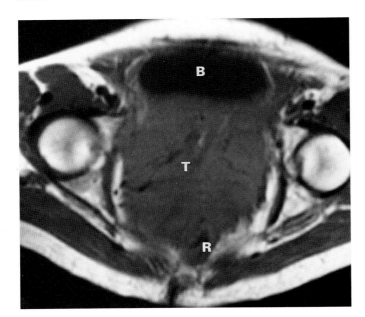

a

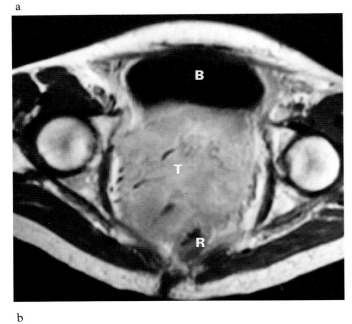

b

Figure 6.31

Disseminated lymphoma presenting as an ovarian mass. Transaxial (**a**) T1- and (**b**) Gd-DTPA-enhanced T1-weighted images showing a large, solid lymphomatous tumor mass (T) inseparable from the bladder (B) and rectum (R). The mass enhances after intravenous gadolinium administration.

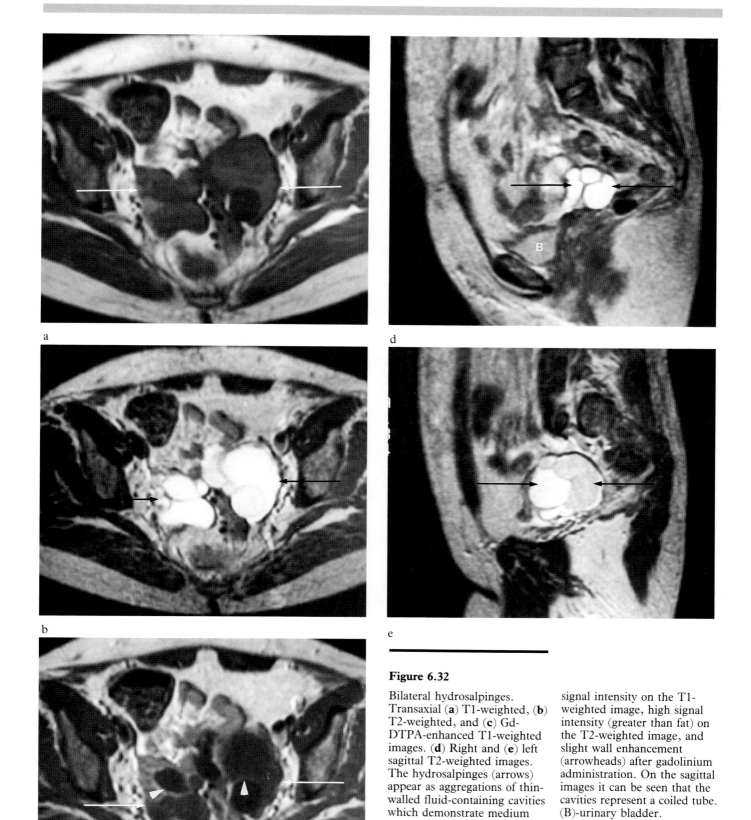

a

d

b

e

Figure 6.32

Bilateral hydrosalpinges. Transaxial (**a**) T1-weighted, (**b**) T2-weighted, and (**c**) Gd-DTPA-enhanced T1-weighted images. (**d**) Right and (**e**) left sagittal T2-weighted images. The hydrosalpinges (arrows) appear as aggregations of thin-walled fluid-containing cavities which demonstrate medium signal intensity on the T1-weighted image, high signal intensity (greater than fat) on the T2-weighted image, and slight wall enhancement (arrowheads) after gadolinium administration. On the sagittal images it can be seen that the cavities represent a coiled tube. (B)-urinary bladder.

c

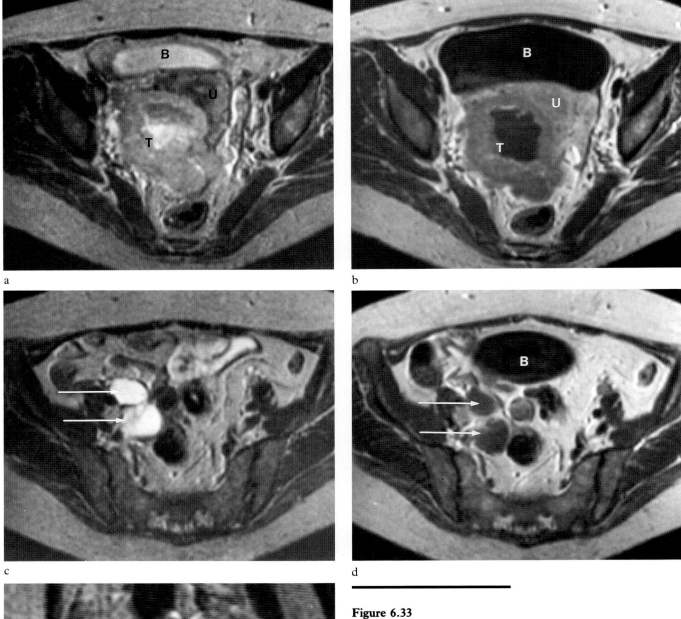

Figure 6.33

Fallopian tube carcinoma.
Transaxial (**a**) T2-weighted and
(**b**) Gd-DTPA-enhanced T1-
weighted images at the same
level. Transaxial (**c**) T2-
weighted and (**d**) Gd-DTPA-
enhanced T1-weighted images
at the same level. (**e**) Sagittal
T2-weighted image. The tumor
(T) is of high signal intensity on
the T2-weighted images and
has a heterogeneous necrotic
center which is well delineated
on the Gd-DTPA-enhanced
image. There is an associated
hydrosalpinx (arrows). (B)-
urinary bladder; (U)-uterus.

7
Pregnancy

Bernadette Carrington

The aim of imaging in the pregnant woman is to recognize normal anatomic and physiologic changes of pregnancy and to distinguish them from maternal disease states. It is also important to identify normal and abnormal fetal development. It is particularly important to achieve both of these goals without causing harm to the developing fetus. Currently the primary screening modality in obstetric radiology is high-resolution ultrasound, which is widely available and provides excellent diagnostic capability without any known adverse effects. MRI offers an alternative to sonography—it is noninvasive, does not involve exposure to ionizing radiation, and has superior contrast resolution and the ability to obtain images in multiple orthogonal planes. Fetal and maternal anatomy are displayed without interference from excess maternal fatty tissue or bowel. MRI does not require a distended bladder for imaging, and it is not impaired by the presence of oligohydramnios, which often degrades ultrasound examinations.

There is no evidence that clinical MR examinations are detrimental to the fetus and no mutagenic or adverse effects have been detected after extensive experimental and clinical studies.[1–7] Nonetheless, as with all new techniques, it is prudent to restrict MRI examination to those patients whose diagnostic problem cannot be solved by ultrasound and who would otherwise require imaging with ionizing radiation. Patients requiring MRI should be informed that there are no known hazards to the fetus, but that as yet unrecognized risks cannot be excluded.

At this time there are three recommended indications for MRI in pregnancy: pelvimetry; evaluation of placenta previa; and imaging of maternal pelvic and abdominal tumors.[8]

Normal pregnancy

Fetal anatomy

The gestation sac, seen in Figure 7.1, can be visualised as early as six weeks, when it is identified as a low signal intensity oval mass within the high signal intensity endometrium. At nine weeks the fetal pole can be seen, and after twelve to sixteen weeks the fetal head and trunk are visualized (Figure 7.2). At this point it is possible to perform biparietal diameter measurements, although obtaining the correct plane of section through the fetal head remains fortuitous.

The morphology of the fetal central nervous system is clearly displayed on MRI scans, and the cardiovascular system and major blood vessels are also easily identified.[9,10] The fetal lungs are extremely well visualized in all cases due to their fluid content, and they demonstrate medium signal intensity on T1-weighted images and high signal intensity on T2-weighted images. It is also possible to identify other fluid-filled structures, such as the stomach or urinary bladder. The lower gastrointestinal tract demonstrates high signal intensity on T1-weighted images due to the presence of intraluminal meconium.[11]

Several reports describe the identification of fetal anomalies and intrauterine growth retardation by MRI,[12–15] but in these situations the primary mode of assessment remains sonography.

Maternal anatomy

Pregnancy changes within the cervix and uterus are clearly visualized on MRI.[16,17] As illustrated in Figure

7.3, the position of the internal and external os are clearly seen, and this facilitates assessment of both fetal and placental position in relation to the cervix. The MR characteristics of the cervix change during pregnancy, and in the third trimester it images with intermediate signal intensity on T1-weighted images. Cervical effacement can also be demonstrated later in pregnancy.

Other maternal changes visible on MRI include lumbar vertebral disc abnormalities. These commonly occur with bulging of the annulus (Figure 7.4), or even herniation of the nucleus pulposus.[16] Disc abnormalities are most frequent in the lower lumbar spine, at L5–S1, and to a lesser extent at L4–5. Generalized pelvic hypervascularity is also seen, with multiple venous collateral vessels resulting from compression of the inferior vena cava by the enlarging uterus. This may lead to the formation of engorged superficial vulvar veins, and even to the development of vulvar varicosities, as depicted in Figure 7.5.

Suggested imaging sequences

In early pregnancy any of the three orthogonal planes may prove useful in image analysis. In the second trimester fetal motion is such that no plane of imaging reliably identifies fetal anatomy. In the third trimester the sagittal plane has been reported as optimal for fetal visualization, as the long axis of the fetus usually parallels the long axis of the mother. Sagittal sections therefore provide a parasagittal or coronal image of the fetus. In addition, there is a relative decrease in amniotic fluid in the third trimester, which tends to reduce fetal motion and improve image quality.

Imaging degradation due to motion is least pronounced on T1-weighted (short TR/short TE) sequences, which also offer the advantage of maximum contrast between the amniotic fluid and both the placenta and fetal subcutaneous fat. However, T2-weighted images are needed to provide optimal delineation of the fetal brain and lungs and for evaluation of the maternal cervix and uterus. Therefore, both T1- and T2-weighted images should be acquired.

Maternal ingestion of sedative drugs, such as diazepam, has been reported to decrease fetal motion and improve image quality.[18] However, sedative administration is not routinely recommended.

Pelvimetry

The most common indication for pelvimetry is a breech presentation.[19] Other indications include face or brow presentation, pelvic deformity, an unusually large fetus, and failure to progress in labor.[20] Conventional radiographic and CT pelvimetry both involve subjecting the fetus to ionizing radiation, and MRI provides an easy, nonionizing alternative for pelvimetry. Scanning in the sagittal and transaxial planes enables measurement of all relevant pelvic diameters, and measurement errors are reported to be less than 1 per cent.[21] The maternal soft tissues can be simultaneously assessed and soft tissue dystocia evaluated. Three measurements are performed in pelvimetry: the **anteroposterior (AP) pelvic inlet** the **transverse pelvic inlet** and the **bispinous diameter.**

The AP inlet measurement is made on a sagittal MR image and is the distance from the sacral promontory to the symphysis pubis. If the AP diameter is measured to the superior aspect of the symphysis, then it is called the **anatomic conjugate** and corresponds to the anatomic division between the true pelvis and the false pelvis. If the diameter is measured to the posterosuperior margin of the symphysis (a few millimeters difference) it is known as the **obstetric (true) conjugate** and is normally greater than or equal to 10 cm.[21]

The transverse pelvic inlet is measured on a transaxial image and is the greatest diameter between the arcuate lines of the iliac bones. It is normally 11.5 cm or greater.

The bispinous diameter is the distance between the ischial spines and is measured on a transaxial image which includes the fovea of the femoral heads. It should measure at least 10.5 cm.[21]

Placental position

As seen in Figure 7.6, the placenta is recognized on MRI early in pregnancy. The placenta demonstrates low to medium signal intensity on T1-weighted images and high signal intensity on T2-weighted images (Figure 7.7). Placental position can be assessed and the distance between the end of the placenta and the internal cervical os can be measured. This is especially useful in the evaluation of **placenta previa.** Hemorrhage due to **abruptio placentae** can be identified as an area of medium or high signal intensity on T1-weighted images, increasing to high signal intensity on T2-weighted images, which is located between the placenta and the uterine wall.

Pathology during pregnancy

Maternal pelvic masses

Because of the limitations imposed on physical examination by the presence of the gravid uterus, evaluation of abdominal or pelvic pathology is difficult in the pregnant female. Radiologic assessment is also limited by a desire to spare the fetus exposure to ionizing radiation. Although sonography therefore remains the initial imaging modality in maternal evaluation, the information obtained may be restricted by the enlarged uterus and lack of tissue specificity. MRI has been shown to be a useful adjunct to ultrasound in the characterization of maternal pelvic masses.[22] Because of superior contrast resolution, a large field-of-view, and multiplanar imaging capability, MRI scans display the anatomy of the maternal abdomen and pelvis, and delineate the extent of any mass lesion.

Leiomyomata in the pregnant uterus are detected more often on MRI scans than on sonograms, and, as seen in Figures 7.8 and 7.9, degenerative leiomyomata can be identified as the source of a suspected adnexal mass or as the cause of pelvic pain. When multiple leiomyomata are found, their location will influence the decision about route of delivery (vaginal versus Caesarean section).

Adnexal lesions are also clearly seen on MRI and simple cysts can be differentiated from more complex lesions, as shown in Figure 7.10. The relationship between a mass lesion and the pregnant uterus is readily established on MRI (Figure 7.11).

Spontaneous abortion

Spontaneous abortion occurs in at least 15–20 per cent of pregnancies, over half during the first trimester. The most important etiological factor in first trimester abortion is chromosomal abnormality, particularly 45 XO and triploidy. Other factors include: (1) maternal infections or systemic illness, such as diabetes mellitus; (2) hormonal imbalance; (3) trauma; (4) uterine pathology, such as submucosal fibroids; and (5) immunological incompatability.[23] In the second trimester, uterine factors such as cervical incompetence and the presence of müllerian duct anomalies play a more important role.

In early pregnancy patients complain of bleeding, pain and the passage of tissue from the vagina. Diagnosis is clinical, based on history and clinical findings. Sonography is performed to confirm the absence of a live fetus and to identify any retained products of conception.

MRI appearance

On MRI scans the enlarged uterus is identified and, in threatened abortion, the gestation sac may be seen (Figure 7.12). Hemorrhage images with high signal intensity on both T1- and T2-weighted scans. Figures 7.13 and 7.14 show the uterus immediately after an

abortion. The uterus remains bulky and the endometrial cavity may be expanded due to bleeding or retained products of conception. The site of previous placental implantation is often identifiable as an area of localized hypervascularity within the myometrium, which demonstrates multiple foci of low signal intensity on both T1- and T2-weighted images.

MR in relation to other imaging modalities

The imaging of patients with suspected abortion is primarily by sonography. MRI is only performed when additional pathology is suspected.

Endometritis

Endometritis, an infection of the endometrium, may be acute or chronic. Acute endometritis most commonly occurs in the puerperium or as a complication of dilatation and curettage. Chronic endometritis is seen secondary to the use of intrauterine devices and in patients with chronic cervicitis. In both acute and chronic disease, infection usually ascends from the lower genital tract and may spread to the adjacent myometrium. In acute disease, patients are symptomatic with pain, pyrexia, or uterine bleeding. Chronic endometritis may be asymptomatic or patients may present with intermittent intermenstrual bleeding or pain.

MRI appearance

The MRI appearance of endometritis is illustrated in Figures 7.14 through to 7.17. The uterus images with medium signal intensity on T1-weighted images and is of high signal intensity on T2-weighted images, with loss of the normal uterine zonal anatomy. After gadolinium-DTPA administration the uterus demonstrates marked uniform enhancement, consistent with hypervascular inflammatory change (Figures 7.14 and 7.15) and zonal anatomy is not appreciated. In puerperal patients (Figures 7.16 and 7.17) the enlarged postpartum uterus can be seen, often demonstrating intraluminal contents with signal characteristics consistent with infected debris.

MRI in relation to other imaging modalities

The diagnosis of endometritis is by clinical history and bacterial cultures of uterine discharge or curettings. MRI findings suggestive of endometritis are often recognized when the examination is requested for another reason, usually to exclude a pelvic abscess.

Gestational trophoblastic disease

The term gestational trophoblastic disease (GTD) includes tumors ranging from benign hydatidiform moles to locally invasive moles and choriocarcinoma. In developed countries it occurs in between 1 in 1000 and 1 in 1200 pregnancies. Its incidence is markedly increased, however, in areas such as Asia and South America, where nutritional factors are thought to play a part. GTD is also associated with increased maternal age, and patients over 40 are up to 12 times more susceptible.

Histologic classification of GTD depends on the degree of differentiation of the trophoblastic tissue within the tumor. Trophoblastic hyperplasia and hydropic villi can be identified in hydatidiform moles, and anaplastic trophoblastic tissue without evidence of villous formation is seen in choriocarcinoma.[24]

Patients with molar pregnancies often present with first trimester bleeding, ectopic pregnancy, or threatened abortion. The uterus may be larger than the patient's dates would suggest, and there is an increased risk of developing toxemia of pregnancy. Occasionally patients expel some of the molar tissue from the uterus. Metastatic disease occurs by hematogenous spread, most commonly to the lungs (80 per cent), vagina (30 per cent), pelvis (20 per cent), liver and brain (10 per cent), and it may be the initial presenting factor.[24]

There is no universally accepted staging system for GTD. Patients are classified according to the presence or absence of metastatic disease and on the basis of risk factors, including (1) uterine and ovarian size (there is an association with theca lutein ovarian cysts), (2) maternal age greater than 40, (3) the presence of toxemia or coagulopathy, and (4) the level of a specific tumor marker called human chorionic gonadotropin (HCG). HCG levels closely correlate with tumor volume and have facilitated management of this condition.

Treatment is by evacuation of the uterine contents followed by dilatation and curettage for hydatidiform moles and single agent chemotherapy or combination chemotherapy for choriocarcinoma.[24] Long-term survival rates are approximately 90 per cent with this treatment.

MRI appearance

Examples of GTD are illustrated in Figures 7.18 through to 7.23. As shown in Figure 7.18, uterine GTD appears as a medium signal intensity tumor mass on T1-weighted images, which changes to heterogeneous high and low signal intensity on T2-weighted images.[25] Tumors are highly vascular and multiple vessels may be identified within the tumor, adjacent myometrium, and adnexae (Figures 7.18–7.21). The vessels are friable and intralesional hemorrhage is fairly common. The uterine zones are distorted or obliterated, and the boundary between the tumor and the myometrium is irregular (Figures 7.19 and 7.21). Figures 7.21 and 7.22 show tumor penetration through the uterine wall. Adnexal cysts (Figures 7.20 and 7.23), which are presumed theca lutein in origin, are seen in over 50 per cent of patients.[25]

After chemotherapy, response is indicated by reduction in serum HCG levels. Concomitant MRI changes involve the return of uterine zonal anatomy (Figure 7.23) which antedates reduction in tumor volume, regression of pelvic vascularity, and the development of intralesional hemorrhage.[25] Theca lutein cysts may persist throughout therapy and for some months afterwards.

MRI in relation to other imaging modalities

When GTD is diagnosed, CT is the imaging procedure of choice for the detection of extrapelvic metastases. Response to therapy is monitored by HCG immunoassay and the HCG level is directly related to residual tumor volume. MRI may be used to evaluate the primary uterine disease, and to assess residual abnormality in those patients in whom the HCG level is static or rising and the uterus remains enlarged.

References

1 BUDINGER JR, Nuclear magnetic resonance (NMR) in vivo studies: known thresholds for health effects, *J Comput Assist Tomogr* (1981) **5**:800–11.

2 COOK P, MORRIS PG, The effects of NMR exposure on living organisms II. A genetic study of human lymphocytes, *Br J Radiol* (1981) **54**:622–4.

3 MCROBBIE D, FOSTER MA, Pulsed magnetic field exposure during pregnancy and implications for NMR imaging: a study with mice, *Magn Reson Imaging* (1985) **3**:231–4.

4 REID A, SMITH PW, HUTCHINSON MJS, Nuclear magnetic resonance imaging and its safety implications: follow-up of 181 patients, *Br J Radiol* (1982) **55**:784–6.

5 WOLFF S, CROOKS LE, BROWN P et al, Tests for DNA and chromosomal damage induced by nuclear magnetic resonance imaging, *Radiology* (1980) **136**:707–10.

6 SCHWARTZ JL, CROOKS LE, NMR produces no observable mutations or cytotoxicity in mammalian cells, *AJR* (1982) **136**:583–5.

7 NATIONAL RADIOLOGICAL PROTECTION BOARD: Revised guidance on acceptable limits of exposure during nuclear magnetic resonance imaging, *Br J Radiol* (1983) **56**:974–7.

8 HRICAK H, Guidelines for magnetic resonance imaging in obstetrics and gynecology. American College of Radiology, *Clinical Applications of Magnetic Resonance Imaging* (1989), 31–5.

9 MCCARTHY SM, FILLY RA, STARK DD et al, Obstetrical magnetic resonance imaging: fetal anatomy, *Radiology* (1985) **154**:427–32.

10 POWELL MC, WORTHINGTON BS, BUCKLEY JM et al, Magnetic resonance imaging (MRI) in obstetrics II: fetal anatomy, *Br J Obstet Gynaecol* (1988) **95**:38–46.

11 COLLETTI PM, PLATT LD, Obstetric MRI acceptable under specific criteria, *Diagnostic Imaging* (1989) **5**:32–6.

12 WEINREB JC, LOWE TW, SANTOS-RAMOS R et al, Magnetic resonance imaging in obstetric diagnosis, *Radiology* (1985) **154**:157–61.

13 MCCARTHY SM, FILLY RA, STARK DD et al, Magnetic resonance imaging of fetal anomalies in utero: early experience, *AJR* (1985) **145**:677–82.

14 STARK DD, MCCARTHY SM, FILLY RA et al, Intrauterine growth retardation; evaluation by magnetic resonance, *Radiology* (1985) **155**:425–7.

15 BROWN CEL, WEINREB JC, Magnetic resonance imaging appearance of growth retardation in a twin pregnancy, *Obstet Gynecol* (1988) **71**:987–8.

16 MCCARTHY SM, STARK DD, FILLY RA et al, Obstetrical magnetic resonance imaging: maternal anatomy, *Radiology* (1985) **154**:421–5.

17 POWELL MC, WORTHINGTON BS, BUCKLEY JM et al, Magnetic resonance imaging (MRI) in obstetrics I: maternal anatomy, *Br J Obstet Gynaecol* (1988) **95**:31–7.

18 WEINREB JC, Human fetal anatomy: MR imaging, *Radiology* (1985) **157**:715–20.

19 VARNER MW, CRUIKSHANK DP, LANKE DW, X-ray pelvimetry in clinical obstetrics, *Obstet Gynecol* (1980) **56**:296–8.

20 BEAN WJ, RODAN BA, Pelvimetry revisited, *Semin Roentgenol* (1982) **3**:164–71.

21 STARK DD, MCCARTHY SM, FILLY RA et al, Pelvimetry by magnetic resonance imaging, *AJR* (1985) **144**:947–50.

22 WEINREB JC, BROWN CE, LOWE TW, Pelvic masses in pregnant patients: MR and US imaging, *Radiology* (1986) **159**:717–24.

23 BIGELOW B, Abortion. In: Blausein A, ed. *Pathology of the female genital tract*, (Springer-Verlag: New York 1982) 785–90.

24 HOSKINS WH, PEREZ C, YOUNG RC, Gynecologic tumors. In: DeVita VT, Hellman S, Rosenberg SA, eds. *Cancer Principles and Practice of Oncology*, (Lippincott: Philadelphia 1989) 1099–161.

25 HRICAK H, DEMAS BE, BRAGA CA et al, Gestational trophoblastic neoplasm of the uterus: MR assessment, *Radiology* (1986) **161**:11–16.

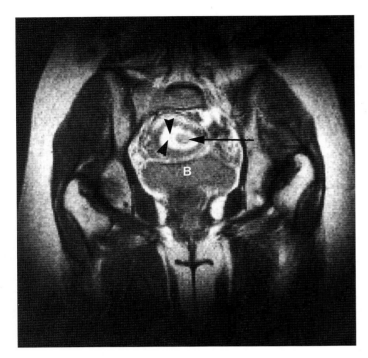

Figure 7.1

Early gestation sac. Coronal T2-weighted image showing low signal intensity gestation sac (arrow) and high signal intensity decidua (arrowheads). (B)-urinary bladder. (0.35T.)

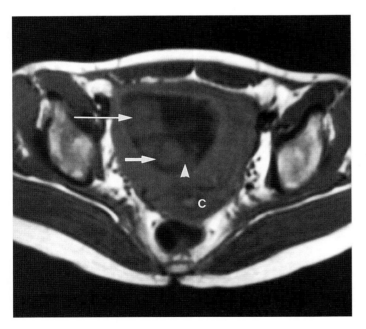

Figure 7.2

Fourteen week pregnancy. Transaxial T1-weighted image showing the fetal head (long arrow), trunk (short arrow), and lower limb (arrowhead). (C)-cervix. (0.35T.)

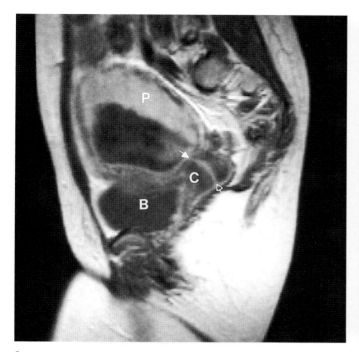

a

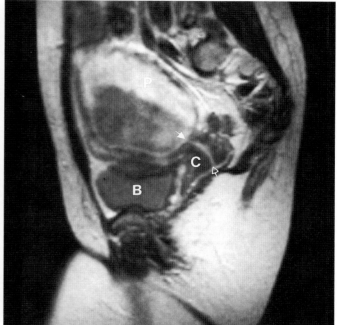

b

Figure 7.3

Visualization of the cervix in the pregnant uterus. Sagittal (**a**) proton density and (**b**) T2-weighted images showing the cervix (C) with visualization of both the internal os (white arrows) and external os (open arrows). The placenta (P) is clearly separated from the internal os. (B)-urinary bladder. (0.35T.)

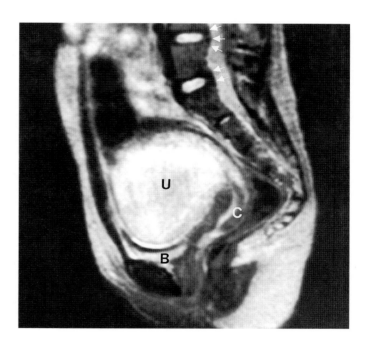

Figure 7.4

Vertebral disc changes in pregnancy. Sagittal T2-weighted image illustrating localized bulging of the annulus fibrosis (small arrows) at L4–5 and to a lesser extent at L5–S1. (B)-urinary bladder; (U)-uterus; (C)-cervix.

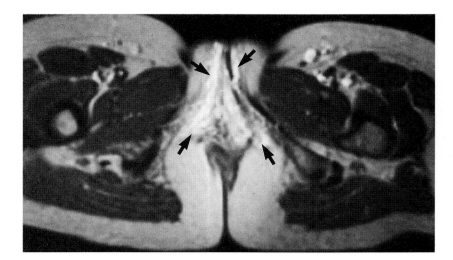

Figure 7.5

Vulvar varicosities in pregnancy. Transaxial T2-weighted image showing multiple tortuous high signal intensity vulvar varicosities (arrows) which demonstrate high signal intensity due to slow flow.

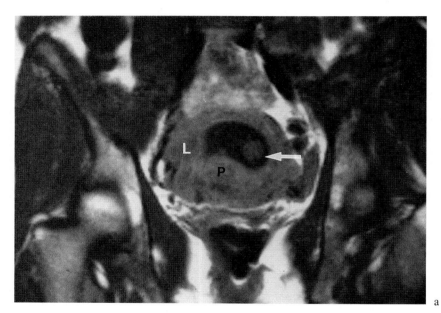

a

Figure 7.6

The placenta in twelve week pregnancy. Coronal (**a**) proton density and (**b**) T2-weighted images depicting the placenta (P) which is of medium signal intensity on the proton density image and increases in signal intensity on the T2-weighted image. The fetal pole (arrow) is identified. (L)-intramural leiomyoma.

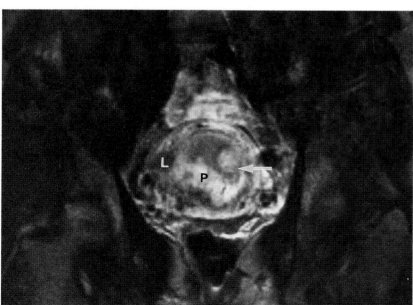

b

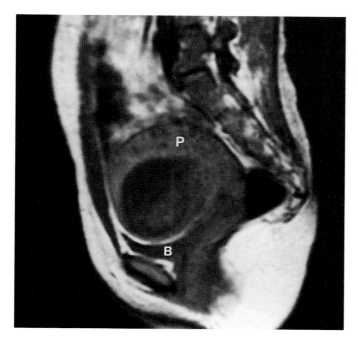

a

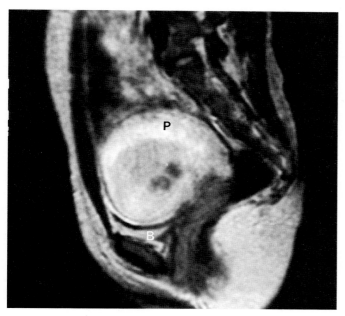

b

Figure 7.7

Normal placenta on MRI. Sagittal (**a**) T1- and (**b**) T2-weighted images demonstrating the placenta (P) in a posterior position. Placental tissue is of medium signal intensity on T1-weighted images and high signal intensity on T2-weighted images. (B)-urinary bladder.

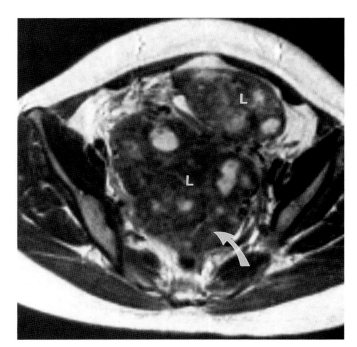

a

Figure 7.8

Multiple intramural leiomyomata and nine week pregnancy. (**a**) Transaxial T2-weighted image and sagittal (**b**) proton density and (**c**) T2-weighted images. There are multiple well defined degenerative leiomyomata (L), the largest of which (curved arrow) had grown rapidly and was felt clinically to represent an adnexal mass. The fetal pole (arrowhead) is identified within the lower signal intensity gestation sac. (D)-decidua. (0.35T.)

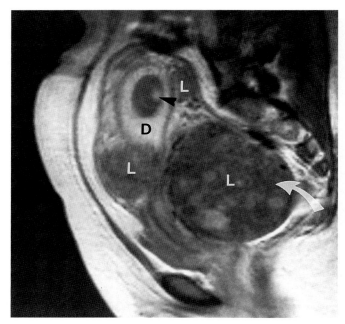

b

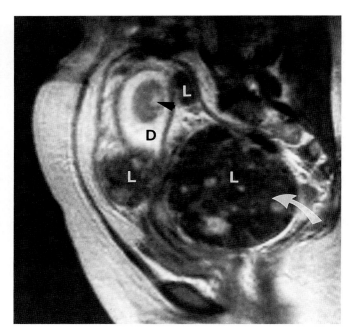

c

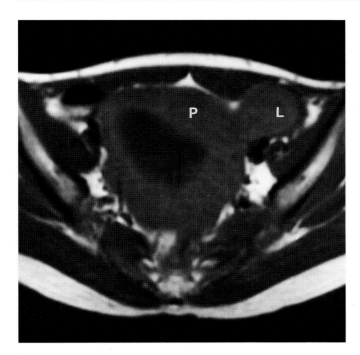

a

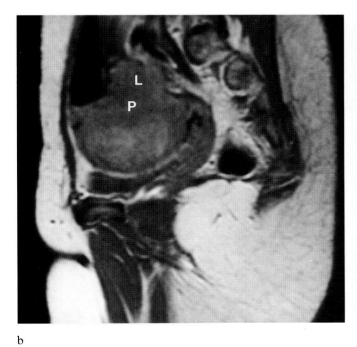

b

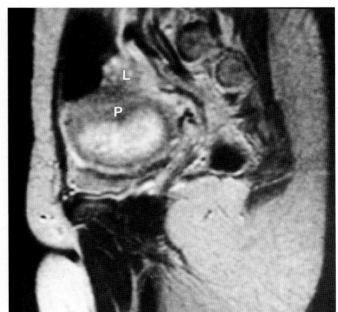

c

Figure 7.9

Subserosal leiomyoma. (**a**) Transaxial T1-weighted image and sagittal (**b**) proton density and (**c**) T2-weighted images. The subserosal degenerative leiomyoma (L) is of medium signal intensity on the T1-weighted image and high signal intensity on the T2-weighted image. (P)-placenta.

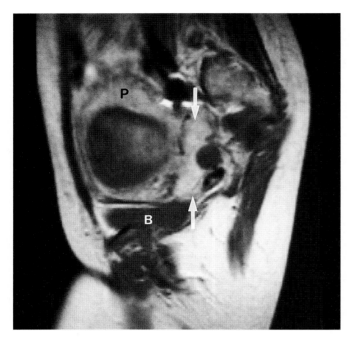

a

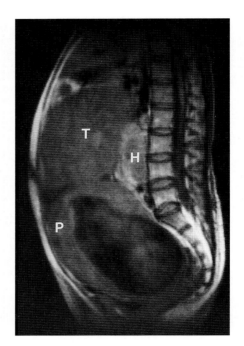

a

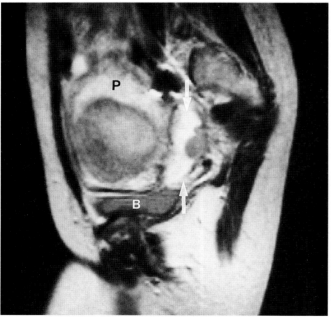

b

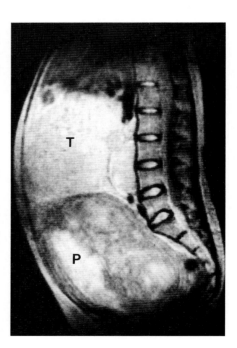

b

Figure 7.10

Adnexal ovarian cyst in pregnant patient. Sagittal (**a**) proton density and (**b**) T2-weighted images showing a complex adnexal cyst (arrows). (P)-placenta; (B)-urinary bladder. (0.35T.)

Figure 7.11

Intra-abdominal tumor mass in pregnant patient. Sagittal (**a**) proton density and (**b**) T2-weighted images illustrating that the large tumor (T) is separate from the gravid uterus and that there is hydronephrosis (H) of the kidney. (P)-placenta. (0.35T.)

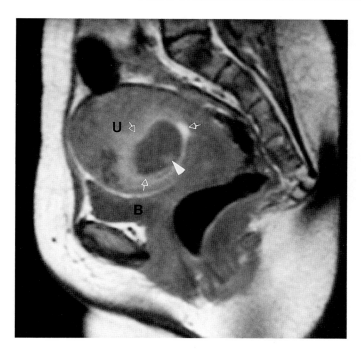

a

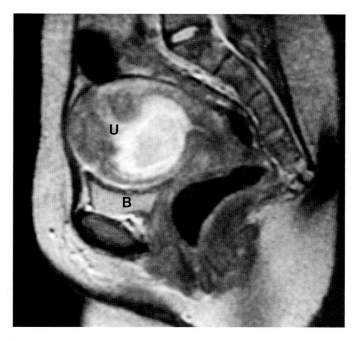

b

Figure 7.12

Threatened abortion. Sagittal (**a**) proton density and (**b**) T2-weighted images showing an enlarged uterus (U) containing a gestation sac with a fetal pole (arrowhead). There is high signal intensity around the gestation sac (arrows) on both images, consistent with hemorrhage. (B)-urinary bladder.

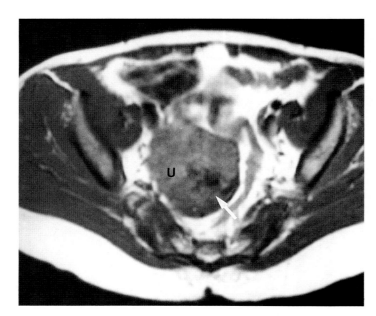

a

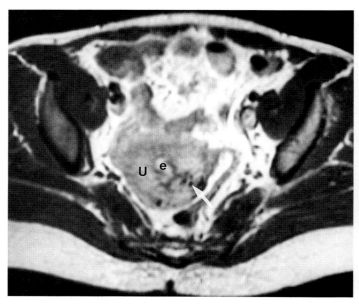

b

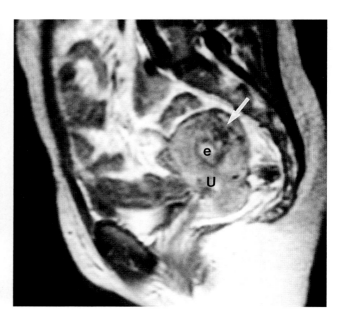

c

Figure 7.13

Uterus after spontaneous abortion. Transaxial (**a**) T1- and (**b**) T2-weighted images and (**c**) sagittal T2-weighted image. The uterus (U) is bulky, with a slightly expanded endometrial cavity (e). The site of prior placental implantation is seen (arrows) as an area of multiple low signal intensity foci consistent with dilated myometrial blood vessels.

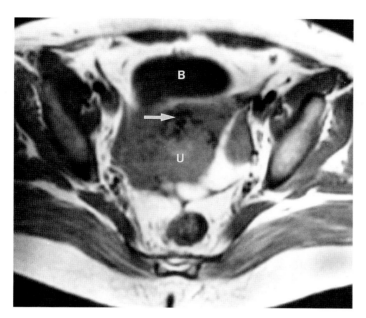

a

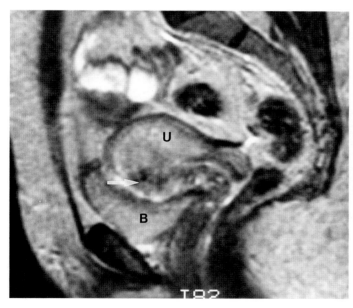

b

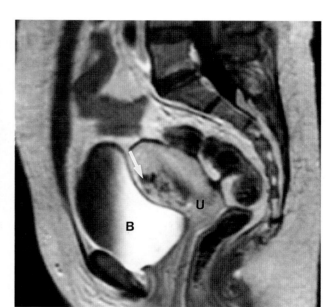

c

Figure 7.14

Recent abortion and endometritis. (**a**) Transaxial T1-weighted image and sagittal (**b**) T2-weighted and (**c**) Gd-DTPA-enhanced T1-weighted images. The implantation site of the placenta is identified as low signal intensity foci within the myometrium (arrows). The uterus (U) shows loss of zonal anatomy on both T2- and gadolinium T1-weighted images with enhancement of the myometrium after gadolinium. (B)-urinary bladder.

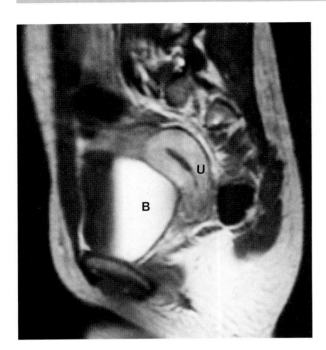

Figure 7.15

Endometritis. Sagittal T1-weighted Gd-DTPA-enhanced image displaying marked enhancement of the uterus (U) with loss of the normal zonal anatomy. (B)-urinary bladder.

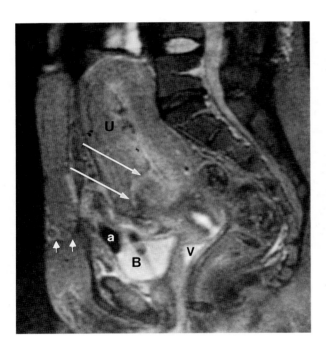

Figure 7.16

Post-Caesarian section endometritis. Sagittal T2-weighted image demonstrating an enlarged uterus (U) with medium to high signal intensity throughout its wall. The lower uterine segment scar is visible (arrows) as is the site of the abdominal wall incision (small arrows). There is air (a) within the bladder (B) after a Foley catheter insertion, and high signal intensity fluid in the endocervical canal and vaginal vault (V).

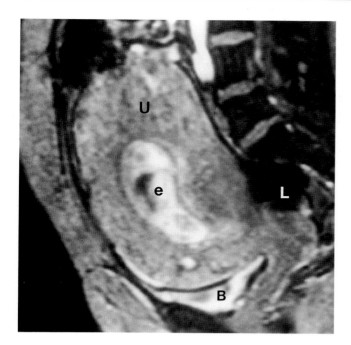

Figure 7.17

Postpartum endometritis. Sagittal T2-weighted image showing a postpartum uterus (U) with abnormal uniform high signal intensity throughout the wall. The endometrial cavity contents (e) are heterogeneous and could represent hemorrhage or retained products. (B)-urinary bladder; (L)-calcified leiomyoma.

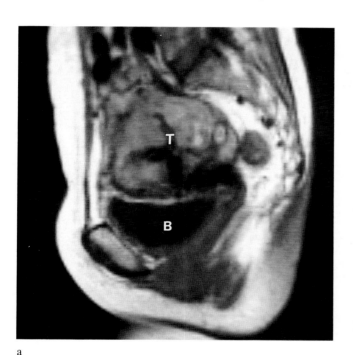

a

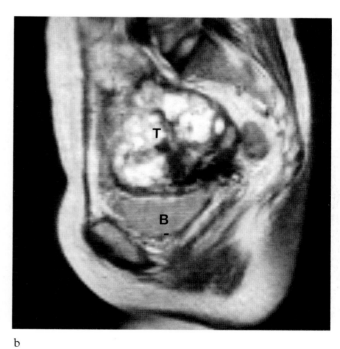

b

Figure 7.18

Gestational trophoblastic disease. Sagittal (**a**) T1- and (**b**) T2-weighted images demonstrating a predominantly medium signal intensity mass on the T1-weighted image (T) which becomes of heterogeneous high signal intensity on the T2-weighted image. (B)-urinary bladder. (0.35T.)

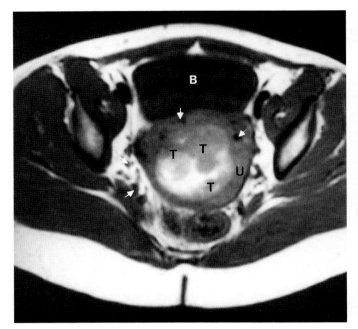

a

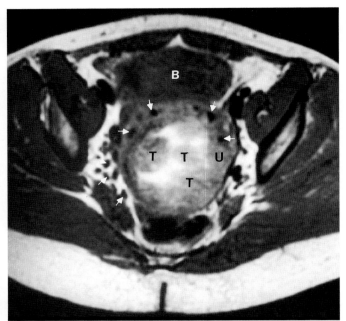

b

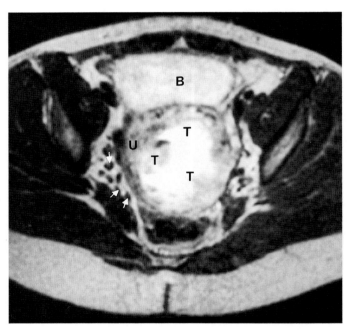

c

Figure 7.19

Gestational trophoblastic neoplasia. Transaxial (**a**) T1-weighted, (**b**) proton density and (**c**) T2-weighted images showing an expanded uterus (U) filled by tumor (T). The tumor is heterogeneous on all sequences and has high signal intensity on the T1-weighted images consistent with hemorrhage. The uterine zonal anatomy is obliterated and the tumor/myometrial interface is indistinct. Multiple engorged blood vessels (small arrows) are seen in the myometrium and adnexae. (B)-urinary bladder.

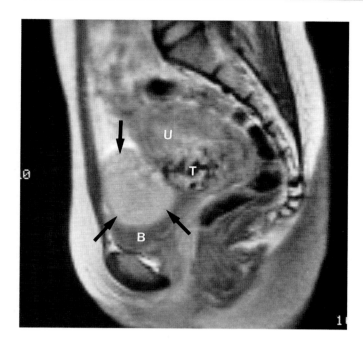

Figure 7.20

Gestational trophoblastic disease with theca lutein cyst. Sagittal proton density image showing a vascular trophoblastic tumor (T) in the anteroinferior uterus (U). There is a rounded high signal intensity ovarian cyst (arrows) above the bladder (B).

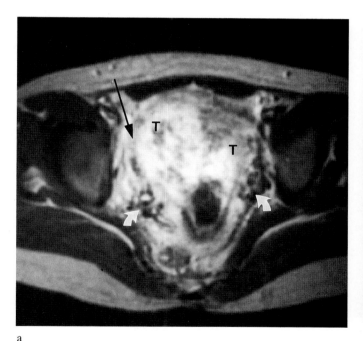

a

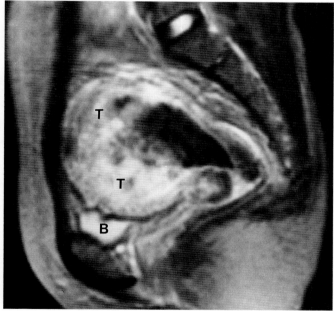

b

Figure 7.21

Gestational trophoblastic disease with transmyometrial extension. (**a**) Transaxial and (**b**) sagittal T2-weighted images illustrating complete penetration through the uterine fundus (arrow) by a large trophoblastic tumor (T). Pelvic hypervascularity is noted (curved arrows). (B)-urinary bladder.

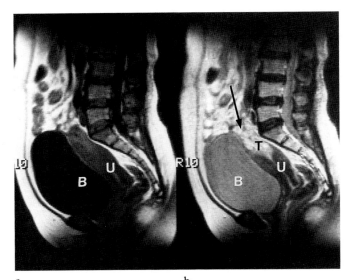

a   b

Figure 7.22

Gestational trophoblastic neoplasia with extension through the myometrium. Sagittal (**a**) T1- and (**b**) T2-weighted images showing a fundal tumor (T) penetrating through the entire myometrium (arrow). (U)-uterus; (B)-urinary bladder. (0.35T.)

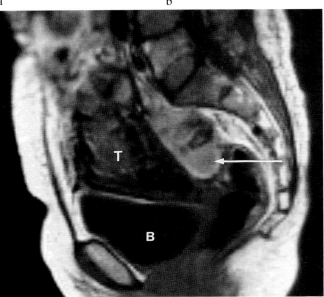

a

Figure 7.23

Gestational trophoblastic neoplasia before and after chemotherapy. Sagittal (**a**) T1-, (**b**) T2-weighted images pretreatment and (**c**) proton density image after chemotherapy. The vascular tumor mass (T) involves the entire uterus and there is a hemorrhagic theca lutein cyst (arrows). After chemotherapy there is a normal uterus (U) with visualization of the uterine zonal anatomy. (B)-urinary bladder; (asterisk)-fluid in the cul-de-sac. (0.35T.)

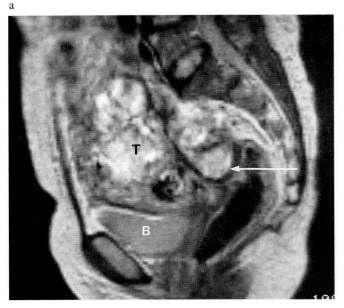

b

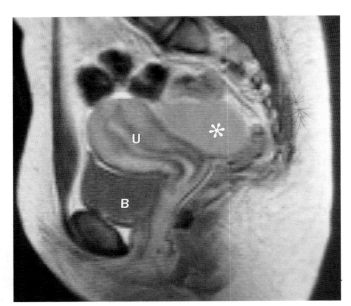

c

8

The Prostate Gland

Hedvig Hricak

The ability to evaluate prostate anatomy and to depict intraprostatic disease has markedly improved with the advent of cross-sectional imaging modalities, such as transrectal ultrasound (TRUS), CT, and MRI. Conventional radiologic techniques—intravenous urogram (IVU), voiding cystourethrogram (VCUG), and retrograde urethrogram—depend on evidence of prostate enlargement or contour distortion to identify prostatic pathology, and thus have a very limited role in the evaluation of prostatic disease. The cross-sectional techniques provide better anatomic evaluation and permit direct visualization of prostate disease.

For benign prostatic disease, TRUS is considered the primary imaging modality. In the evaluation of prostatic malignancy, the relative merits of the cross-sectional imaging modalities are presently being assessed. The undisputed advantages of MRI include excellent tissue contrast, large field-of-view and direct multiplanar imaging allowing detailed evaluation of the prostate.

Normal anatomy of the prostate gland

The prostate is an exocrine gland composed of both glandular and nonglandular tissue. It develops primarily from the mesenchyme of the urogenital sinus, but also contains tissue from both wolffian and müllerian duct origin.[1] In utero, the prostate has five lobular divisions—an anterior lobe, a middle or median lobe, a posterior lobe, and two lateral lobes. The anterior and posterior lobes atrophy during late fetal life (twenty weeks and later). Historically the adult prostate was described as consisting of two lateral lobes and the median lobe.[1] This lobar anatomical description is incorrect in the adult gland and should be applied only

to the anatomy of the fetal gland.[2] The misconception of lobar divisions was caused by the original description by Lowsley, whose anatomic division of an adult gland was based on fetal gland sections.[3] After birth, the prostate decreases in size over the first two months of life and shows no significant change in size (childhood resting phase) until puberty. During the pubertal differentiation phase which lasts six to twelve months, the gland almost doubles in size.[1]

In the mature prostate gland, the lobes have fused and the prostate is composed of glandular and nonglandular tissue. The glandular tissue is divided into three major zones—the peripheral (70 per cent), the central (25 per cent), and the transition (5 per cent) zone.[2] There is also a small area of glandular tissue composed of periurethral glands. Distinction of the prostate glandular zones has clinical significance because the majority of prostate carcinomas (68 per cent) originate in the peripheral zone, whereas only 32 per cent arise in the transition and central zones.[4] Benign nodular hyperplasia, however, usually originates in the transition zone and the periurethral glands.[2] Nonglandular elements of the prostate include the anterior fibromuscular band and the urethra.

Relations of the prostate

The base of the prostate abuts the base of the urinary bladder, and the apex is in contact with the external urethral sphincter, which forms part of the urogenital diaphragm (Figure 8.1). As illustrated in Figure 8.2, the symphysis pubis lies ventral to the prostate, and the two are separated by the retropubic space. The retropubic space is composed of loose aerolar tissue, a rich prostatic venous plexus (plexus of Santorini) and the puboprostatic ligament. The rectum is dorsal to the prostate and is separated from it by Denonvilliers' fascia.[5] The levator ani muscles lie lateral to the prostate, as shown in Figure 8.3.

Vascular supply

The prostate is supplied primarily via the branches of the internal iliac arteries (the obturator, umbilical, and superior and inferior vesical arteries) and a third of its blood supply is from the inferior mesenteric artery via the superior and middle rectal arteries. The arterial supply to the prostate can be divided into two major groups—capsular parenchymal branches with arterial anastomosis, and periurethral branches.[1]

The prostate is drained by the large caliber veins of the vesicoprostatic plexus (also called the periprostatic venous plexus) located lateroposteriorly to the gland (Figure 8.4).[5] The vesicoprostatic plexus communicates with the internal iliac vein and the venous network which lies on the sacrum. This presacral venous plexus communicates with veins in the anterior sacral foramina and with the veins of the sacral canal. The latter play an important role in the blood-borne metastasis of prostatic carcinoma.

Lymphatic drainage

The lymphatic drainage of the prostate accompanies the neurovascular bundle of the bladder, but can also be seen running along the ductus deferens. The regional nodes of the prostate gland include the obturator lymph nodes, internal iliac lymph nodes, external iliac lymph nodes, and common iliac lymph nodes.[1,6] The paraaortic nodes, the inguinal nodes and the presacral nodes are considered juxtaregional nodes, and are involved later in the course of the disease.[6]

MRI appearance of the prostate

On T1-weighted images, regardless of field of strength or patient age, the prostate demonstrates a homogeneous signal of intermediate intensity, and the zones cannot be differentiated. As seen in Figure 8.5, the neonatal prostate shows differentiation between the urethra and the glandular tissue, but zonal anatomy is not seen. The prepubertal gland is small, with a paucity of glandular tissue and a relative increase in periurethral glandular tissue, as shown in Figure 8.6. Zonal differentiation is not present. In an adult, on T2-weighted images, the **zonal anatomy** is well demonstrated, as seen in Figure 8.7. The signal intensity of the peripheral zone increases and is equal to or greater than that of adjacent adipose tissue. The central zone has a lower signal intensity than the surrounding peripheral zone (Figure 8.8).[7–9] It is postulated that the compact striated muscle and fewer glandular elements within the central zone result in a T2-shortening effect and account for the lower signal intensity.[5,7] The transition zone also has a lower signal intensity than the peripheral zone (Figures 8.7, 8.8). Although the transition zone glands are identical to the peripheral zone glands histologically, they are less numerous and are surrounded by a more dense stroma.[5] These two features result in shortening of T2 values and a lower signal intensity on T2-weighted images. The signal intensity of the transition zone is similar to that of the central zone, and the two can be differentiated only by knowledge of their respective anatomic locations (Figure 8.8c).[7] As seen in Figure 8.9, the central zone is most commonly conical in shape with its apex at the verumontanum and base extending posteriorly to the base of the gland.[2] Variations of the shape and the volume of the central zone in young males, however, do exist (Figure 8.10). The transition zone has a horseshoe configuration (Figure 8.7), and is located lateral to the periurethral glands extending from the verumontanum to the bladder neck (Figure 8.8b). Although the transition zone has a uniformly low signal intensity in young subjects, it becomes heterogeneous with development of benign prostatic hyperplasia (BPH).[7] Hyperplastic changes in the periurethral glands cause midline enlargement and elevation of the bladder base.

The nonglandular tissue of the **anterior fibromuscular band** (shown in Figures 8.7 and 8.8c) covers the anterolateral surface of the prostate and demonstrates low signal intensity on both T1- and T2-weighted images.[7] This allows distinction between the prostate and the anterior vascular aerolar tissue within the preprostatic space.

The **urethra** can be used as a key reference point for the prostate. The proximal portion of the urethra extends from the bladder neck through the anterior third of the prostate, to the base of the verumontanum. It is in contact with the periurethral glands laterally and the preprostatic sphincter anteriorly. This part of the urethra is rarely visualized on MRI scans unless a Foley catheter has been placed, or there is dilatation of the urethra due to previous resection of benign prostatic hyperplasia. At the level of the base of the verumontanum, the urethra forms an anterior angle of 35°. The distal prostatic urethra extends from the base of the verumontanum to the apex of the prostate. The **verumontanum** is therefore located in the distal prostatic urethra and is often visualized on MRI scans demonstrating high signal intensity on T2-weighted images as shown in Figure 8.9. Below the level of the verumontanum, the distal prostatic urethra has an additional muscle layer surrounding it.[2,5] On T2-

weighted images, the distal prostatic urethra is visualized as a low signal intensity ring within the peripheral zone. The muscle fibers of the distal urethra radiate laterally and posteriorly into the peripheral zone of the prostate gland and anteriorly into the fibromuscular band.

The appearance of the prostate gland has been described mostly using conventional spin-echo images. Fat saturation spin-echo sequences can also be used. As illustrated in Figure 8.11, the visualization of zonal anatomy is similar to conventional spin-echo sequences, but due to decreased noise, the zonal anatomy can be appreciated even on proton density images. On T2-weighted fat saturation images, the contrast between the high signal intensity peripheral zone and low signal intensity periprostatic fat is excellent, but the structures within the periprostatic fat, such as the neurovascular bundles, are better seen on conventional than on fat saturation images. Unless specified, the remainder of the chapter will refer to conventional spin-echo images only.

The appearance of the prostate following Gd-DTPA injection has not been described in detail. The degree of enhancement is variable and related to age and the time interval between injection and scanning. On early scans enhancement can be seen in the periurethral region as demonstrated in Figure 8.12. On late scans, the gland enhances homogeneously. Because of the variability in glandular appearance, the use of Gd-DTPA has not been advocated routinely.

The relationship of the different zones of the prostate gland changes with age. The volume of the central zone is greatest in the young individual, but with advancing age there is progressive atrophy.[2] In contrast, the transition zone frequently enlarges with age due to BPH. With the development of BPH there is often a low signal intensity stripe at the margin between the transition and the peripheral zone. This represents a **surgical pseudocapsule.** The low intensity is due to compressed/compacted peripheral zone tissue. In addition to the surgical pseudocapsule, there is also a **prostatic capsule** proper. It is approximately 1 mm thick, consists of fibromuscular tissue, and closely invests the glandular tissue of the peripheral zone.[1,2,5] As depicted in Figure 8.13, on T2-weighted images, both the surgical pseudocapsule at the transition/peripheral zone interface and the anatomic capsule at the interface between the peripheral zone and adjacent adipose tissue can be visualized. The prostate is also enveloped by **visceral fascia** which covers the gland with the exception of the ventral surface, apex and the base.[1] The fascia, which is only rarely seen on MRI, appears as a low intensity line on T1-weighted images.

The ability of MR to provide multiplanar imaging allows accurate **volumetric measurement** of the enlarged gland.[10] Because the specific gravity of the prostatic tissue is 1.022, the volume measurements of the prostate can be transferred into grams.[1] The formula for volume measurements ($V = L \times AP \times W \times 0.5$ where L = length, AP = anteroposterior, W = width) is accepted and gives accurate, clinically useful, volumetric measurements.[10]

Suggested imaging sequences

Both T1- and T2-weighted images are needed to evaluate the prostate gland. T1-weighted images are important for tissue characterization (eg, diagnosis of prostatic cyst, abscess, and postbiopsy changes) and are essential in the assessment of periprostatic tumor extension. T2-weighted images allow demonstration of zonal anatomy and depiction of intraprostatic disease. T2-weighted images in two planes of imaging are advocated, one of which should be transaxial. Fat suppression images, because of the high signal-to-noise ratio, are suggested when the quality of conventional spin-echo sequences is suboptimal.

MR offers direct imaging in three orthogonal planes, and each plane has advantages and limitations. Due to the complexity of the prostate zonal anatomy, MRI scans and accompanying serial drawings in the transaxial and sagittal planes are shown. Imaging in the transverse plane allows evaluation of all zonal architecture. As illustrated in Figure 8.14, differentiation between the peripheral and transition zones is best demonstrated in the transverse plane.[3] However, in the transverse plane of imaging, the difficulties may arise in depiction of the central zone at the base of the prostate. The normal central zone demonstrates low signal intensity (Figures 8.14d and 8.15) and this should not be mistaken for prostatic pathology in that location. Another important anatomical landmark is the depiction of the interface between the apex of the prostate and the membranous urethra (Figure 8.16). Tumor extension in this area is of utmost importance as tumor resection is no longer possible. The transverse plane also complements other planes in the demonstration of its relationship to the seminal vesicles, the levator ani and obturator internus muscles, and in depiction of the relationship of the prostate gland to the rectum.

As depicted in Figure 8.17, the sagittal plane is optimal for assessing the relationship between the prostate, bladder base, seminal vesicles and rectum. The coronal plane is complementary in the evaluation of the seminal vesicles as well as the symmetry of the levator ani muscles (Figure 8.18). Differentiation between the peripheral and central zones is best seen in the coronal plane (Figure 8.9).

Pathology of the prostate gland

Congenital anomalies

Congenital anomalies of the prostate—**agenesis** and **hypoplasia**—are frequently associated with other anomalies of the urogenital system. Congenital hypoplasia is most often due to a mesenchymal defect and is often seen in conjunction with prune belly syndrome.[11] Rarely, hypoplasia may be due to in utero distal urethral obstruction.[11]

Congenital cystic anomalies of the prostate

Congenital prostatic cysts are rare and are usually found in middle-aged adults. These cysts may be caused by failure of communication between wolffian ducts and the vesicourethral anlage and occur to either side of the midline. Prostatic utricle cysts and müllerian duct cysts may result from abnormal regression of the müllerian system. Their mechanisms of occurrence may be different. Prostatic utricle cysts are associated with other genital anomalies (such as hypospadias, ambiguous genitalia, undescended testis, or congenital urethral polyp), and are thought to be due to a lack of 5-alpha-reductase in utero. The müllerian duct cyst is not associated with anomalies of the external genitalia, and is caused by blockage of the ducts and acini that arise from the sinoutricular plate.[12] However, imaging findings for both are similar, and the distinction between the two may be arbitrary.

Because it is associated with other genital abnormalities, the prostatic utricle cyst is often discovered in childhood. Clinical symptoms are rare, but persistent infection or stones may develop. Depending on the clinical symptoms, the utricle is usually excised if intervention is needed. The müllerian duct cyst, however, is usually discovered in adulthood as a consequence of clinical symptoms. The symptoms most commonly mimic those of benign prostatic hyperplasia, including complaints of frequency and decrease in the urinary stream. Acute urinary retention due to large müllerian cysts has been reported. Although a midline mass may be palpated clinically, it is often difficult to make a definitive clinical diagnosis. Stones have been reported within these cysts, as has an increased incidence of squamous cell and adenocarcinoma. Treatment is by surgical removal, but often the large size of the müllerian duct cyst makes surgery difficult.

Other prostatic cysts are acquired and are more commonly the result of inflammation, trauma, or retention.

MRI appearance

Prostatic **agenesis** is diagnosed when the only tissue recognized anterior to the rectum is the urethra, often with a thickened periurethral muscle. Prostatic hypoplasia is a difficult diagnosis before puberty as the normal prepubertal gland is very small. An abnormally developed prostate gland is often found in association with other congenital anomalies as seen in Figure 8.19. In an adult (Figure 8.20), a gland of less than 4 gm is considered hypoplastic. On MRI, in addition to small size, zonal anatomy as seen in Figure 8.10 is distorted.

Prostatic cysts are well depicted on MR images, and their location (such as the typical midline location of a prostatic utricle as shown in Figure 8.21, or a müllerian duct cyst as shown in Figure 8.22) is well displayed.[13] Multiplanar imaging allows precise cyst location, helping to differentiate between midline müllerian duct cysts, prostatic parenchymal cysts, and cysts of the seminal vesicles. The signal intensity of a cyst is nonspecific and depends on its fluid content.[13,14] Cysts filled with serous fluid, similar to urine, image with a low signal intensity on T1-weighted images and increase in signal intensity on T2-weighted images. When cysts become infected or hemorrhagic as seen in Figures 8.22 and 8.23, they demonstrate a range of signal intensity on both T1- and T2-weighted images.[13]

MRI in relation to other imaging modalities

An array of radiologic modalities has been applied to the diagnosis of congenital prostatic cysts, especially müllerian duct cysts. On intravenous urography (IVU), the findings are usually indistinguishable from benign enlargement of the prostate gland. Transrectal ultrasonography (TRUS) demonstrates a midline, pear-shaped cystic mass extending cephalad from the verumontanum. A müllerian duct cyst is also visible on CT scans.

The recommended approach to imaging is that transrectal ultrasound be used initially. If TRUS is nondiagnostic, MRI is the next preferred imaging method. However, in patients with complex congenital anomalies, or when a large cul-de-sac mass is felt clinically, MRI should be obtained as an initial examination. Such an example is shown in Figure 8.24, where clinical and US findings diagnosed a müllerian duct cyst, yet on MRI the lesion is seen to be separated from the prostate and is intraperitoneal in location. MRI findings assisted in the choice of surgical approach. At surgery, a mucocele of the appendix was found.

Infectious disease of the prostate

Inflammation of the prostate is customarily grouped into three categories—**bacterial prostatitis** (acute and chronic), **nonbacterial prostatitis**, and **prostadynia** (prostate pain without identifiable infection).[15]

Gram negative organisms (such as *Escherichia coli* and *Klebsiella*) are the most common organisms found in bacterial prostatitis. Gram positive organisms (such as enterococcus or staphylococcus) are found in approximately 5 per cent of cases.[16] Historically, it was thought that prostatitis affected the entire gland. However, recent studies demonstrate that prostatitis is most commonly caused by a local inflammatory process of the peripheral acinar glandular tissue. Symptoms and signs of acute prostatitis include: chills; fever; perineal and low back pain; pain with defecation or after ejaculation; urethral discharge; and decreased size and force of urinary stream associated with dysuria, urgency, frequency, or retention. On clinical examination, the prostate gland is swollen, boggy and tender. Analysis of the expressed prostate secretion is helpful in determining the type of prostatitis.

The clinical symptoms of a **prostatic abscess** are similar to those of acute prostatitis.[17] A prostatic abscess is usually secondary to prostatitis, but rarely it may develop as a result of hematogenous spread.[17] The prostate is usually diffusely enlarged and may have fluctuant tender areas on palpation. If untreated, a prostate abscess may rupture into the urethra, the rectum, the perineum, or, less frequently, into the peritoneum, producing an array of findings.[17]

Unless there is an abscess requiring drainage, the treatment of prostatitis is usually conservative.

MRI appearance

In **acute prostatitis** MR imaging demonstrates the enlarged gland. On T1-weighted images, the peripheral zone may demonstrate normal signal intensity, or as illustrated in Figure 8.25, it may be of lower signal intensity than the adjacent transition zone.[18] On T2-weighted images, the area of prostatitis exhibits high signal intensity and, except for the finding of enlargement, it is difficult to differentiate from the normal peripheral zone. Associated periprostatic fat infiltration and acute inflammatory disease extending to the seminal vesicles are often identified.[18] Prostatitis secondary to long-term Foley catheter placement is identified as a halo of high signal intensity in the periurethral glandular tissue on T2-weighted images (Figures 8.26 and 8.27). Following intravenous gadolinium-DTPA, the area of inflammation shows diffuse increase in signal intensity as seen in Figure 8.27c.

Little information is available on the MRI appearance of **prostatic abscess**.[18,19] On T1-weighted images the findings may be limited to localized enlargement with or without a decrease in signal intensity. The periprostatic fat tissue is usually obliterated. On T2-weighted images the abscess exhibits high signal intensity, often higher than the adjacent peripheral zone (Figure 8.28). The margin between the abscess and the unaffected gland is also often indistinct.[18]

MRI in relation to other imaging modalities

Prostatitis is usually a clinical diagnosis and radiologic evaluation is requested only in difficult cases. Either transrectal ultrasound, CT or MRI can be used.[18,19] Transrectal ultrasound is considered the easiest, highly diagnostic modality and is the initial procedure of choice. It demonstrates ill-defined diffuse hypoechoic areas within the peripheral zone.

More frequently, radiologic evaluation is requested to confirm a prostatic abscess. In these cases, CT is the procedure of choice, and the liquified portion within the inflammatory gland is characteristically demonstrated on CT scans,[20] as depicted in Figure 8.29. When abscess drainage is requested, however, transrectal ultrasound is the recommended approach.

MRI can be used in the evaluation of prostatitis or prostate abscess, but at present does not demonstrate any advantages over ultrasound or CT.

Prostatic calcifications

Prostatic calculi are most commonly seen in the fifth to seventh decade of life and are very rarely found in children. True (primary) prostatic calculi develop in the acini and the ducts of the prostate gland. They differ from urinary calculi which lodge in the prostatic urethra and form secondary dystrophic calculi.[21] Primary calculi are usually multiple and small, varying in size from 1–5 mm. They are rarely symptomatic, although they may pass into the more centrally located prostatic ducts and empty into the urethra on either side of the verumontanum.

Secondary dystrophic calculi are associated with infection, obstruction, necrosis in a prostatic adenoma, or radiation therapy.[21] Dystrophic calcifications are usually larger and more irregular in outline than primary calculi, and severe, symptomatic prostatic calcification has been reported in patients with prostatic cancer receiving radiation therapy. It needs to be emphasized that dystrophic prostatic calculi are not precancerous. Although they have been reported in conjunction with carcinoma, they are neither caused by nor the result of that malignancy.

MRI appearance

Prostatic calculi can be seen on both T1- and T2-weighted MR images as areas of signal void. The characteristic horseshoe configuration of primary prostatic calculi is shown in Figure 8.30. Because of increased noise on T2-weighted images, small calculi may be indistinct in appearance, showing low to medium signal intensity. The MRI finding of prostatic calculi is not specific.

MRI in relation to other imaging modalities

Radiologic examination of calculi is rarely requested, and they are usually an incidental finding. Radiographs of the pelvis demonstrate prostatic calculi in the majority of cases because the calculi most commonly contain calcium phosphate. On both suprapubic and transrectal ultrasound calculi demonstrate bright echogenic foci, which may or may not cause acoustic shadowing. The most sensitive modality for identification of prostate calcification is CT.

On plain films dystrophic calcifications are large, irregular, and may project a considerable distance above the symphysis pubis. In this case, further radiologic examination may be requested to identify their location in the prostate, seminal vesicles, or bladder. Ultrasound is recommended as the primary approach for making this evaluation.

Benign prostatic hyperplasia

Benign prostatic hyperplasia (BPH) is benign enlargement of the prostate gland, most commonly occurring in the transition zone.[2] Histologically, changes of BPH are due to glandular proliferation or, less commonly, proliferation of the interstitium.[2] Changes may be diffuse or focal, forming a prostatic adenoma. Pathological specimens showing an example of glandular (Figure 8.31), interstitial (Figure 8.32) and focal (adenomyoma) (Figure 8.33) BPH with accompanying MRI scans are shown. As illustrated in Figure 8.31, the benign hyperplastic tissue is separated from the often compressed peripheral zone by the surgical pseudocapsule.[2,5]

When BPH is caused predominantly by hyperplasia of the periurethral glands, the median part of the gland is enlarged, and the prostate elevates the bladder trigone. The subvesical (medial lobe) portion may protrude into the bladder (Figure 8.34).[2] Progressive

hypertrophy of the prostate, together with hyperplasia of the musculature of the trigone, gradually causes partial obstruction of the bladder outlet.

The clinical symptoms of BPH are mostly related to the effects of the enlarged gland on the urethra, causing narrowing, elongation, and compression at the bladder neck (Figure 8.35). Symptoms include urgency, frequency, and inability to empty the urinary bladder. Treatment is surgical using a transurethral, suprapubic transvesical, or retropubic extravesical approach.[1] A perineal approach has been used in the past for resection of prostatic adenoma.

MRI appearance

The varied MR appearance of BPH reflects its varying histologic composition.[22-27] Diffuse glandular hyperplasia demonstrates an enlarged prostate gland which images with a homogeneous low intensity signal on T1-weighted images and a homogeneous or heterogeneous medium to high intensity signal on T2-weighted images. As depicted in Figure 8.31, on T2-weighted images the surgical pseudocapsule can be seen at the interface between the transition and the peripheral zones as a low signal intensity stripe.

The predominantly interstitial form of hyperplasia (Figure 8.32) demonstrates glandular enlargement with heterogeneous but usually low signal intensity on T2-weighted images.[23] Infarction is common in this type of BPH, and, depending on the age of the infarct, various ill-defined signal intensities can be demonstrated. Due to the type of growth, interstitial BPH rarely demonstrates a surgical pseudocapsule on T2-weighted images.

In asymmetric nodular hyperplasia (adenoma), the main MRI feature is contour abnormality with nodular enlargement. The signal intensity of the nodules varies on T2-weighted images. An example of low signal intensity adenoma on a T2-weighted image is shown in Figure 8.33.

Following Gd-DTPA injection, various patterns of enhancement can be seen. The finding is not specific, but as seen in Figure 8.34, offers demonstration of zonal anatomy on T1-weighted images. In patients in whom only morphologic display is important and who are not able to cooperate and remain still for the T2-weighted images, Gd-DTPA-enhanced T1-weighted images can be used as an alternative. MRI is excellent for the demonstration of prostatic enlargement. The intravesicular portion of hyperplastic nodules is well displayed on MRI scans (Figure 8.35), and the effects of hypertrophy on the bladder neck can be demonstrated. Volumetric measurement can separately evaluate the degree of enlarged hyperplastic glandular tissue and the volume of the compressed peripheral zone.[10]

Evaluation of the gland following resection for BPH

can be performed. Benign hyperplastic changes involve the periurethral glands and the transition zone. Regardless of the type of surgery (TURP, suprapubic or retropubic prostatectomy) the periurethral tissue is removed and the proximal prostatic urethra expands to fill the defect. Surgical removal extends to the base of the verumontanum (which is the anatomical landmark for the caudal margin of the transition zone) and, as demonstrated in Figure 8.36, this results in a typical postsurgical conical (spinning top) appearance to the proximal urethra. In contrast to previous beliefs, often not all of the adenomatous tissue is removed. As illustrated in Figure 8.37, the residual hyperplastic tissue demonstrates heterogeneous medium to low signal intensity on T2-weighted images. Sometimes only a small volume of the tissue is removed in an asymmetrical fashion (Figure 8.38). When the transition zone is enlarged, it compresses the peripheral zone. As illustrated in Figure 8.39, the peripheral zone will expand following enucleation of the benign tissue.

MRI in relation to other imaging modalities

Clinical examination is often all that is needed for the evaluation of BPH. When radiologic assessment is requested, transrectal ultrasound is the modality of choice. At the same time, transabdominal ultrasound is recommended for evaluation of the kidneys, for assessment of residual bladder volume in suspected bladder outlet obstruction and for determination of prostate size. If the prostate is 50 gm or less, it is customarily removed through a transurethral approach. Open prostatectomy is required for larger glands. MRI is rarely requested for the evaluation of benign disease. It is used only in markedly enlarged glands when ultrasound is limited. It has been shown that there is no significant difference between MRI and US in the estimation of prostate size, where the gland is less than 100 gm but that MRI is superior to US in the assessment of glands greater than 100 gm. This difference reaches statistical significance when the prostate is greater than 150 gm (Figure 8.36). Although the morphologic features of BPH are well displayed on MRI scans, it is not possible to differentiate benign from malignant prostatic disease.[23,24]

Prostatic malignancies

More than 95 per cent of prostatic malignancies are adenocarcinomas.[4] Rarely, a squamous or transitional cell neoplasm is found and very rarely, a sarcoma (0.2–0.5 per cent).[2]

Carcinoma of the prostate (PCa) is the most common human cancer. It is found at autopsy in 30 per cent of men at 50 years of age and in almost 90 per cent at 90 years of age.[28,29] Unlike lung and colon cancer, prostatic cancer is predominantly latent. Even so, approximately 100 000 new cases are diagnosed a year.[28] It is the third most common cause of cancer death in American men over 55 years of age, and it becomes the second leading cause of cancer death in men after 75 years of age.[29] Although the malignant potential in PCa generally correlates with histologic grade, tumor volume, and stage, exceptions do exist and many aspects of the pathobiology of PCa are not understood at present.[28,30] Thus, controversy persists regarding the diagnosis and preferred treatment options.[28,30–32]

Carcinoma of the prostate usually begins in the peripheral zone, often as an adenocarcinoma with varying grades of differentiation (68 per cent of prostate carcinomas originate in the peripheral zone, 24 per cent in the transition zone, and 8 per cent in the central zone). Carcinomas located in the transition zone are most commonly found incidentally during open enucleation or transurethral resection for presumed benign disease[30,31] and foci of carcinoma are found in the prostatic tissue removed in approximately 10 per cent of patients undergoing surgery for benign disease.[30,31]

The accepted approach to diagnosis of PCa is rectal examination followed by biopsy of suspicious lesions. The efficacy of transrectal ultrasound as a screening tool is a controversial topic, at present not resolved.[33] Similarly, prostate-specific antigen (PSA) has received much publicity as a tissue tumor marker, but its true value remains controversial.[34] Although neither transrectal ultrasound nor PSA have proven acceptable for widespread screening, their use in the high risk patient population appears to be justified.

Once prostate carcinoma is histologically diagnosed, accurate staging is essential for selecting the best possible mode of therapy.[32] When carcinoma is confined to the prostate gland, it is theoretically curable by surgical removal of the entire prostate gland and seminal vesicles (radical prostatectomy). However, if the tumor has spread beyond the gland, radiation therapy is generally recommended. Clinical staging by digital rectal examination is subjective and hard to record accurately. It is estimated that understaging occurs in as many as 56 per cent of patients thought clinically to have localized disease.[35] Radiologic examination can be helpful for both local tumor staging as well as evaluation of nodal or distant metastasis.

MRI appearance

The appearance and detection of PCa depend on the location of the tumor and the type of MR imaging sequence used.[28,36–41]

The MRI **appearance** of prostate carcinoma demonstrates different signal intensity patterns. On T1-weighted images, prostate carcinoma may demonstrate a signal intensity similar to or lower than adjacent prostatic tissue (Figure 8.40). As illustrated in Figure 8.40, on T2-weighted images, prostatic carcinoma most commonly demonstrates decreased signal intensity, as compared with the high signal intensity of the normal peripheral zone.[36–41] Rarely, high signal intensity tumors (higher than the surrounding peripheral zone) can be seen.[36–38] Only tumors located in the peripheral zone can be detected on MRI scans.[39–41] The normal heterogeneous signal intensity of the transition zone precludes detection of tumors in this location, since both tumor and changes of BPH can exhibit similar low signal intensity (Figure 8.41).[41] Similar to the appearance in the peripheral zone, high signal intensity tumors can be seen in the transition zone as well (Figure 8.42). Following Gd-DTPA injection, various appearances of prostate carcinoma have been reported, depending on the time interval between injection and imaging. In the early postinjection period, a tumor may exhibit more enhancement than the adjacent peripheral zone, but on more delayed scans, the signal intensity of the tumor becomes similar to the adjacent prostatic tissue (Figure 8.43). Just as MRI cannot differentiate between benign and malignant prostate pathology (Figure 8.44), so it cannot distinguish between the different histologic subtypes of prostate malignancies. Prostatic sarcoma as seen in Figure 8.45 shows nonspecific diffuse prostatic enlargement of heterogeneous signal intensity.

Tumor detection can be hampered by postbiopsy changes. The appearance of **postbiopsy changes** in the gland is related to the time interval between the biopsy and MR examination.[39,41] Hemorrhage is a common consequence of biopsy and has variable MRI appearances. In the immediate postbiopsy period, the biopsy site may demonstrate low signal intensity on T1-weighted images and high signal intensity on T2-weighted images. As shown in Figure 8.46, after approximately seven days, due to the presence of extracellular methemoglobin (subacute hemorrhage), high signal intensity is seen on both T1- and T2-weighted images. Postbiopsy changes demonstrating high signal intensity on T1-weighted images and low signal intensity on T2-weighted images (intracellular deoxy- or methemoglobin) have also been reported. Occasionally, hemorrhage can be visualized along the needle track (Figure 8.47), or hemorrhage can involve a large portion of the gland (Figure 8.48). In addition to postbiopsy hemorrhage, interstitial edema may be present. In these cases, the biopsy area images with low signal intensity on T1-weighted images and high signal intensity on T2-weighted images (Figure 8.49). Postbiopsy hemorrhage may also result in a peri-prostatic hematoma, identifiable on MRI. In this situation clinical examination is limited and cannot differentiate between hematoma and periprostatic tumor extension, making MRI study a very valuable adjunct (Figure 8.50).

Attempts have been made to measure tumor volume by MRI. Because of inconsistency in tumor visualization and a wide range of postbiopsy changes, both overestimation and underestimation of tumor volume may occur. Smaller lesions are overestimated in 44 per cent of cases and larger lesions are underestimated in 55 per cent of cases.[40] In up to 60 per cent of cases, the tumor is multifocal, as seen in Figure 8.51, and thus makes estimation of total tumor volume difficult.

Staging of PCa   Accurate **staging** of prostatic carcinoma is crucial to the treatment decision, and, although controversial, staging of prostate cancer appears to be the strength of MRI. As shown in Table 8.1, staging by MRI can follow a modified Jewett[42] or the TNM[6] classification.

Table 8.1 MRI staging criteria following Jewett and TNM classification of prostate cancer

Jewett	TNM	System description T-primary tumor
A	T1	Tumor is incidental histological finding
A1	T1A	3 or fewer microscopic foci of carcinoma
A2	T1B	More than 3 microscopic foci of carcinoma
B	T2	Tumor present clinically, but grossly limited to the gland
B1	T2A	Tumor 1.5 cm or less in greatest dimension with normal tissue on a least 2 sides
B2	T2B	Tumor more than 1.5 cm in greatest dimension or in more than one lobe
C	T3	Tumor invades into the prostatic apex or into or beyond the prostatic capsule, bladder neck or seminal vesicle but is not fixed
	T3A	Tumor invasion is transcapsular
	T3B	Tumor invades seminal vesicles, bladder neck
	T4	Tumor is fixed or invades adjacent structures other than those listed in T3
D	T (any) N (any) M (any)	Any size of local tumor plus lymph nodes and systemic metastasis
D1	T (any) N1 M0	Metastasis in a single pelvic lymph node, 2 cm or less in greatest dimension
D2	T (any) N (any) M1	Distant metastasis

Stage A (T1) prostatic carcinomas are nonpalpable lesions discovered incidentally during surgery for presumed benign disease. Most of stage A carcinomas are located in the transition zone.[30] When the residual cancer is of small volume and confined to the transition zone, it cannot be detected by MRI.[41] However, although incidentally detected, the cancer can be of larger volume (stage A2) and extend into the peripheral zone. As seen in Figure 8.52, MRI will detect tumor extension to the peripheral zone. In this patient group, the main role of MRI is to assess the local (Figure 8.42) and nodal spread of cancer, as 35 per cent of these patients will have tumor-positive lymph nodes at surgery.[32] Therefore, MRI evaluation of tumor extent is important, and it complements clinical assessment in reaching therapeutic decisions.

Prostatic carcinoma is classified as **stage B (T2)** when the signal abnormality is confined to the gland proper. Based on visualized tumor volume, differentiation between stage B1 (T2A) (Figure 8.53) and stage B2 (T2B) (Figure 8.54) can be made.

The tumor is diagnosed as **stage C (T3)** when it spreads outside the gland. Periprostatic spread is indicated by: (1) abnormal signal intensity within periprostatic fat (with or without involvement of the levator ani muscle) and/or the periprostatic venous plexus; (2) asymmetry in size and intensity of the seminal vesicles; and (3) abnormal intensity within the invaded bladder and urethra.

Although change in the periprostatic fat signal has been reported as the least sensitive indicator of tumor extension, these reports were often based on images obtained with thick sections. With thin (5 mm) contiguous sections, the accuracy of detection of periprostatic tumor extension may improve. At present, the most reliable finding in transcapsular tumor invasion is a localized tumor bulge extending beyond the expected outline of the gland as illustrated in Figure 8.55. MRI offers direct visualization of tumor site and permits identification of tumor proximity to, and involvement of, the dorsolateral neurovascular bundles (Figure 8.55). Surgical preservation of the neurovascular bundles is essential to maintain potency. On MRI, it is also possible to evaluate tumor extension to the apex of the gland, the presence of which precludes successful surgical resection. Tumor extension into the apical region is demonstrated in Figure 8.56.

Identification of tumor extension into the seminal vesicles is well evaluated by MR imaging.[18,37–39] Both size and configuration of the seminal vesicles are demonstrated, as are changes in signal intensity caused by tumor invasion.[37–39] Unless the seminal vesicles contain blood, direct tumor extension demonstrates lower signal intensity than the uninvolved portion of the seminal vesicle. As shown in Figure 8.57, tumor invasion may be localized,[19] involving only the medial aspect of the gland, or as seen in Figure 8.58, it can

be diffuse. When bleeding is present within the seminal vesicles (Figure 8.57), the differentiation between bleeding caused by tumor extension or postbiopsy hemorrhage is not possible, lowering the accuracy of MRI in the depiction of tumor extension. An accuracy of 78 per cent of seminal vesicle tumor extension has been reported.[18] The introduction of endorectal MRI surface coils (Figure 8.59) may further improve the evaluation of periprostatic tumor invasion.[43–45]

Tumor invasion of the bladder is diagnosed when on T2-weighted images, the normal low signal intensity bladder wall is no longer seen, perivesical fat at the bladder base is obliterated and direct tumor spread can be demonstrated (Figure 8.60). Similar guidelines are used for the diagnosis of direct tumor extension into the rectum, which in PCa is a late finding. Detection of tumor extension into the bladder and rectum is facilitated by use of the sagittal plane of imaging (Figure 8.61).

Prostatic cancer is considered to be **stage D1** (any stage T, N, M) when pelvic lymph nodes greater than 1 cm in size are detected (Figure 8.62). Lymph nodes in the pelvis (Figure 8.63) should not be confused with the vesicoprostatic plexus (Figure 8.64). The knowledge of anatomic location in addition to the ability of MRI to detect the vessels will obviate this mistake. In the diagnosis of **stage D1** disease, the knowledge of lymphatic drainage is essential. As illustrated in Figure 8.65, the detection of nodes located in the cul-de-sac (it is very unlikely that these would be of prostatic origin), mandates the search for a second (most nodes in this location probably gastrointestinal) malignancy.

A classification of **stage D2** is assigned when there is abnormal signal intensity within the pelvic bones or other distant metastases are present. Because bony metastases in prostatic cancer are almost invariably osteoblastic, they exhibit low signal intensity on both T1- and T2-weighted images (Figure 8.66).

MRI in relation to other imaging modalities

There is no set protocol for imaging in prostatic carcinoma, and selection of a particular technique (transrectal ultrasound, computed tomography, or MRI) depends on the expertise of personnel at the institution and the modalities available. None of the methods are flawless, each has advantages and disadvantages; and a judicious combination probably provides the best results.

In the detection of PCa, rates as high as 92 per cent have been reported,[39] but the results of multicenter studies are disappointingly low, with only 60 per cent of lesions greater than 5 mm in any one dimension being detected on MRI scans.[40] Signal intensity changes in the prostate are not specific, and various benign or malignant conditions can mimic one another. Therefore, MRI cannot be used for diagnosis, and histologic diagnosis based on prostatic biopsy is essential.[23,24] In the staging of PCa, evaluation by TRUS is restricted to local staging only, whereas both CT and MRI allow detection of local, nodal, and distant metastatic invasion. Although reported accuracy figures vary widely, the latest study indicates that the overall accuracy for staging PCa is 58 per cent for US, 65 per cent for CT, and 69 per cent for MRI.[40]

Either TRUS or MRI can be used in the identification of early transcapsular invasion, but at present neither is accurate or sensitive enough to use as the basis for therapy decisions. TRUS, however, is advocated as a more accurate modality for transcapsular tumor invasion (Figure 8.67). However, it is thought that MRI is the better modality for identifying invasion of the seminal vesicles (Figure 8.68). In the evaluation of lymph node metastases, both CT and MRI rely upon size of the nodes, and accuracy for the two methods is similar.

Recurrent prostatic cancer

The subject of recurrent prostatic cancer needs to be considered in the light of the initial therapy, which is either radical prostatectomy or radiation therapy. Both hormonal therapy and chemotherapy are usually given for systemic tumor spread and therefore will not be discussed in relation to local recurrence.

Monitoring patients after radical prostatectomy

For monitoring patients after radical prostatectomy, prostate-specific antigen (PSA) is emerging as the most important tool for the detection of recurrent prostate cancer.[46] Detectable PSA levels three to six months after radical prostatectomy indicate the presence of disease.[47] The recurrent disease, however, may be local or systemic, a finding that affects the treatment options. Locally, recurrent prostate cancer can be present from 20 to 78 months postsurgery, with a median interval of 58 months to 4.8 years.[46] The approach to the management of local recurrent prostate cancer is radiation therapy in the absence of evidence of other metastatic sites. Hormone therapy is recommended for patients with evidence of systemic disease. It has been reported that in patients with elevated PSA, local recurrence is present in 30 to 40 per cent.[46] Occasionally, tumor recurrence will be present in the absence of an elevated PSA. These cases come to attention during physical examination or unrelated clinical presentation. When local tumor

recurrence is suspected further evaluation by imaging is suggested.

MRI appearance

In the case of recurrent tumor following radical prostatectomy, most commonly tumor arises from a positive surgical margin and will be located in close proximity to the resection site. As illustrated in Figure 8.69, the tumor's signal intensity is usually low on a T2-weighted image, making tissue characterization between scar and tumor limited, and the diagnosis of tumor recurrence mainly lies on the finding of a tumor mass, often deforming or protruding into the urinary bladder.

MRI in relation to other modalities

The use of CT for the evaluation of pelvic recurrence is limited, not only due to image degradation by clip artifacts, but also because CT lacks tissue contrast sufficient to differentiate between fibrous scar and recurrent tumor. Transrectal ultrasound has been advocated for the evaluation of the recurrent prostate cancer, but assessment is limited by a lack of normal tissue standards for comparison. While MRI allows large field-of-view imaging and has excellent soft tissue contrast, the tumor's low signal intensity on T2-weighted images limits its diagnostic usefulness. Because of limited evaluation by imaging, blind biopsies of the prostatic bed have been advocated, but ultrasound-guided biopsy may be a more effective approach. If local recurrence is not demonstrated, then a search for systemic metastases is needed. Radionuclide scanning is the most practical recommended method for identifying bony metastases. Other metastatic sites, such as the liver and brain, can be evaluated by either CT or MRI, while for lung metastases, chest film and CT are recommended.

Monitoring patients after prostate radiation therapy

Monitoring patients after radiation therapy remains one of the most difficult areas in patient management and follow-up. While PSA is of proven value following radical prostatectomy, radiation therapy may or may not result in decrease of the PSA levels. However, it is generally agreed that an increase in PSA levels indicates active disease. Because the radiation therapy itself induces tissue changes (see Chapter 14), the evaluation of the postradiation prostate gland by MRI is very limited.

References

1 LIERSE W, *Applied Anatomy of the Pelvis* (Springer-Verlag: Berlin 1984) 160–8.

2 MCNEAL JE, The prostate gland: morphology and pathobiology, *Monogr Urol* (1983) **4**:5–13.

3 LOWSLEY OS, The development of the prostate gland with reference to the development of other structures at the neck of the urinary bladder, *Am J Anat* (1912) **13**:299–349.

4 STAMEY TA, MCNEAL JE, FREIHA FS et al, Morphometric and clinical studies on 68 consecutive prostatectomies, *J Urol* (1988) **139**:1235–41.

5 VILLERS A, TERRIS MK, MCNEAL JE et al, Ultrasound anatomy of the prostate: the normal gland and anatomical variations, *J Urol* (1990) **143**:732–8.

6 SPIESSL B, BEAHRS OH, HERMANEK P et al, *TNM Atlas: Illustrated Guide to the TNM/pTNM-classification of Malignant Tumors*, 3rd edn. (Springer-Verlag: Berlin 1989).

7 HRICAK H, DOOMS GC, MCNEAL JE et al, MR imaging of the prostate gland: normal anatomy, *AJR* (1987) **148**:51–8.

8 PHILLIPS ME, KRESSEL HY, SPRITZER CE et al, Normal prostate and adjacent structures: MR imaging at 1.5 T, *Radiology* (1987) **164**:381–5.

9 KOSLIN DB, KENNEY PJ, KOEHLER RE et al, Magnetic resonance imaging of the internal anatomy of the prostate gland, *Invest Radiol* (1987) **22**:947–53.

10 HRICAK H, JEFFREY RB, DOOMS GC et al, Evaluation of prostate size: a comparison of ultrasound and magnetic resonance imaging, *Urol Radiol* (1987) **9**:1–8.

11 GRESKOVICH FJ III, NYBERG LM JR, The prune-belly syndrome: a review of its etiology, defects, treatment and prognosis, *J Urol* (1988) **140**:707–12.

12 DONOHOE PK, BUDZIK GP, TRETSLAD R et al, Müllerian-inhibiting substance: an update, *Recent Prog Hormone Res* (1982) 279–330.

13 THURNHER S, HRICAK H, TANAGHO EA, Müllerian duct cyst: diagnosis with MR imaging, *Radiology* (1988) **167**:631–6.

14 KNEELAND JB, AUH YH, MCCARRON JP et al, Computed tomography, sonography, vesiculography, and MR imaging of a seminal vesicle cyst, *J Comp Asst Tomogr* (1985) **9(5)**:964–6.

15 PFAV A, Prostatitis: a continuing enigma, *Urol Clin North Am* (1986) **13**:695–715.

16 MEARES EM, Prostatitis and related disorders. In: *Campbell's Urology*, 5th edn. (W B Saunders: Philadelphia 1986).

17 BECKER LE, SHERRIB WR, Prostatic abscess: a diagnostic and therapentic approach, *J Urol* (1964) **91**:582–4.

18 NURUDDIN RN, HRICAK H, MCCLURE RD et al, Magnetic resonance imaging of the seminal vesicles, *AJR* (submitted).

19 PAPANICOLAOU N, PFISTER LC, STAFFORD S et al, Prostatic abscess: imaging with transrectal sonography and MR, *AJR* (1987) **149**:981–3.

20 DENNIS MA, DONOHUE RE, Computer tomography of prostatic abscess, *J Comput Assist Tomogr* (1985) **9(1)**:201–2.

21 HRICAK H, Radiologic evaluation of the urinary bladder and prostate. In: Allison DJ, Grainger RG, eds. *Diagnostic Radiology*, 2nd edn. (Churchill Livingstone: London 1990).

22 CARROL CL, SOMMER FG, MCNEAL JE et al, The abnormal prostate: MR imaging at 1.5 T with histopathologic correlation, *Radiology* (1987) **163**:521–5.

23 HRICAK H, TANAGHO EA, MCNEAL JE, Prostatic pathology: correlation between MRI and histologic findings, Presented at the fifth annual meeting of Society of Magnetic Resonance in Medicine (1985) Montreal, Canada.

24 LING D, LEE JKT, HEIKEN JP et al, Prostate carcinoma and benign prostatic hyperplasia: inability of MR imaging to distinguish between the two diseases, *Radiology* (1986) **158**:103–7.

25 PHILLIPS ME, KRESSEL HY, SPRITZER CE et al, Prostatic disorders: MR imaging at 1.5 T. *Radiology* (1987) **164**:386–92.

26 ALLEN KS, KRESSEL HY, ARGER PH et al, Age-related changes of the prostate: evaluation by MR imaging, *AJR* (1989) **152**:77–81.

27 SCHIEBLER ML, TOMASZEWSKI JE, BEZZI M et al, Prostatic carcinoma and benign prostate hyperplasia: correlation of high-resolution MR and histopathologic findings, *Radiology* (1989) **172**:131–7.

28 HRICAK H, Editorial on imaging prostate carcinoma, *Radiology* (1988) **169**:569–71.

29 *Cancer Facts and Figures-1989*, American Cancer Society, Atlanta.

30 MCNEAL JE, PRICE HM, REDWINE E et al, Stage A versus stage B adenocarcinoma of the prostate: morphological comparison and biological significance, *J Urol* (1988) **139**:61–5.

31 KABALIN JN, MCNEAL JE, PRICE HM et al, Unsuspected adenocarcinoma of the prostate in patients undergoing cystoprostatectomy for other causes: incidence, histology and morphometric observations, *J Urol* (1989) **141**:1091–4.

32 SCHMIDT JD, METTLIN CJ, NATARAJAN N et al, Trends in patterns of care for prostatic cancer, 1974–1983: results of surveys by the American College of Surgeons, *J Urol* (1986) **136**:416–21.

33 LEE F, GRAY JM, MCLEARY RD et al, Transrectal ultrasound in the diagnosis of prostate cancer: location, echogenicity, histopathology and staging, *Prostate* (1985) **7**:117–29.

34 STAMEY TA, YANG N, HAY AR et al, Prostate specific antigen as a serum marker for adenocarcinoma of the prostate, *N Engl J Med* (1987) **317**:909–16.

35 WALSH PC, JEWETT HJ, Radical surgery for prostatic cancer, *Cancer* (1980) **45**:1906–11.

36 BRYAN PJ, BUTLER HE, NELSON AD et al, Magnetic resonance imaging of the prostate, *AJR* (1986) **146**:543–48.

37 HRICAK H, DOOMS GC, JEFFREY RB et al, Prostate carcinoma: staging by clinical assessment, CT, and MR imaging, *Radiology* (1987) **162**:331–6.

38 BIONDETTI PR, LEE JKT, LING D et al, Clinical stage B prostate carcinoma: staging with MR imaging, *Radiology* (1987) **162**:325.

39 BEZZI M, KRESSEL HY, ALLEN KS et al, Prostatic carcinoma: staging with MR imaging at 1.5 T, *Radiology* (1988) **169**:339–46.

40 RIFKIN MD, GATSONIS CA, ZERHOUNI EA et al, Endorectal US and MR imaging: accuracy for staging prostate cancer. RSNA 1989, Chicago. (Abst), *Radiology* (1989) **173(P)** (Suppl):143.

41 SUGIMURA K, HRICAK H, CARROL P, Value of MR imaging in the detection of stage A prostate carcinoma. RSNA 1989, Chicago. (Abst), *Radiology* (1989) **173(P)** (Suppl):143.

42 JEWETT HJ, The present status of radical prostatectomy for stages A and B prostatic cancer, *Urol Clin* (1975) **2**:105–24.

43 BERTHOTY DP, MATTREY RF, MARTIN JF et al, Role of transrectal MR imaging in prostatic carcinoma. RSNA 1989, Chicago. (Abst), *Radiology* (1989) **173(P)** (Suppl):143.

44 MARTIN JF, HAJEK P, BAKER L et al, Inflatable surface coil for MR imaging of the prostate, *Radiology* (1988) **167**:268–70.

45 SCHNALL MD, LENKINSKI RE, POLLACK HM et al, Prostate: MR imaging with an endorectal surface coil, *Radiology* (1989) **172**:570–4.

46 KALO K, LANGE P, Open discussion: monitoring response to therapy. In: Resnick M, Watanabe W, Karr JP, eds. *Diagnostic Ultrasound of the Prostate* (Elsevier Science Publishing Co: New York 1989).

47 CATALONA WJ, MILLER DR, KAVOUSSI LR, Intermediate term survival results in clinically understaged prostate cancer patients following radical prostatectomy, *J Urol* (1988) **140**:540–3.

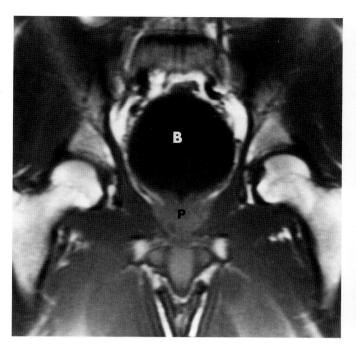

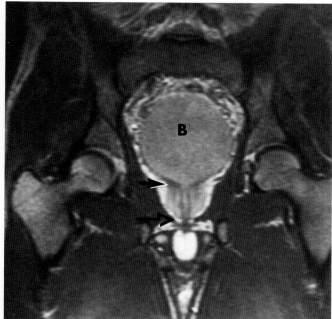

a

b

Figure 8.1

Superoinferior relations of the prostate. Coronal (**a**) T1- and (**b**) T2-weighted images demonstrating that the base of the prostate (black arrow) abuts the base of the bladder (B). The apex of the prostate is in contact with the membranous urethra—the external urethral sphincter (open arrow). (P)-prostate.

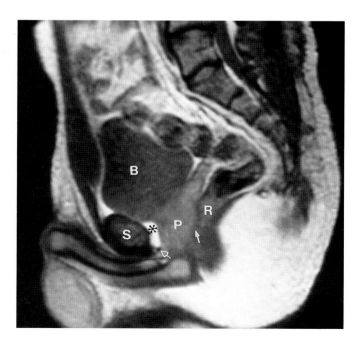

Figure 8.2

Anteroposterior relations of the prostate. Sagittal proton density image illustrating that the retropubic space (asterisk) separates the prostate (P) from the symphysis pubis (S). Puboprostatic ligament (open arrowhead). Posteriorly, the prostate is separated from the rectum (R) by Denonvilliers' fascia (arrow). (B)-urinary bladder.

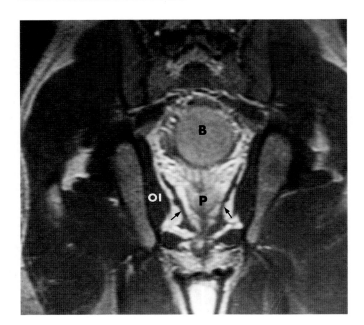

Figure 8.3

Lateral relations of the prostate. Coronal T2-weighted image showing that the levator ani muscles (small solid arrows) are lateral to the prostate (P) and medial to the obturator internus muscles (OI). (B)-urinary bladder.

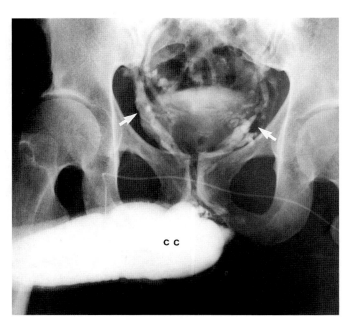

a

Figure 8.4

Vesicoprostatic plexus. (**a**) is a corpora cavernosogram. (**b**) and (**c**) are two consecutive coronal T1-weighted images. (**d**) and (**e**) are transaxial T2-weighted images. Large vesicoprostatic veins (arrows) seen lateral and posterior to the prostate are well filled during the corpora cavernosogram due to the patient's venogenic impotence. (CC)-Corpora cavernosa. The vesicoprostatic venous plexus (arrows) demonstrates medium signal intensity on the T1-weighted images and shows marked enhancement on the T2-weighted images. (P)-prostate gland; (R)-rectum; (B)-bladder; (SV)-seminal vesicles.

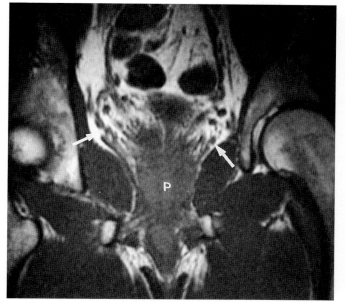

b

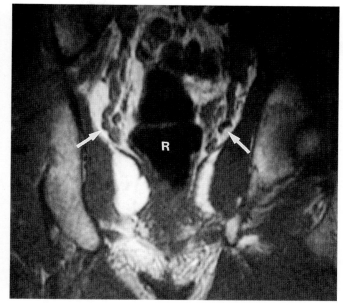

c

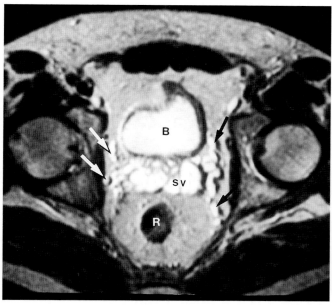

d

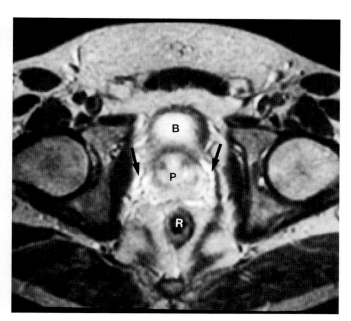

e

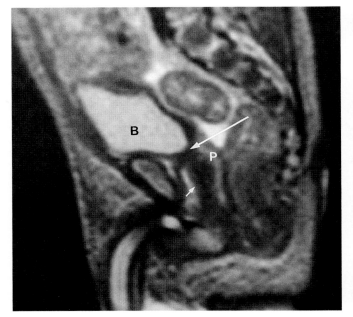

a

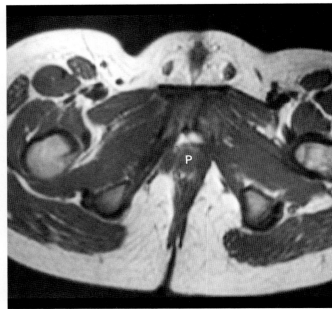

a

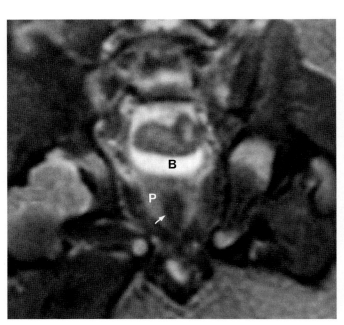

b

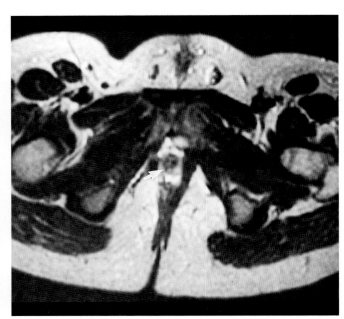

b

Figure 8.5

Neonatal prostate. (**a**) Sagittal and (**b**) coronal T2-weighted images. The relative size of the prostate (P) is comparable to the adult gland, with the base of the prostate (long arrow) being at the level of the upper two-thirds of the symphysis pubis. The zonal anatomy is not identified. However, the urethra (short arrow) is seen. (B)-urinary bladder.

Figure 8.6

Prepubertal prostate. Transaxial (**a**) T1- and (**b**) T2-weighted images demonstrating that the prostate (P) is relatively small and without zonal differentiation. The largest component of the gland is periurethral tissue (arrow).

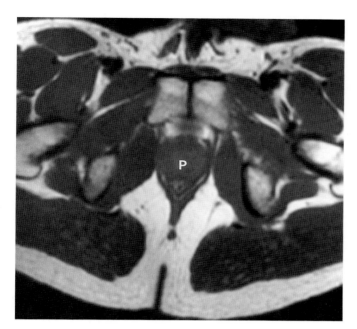

a

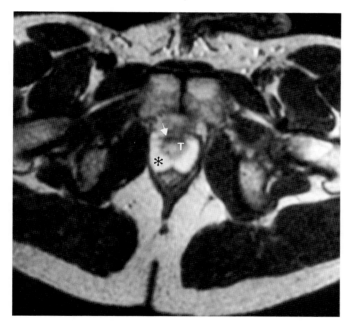

b

Figure 8.7

Adult prostate. Transaxial (**a**)
T1-, (**b**) T2-weighted images.
On the T2-weighted image,
there is differentiation into a
peripheral zone (asterisk),
transition zone (T), and
anterior fibromuscular band
(short white arrow).

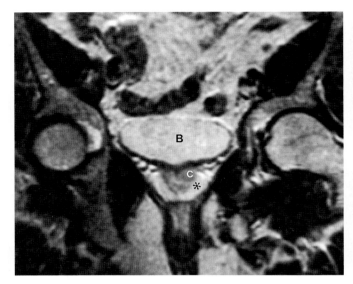

a

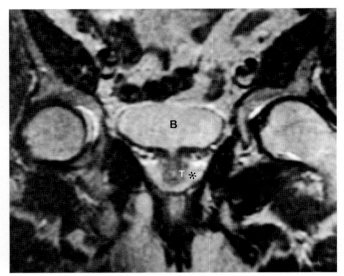

b

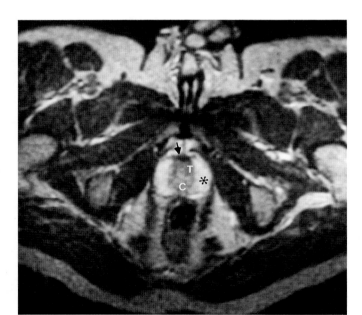

c

Figure 8.8

Similar signal intensity between the central and transition zones on T2-weighted images. 35° oblique coronal (**a**) posterior section, (**b**) section at the bladder neck, and (**c**) transaxial oblique section. On the posterior coronal image, the central zone (C) is imaged with lower signal intensity than the peripheral zone (asterisk). At the level of the bladder neck, however, the low signal intensity area represents the transition zone (T). On the oblique axial images the central zone (C) and transition zone (T) can only be differentiated by the knowledge of their relative positions. (Arrow)-anterior fibromuscular band.

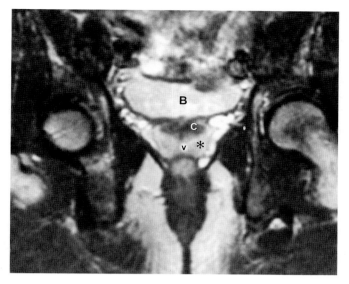

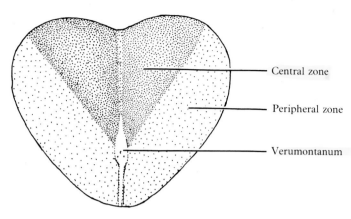

a

b

Central zone

Peripheral zone

Verumontanum

Figure 8.9

The central zone of the prostate. (**a**) Oblique coronal T2-weighted image. (**b**) Schematic drawing. The central zone (C) is conical in shape, with its apex at the verumontanum (V). (Asterisk)-peripheral zone; (B)-urinary bladder.

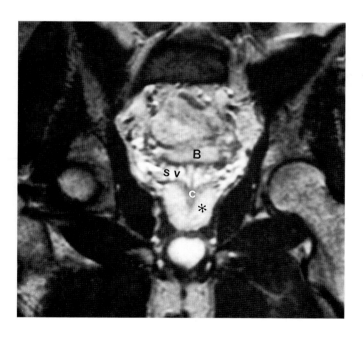

Figure 8.10

Small 'heart-shaped' central zone (C) in normal young adult. Coronal T2-weighted image. (Asterisk)-peripheral zone; (SV)-seminal vesicles; (B)-urinary bladder.

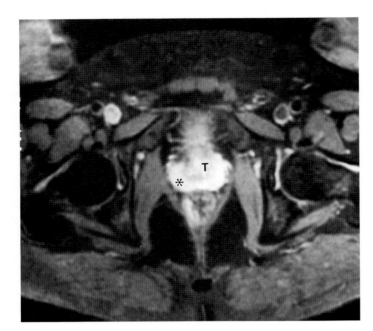

a

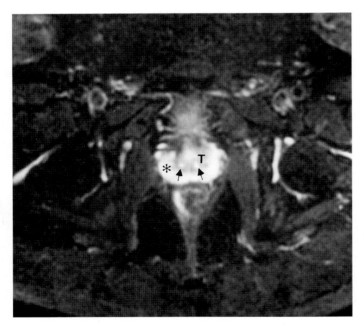

b

Figure 8.11

Fat saturation transaxial images of the prostate. (**a**) Proton density and (**b**) T2-weighted fat saturation images showing that zonal anatomy with the differentiation between high signal intensity peripheral zone (asterisk) and lower signal intensity transition zone (T) can be appreciated on the proton density fat saturation image. (Arrows)-ejaculatory ducts in the central zone.

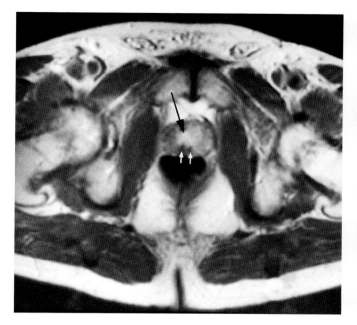

a

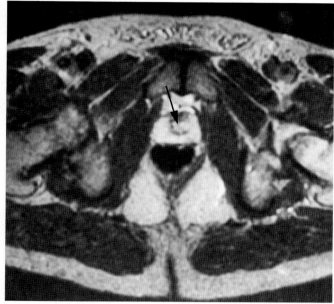

b

Figure 8.12

The appearance of the prostate after intravenous gadolinium-DTPA. (**a**) Gadolinium-enhanced transaxial T1-weighted image showing enhancement of the periurethral region (arrow). The ejaculatory ducts (small white arrows) are seen due to enhancement of the adjacent central zone. (**b**) T2-weighted image, where the periurethral tissue is of heterogeneous mostly high signal intensity, indicating benign prostatic hypertrophic changes.

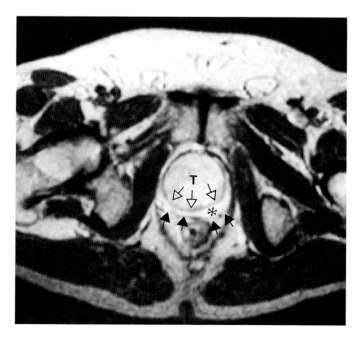

Figure 8.13

The prostate capsules. Transaxial T2-weighted image demonstrating the surgical pseudocapsule (open arrowhead) between the transition (T) and peripheral (asterisk) zones. The prostatic capsule proper (small black arrows) is seen around the periphery of the gland.

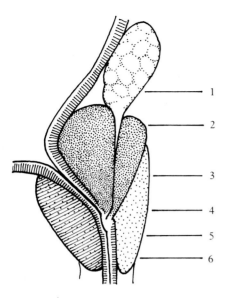

a

Figure 8.14

Serial transaxial T2-weighted images through the prostate with accompanying schematic drawings at the same anatomical level. (**a**) Sagittal drawing demonstrating planes of section for accompanying transaxial planes; 1-(**b**)(**c**) at the level of the seminal vesicles; 2-(**d**)(**e**) at the level of the base of the prostate; 3-(**f**)(**g**) below the level of the bladder neck; 4-(**h**)(**i**) at the level of the verumontanum; 5-(**j**)(**k**) below the level of the verumontanum; 6-(**l**)(**m**) at the apex of the prostate.

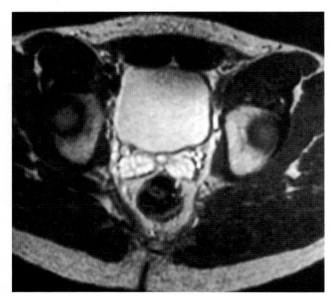

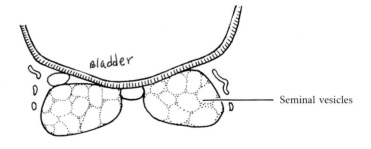

1-(b) (c)

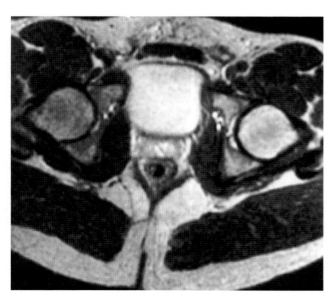

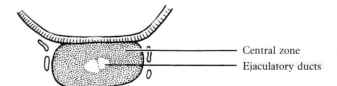

2-(d) (e)

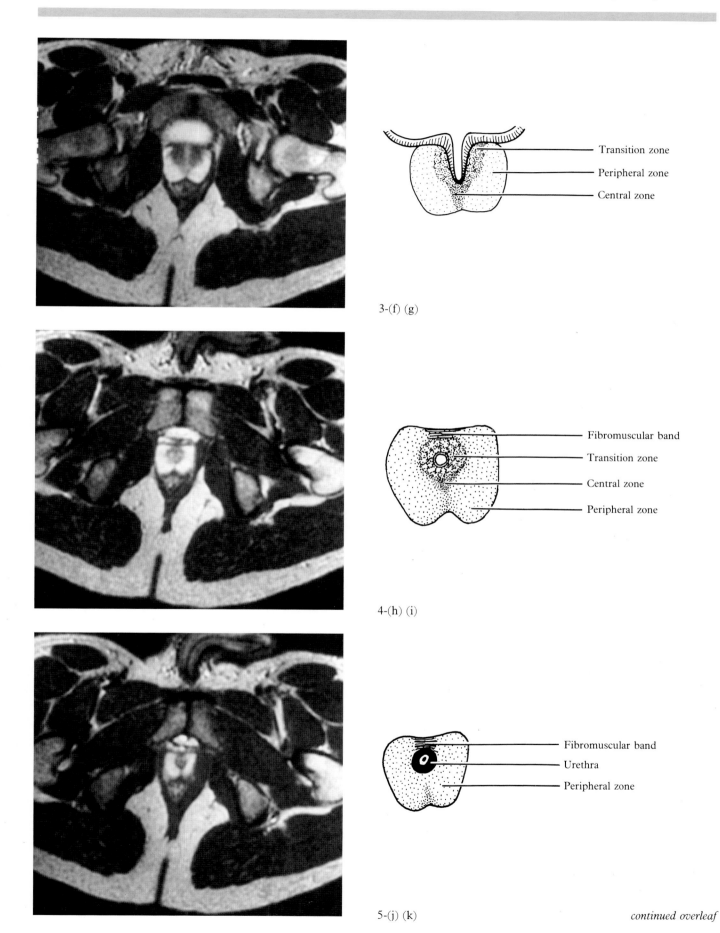

3-(f) (g)

Transition zone
Peripheral zone
Central zone

4-(h) (i)

Fibromuscular band
Transition zone
Central zone
Peripheral zone

5-(j) (k)

Fibromuscular band
Urethra
Peripheral zone

continued overleaf

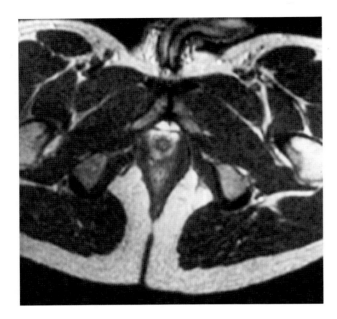

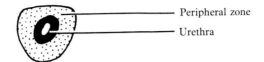

——— Peripheral zone
——— Urethra

Figure 8.14 (*continued*) 6-(1) (m)

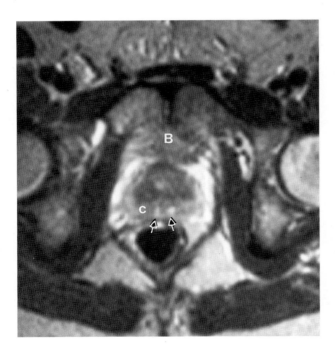

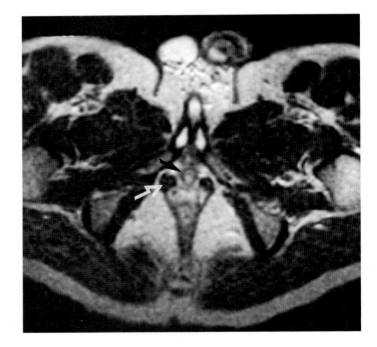

Figure 8.15

Central zone with identification of the ejaculatory ducts. Transaxial T2-weighted image at the level of the prostate base. Note, low signal intensity of the normal central zone (C) surrounding the ejaculatory ducts (arrows). (B)-urinary bladder.

Figure 8.16

Membranous urethra. Oblique transaxial T2-weighted image at the level of the membranous urethra (arrow). (Open arrow)-levator ani muscle.

1-(b) (c) (d)

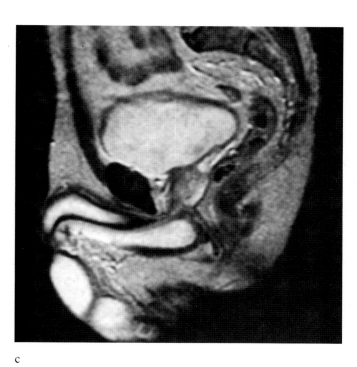

a

b

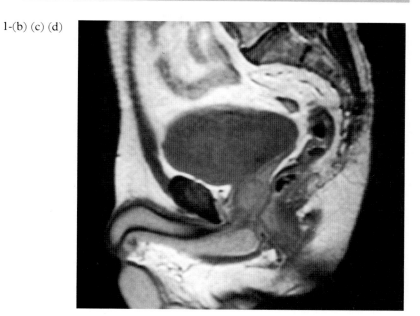

Ejaculatory duct

Central zone

Peripheral zone

Fibromuscular band

c

d

Figure 8.17

Sagittal proton density (**b**), (**e**) and (**h**) and T2-weighted (**c**), (**f**) and (**i**) images through the prostate with accompanying schematic drawings at the same anatomical level, demonstrating the relation of the zonal anatomy. (**a**) Transaxial schematic drawing illustrating the planes of section; 1-(**b**)(**c**)(**d**) midline; 2-(**e**)(**f**)(**g**) 1.0 cm lateral; 3-(**h**)(**i**)(**j**) 1.5 cm lateral. Proton density images have been included for ease of anatomical identification.

continued overleaf

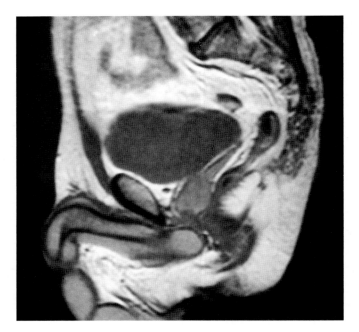

e

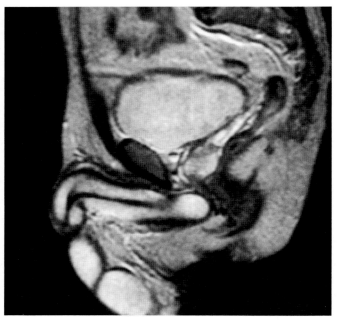

f

Figure 8.17 (*continued*) 2-(e) (f) (g)

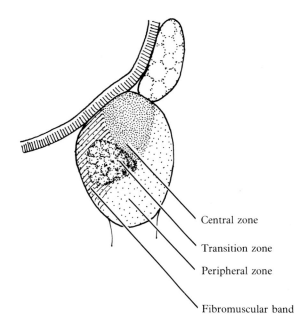

g

Central zone

Transition zone

Peripheral zone

Fibromuscular band

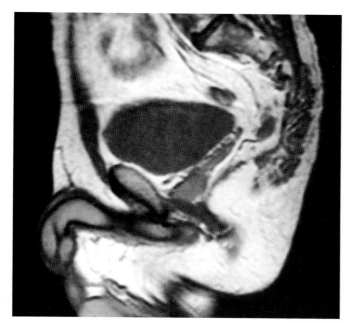

h

3-(h) (i) (j)

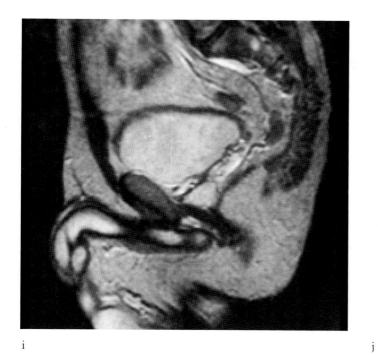

i

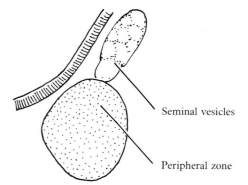

j

Seminal vesicles

Peripheral zone

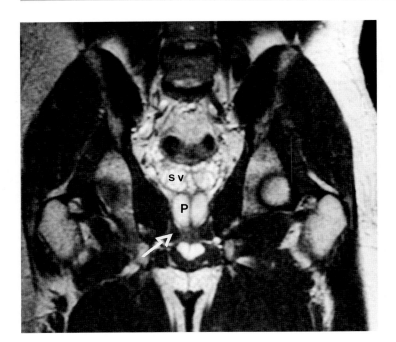

Figure 8.18

Coronal plane demonstrating the prostate (P), seminal vesicles (SV) superiorly, and levator ani muscle (open arrow) laterally.

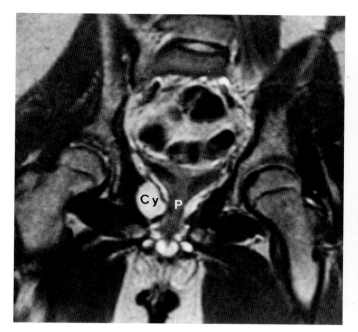

a

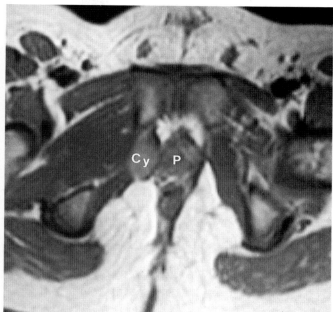

b

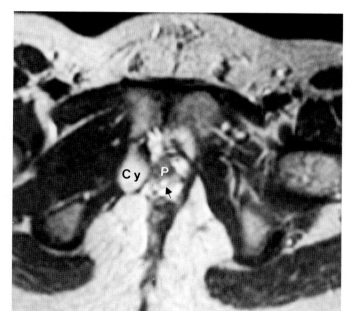

c

Figure 8.19

Prostate hypoplasia in a patient (age 25 years) with true hermaphroditism. (**a**) T2-weighted coronal, (**b**) proton density and (**c**) T2-weighted transaxial images. The prostate (P) is not only small in size but zonal anatomy is not seen. (Arrow)-utricle; (CY)-incidental finding sebaceous cyst.

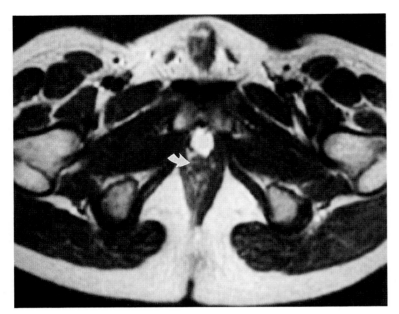

a

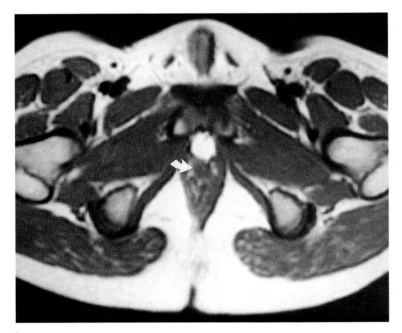

b

Figure 8.20

Prostate hypoplasia. Transaxial (**a**) proton density and (**b**) T2-weighted images showing a small prostate (less than 1 cm in any diameter). The zonal anatomy is not displayed, and the prostatic glandular tissue (arrow) is of low signal intensity.

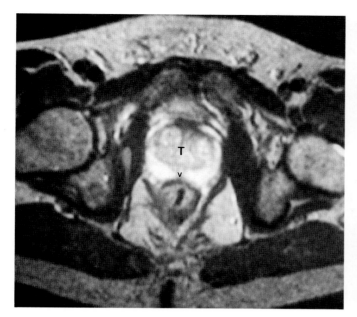

a

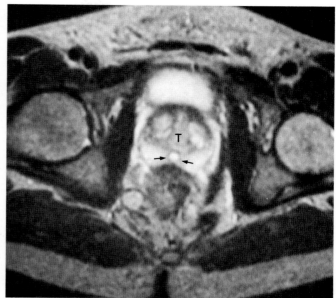

b

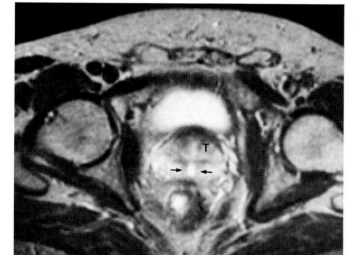

c

Figure 8.21

Prostatic utricle in an
asymptomatic patient.
Transaxial T2-weighted
images. Image located: (**a**) at
the verumontanum; (**b**) above
the verumontanum; (**c**) at the
bladder neck. The gland is
enlarged due to benign
hyperplastic changes in the
transition zone (T). The utricle
(arrows) is seen only above the
level of the verumontanum (V).

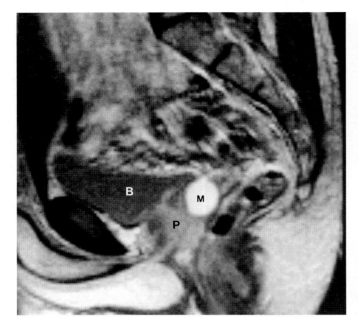

a

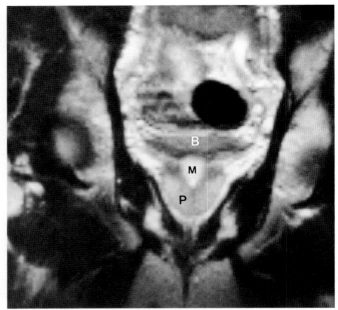

b

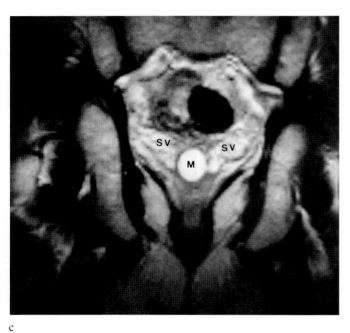

c

Figure 8.22

Müllerian duct cyst. T2-weighted (**a**) sagittal, (**b**) and (**c**) coronal images. The midline müllerian duct cyst (M) arises at the level of the verumontanum and passes superiorly and posteriorly above the base of the prostate gland (P). The midline cyst (M) is distinct from the normal seminal vesicles (SV). (B)-urinary bladder.

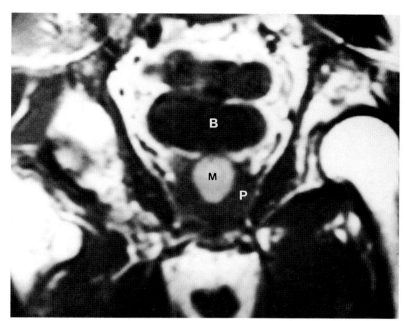

a

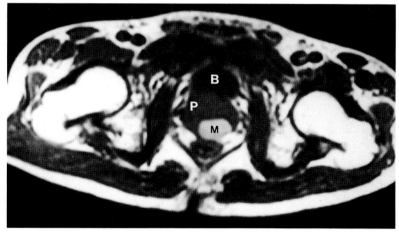

b

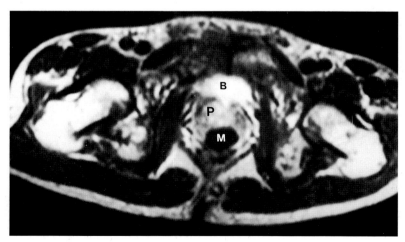

c

Figure 8.23

Hemorrhagic müllerian duct cyst. (**a**) T1 coronal, (**b**) T1 transaxial and (**c**) T2 transaxial images. The müllerian duct cyst (M) is of high signal intensity on the T1-weighted image and of low signal intensity on the T2-weighted image due to the presence of intracellular methemoglobin. (B)-urinary bladder; (P)-prostate. (Courtesy of Dr Kim Seul, University of Korea.)

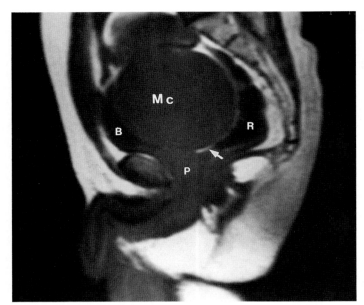

a

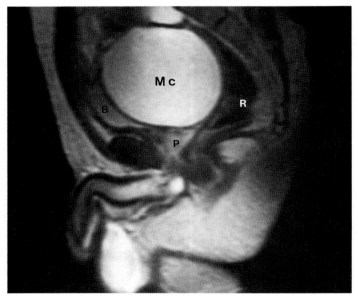

b

Figure 8.24

Mucocele of the appendix misdiagnosed clinically and on TRUS as a müllerian duct cyst, (**a**) T1- and (**b**) T2-weighted images. The mucocele (Mc) is separated from the prostate (P) by a fat plane (arrow). (B)-urinary bladder; (R)-rectum.

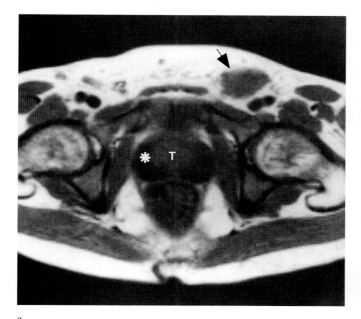

a

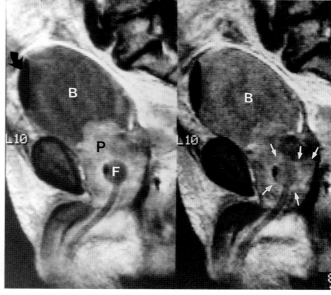

a   b

b

Figure 8.26

Acute prostatitis secondary to placement of the Foley. Sagittal (**a**) proton density, and (**b**) T2-weighted images. The prostate gland (P) is enlarged due to benign prostatic hyperplasia. A Foley catheter balloon (F) is wrongly (by omission) inflated within the prostatic urethra. Inflammatory change demonstrates diffuse high signal intensity of the gland on the T2-weighted image (arrow). (B)-urinary bladder; (curved arrow)-air in the bladder. (0.35T.)

Figure 8.25

Acute prostatitis. Transaxial (**a**) T1- and (**b**) T2-weighted images. The prostate is enlarged and the peripheral zone (asterisk) is of lower signal intensity than the adjacent transition zone (T). The peripheral zone markedly increases in signal intensity on T2-weighted images. In this patient, prostatitis was the sequel to acute epididymitis. Ascending inflammation causing the enlargement of the spermatic cord (arrow) is seen. (0.35T.)

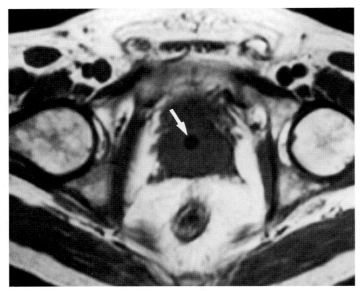

a

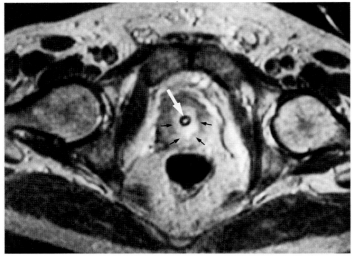

b

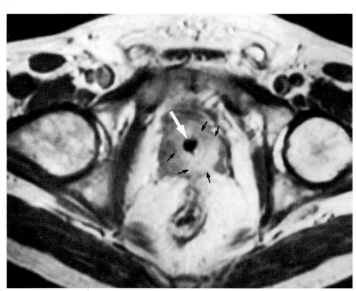

c

Figure 8.27

Acute prostatitis secondary to long-term indwelling catheter. Transaxial (**a**) T1-, (**b**) T2-, and (**c**) Gd-DTPA-enhanced T1-weighted images. On the T2-weighted and Gd-enhanced T1-weighted images, the periurethral region shows an increase in signal intensity (small black arrows), but the enhancing tissue on the gadolinium image is of greater volume (than seen on the T2-weighted image) and extends into the peripheral zone. (White arrow)-urethral catheter.

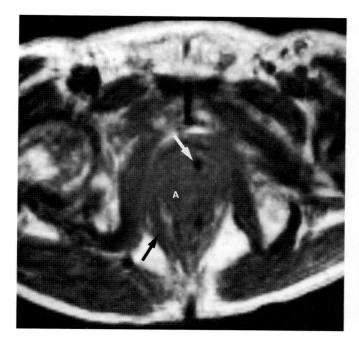

a

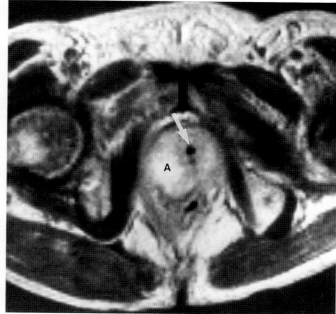

b

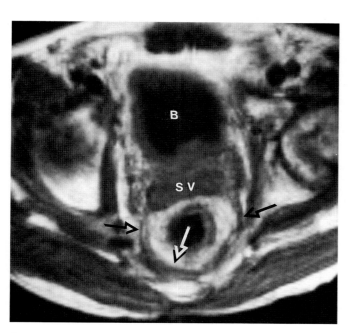

c

Figure 8.28

Prostatic abscess. Transaxial (**a**) T1-, and (**b**) T2-weighted images through the prostate with (**c**) T1-weighted transaxial image at the level of the seminal vesicles. On the T1-weighted image, the prostate shows asymmetrical enlargement and infiltration of the periprostatic fat (black arrow). The urethra (arrow) is displaced. The abscess (A) is of medium signal intensity on T1-weighted images but markedly increases in signal intensity on T2-weighted images, where it displays an indistinct margin. Inflammation has spread to the seminal vesicles (SV) (which are enlarged and demonstrate an ill-defined margin), perirectal fascia (black open arrows) and presacral space (white open arrow). (White arrow)-Foley catheter in the urethra.

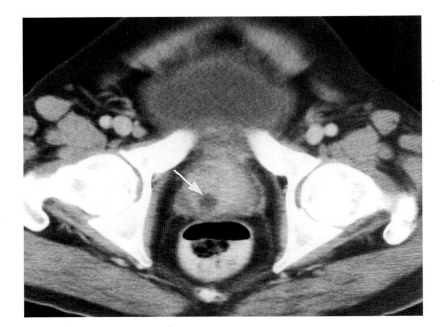

Figure 8.29

Prostate abscess demonstrated on CT as ill-defined low density region (arrow) within the prostate gland.

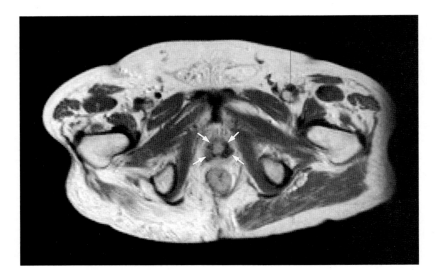

Figure 8.30

Prostatic calcification. T2-weighted transaxial image demonstrating characteristic horseshoe-shaped low signal intensity punctuate calcifications in the periurethral region (arrows). (0.35T.)

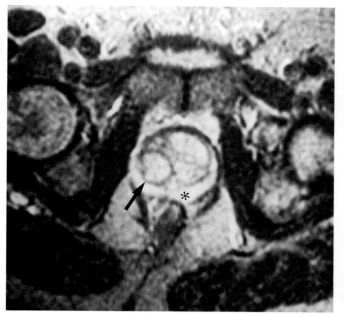

a

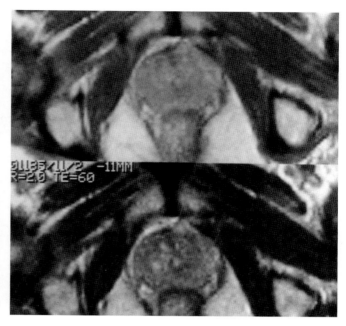

a

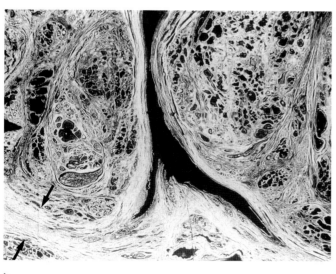

b

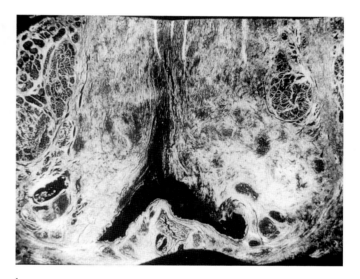

b

Figure 8.31

Glandular benign prostatic hyperplasia. (**a**) T2-weighted MR image, (**b**) thick section histologic specimen. On the MR image, the glandular portion of BPH exhibits heterogeneous signal intensity with a well-defined surgical pseudocapsule (arrow). (Asterisk)-normal peripheral zone. The surgical pseudocapsule (arrows) is also seen on the histologic section. (Courtesy of JE McNeal, MD.)

Figure 8.32

Predominantly interstitial type benign prostatic hyperplasia. (**a**) Proton density and T2-weighted MR image, (**b**) thick section histologic specimen. Note marked difference in the MRI and histologic appearance of interstitial versus glandular type (Figure 8.31) of BPH. No surgical pseudocapsule is demonstrated. (0.35T.) (Courtesy of JE McNeal, MD.)

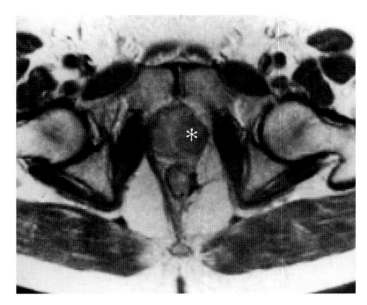

a

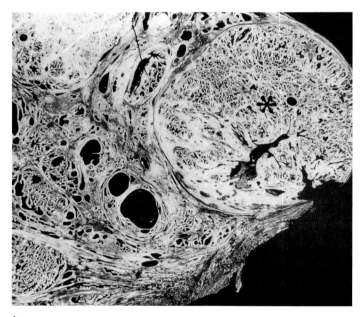

b

Figure 8.33

Focal benign prostatic hyperplasia. (**a**) T2-weighted MR image, (**b**) thick section histologic specimen. Prostatic nodule (asterisk) on MRI scan is of low signal intensity and is indistinguishable from prostate cancer. (0.35T.)
(Courtesy of JE McNeal, MD.)

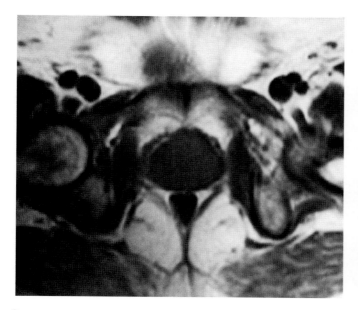

a

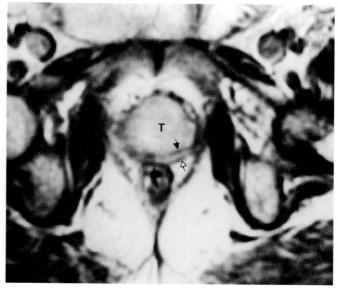

b

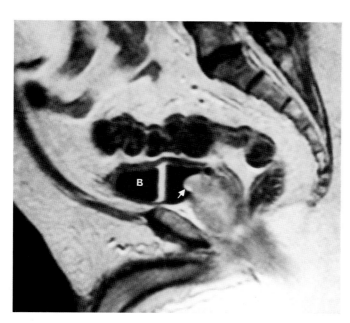

c

Figure 8.34

Appearance of BPH following Gd-DTPA injection. Transaxial T1-weighted image, (**a**) before, (**b**) immediately following Gd-DTPA injection and (**c**) sagittal delayed postGd-DTPA-enhanced T1-weighted image. Following Gd-DTPA injection, both the enlarged transition zone (T) and the peripheral zone show enhancement, while the surgical pseudocapsule (black arrow) and the capsule proper (open arrow) do not. On the delay-enhanced scan, the hyperplastic tissue is of heterogeneous signal intensity. Large subvesicular nodule (arrow) protrudes into the urinary bladder (B).

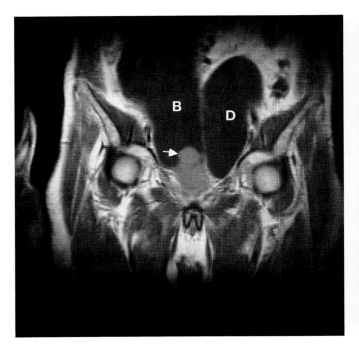

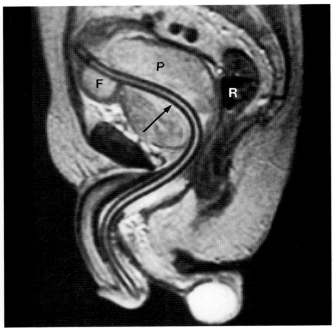

a

Figure 8.35

Benign prostatic hyperplasia with enlargement of the subvesicular glandular tissue which protrudes into the urinary bladder (B). The patient has a large bladder diverticulum (D). Coronal T1-weighted image. (Arrow)-median lobe. (0.35T.)

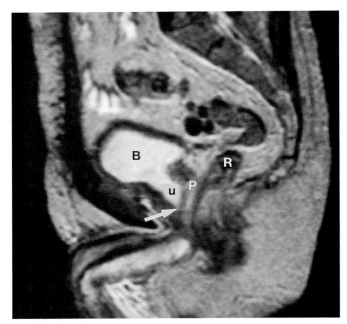

b

Figure 8.36

Benign prostatic hyperplasia. Sagittal T2-weighted image (**a**) pre- and (**b**) post-open enucleation (retropubic prostatectomy). Before surgery, the prostate gland (P) is markedly enlarged, elevating the bladder base. (F)-Foley catheter balloon; (black arrow)-Foley catheter. Following surgery, the proximal prostatic urethra demonstrates a conical urine-filled defect extending to the level of the verumontanum (arrow). (U)-urethra; (B)-urinary bladder; (R)-rectum; (P)-residual prostatic tissue.

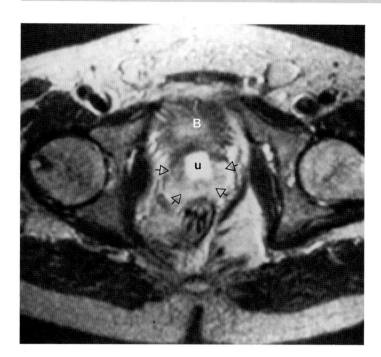

Figure 8.37

Large post-TURP urethral defect (U) on transaxial T2-weighted image with residual adenomatous tissue (open arrows). (B)-urinary bladder.

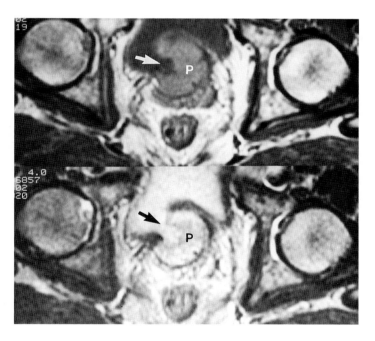

a

b

Figure 8.38

Small, asymmetrical TURP defect (arrow) within an otherwise enlarged intravesical portion of the prostate (P). Transaxial (**a**) proton density, (**b**) T2-weighted images.

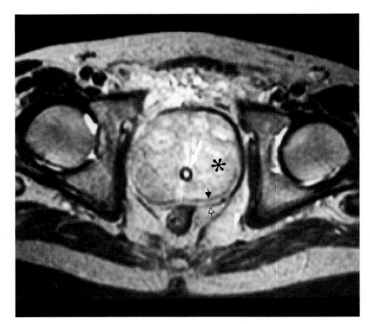

a

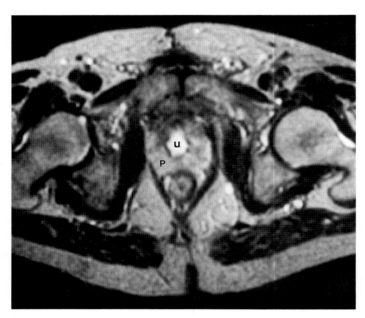

b

Figure 8.39

Compression of the peripheral zone by large transition zone BPH, T2-weighted transaxial image (**a**) before and (**b**) after open enucleation. The large BPH (asterisk) is compressing the peripheral zone seen between the surgical pseudocapsule (solid black arrow) and prostate capsule proper (open black arrow). A Foley catheter is present within the prostatic urethra (white arrow). Following surgery, the prostatic urethra is dilated (U). The peripheral zone (P) has expanded.

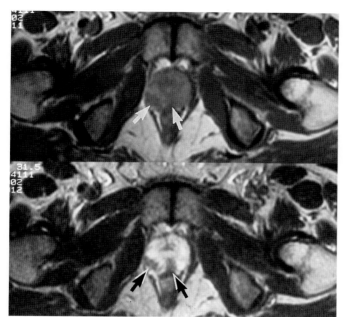

a

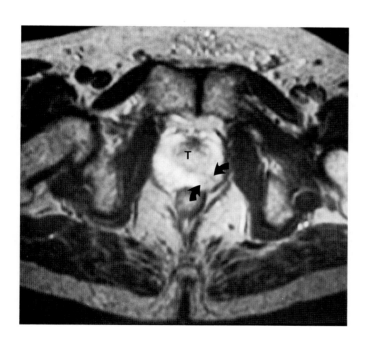

b

Figure 8.40

Prostatic carcinoma. Transaxial (**a**) proton density, (**b**) T2-weighted images. Two small peripheral zone tumors are present, both of which are of medium signal intensity on the proton density image and of low signal intensity on the T2-weighted image (arrows).

Figure 8.41

Prostatic carcinoma with tumor in the peripheral and the transition zone. T2-weighted transaxial image showing the low signal intensity nodule in the peripheral zone (curved arrows). The transition zone (T) is of low signal intensity, but the signal intensity changes are similar to those found in benign prostatic hyperplasia. Tumor, however, was present at surgery.

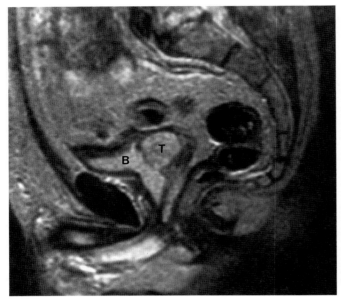

a

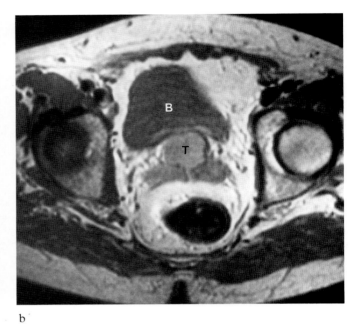

b

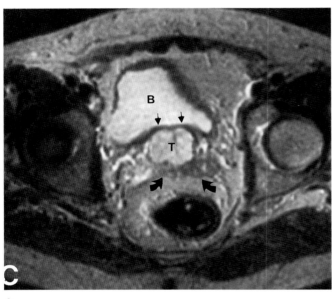

c

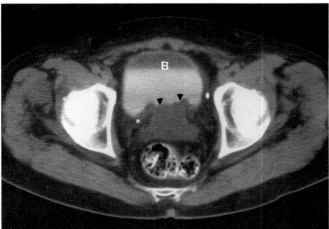

d

Figure 8.42

A prostatic carcinoma located in the transition zone imaged with high signal intensity. Stage A prostate cancer was found during TURP, but following MRI study and surgery, the patient was classified as stage T3B. (**a**) Sagittal T2-weighted image; (**b**) transaxial proton density image; (**c**) transaxial T2-weighted image and (**d**) CT scan at same anatomical level. Status post-TURP tumor mass (T) exhibits high signal intensity on the T2-weighted image. The seminal vesicles (curved arrows) are of abnormal low signal intensity on the T2-weighted image, indicating invasion. On CT the urinary bladder (B) appeared invaded (black arrows), but the bladder wall was intact on MRI and surgery.

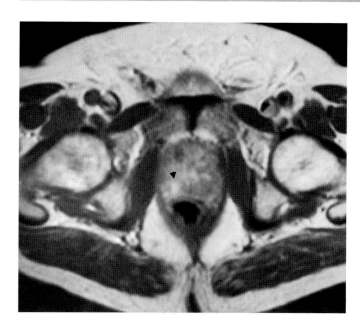

Figure 8.43

Prostatic carcinoma appearance after Gd-DTPA injection. Transaxial T1-weighted gadolinium-enhanced image in the early postinjection period showing localized enhancement in the peripheral zone (arrows) corresponding to carcinoma found at surgery.

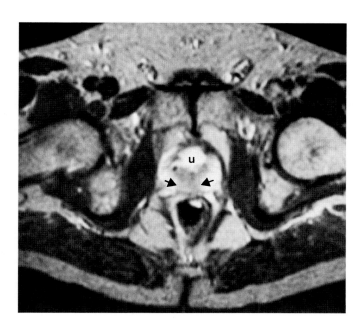

Figure 8.44

Prostatic dysplasia, the signal intensity of which mimics carcinoma on MRI. Transaxial T2-weighted image showing a focus of low signal intensity in the peripheral zone (arrows) indistinguishable from a tumor. However, on histology, this represented dysplastic changes. A dilated prostatic urethra (U) is seen post-TURP.

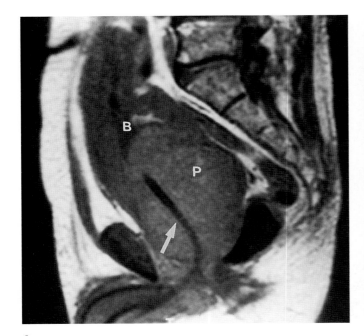

a

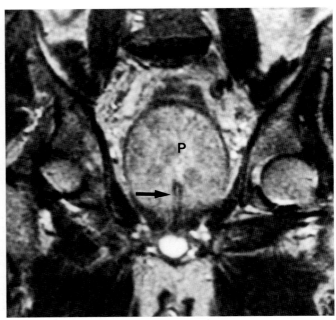

b

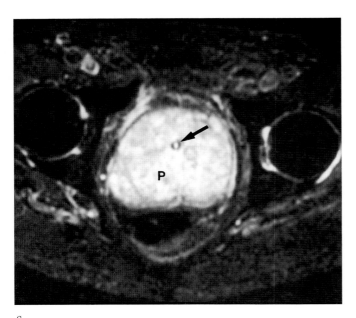

c

Figure 8.45

Prostatic sarcoma. (**a**) Sagittal
T1-weighted image, (**b**) coronal
T2-weighted image and (**c**)
transaxial fat suppression T2-
weighted image. The prostate
(P) is markedly enlarged and of
heterogeneous signal intensity
on the T2-weighted image. (B)-
urinary bladder; (arrow)-Foley
catheter. The prostate signal
intensity is nonspecific. Diffuse
sarcoma was found at surgery.
Because the conventional T2-
weighted image was of
suboptimal quality, a fat
suppression image was chosen
for the transaxial plane.

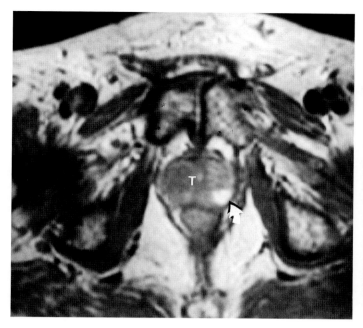

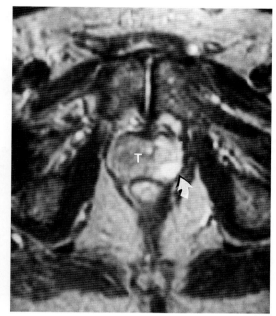

a

b

Figure 8.46

Subacute postbiopsy hemorrhage. Transaxial (**a**) T1-weighted and (**b**) T2-weighted images demonstrating postbiopsy hemorrhage (arrow) which is of high signal intensity on both T1- and T2-weighted images. The hemorrhage masks the presence of a tumor in that region of the peripheral zone. The tumor (T) in the remainder of the gland can be detected.

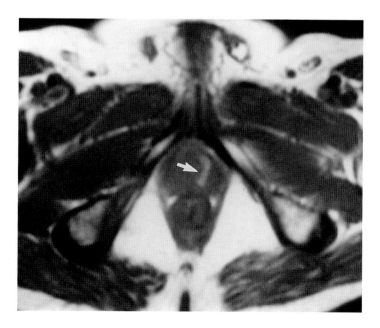

Figure 8.47

Intraprostatic hemorrhage along the needle track (arrow) on a transaxial T1-weighted image.

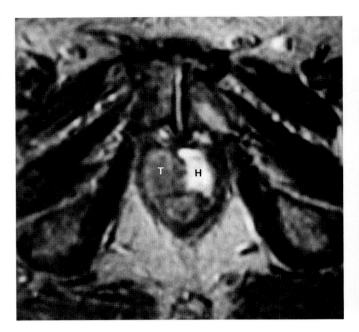

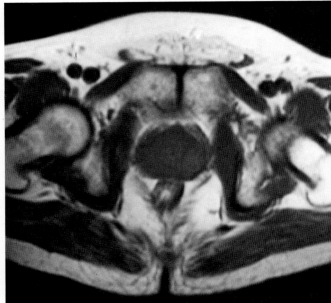

a

Figure 8.48

Large intraprostatic
hemorrhage (H) on a transaxial
T2-weighted image involving
half of the gland. At surgery,
the tumor (T) extended
throughout the entire prostate.

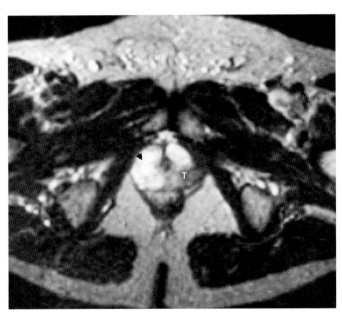

b

Figure 8.49

Interstitial edema postprostatic
biopsy. Transaxial (**a**) T1- and
(**b**) T2-weighted images. The
biopsy area (arrow) is not
detected on the T1-weighted
image and demonstrates high
signal intensity on the T2-
weighted image (black arrow).

At histology, interstitial edema
mixed with cancer was present.
The edematous changes are
probably responsible for
masking the tumor signal
intensity, which was involving
the entire gland. Tumor (T) can
be seen in the left gland.

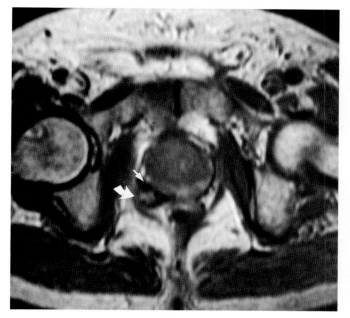

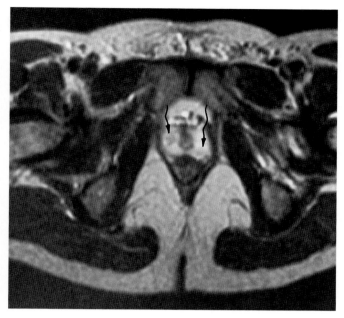

a

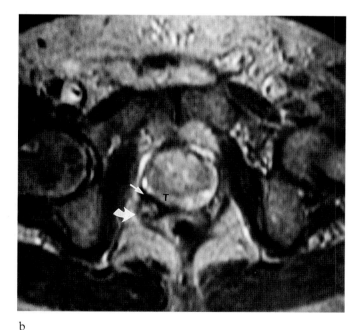

b

Figure 8.51

Multifocal prostatic carcinoma. Transaxial T2-weighted image demonstrating two peripheral zone tumors (arrows).

Figure 8.50

Periprostatic hematoma postbiopsy. Transaxial (**a**) T1-, and (**b**) T2-weighted images showing a periprostatic hematoma (white curved arrow) of medium signal intensity on the T1-weighted and heterogeneous signal on the T2-weighted image. The hematoma is separated from the adjacent peripheral zone tumor (T) by the thick low signal intensity band (straight arrow).

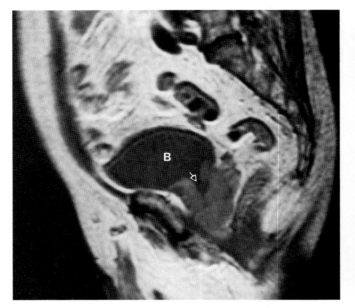

a

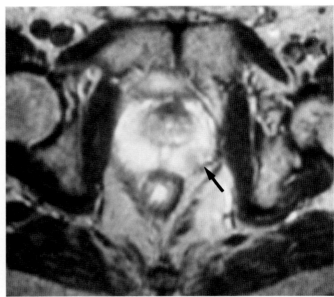

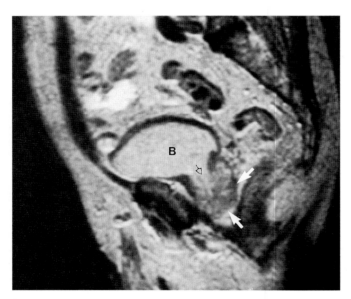

b

Figure 8.53

Prostate carcinoma stage B1. Transaxial T2-weighted image showing a localized low signal intensity tumor (arrow) measuring less than 1.5 cm in diameter and confined to one side of the gland.

Figure 8.52

Prostate carcinoma stage A2. Sagittal (**a**) proton density, and (**b**) T2-weighted images showing previous TURP defect (open arrow) and the presence of a tumor (arrows) within the peripheral zone. (B)-urinary bladder.

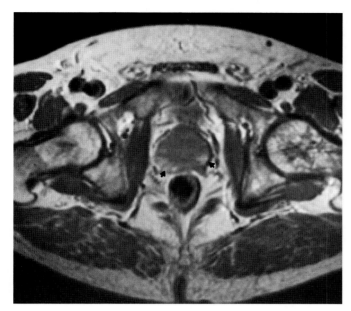

a

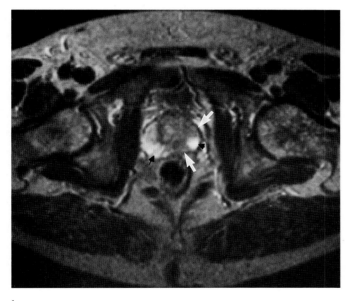

b

Figure 8.54

Prostate carcinoma stage B2. Transaxial (**a**) proton density and (**b**) T2-weighted images showing a low signal tumor (white arrows) measuring greater than 1.5 cm and involving the entire left side of the gland. High signal intensity areas (black arrows) are due to postbiopsy hemorrhage. At surgery, the tumor involved both sides of the gland.

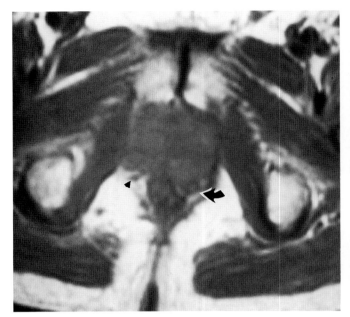

a

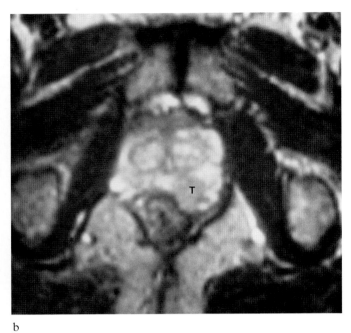

b

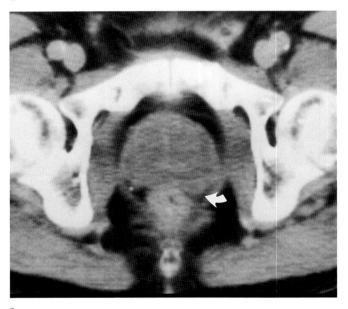

c

Figure 8.55

Prostatic carcinoma, stage C.
Transaxial (**a**) T1- and (**b**) T2-
weighted images. (**c**) CT scan
of the same level. There is a
localized bulge at the left
posterolateral margin of the
gland (arrow) which
demonstrates abnormal low
signal on the T2-weighted
image due to a tumor (T). The
nodule extends into the location
of the left neurovascular
bundle, consistent with nerve
infiltration. The right
neurovascular bundle is not
invaded (small black arrow).
The same bulge is identified on
CT but CT density difference
does not allow the direct tumor
visualization.

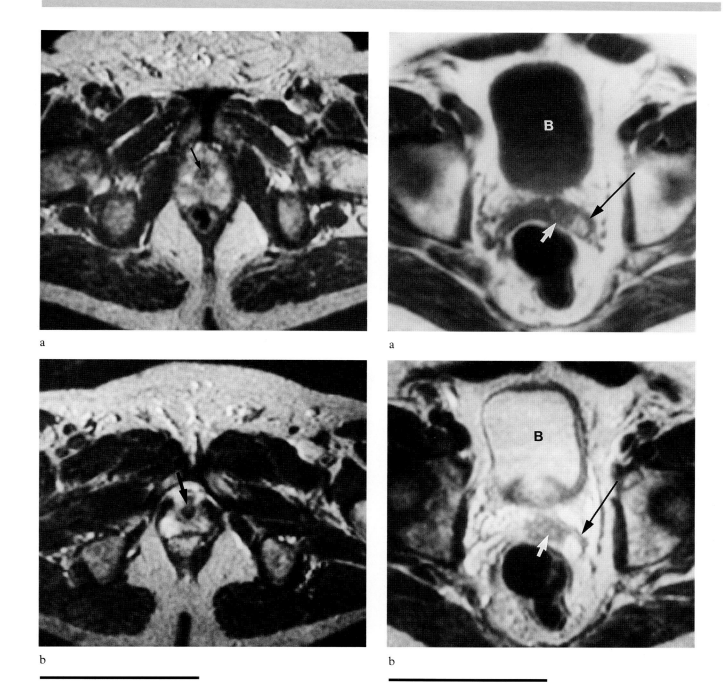

Figure 8.56

Prostatic carcinoma extending into the apex of the gland—stage B2. Transaxial T2-weighted images (**a**) below the level of the verumontanum and (**b**) at the apex of the gland. A low signal intensity tumor is seen diffusely involving the apex of the gland. (Arrow)-urethra.

Figure 8.57

Prostatic carcinoma with localized invasion of the left seminal vesicle stage C/T3B. Transaxial (**a**) proton density and (**b**) T2-weighted images illustrating abnormal low signal intensity area (white arrow) within the proximal portion of the seminal vesicles due to prostate carcinoma tumor infiltration. Hemorrhage seen at the tip of the left seminal vesicle (long black arrow) was due to vascular erosion by the tumor. (B)-urinary bladder.

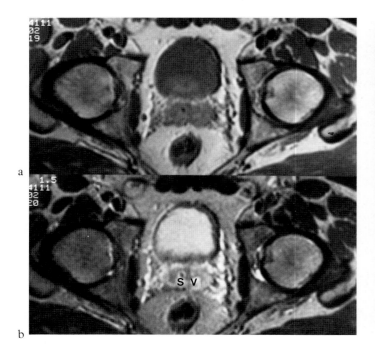

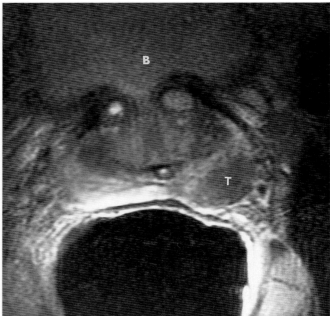

a

Figure 8.58

Prostatic carcinoma with diffuse involvement of the seminal vesicles. Stage C/T3B. Transaxial (**a**) T1- and (**b**) T2-weighted images illustrating abnormal low signal intensity foci throughout the seminal vesicles (SV) on the T2-weighted image due to prostate tumor invasion.

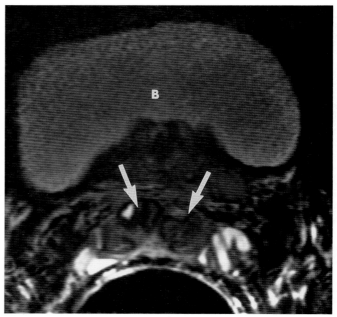

b

Figure 8.59

Stage C/T3B, prostate carcinoma; endorectal surface coil T2-weighted transaxial image at the level of (**a**) the base of the prostate gland, (**b**) seminal vesicles. Tumor (T) in the left peripheral zone demonstrates early transcapsular invasion. Low signal intensity tumor is extending into both seminal vesicles (long white arrows). (B)-urinary bladder. (Courtesy of Dr Herbert Kressel.)

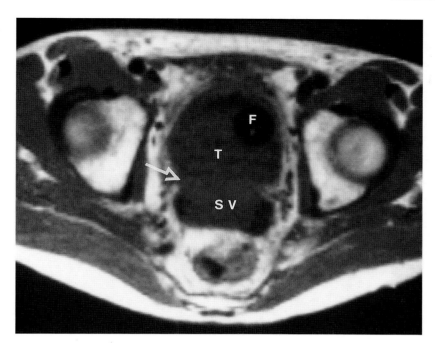

a

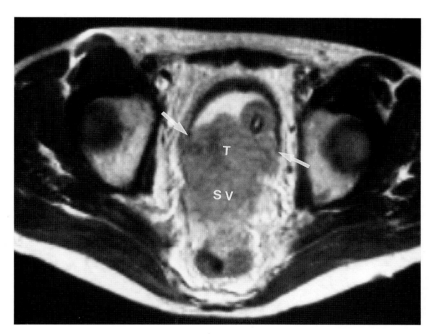

b

Figure 8.60

Prostatic carcinoma invading the urinary bladder. Stage C/T3B. Transaxial (**a**) T1-weighted image, and (**b**) T2-weighted image. A large prostate tumor (T) is invading the bladder, with loss of the normal low signal intensity bladder wall (arrows) on the T2-weighted image. The seminal vesicles (SV) are also replaced by tumor. The angle between the seminal vesicles and bladder is lost (open arrow), a late finding. (F)-Foley catheter balloon. (0.35T.)

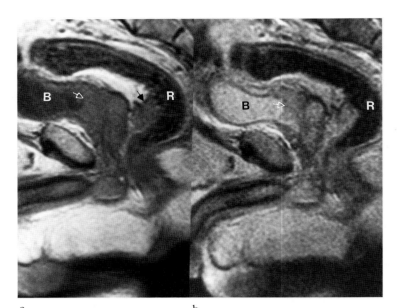

a   b

Figure 8.61

Prostatic carcinoma extending into the bladder and rectum. Stage C/T4. Sagittal (**a**) proton density, and (**b**) T2-weighted images showing tumor invasion of the bladder (white open arrow) and rectum (black arrow). (B)-urinary bladder; (R)-rectum.

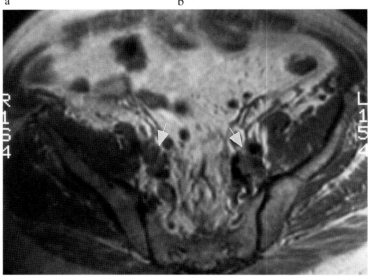

Figure 8.62

Prostatic carcinoma with lymphadenopathy. Stage D1. Transaxial proton density image showing bilateral lymphadenopathy (arrows) at the bifurcation of the common iliac arteries due to metastatic prostate carcinoma.

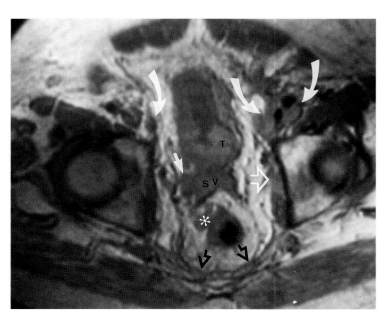

Figure 8.63

Prostatic carcinoma, stage D. Transaxial T1-weighted image showing extensive local spread of the disease with tumor extension into the urinary bladder (T), perirectal space (asterisk), presacral space (black open arrowheads), and pelvic sidewall (white open arrow). Enlarged lymph nodes in the inguinal (curved arrows) region and adjacent to (straight arrow) the seminal vesicles (SV) are seen.

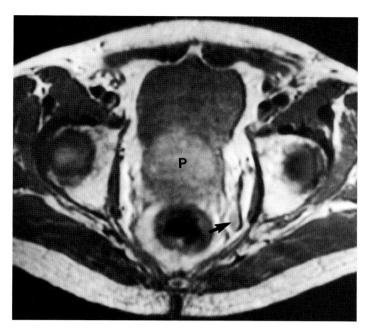

a

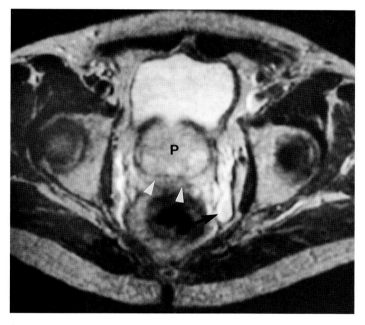

b

Figure 8.64

Vesicoprostatic plexus (black arrow) mimicking a lymph node on a transaxial (**a**) T1-weighted image but shown to be a blood vessel on the (**b**) T2-weighted image. Prostate (P) is enlarged due to benign prostatic hypertrophy. (Small white arrows)-peripheral zone carcinoma.

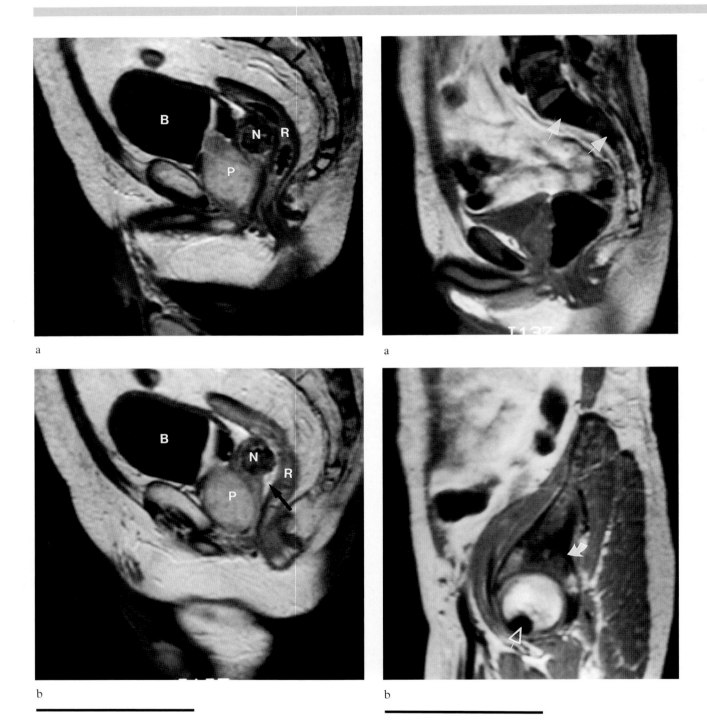

a

b

a

b

Figure 8.65

Enlarged lymph node in vesicorectal pouch (cul-de-sac). (**a**) and (**b**) Gd-DTPA-enhanced T1-weighted sagittal images. Because of its location ('drop metastasis'), the node (N) is unlikely to be due to prostate carcinoma. A subsequent barium enema revealed carcinoma of the cecum. (Arrow)-fat in the cul-de-sac; (B)-urinary bladder; (P)-prostate; (R)-rectum.

Figure 8.66

Bony metastases from prostate carcinoma. Stage D2. (**a**) and (**b**) T1-weighted sagittal images showing widespread low signal intensity bony metastases involving the sacrum (arrows), femoral head (open arrow) and ilium (curved arrow).

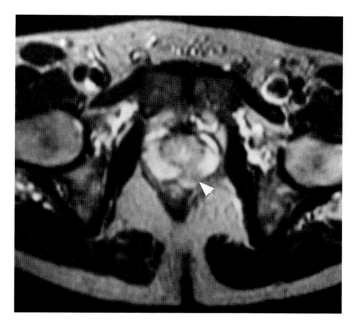

a

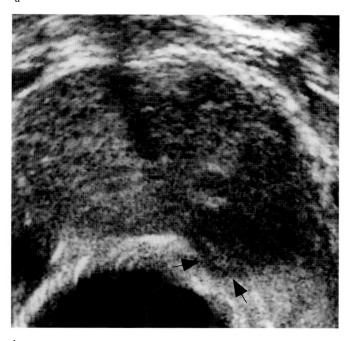

b

Figure 8.67

Early transcapsular tumor extension detected by TRUS but not by MRI. (**a**) MRI transaxial T2-weighted image and (**b**) TRUS. On MRI, the tumor (white arrow) appears to be confined to the gland but on the TRUS a localized bulge (arrows) is seen indicating transcapsular extension.

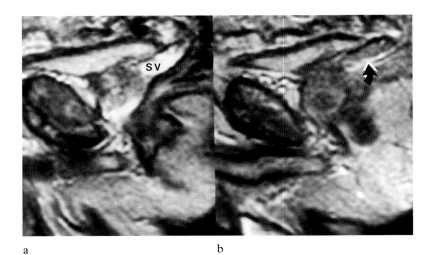

a   b

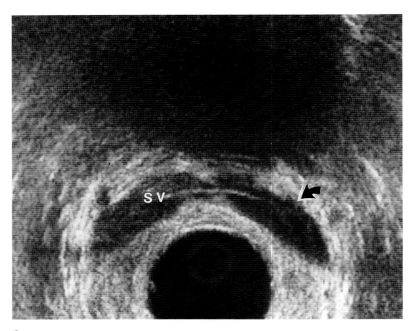

c

Figure 8.68

Prostatic tumor involvement of the seminal vesicles detected by MRI but not by ultrasound. (**a**) and (**b**) are sagittal T2-weighted images. (**c**) Transaxial TRUS. The right seminal vesicle (SV) in (**a**) is of normal high signal intensity but the left seminal vesicle (arrow) in (**b**) is of abnormal low signal intensity due to tumor involvement. The seminal vesicles appear symmetrical on TRUS and invasion of the left side seminal vesicle is not detected.

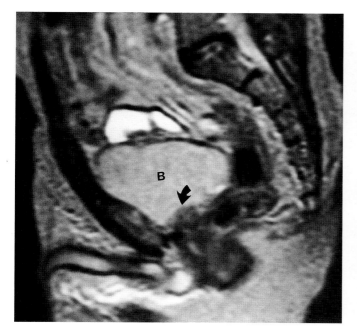

a

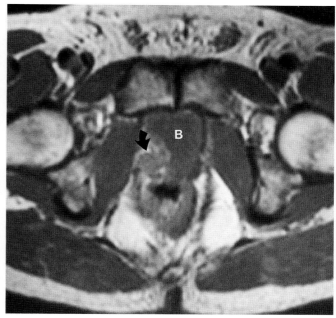

b

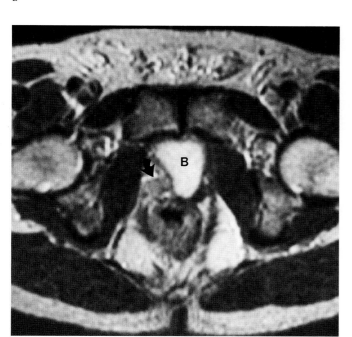

c

Figure 8.69

Recurrent prostate carcinoma after radical prostatectomy. sagittal (**a**) T2-weighted image, transaxial (**b**) proton density and (**c**) T2-weighted images. A tumor mass (curved arrow) is seen lateral and inferior to the urinary bladder (B). The tumor is of medium signal intensity on the T1-weighted image and low signal intensity on the T2-weighted image. The diagnosis of tumor is made by the size and shape of the lesion, and by the mass effect on the adjacent bladder.

9

The Seminal Vesicles

Hedvig Hricak

The seminal vesicles, situated 12 to 15 cm from the anal verge, are difficult to palpate digitally, and radiologic assessment is an important tool in clinical evaluation.[1] Radiologic studies are appropriate in the investigation of suspected congenital anomalies, in selected cases of infertility with low ejaculatory volume and/or azoospermia, in hemospermia, and in the assessment of primary or metastatic neoplasms. All of the cross-sectional imaging modalities—computed tomography (CT),[2] transrectal ultrasound (TRUS),[3] and magnetic resonance imaging (MRI)[4–12]— provide morphologic display of the seminal vesicles. Seminal vesiculography is frequently used for demonstration of seminal vesicle architecture,[1] but this invasive procedure involves cannulation of the ductus deferens, and may be complicated by infection and cicatrization.[4] MRI provides excellent display of the seminal vesicles in axial, coronal and sagittal planes without the risks attendant on an invasive study. As the technology of MRI becomes more advanced, and as the technique becomes more widely used, MRI is likely to play a dominant role in the evaluation of the anatomy and pathology of seminal vesicles.

Normal anatomy of the seminal vesicles

The seminal vesicles are paired, androgen-dependent, accessory glands which, together with the ductus deferens, ejaculatory duct and the epididymis, develop from the mesonephric–wolffian duct. The seminal vesicles and the ampulla of the ductus deferens appear as a common swelling at the termination of the mesonephric duct during the end of the third month of development. The seminal vesicles then elongate to form a duct from which hollow diverticula bud.

The seminal vesicles are located cephalad to the prostate gland, dorsal to the urinary bladder, and ventral to the rectum (Figure 9.1). In children, the seminal vesicles are entirely covered by the peritoneum. In adults, however, they are mostly extraperitoneal, and only the lateral tips are covered by the peritoneum. The anterior surface of the seminal vesicles is in close contact with the posterior surface of the urinary bladder, and the rectovesical fascia is interposed between the seminal vesicles and the rectum. At the point where the seminal vesicles diverge, forming an angle to the horizontal plane of 50–60°, the tips of the glands are approximately 7–8 cm apart. As illustrated in Figure 9.1, the ampulla of the ductus deferens runs along the medial margin of the vesicle, the ureters are anterior, and the veins of the vesicoprostatic venous plexus lie laterally to each seminal vesicle.[1,11]

Each seminal vesicle consists of a single tube coiled upon itself, giving rise to 10–12 irregular diverticula. The diameter of the tube is 3–4 mm and the length is 3–6 cm. When the tube is uncoiled, the length varies from 10–15 cm. The width of the seminal vesicles is 8–20 mm. Each seminal vesicle is enveloped in a dense fibromuscular sheet. In its medial portion, the tube is constricted and forms a narrow, straight, short duct with an internal diameter of approximately 1.5 mm. This is called the excretory duct of the seminal vesicle and it joins at a variable point with the ductus deferens to form the ejaculatory duct.[11]

Goblet cells in the diverticula of the seminal vesicles produce secretions which form a large part of the seminal vesicle fluid. The vesicles contract during ejaculation, and the seminal vesicle fluid forms the bulk of the ejaculatory fluid. The seminal vesicles are

313

not, however, a reservoir for spermatozoa. The arterial supply of the seminal vesicles is derived from the inferior vesical and middle rectal arteries, and from the artery of the ductus deferens. The veins accompany the arteries, and lymphatic drainage is to the internal and external iliac chains.

MRI appearance

The size, configuration, and fluid content of the seminal vesicles can be evaluated with MRI.[4,6,7] As shown in Figure 9.2, on T1-weighted images, normal seminal vesicles demonstrate homogeneous and symmetrical signal intensity similar to, or slightly higher than, that of the adjacent obturator internus muscle. Because the seminal vesicles are secretory as well as excretory organs, signal intensities on T2-weighted images may vary without indicating any pathology.[7] On T2-weighted images, normal seminal vesicles may demonstrate a signal intensity lower than, similar to, or higher than adjacent fat.[7] The grape-like configuration of the seminal vesicles is best appreciated on T2-weighted images (Figure 9.2), where the low signal intensity outer fibromuscular sheet and the inner convolutions can be differentiated from the high signal intensity fluid.

The ductus deferens, located medial to the seminal vesicles, demonstrates medium to low signal intensity on T1-weighted images, and a low signal intensity ring corresponding to the outer fibromuscular band can be seen on T2-weighted images (Figure 9.3). The vessels of the vesicoprostatic venous plexus can be seen surrounding the tips of the seminal vesicles, and as illustrated in Figure 9.4, are most prominent laterally.

On gadolinium-DTPA-enhanced T1-weighted images as depicted in Figure 9.5, the walls of the seminal vesicle convolutions demonstrate enhancement, while the fluid remains of low signal intensity.

With fat saturation techniques, the grape-like configuration of the seminal vesicles can be seen even on T1-weighted images (Figure 9.6). The high signal intensity is due to computer contrast adjustment, compensating for the loss of brightness of the surrounding fat. On Gd-DTPA-enhanced T1-weighted fat saturation images, as seen in Figure 9.7, the wall of the seminal vesicles is of higher signal intensity than their fluid content, which does not enhance. In spite of the suppression of the high signal intensity of fat with this technique, the high signal intensity of contrast-enhanced urine in the bladder produces a different gray scale (readjustment by the computer), making the fluid in the seminal vesicles image with lower signal intensity.

The average length of the seminal vesicle, as measured on MRI scans, is 3.1 ± 0.7 cm.[7] This figure is less than that reported in the anatomy literature (4 to 6 cm),[12] probably because of the oblique orientation of the seminal vesicles in relation to the orthogonal axis of the body. With this angle of orientation, as shown in Figure 9.8, it is unlikely that both the medial and lateral ends of the seminal vesicles are included in a single 5 mm or 10 mm slice, and their length is therefore systematically underestimated. The width of the seminal vesicles is reported to be 17 ± 4 mm, similar to that reported from autopsy studies.[7,12] Because the seminal vesicles are androgen-dependent sex accessory glands, there is a complex relationship between size and chronologic age.[1] Before puberty, very little, if any, fluid is present within the seminal vesicles. As shown in Figure 9.9, the width of seminal vesicles is smaller in pediatric patients, and on T2-weighted images the seminal vesicles demonstrate symmetrical lower signal intensity. Although no statistically significant correlation between chronological age and the size of the adult seminal vesicles has been reported in the MRI literature, there is a tendency for the seminal vesicles to be wider in the fifth and sixth decades of life (probably due to concomitant prostatic enlargement) and smaller after the sixth decade (probably due to decreased androgen stimulation and resultant smaller volumes of seminal vesicle fluid).[7] Great variations in the size of seminal vesicles can occur in men of the same age group (Figures 9.10 and 9.11). The seminal vesicles are usually symmetrical in size, but asymmetry has been reported in up to 10 per cent of patients. As illustrated in Figure 9.12, even when asymmetrical in size, the normal seminal vesicles are symmetrical in signal intensity on T1- and T2-weighted images.[7]

The location of the seminal vesicles—posterior to the urinary bladder, anterior to the rectum, and superior to the prostate gland— is well displayed on MRI. The location of the seminal vesicles, however, is influenced by urinary bladder or rectal distention, patient position, or as seen in Figure 9.13, by the presence of an adjacent pelvic mass. Furthermore, the location and orientation of the glands change in patients who have had previous abdominoperineal resection. In these patients the seminal vesicles (Figure 9.14), are displaced posteriorly. In addition, the orientation of the seminal vesicles can be affected by scarring (Figure 9.15). Change in the orientation of the seminal vesicles (being more vertical and the angle between them more acute) can also be seen in patients with pelvic lipomatosis[13] (Figure 9.16).

Appearance of the seminal vesicles following endocrine or radiation therapy

Production of seminal vesicle fluid, which is androgen dependent and requires intact glandular elements of the goblet cells, is affected by both hormones[7] and radiation therapy.[14] It is diminished in patients receiving estrogen therapy (Figure 9.17), in patients who have had bilateral orchiectomy, in severe alcoholics (Figure 9.14), and in older patients. It is generally agreed that androgen secretion decreases after the age of 70 years,[7] and variations in the appearance of the seminal vesicles will be noted (Figure 9.11). Radiation therapy causes direct epithelial injury resulting in glandular atrophy and decreased fluid production. Seminal vesicle tissue toxicity has been reported with radiation doses of 5000 cGy or greater.[14]

When seminal fluid production is reduced by either endocrine (Figure 9.17) or radiation (Figure 9.18) causes, there is a global and symmetrical effect on the MR appearance of the seminal vesicles.[7] On T2-weighted images the seminal vesicles appear small and demonstrate low signal intensity. When seminal vesicle signal intensity is decreased due to androgen depletion it may be similar to or lower than adjacent adipose tissue, but not as low as that of the skeletal muscle (Figure 9.17). This finding is important in diagnosing seminal vesicle tumor invasion. Following radiation therapy, however, the seminal vesicles may demonstrate very low signal intensity, making the distinction between radiation changes and tumor invasion difficult (Figure 9.19).

Recommended imaging sequences

Both T1- and T2-weighted images are recommended for the complete evaluation of the seminal vesicles. T1-weighted images are necessary for the demonstration of the presence of the seminal vesicles, for fluid characterization, and for assessment of perivesicular tumor extension. T2-weighted images are required to demonstrate the internal architecture of the seminal vesicles, and are helpful in the assessment of fluid characterization and in tumor detection.

The value of the use of Gd-DTPA in assessing the seminal vesicles is still being explored.

Conventional spin-echo images have provided the bulk of the information about this organ to date. Fat saturation sequences, though promising because of excellent contrast resolution between the seminal vesicles and surrounding adipose tissue, need more extensive studies.

Transaxial imaging is recommended in all patients. Sagittal imaging, as illustrated in Figure 9.20, allows demonstration of the relationships among the seminal vesicles, the prostate gland, the urinary bladder, and the rectum. The addition of the sagittal plane is helpful in the assessment of congenital anomalies and tumor extension. Coronal imaging (Figure 9.3) demonstrates the relationships among the seminal vesicles, the ampulla of the ductus deferens and the prostate gland, and is also useful in the assessment of congenital anomalies and tumor extension.

Pathology of the seminal vesicles

Congenital anomalies

Congenital anomalies of the seminal vesicles include abnormalities in number (agenesis or duplication), abnormalities in position (ectopia), and congenital seminal vesicle cysts.[11] **Agenesis** of the seminal vesicles can be unilateral or bilateral. When unilateral, agenesis is often an incidental finding, commonly associated with ipsilateral renal agenesis and congenital absence of the ductus deferens. Bilateral seminal vesicle agenesis, in which the volume of the ejaculate is very small (less than 1.5 ml), usually comes to the clinician's attention as one of the causes of infertility. **Ectopia** (abnormality in position) is also often associated with renal agenesis.

The most common congenital anomaly of the seminal vesicles are **seminal vesicle cysts**.[15] They may be unilateral or, less commonly, bilateral; unilocular or multilocular; and can involve one or more convolutions of the seminal vesicles. Seminal vesicle cysts may be acquired, in which case they are often related to partial or complete obstruction of the ejaculatory duct.[15] Clinical symptoms usually parallel the size of the cyst. Small seminal vesicle cysts are usually an incidental finding during US, CT, or MRI evaluation of the pelvis. A large cyst, however, may irritate the bladder causing dysuria, frequency, perineal pain, and painful ejaculation. Bladder outlet obstruction by seminal vesicle cysts has been reported. Although rectal examination may reveal the presence of a cystic mass above the prostate, the high position of the seminal vesicles makes rectal examination difficult.

Pelvic **arteriovenous malformations** (AVMs) are rare lesions. They are characterized by the presence of many feeding arteries and lack of confinement to a single anatomical region. The incidence of AVMs in the pelvis is higher in females. In males, due to the presence of the rich vesicoprostatic venous plexus, AVMs are commonly seen in the vicinity of the seminal vesicles and can be a cause of hemospermia.

MRI appearance

Agenesis of the seminal vesicles is best identified on T1-weighted transaxial MR images. As depicted in Figure 9.21, in bilateral seminal vesicle agenesis the only structure seen between the rectum and the bladder base is areolar tissue.[7] Since many of the vessels of the vesicoprostatic venous plexus are present in that location, caution must be exercised to avoid mistaking the vesicoprostatic venous plexus for small seminal vesicles. Characteristically, these vessels will exhibit very high signal intensity on a second echo image. With unilateral seminal vesicle agenesis, the existing side is seldom normally developed. As seen in Figure 9.22, the developed seminal vesicle is small or can be hypoplastic (Figure 9.23). In addition to the transaxial plane of imaging, which is essential, agenesis of seminal vesicles may also be diagnosed from scans in the sagittal or coronal planes.

Hypoplasia of the seminal vesicles, which causes a decreased amount of seminal vesicle fluid, is a clinical entity often discussed in assessment of male infertility. It is difficult to establish this diagnosis because of the wide variations in the size of normal seminal vesicles. However, it is generally accepted that seminal vesicles which are less than 2 cm in length and less than 0.5 cm in width, and which lack normal convolutions are hypoplastic.

Seminal vesicle cysts can be identified and differentiated from prostatic cysts on MRI scans. In contrast to müllerian duct cysts, seminal vesicle cysts (Figure 9.24) are lateral in location and often cause obstruction of the ipsilateral seminal vesicle.[6,7,16] Seminal vesicle cysts can be medial in location (Figure 9.25), but unlike müllerian duct cysts they never communicate with the prostate. The fluid in seminal vesicle cysts varies in signal intensity depending on its composition. Since hemorrhage is a common complication, the cyst's fluid content may image with high signal intensity on both T1- and T2-weighted scans (Figure 9.24).

Because of MRI's unique ability to discern vascular structures without the need for any contrast media, it can be used in the diagnosis of **AV malformations** as well. The diagnosis is based on the finding of abundant amounts of vessels in the vesicoprostatic plexus. Other modalities, such as CT (Figure 9.26) and ultrasound are less reliable for the characterization of pelvic AVMs.

MRI in relation to other imaging modalities

Congenital anomalies, including agenesis and ectopia, have historically been evaluated by seminal vesiculography.[1] Currently, however, cross-sectional imaging (ultrasound, CT and MRI) has replaced the seminal vesiculogram in the evaluation of agenesis or hypoplasia of the seminal vesicles. For the diagnosis of seminal vesicle ectopia, however, a vesiculogram is still the most accurate approach. Seminal vesicle cysts can be depicted with either transrectal ultrasound, CT,

or MRI. Although TRUS is now advocated as the primary imaging modality, results may be compromised because of the high position of the seminal vesicles, and evaluation is difficult when the cyst is large. CT, which has a larger field-of-view and is not as operator dependent as TRUS, has been advocated as an alternative when TRUS is not satisfactory. However, CT is limited to direct transaxial imaging; the origin of large cysts is sometimes difficult to assign, and multiplanar imaging with MRI offers a significant advantage. Presently ultrasound is recommended as the primary approach in the evaluation of the seminal vesicles and, if equivocal, MRI is the next study for further evaluation. CT is used for those patients in whom an ultrasound guided biopsy or cyst puncture is not technically feasible. Because congenital anomalies of the seminal vesicles are frequently associated with renal agenesis, examination of the kidneys is always advised.

Inflammatory disease

Inflammation of the seminal vesicles—seminal vesiculitis—is a very difficult clinical diagnosis.[1,17] Infection usually ascends from the prostate gland or is associated with epididymitis, but isolated seminal vesiculitis can occur and usually presents with hemospermia. Clinical presentation and the imaging findings depend on whether the inflammation is in the acute, subacute or chronic phase.[1,7]

MRI appearance

In the clinical setting of **acute inflammation**, on MRI the seminal vesicles may appear normal or one or both of the seminal vesicles may be enlarged.[7] The signal intensity on either the T1- or T2-weighted images may be normal, or as shown in Figure 9.27, the involved seminal vesicle on T1-weighted MR images may demonstrate a signal intensity lower than the normal contralateral seminal vesicle or the adjacent obturator internus muscle. Similarly, on T2-weighted images, the signal intensity may be normal or lower than normal.

In **subacute infection**, various MRI features can be seen ranging from normal appearing seminal vesicles to evidence of blood within the gland. Hemospermia is the most common clinical finding in subacute infection. Blood within the seminal vesicles produces signal intensity changes which vary depending on the age of the bleeding. The seminal vesicles may demonstrate high signal intensity on both T1- and T2-weighted images (Figure 9.28).[7]

Chronic inflammation results in small, often fibrotic seminal vesicles that produce less vesicular fluid and consequently image with lower than normal signal intensity on T2-weighted images. As illustrated in Figure 9.29, the small seminal vesicles seen on the T1-weighted image can be correlated with a fibrotic gland seen on seminal vesiculography.

Abscess of the seminal vesicle is demonstrated as a mass lesion of low signal intensity on the T1-weighted image. The margins of the abscess are ill-defined, and the adjacent fat is usually infiltrated. On T1-weighted images, perivesicular adipose tissue demonstrates low signal intensity stranding. Extension of the inflammatory process along the perirectal fascia into the presacral region can also be seen (Figure 9.30).

MRI in relation to other imaging modalities

Inflammatory disease of the seminal vesicles is usually a clinical diagnosis not requiring any imaging procedures. However, the evaluation of unexplained hemospermia or suspected obstruction of the seminal vesicles by calculus in the ejaculatory duct may be facilitated by TRUS or MRI. MRI is superior to TRUS for the detection of blood in the seminal vesicles. However, if a calculus in the ejaculatory duct is suspected, TRUS is the modality of choice. CT, TRUS, and MRI are appropriate in the evaluation of an abscess, but the CT finding of a low- or fluid-density ill-defined mass is the most specific. If abscess drainage is required, TRUS is the recommended procedure.

Tumors of the seminal vesicles

Primary tumors of the seminal vesicles, benign or malignant, are rare.[1] They are mostly asymptomatic and found incidentally. Infrequently, they may cause hemospermia, and benign tumors do so more often than malignant tumors.[1] Histologically, the most common benign tumors are leiomyomas; but fibromas, angiomas, and lipomas have also been reported.

Most malignant tumors of the seminal vesicles are metastatic usually due to extension of tumor arising from the prostate gland, the urinary bladder and the rectum. Metastatic tumor invasion from the prostate usually occurs via the ejaculatory duct or by direct tumor extension through the perivesical tissue.[18] Tumor invasion from the bladder and rectum occurs by direct spread through the perivesical adipose tissue.

Primary seminal vesicle cancers are usually adenocarcinomas, most frequently occurring in men of 60–80 years of age. Sarcomas, fibrosarcomas, and leiomyosarcomas may also arise in the seminal vesicles.[19]

MRI appearance

Multiplanar MR imaging facilitates the detection of the tumors of the seminal vesicles.[4,7] As illustrated in Figure 9.31, benign tumors of the seminal vesicles present masses with smooth, sharp outlines and normal adjacent fat.[4] On T1-weighted images, tumors demonstrate nonspecific medium signal intensity and increase in signal intensity on T2-weighted images. Depending on their location, they may cause seminal vesicle obstruction and the glands may be asymmetrically enlarged. When tumors cause hemospermia, the signal intensity of the fluid content of the seminal vesicles is changed and depends on the age of the blood. To date the MRI appearance of a primary malignant tumor of the seminal vesicles has not been described.

The MRI appearance of secondary tumor involvement depends on the route of spread and the degree of seminal vesicle invasion. When tumor invasion due to prostate carcinoma follows the course of the ejaculatory ducts, the seminal vesicles may appear normal on T1-weighted images. As illustrated in Figure 9.32, on T2-weighted images unilateral or bilateral areas of low signal intensity may be seen in the medial part of the gland (the seminal vesicle neck).[7–10]

The diagnosis of direct tumor invasion is facilitated by the use of the sagittal plane of imaging. As seen in Figure 9.33, direct tumor spread is well displayed on sagittal T2-weighted images. This is especially important as on the transaxial plane it is sometimes difficult to differentiate normal low signal intensity of the central zone in the base of the prostate gland (see Chapter 8) from invasion of the medial seminal vesicles. The distal portions of the vesicles may appear normal (Figure 9.33) or distended (Figure 9.34), or may demonstrate hemorrhage. Obstruction of the seminal vesicle is not a definitive sign of invasion, since it may be secondary to extrinsic compression by tumor bulk or caused by a nonmalignant process such as benign prostatic enlargement. Blood within the seminal vesicles (Figure 9.35) can be identified by the presence of high signal intensity fluid on T1-weighted images. Bleeding may be due to tumor invasion or it may be due to a recent biopsy. MR imaging cannot differentiate between these two entities nor can MRI identify tumor microinvasion.

In direct tumor invasion (Figure 9.36) the tissue planes between the seminal vesicles, urinary bladder and the prostate are infiltrated. A contiguous mass of low signal intensity can be seen.

At present, there is no proven value for the use of

either Gd-DTPA or fat saturation images (Figure 9.37) in the diagnosis of seminal vesicle tumor invasion.

MRI in relation to other imaging modalities

All cross-sectional imaging modalities can be used for the evaluation of primary or secondary tumors of the seminal vesicles. Before the advent of TRUS or MRI, CT was considered the modality of choice. CT studies are, however, limited by poor contrast resolution and transaxial planar imaging. CT has been replaced by TRUS and MRI as primary imaging modalities for assessment of seminal vesicle pathology.

The selection of TRUS versus MRI as the primary imaging route is still controversial. With TRUS, asymmetry in the size of seminal vesicles can be detected, but tissue characterization is limited and blood within the seminal vesicles may not be demonstrated. Furthermore, its usefulness in the evaluation of seminal vesicle tumor invasion arising from carcinoma of the bladder or rectum has not been reported. MRI has been shown to be useful in the evaluation of tumor invasion from the prostate (see Chapter 8), bladder (see Chapter 12), or rectum (see Chapter 13). Detection of prostate tumor invasion of the seminal vesicles has been reported with an accuracy of 78 per cent,[7] with a 90 per cent negative predictive value, underscoring the importance of MRI in the evaluation of seminal vesicles.[7]

References

1 BOREAU J, *Images of the Seminal Tracts: Radiological and Clinical Comparisons*, (S Karger: New York 1974).

2 SILVERMAN PM, DUNNICK NR, FORD KK, Computer tomography of the normal seminal vesicles, *Comput Radiol* (1985) 9(6):379–85.

3 LEE SB, LEE F, SOLOMON MH et al, Seminal vesicle abscess: diagnosis by transrectal ultrasound, *J Clin Ultrasound* (1986) 14:546.

4 MCCLURE RD, HRICAK H, Magnetic resonance imaging: its application to male infertility, *Urology* (1986) 27:91–8.

5 EDSON S, HRICAK H, MRI of the seminal vesicles: normal anatomy and pathology. Presented at the Society for Magnetic Resonance Imaging, 1987.

6 KNEELAND JB, AUH YH, MCCARRON JP et al, Computer tomography, sonography, vesiculography, and MR imaging of a seminal vesicle cyst, *J Comp Asst Tomogr* (1985) 9(5):964–6.

7 NURUDDIN RN, HRICAK H, MCCLURE RD et al, Magnetic resonance imaging of the seminal vesicles, *AJR* (submitted).

8 BIONDETTI PR, LEE JKT, LING D et al, Clinical stage B prostate carcinoma: staging with MR imaging, *Radiology* (1987) 162:325–9.

9 HRICAK H, DOOMS GC, JEFFREY RB et al, Prostate carcinoma: staging by clinical assessment, CT and MR imaging, *Radiology* (1987) 162:331–6.

10 BEZZI M, KRESSEL HY, ALLEN KS et al, Prostatic carcinoma: staging with MR imaging at 1.5 T, *Radiology* (1988) 169:339–46.

11 LIERSE W, *Applied Anatomy of the Pelvis* (Springer-Verlag: Heidelberg 1984) 169–70.

12 NISSON S, The human seminal vesicles, *Acta Chir Scan* (Supplement) (1962) 296:36–42 and 50–63.

13 DEMAS BE, AVALLONE A, HRICAK H, Pelvic lipomatosis: diagnosis and characterization by magnetic resonance imaging, *Urol Radiol* (1988) 10:198–202.

14 SUGIMURA K, CARRINGTON B, QUIVEY J et al, Postirradiation changes in the pelvis: assessment with MR imaging, *Radiology* (1990) 175:805–13.

15 ROEHOBORN CG, SCHNEIDER HJ, RUGENDERF EW et al, Embryological and diagnostic aspects of seminal vesicle cysts associated with upper urinary tract malformations, *J Urol* (1986) 135:1029–32.

16 THURNER S, HRICAK H, TANAGHO EA, Müllerian duct cyst: diagnosis with MR imaging, *Radiology* (1988) 167:631–6.

17 MEARES EM, Prostatalis and related disorder. In: Walsh PC, Gittes RF, Perlmutter AD et al, *Campbell's Urology* (WB Saunders: Philadelphia 1986) 868–85.

18 STAMEY TA, MCNEAL JE, FREIHA FS et al, Morphometric and clinical studies on 68 consecutive radical prostatectomies, *J Urol* (1988) 139:1253.

19 MURPHY GP, GEATA JF, Tumors of testicular adnexal structures and seminal vesicles. In: Walsh PC, Gittes RF, Perlmutter AD et al, *Campbell's Urology* (WB Saunders: Philadelphia 1986) 1607–14.

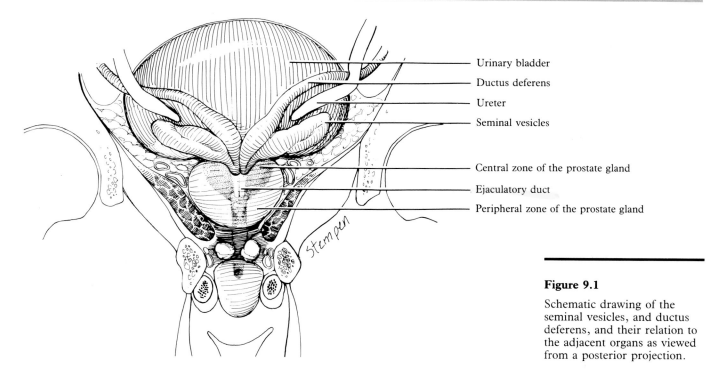

Figure 9.1

Schematic drawing of the seminal vesicles, and ductus deferens, and their relation to the adjacent organs as viewed from a posterior projection.

In the schematic drawing, the following are labeled:
Urinary bladder
Ductus deferens
Ureter
Seminal vesicles
Central zone of the prostate gland
Ejaculatory duct
Peripheral zone of the prostate gland

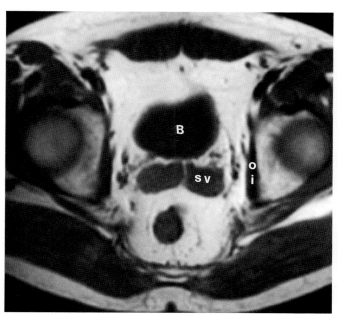

a

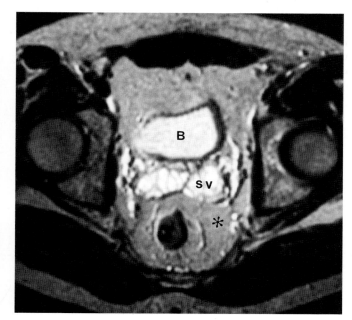

b

Figure 9.2

Normal seminal vesicles in the transaxial plane, (**a**) T1- and (**b**) T2-weighted images. On the T1-weighted image, the signal intensity of the seminal vesicle (SV) is slightly higher than that of the adjacent obturator internus muscle (Oi) or urine within the urinary bladder (B). On the T2-weighted image, the seminal vesicles (SV) show increase in signal intensity [their signal intensity is higher than that of the adjacent fat (asterisk)]. They demonstrate a grape-like configuration, with differentiation between low signal intensity septa and high signal intensity fluid.

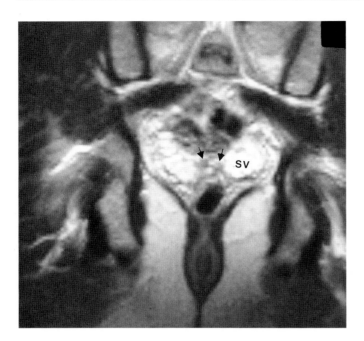

Figure 9.3

Normal seminal vesicles and ductus deferens in a coronal plane, T2-weighted image. The seminal vesicles (SV) demonstrate a grape-like configuration and are of high signal intensity. The ductus deferens, in contrast, are shown as two low signal intensity dots (arrows) in the medial part of the seminal vesicles. (0.35T.)

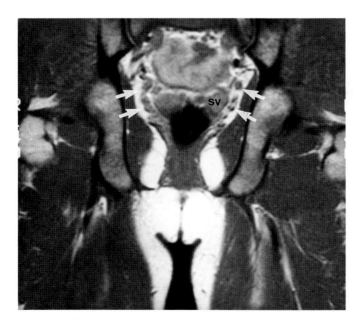

Figure 9.4

Demonstration of the vesicoprostatic plexus and its relation to the seminal vesicles. Coronal plane, proton density image. Lateral to the tips of the vesicles (SV) is the vesicoprostatic plexus (arrows).

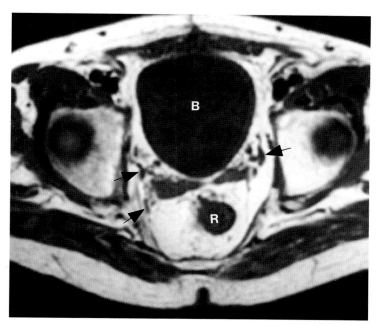

a

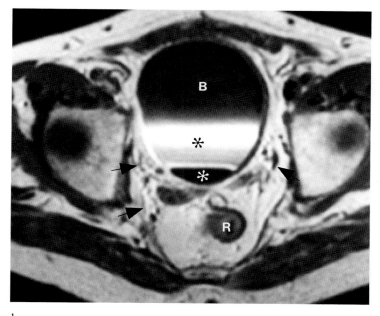

b

Figure 9.5

Appearance of the normal seminal vesicles following Gd-DTPA injection. Transaxial T1-weighted (**a**) noncontrast, and (**b**) contrast-enhanced images. On the nonenhanced image, the seminal vesicles demonstrate a homogeneous medium signal intensity. Following Gd-DTPA injection, the septa show an increase in signal intensity while the fluid within the seminal vesicles remains of low signal intensity, resulting in a grape-like appearance. (Arrows)-vesicoprostatic plexus; (B)-urinary bladder; (R)-rectum. Note the different layers of signal intensity of Gd-DTPA in the bladder, corresponding to the degree of concentration of the contrast material. Urine (B) not mixed with Gd-DTPA is of low signal intensity, dilute Gd-DTPA in the urine (black asterisk) is of high signal intensity, and concentrated Gd-DTPA in the dependent portion of the bladder (white asterisk) shows low signal intensity due to great shortening of T2 value.

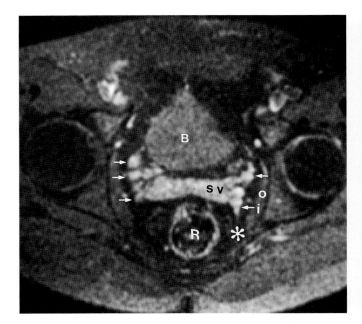

a

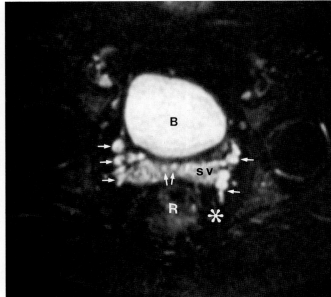

c

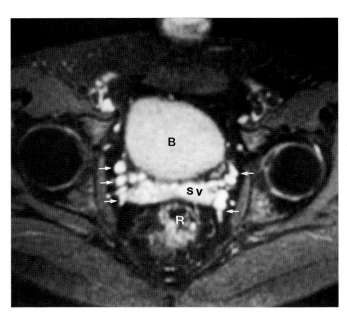

b

Figure 9.6

Appearance of the seminal vesicles using spin-echo fat saturation technique. Transaxial (**a**) T1- weighted, (**b**) proton density and (**c**) T2-weighted images. The seminal vesicles (SV), even on the T1-weighted image, demonstrate a grape-like configuration and are of higher signal intensity than the adjacent fat (asterisk), obturator internus muscle (Oi) or urine in the bladder (B). Marked increase in signal intensity of the seminal vesicles (SV) is seen on the T2-weighted image. The ring-like appearance of the ductus deferens is visible (double vertical white arrows). The vesicoprostatic plexus (horizontal white arrows) is seen lateral to the tips of the seminal vesicles (SV). The veins of the plexus show high signal intensity. A flow compensation technique was employed. (R)-rectum.

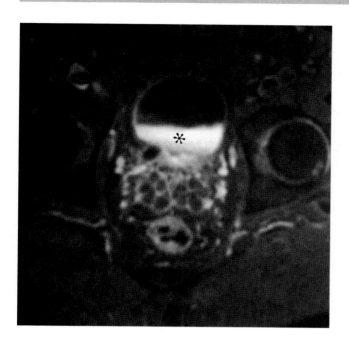

Figure 9.7

Appearance of the normal seminal vesicles on a Gd-DTPA-enhanced T1-weighted fat saturation image. Enhanced wall of the seminal vesicles contrasts with the lower signal intensity fluid, retaining the grape-like configuration. Note the high signal intensity of the Gd-DTPA-enhanced urine (asterisk) responsible for the setting of the computer gray scale as compared to Figure 9.6.

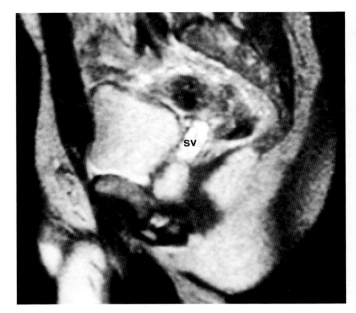

a

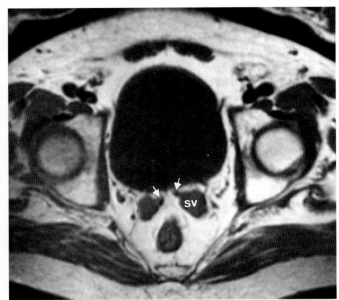

b

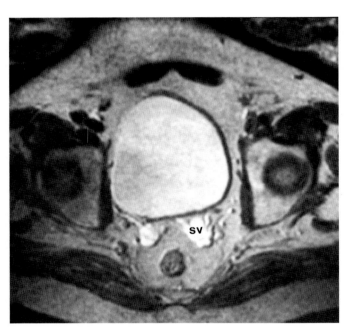

c

Figure 9.8

Normal seminal vesicles with their oblique orientation limiting accurate measurements of their length. (**a**) Sagittal T2-weighted image, (**b**) transaxial T1-weighted image, and (**c**) transaxial T2-weighted image. The oblique vertical orientation of the seminal vesicles (SV) as seen in the sagittal plane precludes accurate assessment of their length. In the transaxial plane, only the tips of the seminal vesicles (SV) are seen at this level. (Arrows)-ductus deferens.

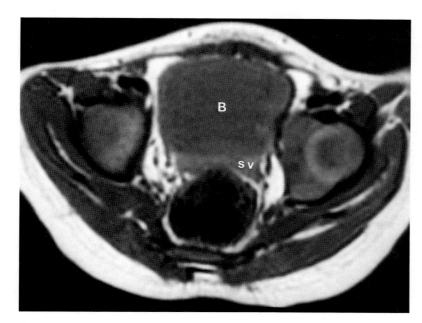

a

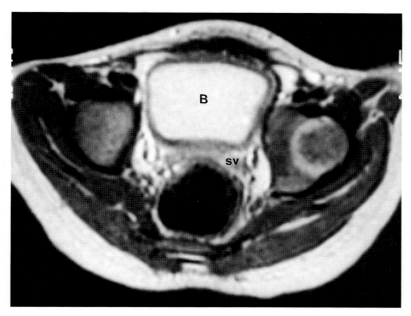

b

Figure 9.9

Seminal vesicles in a prepubertal boy. Transaxial (**a**) T1-weighted and (**b**) T2-weighted images. On the T1-weighted image, the seminal vesicles (SV) are small and demonstrate signal intensity slightly higher than urine within the urinary bladder (B). On a T2-weighted image, the seminal vesicles remain of low signal intensity. The small size and low signal intensity of the seminal vesicles is a normal finding before puberty.

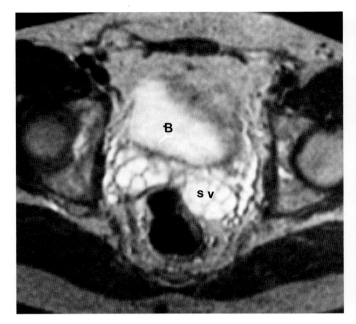

a

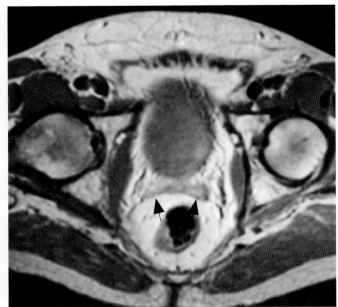

b

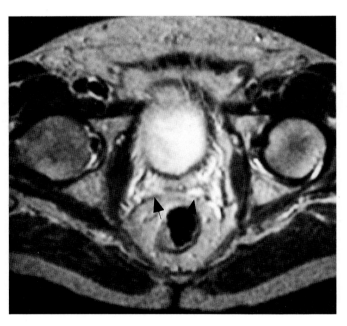

c

Figure 9.10

Difference in the size of normal seminal vesicles in two 35-year-old subjects, (**a**) transaxial T2-weighted image. In this patient, the seminal vesicles (SV) are prominent and of high signal intensity. (B)-urinary bladder. (**b**) Proton density and (**c**) T2-weighted images in a different man. The seminal vesicles (arrows) are small, but on the T2-weighted image, they exhibit higher signal intensity than the adjacent fat.

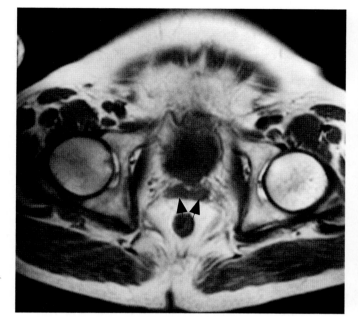

a

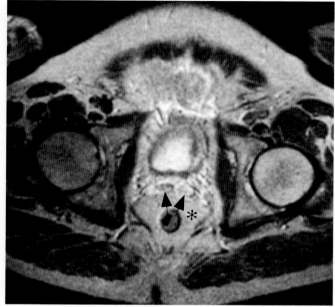

b

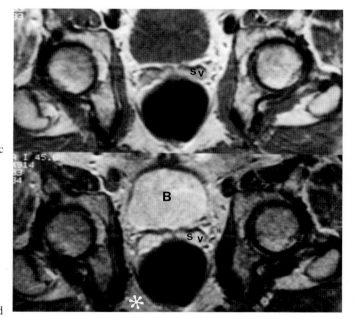

c

d

Figure 9.11

Difference in the size and MRI appearance of the seminal vesicles in two age matched 75-year-old men. Transaxial (**a**) and (**b**) are proton density and T2-weighted images in a man whose seminal vesicles (arrows) are small, and on the T2-weighted image, demonstrate a signal intensity lower than that of the adjacent fat (asterisk). In the other 75-year-old patient, as seen on the transaxial (**c**) proton density and (**d**) T2-weighted images, the seminal vesicles (SV) are of larger size, and their signal intensity is higher than fat (asterisk) but similar to the urine in the urinary bladder (B).

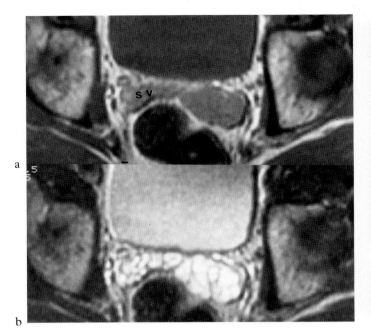

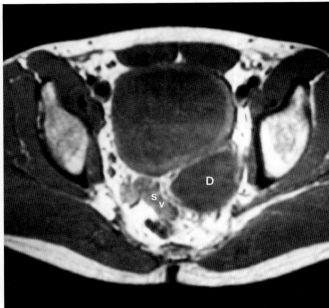

a

Figure 9.12

Asymmetry in size of the normal seminal vesicles. (**a**) Proton density and (**b**) T2-weighted images. The right seminal vesicle (SV) is considerably smaller than the left one. However, on a T2-weighted image, both seminal vesicles demonstrate symmetrical increase in signal intensity.

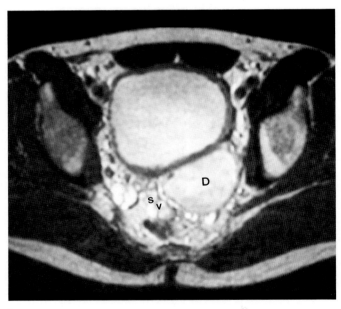

b

Figure 9.13

Displacement of the seminal vesicles by a large bladder diverticulum. (**a**) T1-weighted image and (**b**) T2-weighted image. The left seminal vesicle (SV) is of normal size and signal intensity but it is displaced by a large bladder diverticulum (D).

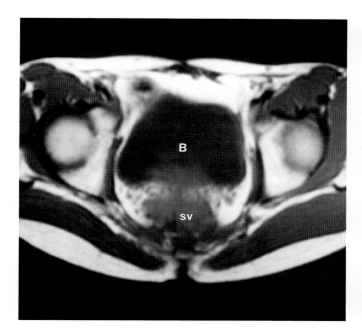

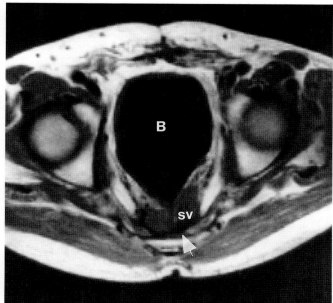

a

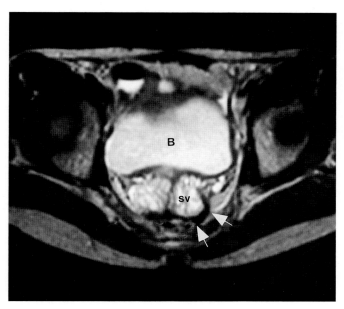

b

Figure 9.14

Position of the seminal vesicles following abdominoperineal resection, (**a**) T1- and (**b**) T2-weighted images. The seminal vesicles (SV) are displaced posteriorly. The low signal intensity stripe in the presacral region (arrows) represents scarring. (B)-urinary bladder.

Figure 9.15

Change in the orientation of the seminal vesicles, following abdominoperineal resection, transaxial T1-weighted image. The orientation of the seminal vesicles (SV) and the angle between them is reversed due to previous surgery and scarring (arrow). (B)-urinary bladder.

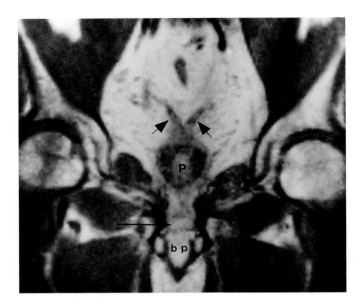

Figure 9.16

Position of the seminal vesicles in a patient with pelvic lipomatosis, coronal T2-weighted image. The orientation of the seminal vesicles (arrows) is more vertical and the angle between them is more acute than normal. The seminal vesicles are also of low signal intensity, in this patient, probably due to known severe alcoholism. The apex of the prostate gland (P) is high in position, part of morphologic changes in pelvic lipomatosis. (Arrow)-the level of the membranous urethra; (bp)-bulb penis. (0.35T.)

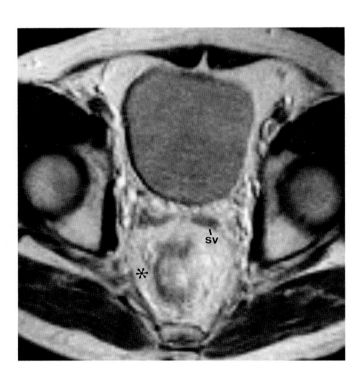

Figure 9.17

Seminal vesicles following estrogen administration (estrogen given for six months). Transaxial T2-weighted image. The seminal vesicles (SV) are small in size and exhibit lower signal intensity than the adjacent adipose tissue (asterisk).

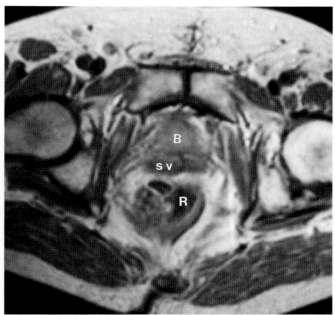

a

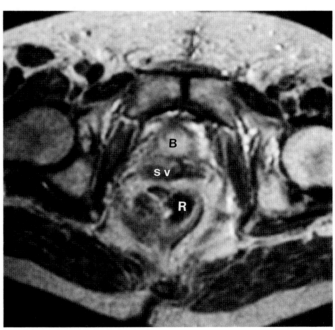

b

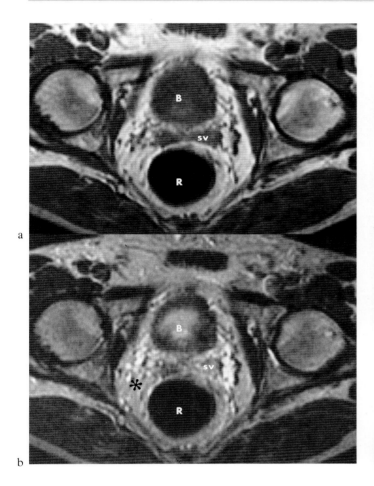

a

b

Figure 9.18

MRI appearance of the seminal vesicles following radiation therapy, transaxial (**a**) proton density image and (**b**) T2-weighted image. The seminal vesicles (SV) are small in size, and on the T2-weighted image, their signal intensity is lower than urine in the urinary bladder (B) and is similar to the adjacent fat (asterisk). (R)-rectum.

Figure 9.19

MRI appearance of the seminal vesicles following radiation therapy, transaxial (**a**) proton density and (**b**) T2-weighted images. The seminal vesicles (SV) are small and of uniformly low signal intensity on the T2-weighted image. Because the seminal vesicles were normal in appearance on the pretreatment scan, it is assumed that the present change in signal intensity is due to radiation. (B)-urinary bladder; (R)-rectum.

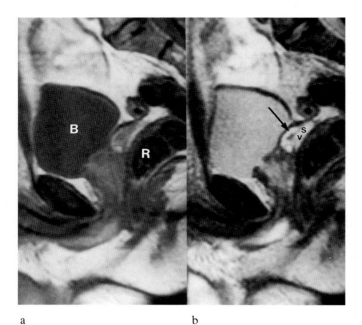

a   b

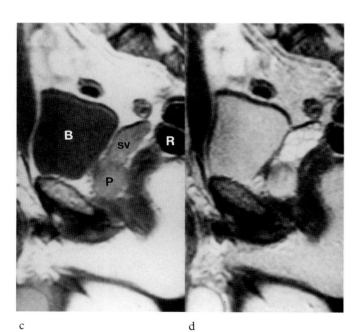

c   d

Figure 9.20

Normal appearance of the ampulla of the ductus deferens and seminal vesicles in the sagittal plane of imaging; images (**a**) and (**b**) are proton density and T2-weighted images in the midline location, and images (**c**) and (**d**) are proton density and T2-weighted images at the more lateral location. The seminal vesicles (SV) are seen posterior to the urinary bladder (B), anterior to the rectum (R) and superior to the prostate gland (P). In the midline section, T2-weighted image, the ampulla ductus deferens (arrow) can be seen anterior to the seminal vesicles (SV). In a more lateral section, the grape-like configuration of the seminal vesicles is appreciated on the T2-weighted image and their relation to the bladder (B), rectum (R) and prostate gland (P) is well displayed. The ampulla of the ductus deferens, being small, is seen only in the midline location.

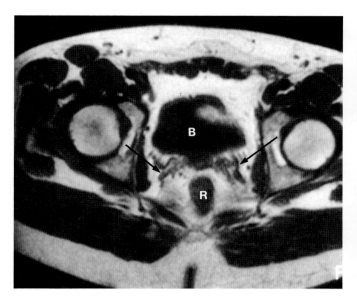

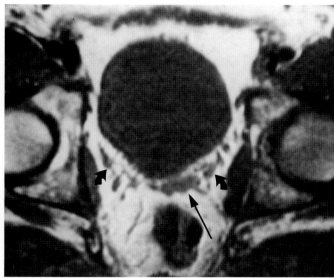

a

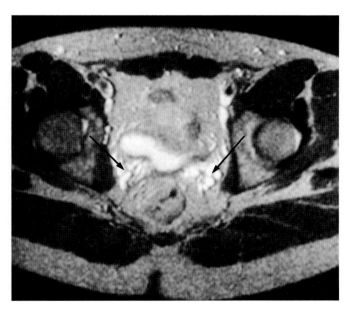

b

Figure 9.22

Unilateral seminal vesicle agenesis with a small contralateral gland, transaxial T1-weighted image. The small seminal vesicle on the left (arrow) is visualized. (Curved arrows)-vesicoprostatic plexus.

Figure 9.21

Bilateral seminal vesicle agenesis. (**a**) T1-weighted image, and (**b**) T2-weighted image. On the T1-weighted image, there are serpiginous tubular structures (long arrows) seen between the urinary bladder (B) anteriorly and rectum (R) posteriorly. On the T2-weighted image, marked signal enhancement is identified indicating that the tissue between the bladder and rectum represents serpiginous veins.

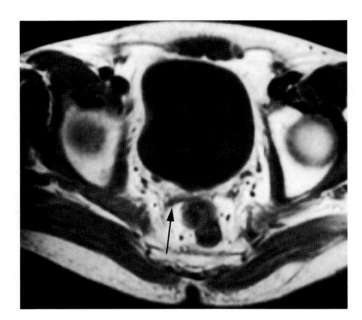

Figure 9.23

Unilateral seminal vesicle
agenesis with hypoplastic
contralateral gland. The small
right seminal vesicle (arrow) is
depicted as a narrow low signal
intensity stripe on the T1-
weighted image.

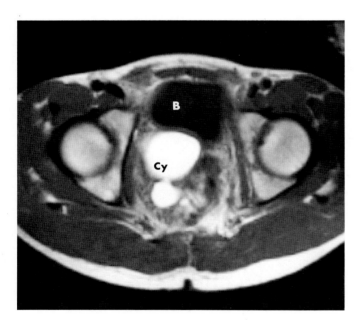

Figure 9.24

Seminal vesicle cyst in its
typical lateral location,
transaxial T1-weighted image.
The high signal intensity of the
seminal vesicle cyst (Cy) in this
T1-weighted image indicates
subacute hemorrhage. (B)-
urinary bladder. (0.35T.)

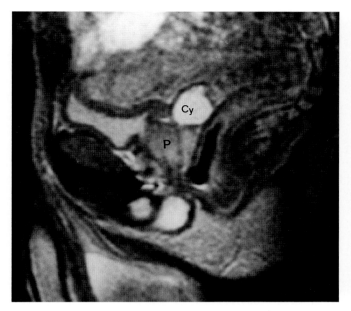

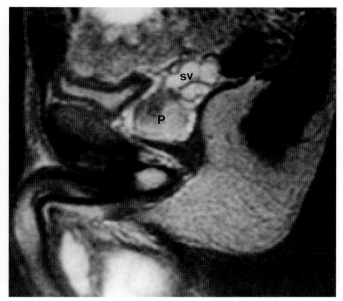

a   b

Figure 9.25

Seminal vesicle cyst, sagittal T2-weighted images: (**a**) more midline and (**b**) lateral sections. While the cyst (Cy) is in the midline location, it does not communicate with the prostate gland (P). The ipsilateral seminal vesicle (SV) is distended.

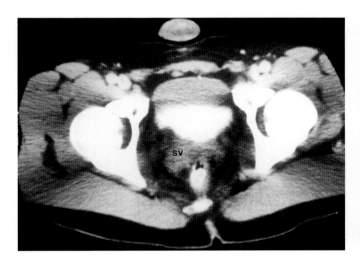

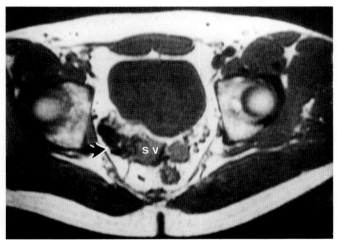

a   b

Figure 9.26

Arteriovenous malformation of the right seminal vesicle. (**a**) CT scan and (**b**) T1-weighted transaxial image. While on CT the only finding is the asymmetrical enlargement of the right seminal vesicle (SV), on MRI the large vessels (curved arrow) can be differentiated from the right seminal vesicle (SV).

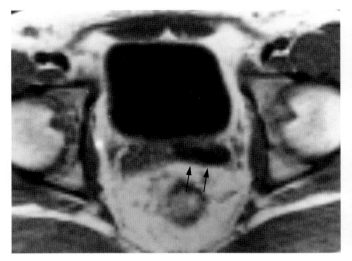

a

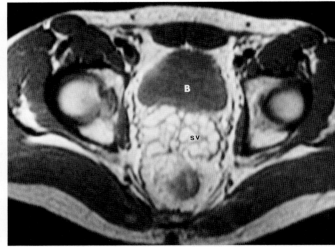

a

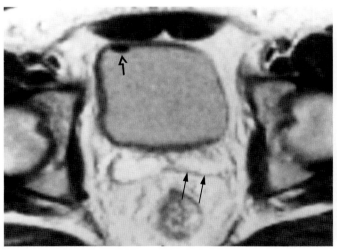

b

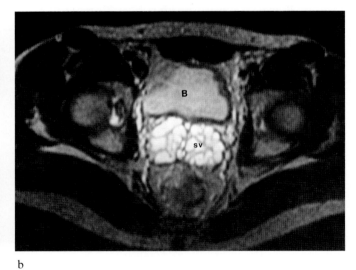

b

Figure 9.27

Acute inflammation of the left seminal vesicle, transaxial (**a**) T1- and (**b**) T2-weighted images. On the T1-weighted image, the signal intensity of the left seminal vesicle (arrows) is similar to urine in the urinary bladder and is of lower signal intensity than the contralateral right gland. On the T2-weighted image, the signal intensity of the left seminal vesicle is, however, unremarkable. The low signal intensity area in the urinary bladder (open arrow) is air due to recent cystoscopy.

Figure 9.28

Subacute infection of the seminal vesicles, transaxial (**a**) T1- and (**b**) T2-weighted images. The seminal vesicles (SV) are markedly enlarged and exhibit high signal intensity of both the T1- and T2-weighted images indicating bleeding. (B)-urinary bladder.

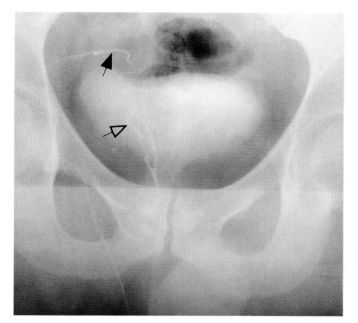

a

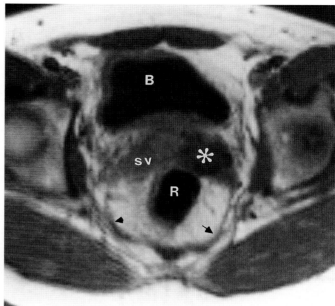

a

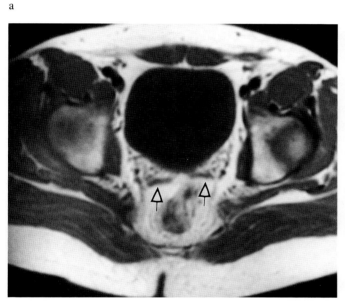

b

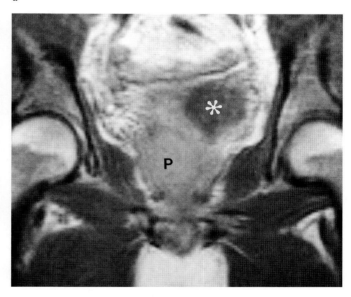

b

Figure 9.29

Chronic infection of the seminal vesicles, (**a**) seminal vesiculogram and (**b**) T1-weighted MRI image. The injection through the right ductus deferens (solid arrow) demonstrate a narrow ampulla ductus deferens with a small fibrotic right seminal vesicle (open arrow). On the T1-weighted MR image, both seminal vesicles (open arrows) are small. They remained of low signal intensity on the T2-weighted image (not shown).

Figure 9.30

Abscess in the left seminal vesicle, (**a**) transaxial T1-weighted image and (**b**) coronal proton density image. The right seminal vesicle (SV) is enlarged and the margins towards the adjacent fat are indistinct indicating inflammation. On the left side, a localized area of lower signal intensity (asterisk) with indistinct margins is identified. The left seminal vesicle abscess was surgically drained. Note the extensive inflammatory reaction extending along the thickened perirectal fascia (small black arrows) into the presacral region. (B)-urinary bladder; (R)-rectum; (P)-prostate. (0.35T.)

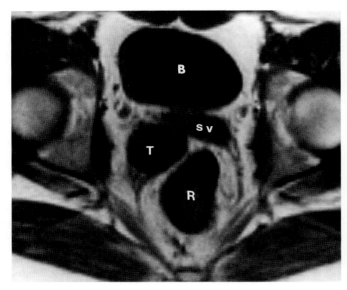

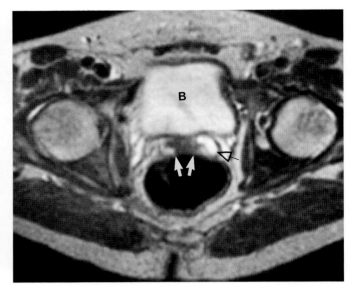

a

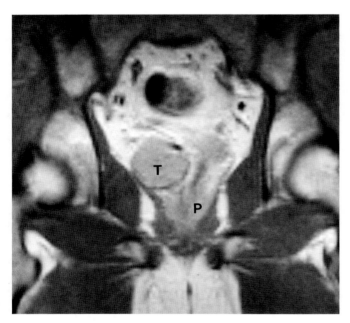

b

Figure 9.32

Prostate carcinoma with extension to the seminal vesicles, transaxial T2-weighted image. Low signal intensity extending into the medial part of both seminal vesicles (arrows) indicates tumor invasion. The distal part of the left seminal vesicles (open arrow) is normal. (B)-urinary bladder.

Figure 9.31

Schwannoma right seminal vesicles, (**a**) transaxial T1- and (**b**) coronal T2-weighted images. A tumor mass (T) is seen arising from the right seminal vesicles. The left seminal vesicle (SV) is normal. The tumor signal intensity is nonspecific but the tumor is sharply marginated and the adjacent fat is not infiltrated, in contrast to the abscess seen in Figure 9.30. (B)-urinary bladder; (R)-rectum. (0.35T.)

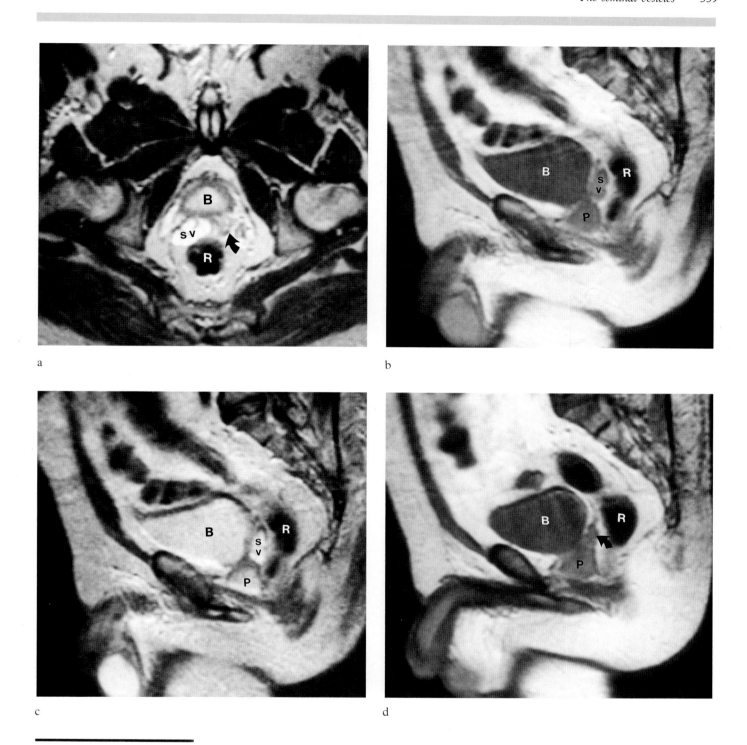

a

b

c

d

Figure 9.33

Prostate carcinoma with direct
tumor extension into the
seminal vesicles. (**a**) Oblique
transaxial T2-weighted image,
(**b**) proton density image and
(**c**) T2-weighted image through
the right seminal vesicle, (**d**)
sagittal proton density image

continued overleaf

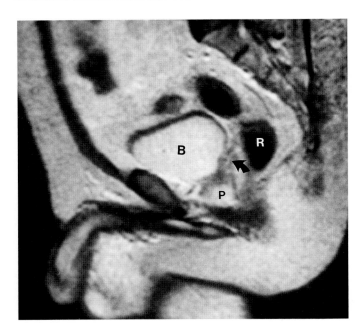

e

Figure 9.33 *continued*

and (**e**) T2-weighted image through the left gland. The right seminal vesicle (SV) is normal. Low signal intensity of the left seminal vesicle (curved arrow) is seen in the transaxial and in the sagittal plane. (B)-urinary bladder; (R)-rectum; (P)-prostate gland.

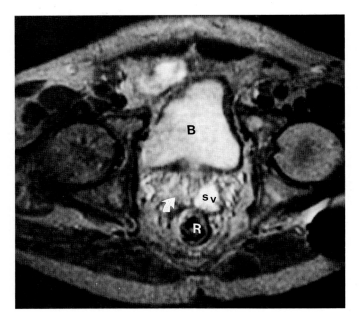

Figure 9.34

Tumor invasion of the seminal vesicles with obstruction of the distal portion (tip of left seminal vesicle), transaxial T2-weighted image. The tumor, demonstrating the low signal intensity, invaded the right (curved arrow) and the medial part of the left seminal vesicles. The tip of the left seminal vesicle (SV) is distended. (B)-urinary bladder; (R)-rectum.

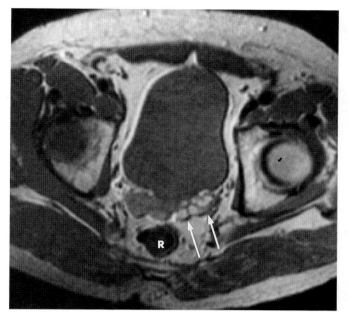

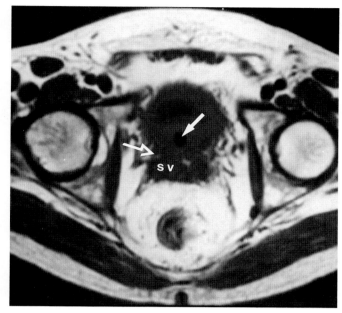

a

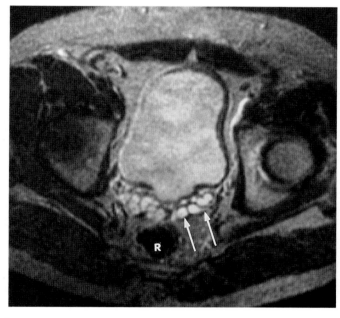

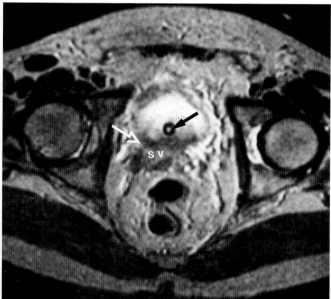

b

Figure 9.35

Bleeding into the left seminal vesicle following biopsy. Transaxial (**a**) proton density and (**b**) T2-weighted images. On the proton density image, the left seminal vesicle is of high signal intensity (long white arrows) indicating bleeding. However, it is not possible to differentiate bleeding secondary to biopsy from bleeding due to direct tumor invasion. (R)-rectum.

Figure 9.36

Direct tumor invasion of the seminal vesicles. Transaxial (**a**) T1- and (**b**) T2-weighted images. On the T1-weighted image, the tissue plane (open arrow) between the seminal vesicles (SV) and the urinary bladder is indistinct. On the T2-weighted image, the seminal vesicles (SV) show low signal intensity indicating tumor invasion. Foley catheter within the enlarged subvesicular portion of the prostate gland (arrow).

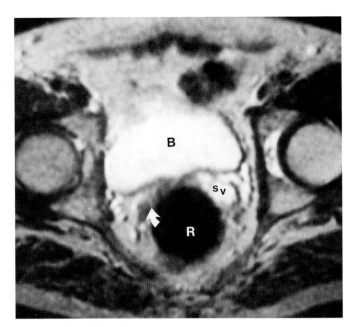

a

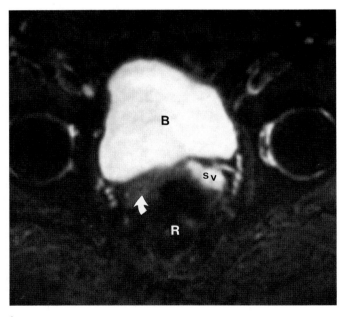

b

Figure 9.37

Seminal vesicle invasion by prostate carcinoma on a fat saturation image. Transaxial T2-weighted images, (**a**) conventional spin-echo and (**b**) fat saturation image. The left seminal vesicle (SV) is normal. The right seminal vesicle (curved arrow) demonstrates low signal intensity indicating tumor invasion. (B)-urinary bladder; (R)-rectum.

10
The Testis

Hedvig Hricak

Bimanual palpation is the primary examination in the evaluation of testicular pathology. However, because clinical signs and symptoms are nonspecific, variable, and commonly misleading, a variety of imaging modalities—including diagnostic ultrasound (US),[1-4] computed tomography (CT),[5,6] testicular arteriography and venography,[7] and technetium-99m (^{99m}Tc) radionuclide scanning[8]—have been described as valuable adjuncts in differentiating scrotal and testicular abnormalities. At present, high resolution, real-time ultrasonography is the imaging modality of choice in the evaluation of the testes.[2,9] Magnetic resonance imaging (MRI) is considered a problem-solving modality when ultrasound is inconclusive or technically inadequate.[9-20] The use of ^{31}P MR spectroscopy (MRS) has recently been reported in the assessment of testicular metabolic integrity.[20-23]

Normal testicular anatomy

The testis develops from an elongated embryonic gonad that lies ventral to the mesonephric ridge.[24] Internal descent brings the testis to the site of the future internal inguinal ring. External descent begins with migration through the inguinal canal into the scrotum. Arrest of testicular descent may occur anywhere along this pathway.

In the normal adult, the testis lies within the scrotum. The wall of the scrotum consists of the scrotal skin, the dartos muscle and fascias including external spermatic, cremasteric, and internal spermatic fascias. The septum (which divides the scrotum into two cavities) contains all the layers of the scrotal wall except the skin.

The testis is 4–5 cm long, approximately 2–3 cm wide, and 2–3 cm in anteroposterior diameter.[24] The weight of the normal adult testis is 15–25 gm. The appendix of the testis, a vestige of the müllerian duct, is found at the upper pole. As illustrated in Figure 10.1, each testis is enveloped by an outpouching of peritoneum called the **tunica vaginalis propria testis**. The visceral lamina of the tunica vaginalis covers the anterior and lateral surfaces of the testis. The postero-lateral border—the bare area of the testis—is covered by the epididymis. The parietal lamina of the tunica vaginalis merges with the visceral layer to enclose a serous cavity, where a small amount of fluid (0.5 ml^3) is normally present. An increase in the amount of fluid is called a hydrocele.

The **tunica albuginea**, a dense fibrous connective tissue capsule approximately 0.6 mm thick, forms a covering for the testis itself.[24] Along the posterior aspect of the testis, the tunica albuginea invaginates into the gland as the **mediastinum testis**. The length of the mediastinum testis varies. Fibrous **septula testes**, which extend radially from the mediastinum testis to the periphery of the tunica albuginea, divide the gland into 200–250 pyramidal **lobular testes**. Each lobular testis is composed of two to four convoluted seminiferous tubules. There are a total of 400–600 seminiferous tubules within the testis, with a rich anastomotic network connecting them. In the region of the mediastinum testis, the tubules straighten to form the **rete testis**. Rete testes are the beginning of the semen conductive system. **Efferent ductules** run from the rete testis to the duct of the epididymis.

The **epididymis**, which lies along the posterior aspect of the testis, is customarily divided into three regions: the head (caput, globus major), the body (corpus), and the tail (caudo, globus minor). From the rete testis, the 10–12 efferent ductules run to the head

343

of the epididymis and open end-to-side into the **duct of the epididymis**. The efferent ductules form the head of the epididymis, and the coiled duct of the epididymis forms the epididymal body (when uncoiled the duct of the epididymis is 7 meters long). As the duct of the epididymis runs towards the periphery it narrows and assumes the characteristic appearance of the ductus deferens.

The **ductus deferens (vas deferens)** is a continuation of the ductus epididymis. It is approximately 30 cm long and extends from the tail of the epididymis to the ejaculatory ducts. Together with vascular and lymphatic vessels, the ductus deferens at the level of the neck of the scrotal sac is encompassed by a connective tissue fascia (each layer of the abdominal wall muscle contributes to the fascia layer of the spermatic cord) and parts of the cremasteric muscle to form the **spermatic cord**. As illustrated in Figure 10.2, the spermatic cord extends from the scrotal sac through the subcutaneous fat and as it passes through the external inguinal ring, it changes its layering coats. The **external inguinal ring** is a triangular opening demarcated medially and laterally by the crura of the aponeurosis of the external oblique muscle and at its base by the pubic crest. The ductus deferens and accompanying vessels and lymphatics then pass through the **inguinal canal** (which is not a true canal but rather a space between the layers of the wall), to reach the internal inguinal ring. The **internal inguinal ring** is bordered medially by the inferior epigastric vessels, laterally and superiorly by the arching muscle fibers of the transversus abdominis muscle and anteriorly by external oblique aponeurosis.[24] After the ductus passes through the internal ring, the ductus deferens separates from the vascular and lymphatic structures, loops behind the inferior epigastric artery, and passes downwards and posteriorly along the lateral pelvic wall.

The testis is an endocrine gland which produces testosterone and is also responsible for spermatocytogenesis. The epididymis serves as a conduit for sperm transport and as a storage organ. It is also essential for the normal maturation of spermatozoa. The ductus deferens serves as a conduit between the epididymis and the ejaculatory duct.

Vascular supply

The major arterial supply to the testis is via the testicular artery, which arises from the aorta or the renal artery. The artery of the vas deferens and the cremastic artery also supply the testis.

The veins of the testes converge on the mediastinum testes and form the **pampiniform plexus**. The pampiniform plexus accompanies the testicular artery in the spermatic cord. At the level of the internal inguinal ring, this plexus joins to form the common spermatic vein and runs upwards following the arterial tree.

Lymphatic drainage

Lymphatic drainage of the testis usually follows its vascular supply and drains directly to the paraaortic (paralumbar) lymph nodes. On the left side the lymphatic vessels follow the testicular artery to the left renal artery and drain into the periaortic and preaortic nodes at the level L_1–L_2.[25] On the right side the lymph node drainage is to the aortocaval, preaortic and precaval nodes at the level L_1–L_3.[25] However, variations in the lymphatic drainage do exist. In addition, the testes may drain to the regional nodes of the **internal, external and common iliac nodes** via the epididymal and cremasteric arteries.

The inguinal lymph nodes are **not** regional nodes of the testis. Invasion of the inguinal lymph nodes by testicular tumor can occur only by retrograde spread from the iliac nodes.

MRI appearance

On T1-weighted MR images, as illustrated in Figure 10.3, the normal testis demonstrates a homogeneous medium signal intensity, similar to the signal intensity of the corpora cavernosa or corpus spongiosum and lower than adjacent adipose tissue.[9–11] On T2-weighted images (Figure 10.3), testicular tissue increases in signal intensity, and is similar to, or more commonly higher than, that of fat. It has been reported that on T2-weighted images the signal intensity of the testis parallels that of the corpora cavernosa. The great variations in the signal intensity of the corpora cavernosa, however, are normally present, limiting the value of that comparison. The tunica albuginea, being collagen tissue, images with low signal intensity on both T1- and T2-weighted scans.[9] As depicted in Figure 10.3, the contrast between the low signal intensity tunica albuginea and the high signal intensity testicular tissue is best depicted on T2-weighted images.[9,10] T2-weighted images (Figure 10.4) are also needed to demonstrate the mediastinum testis, which can be seen as a low signal intensity stripe invaginating into the homogeneous high signal intensity testicular tissue. Often fine low signal intensity septula will be seen extending from the mediastinum testis laterally (Figure 10.5).

On T1-weighted images the signal intensity of the epididymis is similar to or slightly lower than that of the testis.[10] As shown in Figures 10.3 and 10.6 the signal intensities of the epididymis and surrounding fluid are often similar on T1-weighted images. On T2-weighted images the epididymis demonstrates a lower signal intensity than adjacent testicular tissue, or surrounding fluid, making their differentiation possible.

A small amount of normal serous fluid, which demonstrates medium to low signal intensity on T1-weighted images and high signal intensity on T2-weighted images (Figures 10.3 and 10.6), can be detected between the layers of the tunica vaginalis. The skin of the scrotum demonstrates higher signal intensity than the cremasteric muscle or the fascia on the T1-weighted image (Figure 10.3). On the T2-weighted image all the parts of the scrotum decrease in signal intensity. The veins of the pampiniform plexus can be demonstrated as serpiginous tubular structures which, at the level of the scrotal neck, join the ductus deferens, the arteries and the nerves to form the spermatic cord (Figure 10.7). The fascias and the cremasteric muscle within the spermatic cord form an envelope which is seen as a low signal intensity ring on MR scans. Separate structures within the spermatic cord are difficult to recognize on MR imaging (Figure 10.8). However, the anatomical landmarks of the spermatic cord, external inguinal ring, inguinal canal, and internal inguinal ring are well displayed, as illustrated in Figure 10.9. The low signal intensity ring corresponding to the envelope of the spermatic cord is seen within the subcutaneous fat. The level of the external inguinal ring is at or just superior to the upper margin of the symphysis pubis, and crura of the external oblique muscle are seen on each side. The low signal intensity ring is still seen, but the layers of the wall of the spermatic cord start changing. The inguinal canal is oblique in orientation, and although in an adult it is up to 5–7 cm long, its vertical distance between the external and the internal inguinal rings is only 1–2 cm. The internal inguinal ring is demarcated by the inferior epigastric vessels medially (Figure 10.10). After the level of the internal inguinal ring the ductus deferens and the testicular vessels diverge, the former passing downwards towards the seminal vesicles (Figure 10.10b) and the latter ascending into the abdomen. The course of the spermatic cord and the inguinal canal can be demonstrated on either the transaxial, sagittal (Figure 10.11) or coronal planes (Figure 10.12).

Recommended imaging sequences

Both T1- and T2-weighted images are suggested for the complete evaluation of the scrotum. T1-weighted images are helpful for tissue characterization, in determination of the nature of a fluid collection (serous or complicated), and in the diagnosis of hemorrhage. T2-weighted images are necessary to differentiate among the testis, the tunica albuginea, and the epididymis; and to detect intratesticular pathology.

Transaxial (Figure 10.3) and coronal planes (Figure 10.13) or imaging allow the comparison of the signal intensity between the two testicles, and either plane can be used for the demonstration of intratesticular pathology. If pathology of the epididymis is in question, sagittal (Figure 10.6) or transaxial (Figure 10.3) planes are recommended. Both offer visualization of the epididymis, which is located posterior to the testis.

Thin (4 or 5 mm thick) slices are essential in the evaluation of testicular pathology, and the use of a surface coil, which provides a higher signal-to-noise ratio, is recommended.

MRI appearance of testicular prosthesis

The awareness of cosmetic and psychological impact in patients with congenital or surgical absence of the testis has increased the use of prosthetic testicles. Different silicon prostheses are available, rendering different MRI appearances. Older prostheses contain viscous fluid, they are hard on palpation, and as shown in Figure 10.14, on MRI they demonstrate low signal intensity on either T1- or T2-weighted images. Chemical-shift artifacts at the tissue–prosthesis interface are pronounced. Newer prostheses are made of solid elastomer, and they have the consistency similar to normal testicular tissue. As shown in Figure 10.15, on MRI their signal intensity parallels normal testis, being of medium signal intensity on the T1-weighted image and of high signal intensity on the T2-weighted image. The point of differentiation is pronounced chemical-shift artifact and absence of other scrotal or spermatic cord structures.[26]

Pathology of the testis

Congenital anomalies

Congenital anomalies of testicular size result in congenitally small, rudimentary testes. Although the anomaly is usually unilateral, often discovered at puberty on clinical examination, bilateral forms in conjunction with micropenis have been reported.[27] Congenital absence of the testes may be unilateral (**monorchidism**) or bilateral (**anorchidism**). Congenital duplication of the testes—**polyorchia**—is a rare anomaly in which the duplicated testes are usually surrounded by a single tunica albuginea and most commonly have a single epididymis and vas deferens.[28]

Undescended testis

The most common genitourinary anomaly is undescended testis. The causes of the nonpalpable testis (**cryptorchidism**) can be divided into three categories: (1) congenital absence (the cause of cryptorchidism in 3–5 per cent of patients); (2) the retractile or migratory testis (accounting for up to 70 per cent of cases thought to be undescended); and (3) the truly maldescended testis (accounting for 30 per cent of patients presenting with nonpalpable testes).[24] The **retractile (migratory) testis** lies in the scrotum intermittently. Its high position is thought to be due to contraction of the cremasteric muscle. The **truly undescended** testis can be in a high scrotal position (within the expected course of the spermatic cord, usually close to the external inguinal ring), in the cannicular position (in the inguinal canal between the external and internal rings) or in the abdominal position (outside the internal inguinal ring). When the testis is located outside the expected descended position it is referred to as maldescended testis. Only 1 per cent of undescended testes are truly ectopic in location.[24] About 10 per cent of truly undescended testes are bilateral.[29]

Various mechanisms responsible for testicular descent into the scrotum, including different physical and endocrine factors, have been proposed. The process is complex, including many variables among which the role of gubernaculum is important. After development, the testis lies on top of the conically-shaped fibromuscular gubernaculum which acts as a leading edge in its scrotal descent. The testis never lies within the peritoneal cavity during embryological descent, and internal descent starts very close to the internal inguinal ring. It has been reported that the testis is never more than 1.3 mm from the internal ring at any time during its development.[29,30] The testis starts its external descent at about the seventh month of gestation, and this is why the rate of occurrence of undescended testes depends on the maturity and weight of the infant. Incidence at birth in otherwise normal boys is 3.5 per cent, but in premature infants weighing under two pounds, the incidence may be as high as 100 per cent. Many undescended testes spontaneously descend between birth and one year of age, and at that time the prevalence falls to 0.8 per cent. Spontaneous descent after one year of age is unlikely, however, and studies of school children and military recruits demonstrate a 1 per cent incidence of true cryptorchidism.[31]

Cryptorchidism is clinically important because it is associated with a variety of disorders including an increased incidence of malignant neoplasms; testicular torsion; associated congenital anomalies (including agenesis) of the mesonephric duct; urinary tract anomalies (3 per cent); inguinal hernias; and infertility.[32] If untreated, bilateral undescended testes have an infertility rate of 100 per cent. With surgery, the infertility rate decreases to 40 per cent. In unilateral cryptorchidism the mean fertility rate is 60 per cent.[31,33] Surgery is also recommended because of the cosmetic and psychological impact of cryptorchidism. Preoperative localization of testes allows the surgical approach to be planned, reducing the extent of exploration and anesthesia time.

MRI appearance. The MRI diagnosis of undescended testis is based on demonstration of a mass, usually elliptical in configuration (conforming to the contour of the spermatic cord or the inguinal canal), present along the expected path of the testicular descent.[16] Knowledge of the landmarks of the inguinal canal, including the location of the internal and external rings are important in the correct preoperative evaluation of testicular position. Figure 10.16 illustrates the undescended testis in high scrotal position, approximately 2 cm outside the external inguinal ring. Figure 10.17 illustrates the location of the undescended testis just outside the external inguinal ring, and Figure 10.18 shows the intra-abdominal (outside the internal inguinal canal) location of the undescended testis.

MRI is an excellent modality for depicting the undescended testis when the testis is located along the course of the spermatic cord, in the inguinal canal (canalicular) or just outside the internal inguinal ring. However, MRI is less accurate for the detection of high abdominal or ectopic testes. Controversies surround the description of the 'high abdominal' testis. 'High abdominal' testis has been referred to as the position of the maldescended testis along the course of the testicular artery. It is therefore located extraperitoneally, in close proximity to the psoas muscle. This type of maldescended testis can be detected on MRI. However, MRI is not applicable for the detection of the other intra-abdominal locations, which are however often referred to as the ectopic, rather than maldescended intra-abdominal testis. When searching for the undescended testis, the depiction of the inguinal ring or the structure of the spermatic cord proximal to the testis is a helpful landmark. The testes, when located within the spermatic cord (Figure 10.16) can be readily differentiated from inguinal lymph nodes (not easily accomplished with ultrasound). The ductus deferens and vessels can be followed within the spermatic cord to the level of the testes. However, the ductus deferens can be present caudal to the undescended testis and, therefore, the identification of the spermatic cord structures is not always reliable in predicting testis location. In addition, identification of a blind ending ductus deferens does not necessarily imply absence of the testes, since embryological development of the gonads and ductal structures is initially independent. Difficulties have been reported in misdiagnosing the remaining bulbous gubernaculum as an undescended testis.[34] The demonstration of a mediastinum testis (Figure 10.16) is a helpful finding in favor of an undescended testis, but due to the small size of the testis and present overall MRI resolution, the mediastinum testis in a small child is seldom seen. The tissue characterization can be attempted. The gubernaculum testis demonstrates low signal intensity on both T1- and T2-weighted images (Figure 10.16). The testis, when no fibrosis has occurred, will be of high signal intensity (Figure 10.16). However, in testicular atrophy this point of tissue characterization is not helpful as the atrophic undescended testis (Figure 10.19) will demonstrate low signal intensity on a T2-weighted image.

MR imaging can be applied to the differentiation between a retractile testis and a truly undescended testis. The volume and the signal intensity of the retractile testis are normal, and gubernaculum along the pathway of the spermatic cord (Figure 10.20) is well developed. As illustrated in Figure 10.21, the size and the signal intensity of the undescended testis, however, may also be normal, but the gubernaculum is usually not well developed, or as shown in Figure 10.19, the testicular tissue may demonstrate signal intensity lower than normal on T2-weighted images.

The undescended testis can be seen on any orthogonal plane scan. When located in the spermatic cord or the inguinal canal, the undescended testis is elliptical in shape and a scan in the sagittal or coronal plane (Figure 10.16) performed along the testicular long axis is optimal. However, when the testis is located above the inguinal ring its orientation often changes (Figure 10.18), the long axis being horizontal, and the transaxial plane of imaging is therefore preferable.

MRI in relation to other imaging modalities.   Currently CT is very seldom requested for the evaluation of undescended testis. CT has been largely replaced by US and MRI. Sonography has been advocated as the primary imaging modality in the search for undescended testes. However, ultrasound has a small field-of-view, and may be limited by patient physique.[1,2,35] When ultrasound results are inconclusive, MRI should be used as a problem-solving modality.[16] Many clinicians, however, prefer MRI as the initial study. Advantages of MRI include its large field-of-view, operator independence, and demonstra-

tion of the undescended testicle in two views perpendicular to each other (Figure 10.16). Also, with MRI it is possible to differentiate the testis within the spermatic cord from adjacent inguinal lymph nodes, and concomitant pathology as shown in Figure 10.22 will not preclude identification of the testis. The position of the undescended testis can be identified with a high degree of accuracy, and categorized as high scrotal, canalicular, or abdominal (outside the internal inguinal ring). The distance between the undescended testis and the external or internal inguinal ring can be assessed with MRI. When the testis is maldescended or ectopic in location, the role of MRI is more limited. The potential of MRI for tissue characterization and for quantitative assessment of the degree of testicular fibrosis needs to be further explored.

Spermatic cord torsion

Because the diagnosis of torsion continues to represent a clinical challenge, and because clinical differentiation between torsion and epididymitis has been reported to be difficult in as many as 50 per cent of cases,[36] a variety of radiologic modalities has been explored to help in identification of this surgical emergency.

Torsion of the spermatic cord results from faulty development such as absence of or defective fixation by the gubernaculum, a long mesorchium, or an entwined cremasteric muscle.[24] It can be extravaginal (usually seen in a newborn), or intravaginal. Although any degree of spermatic cord torsion can occur, clinical symptoms usually accompany torsion of 360 degrees and greater. The associated pain often occurs when the patient is at rest or asleep. In the newborn, spermatic cord torsion is characterized by swelling and redness of the scrotum, often without symptoms.

MRI appearance.   In an animal model of acute torsion, MRI findings of enlargement of the testis have been reported.[20] The acutely torsed testis demonstrated normal signal intensity on both T1 and T2 SE-weighted images or diffuse heterogeneous signal intensity on T2-weighted images has been seen. In the intermittent torsion (Figure 10.23), diffuse subacute hemorrhage is the histologic hallmark and on MRI the testis is enlarged and demonstrates high signal intensity on both T1- and T2-weighted images. The GRE was not performed. In chronic torsion, a decrease in signal intensity on T2-weighted images is the most consistent feature.[17,20] The additional findings of a torsion knot and whirlpool pattern, resulting from the twisting of the spermatic cord, along with spermatic cord vascularity were found helpful in identifying torsion and in differentiating it from epididymitis.[17] Other features which help to distinguish subacute torsion from epididymitis include small testicular size and decreased vascularity,[17] both of which are seen in chronic torsion. Although initial MRI findings are encouraging, at present they are not specific enough for definite diagnosis of torsion. [31]P MR spectroscopy has shown promise in the evaluation of acute torsion, although larger studies are needed to ascertain its clinical value. As depicted in Figure 10.24, the marked decrease in ATP and PM levels with a concomitant increase in inorganic phosphorus (P_i) are thought to be characteristic of spermatic cord torsion.[23]

MRI in relation to other imaging modalities. If radiologic evaluation of torsion is needed, color Doppler sonography or radionuclide imaging are the most appropriate studies. The exact roles of MR imaging and ^{31}P spectroscopy need to be further explored.

Fluid collections and benign scrotal masses

Hydrocele

Hydrocele is an abnormal accumulation of serous fluid between the visceral and parietal layers of the tunica vaginalis. In congenital hydrocele the funicular process, the tunica vaginalis, fails to close and there is a direct communication between the scrotal sac and the abdominal cavity.[24] A secondary hydrocele may be idiopathic, but more often is associated with epididymitis, orchitis, or chronic or missed spermatic cord torsion. Hydrocele formation may also be associated with scrotal trauma or a neoplasm (less than 10 per cent of cases). An acute hydrocele has a thin wall and always transilluminates. These patients very seldom require radiologic examination. A chronic hydrocele, however, usually has a thick wall and therefore will not transilluminate. In those patients the clinical evaluation of the etiology of the enlarged scrotum is limited and imaging is helpful.

MRI appearance. Since hydrocele is a fluid accumulation, as depicted in Figure 10.25, it images with low signal intensity on T1-weighted scans and increases in signal intensity on T2-weighted scans.[9] Some hydroceles are uniloculated, but multiloculated hydroceles with thick septations may also occur. Similarly, the wall of the hydrocele may be asymmetrically thickened. Differentiation between the testis and hydrocele, as well as the detection of fibrous septa within the hydrocele, are optimal on T2-weighted images.[9-11]

Associated causes of hydrocele, such as orchitis, epididymitis, or tumor, can be concomitantly demonstrated. Scrotal wall thickening, when present, is depicted on both T1- and T2-weighted images. When the thickening of the scrotal wall is due to edema (such as lymphedema or elephantiasis) the signal intensity of the wall on both T1- and T2-weighted images will be similar to the hydrocele. The diagnosis is reinforced by the anatomical landmarks. The hydrocele is the fluid accumulation between the two layers of tunica vaginalis. The tissue outside the parietal layers of the tunica vaginalis is scrotal skin, as illustrated in Figure 10.26.

Hematocele

Hematocele is a hemorrhage between the two layers of the tunica vaginalis. Although some hematoceles develop spontaneously, they usually develop rapidly as the result of trauma. Unlike the hydrocele, the hematocele will not transilluminate even when acute.

MRI appearance. The MR signal intensity of the hematocele depends on the age of the bleeding. A fresh hematocele may exhibit medium signal intensity on T1-weighted images and increase in signal intensity on T2-weighted images. A chronic hematocele, as shown in Figure 10.27, demonstrates high signal intensity on both T1- and T2-weighted images.[18] Use of gradient-echo (GRE) imaging allows specific diagnosis of hematocele.

Spermatocele

Spermatocele is a retention cyst of small tubules within the epididymis, most commonly present in the head.[36] A spermatocele may be unilateral or bilateral, unilocular or multilocular. The serous fluid within a spermatocele may be complicated by sediment, which is composed of cellular debris, fat, or spermatozoa.

MRI appearance. On MRI, spermatoceles are seen as fluid collections in the region of the epididymis.[12] They image with various signal intensities, depending on the protein content of the cystic fluid. A spermatocele may be differentiated from a hydrocele based on its anatomical landmarks.

Varicocele

Dilatation of the testicular vein, known as a varicocele, may be primary, idiopathic, or secondary resulting from pressure on the spermatic vein or its tributaries by enlarged intra-abdominal organs or by the presence of abdominal tumor. Results from earlier clinical studies and physical examinations have indicated that the vast majority of varicoceles are left-sided. Recent reports, however, document a substantially increased incidence of ultrasonographically demonstrable right-sided varicoceles.[37]

In the evaluation of male infertility, radiology is useful in demonstrating varicoceles, in measuring their size, and in identifying any effect on the size of the veins caused by positional change.[36,37]

MRI appearance. On MRI scans a varicocele is imaged as a collection of tubular, seripiginous vessels in the region of the head of the epididymis and spermatic cord.[26] The signal intensity varies, depending on the flow velocity. Often, as illustrated in Figure 10.28, the varicocele demonstrates medium signal intensity on T1- and increased signal intensity on spin-echo T2-weighted images.

Scrotal hernia

The diagnosis of scrotal hernia is usually made on clinical findings alone. Only in rare instances, when physical examination is limited due to patient size, or marked enlargement of the scrotum is accompanied by a sudden onset of testicular pain, is imaging evaluation appropriate.

MRI appearance. The MRI appearance of a scrotal hernia depends on its contents. A complex mass is demonstrated within the scrotum, and the adjacent normal testicular tissue can be visualized. Air within the bowel or fat content of the mesentery are readily displayed on MRI. Descent of the hernia with widening along the inguinal canal, is also easily demonstrated. Meconium hernia (Figure 10.29) was clinically and on US study misdiagnosed as testicular mass.

MRI in relation to other imaging modalities

Ultrasound is the primary imaging modality for evaluating benign scrotal masses and for differentiating between intra- and extratesticular disease. If ultrasound is inconclusive, MRI studies may provide the necessary information. Although MRI is more sensitive than ultrasound for characterizing fluid collections (ie, differentiating serous from hemorrhagic fluid), the diagnosis of hematocele is usually clinical, made in conjunction with a history of testicular trauma. Varicoceles can also be demonstrated on

MRI scans, but the finding is usually incidental. If the presence of varicocele is of clinical importance, ultrasound is the only study required. For the evaluation of benign scrotal masses, MRI should be looked upon as a problem-solving modality.

Epididymitis and orchitis

Acute epididymitis is the most common inflammatory lesion of the scrotum. Associated orchitis is found in up to 20 per cent of patients. Isolated orchitis is rare, unless caused by a viral infection (most often mumps). Orchitis is almost always seen as a diffuse process associated with epididymitis. If edema of the scrotal contents is severe, testicular blood flow may be compromised resulting in focal or diffuse infarction of the testis and/or epididymis. Rarely, testicular rupture may complicate severe acute orchitis. Clinically, it is important to differentiate acute epididymitis from acute torsion of the spermatic cord or testicular tumor. Scrotal abscess and scrotal gangrene may complicate epididymitis and/or orchitis. An infected hydrocele (**pyocele**) occurs in these patients and is usually associated with pyogenic testicular abscess.

MRI appearance

In acute epididymitis, as depicted in Figure 10.30, MR demonstrates an enlarged epididymis which remains of lower signal intensity on T2-weighted images. The inflammatory process often ascends along the spermatic cord. The inflammation of the ductus deferens is shown in Figure 10.31. When orchitis accompanies epididymitis, affected testicular tissue demonstrates heterogeneous or homogeneous (Figure 10.32) decrease in signal intensity on T2-weighted images. Associated thickening of the scrotal skin can be detected. The presence of air (Figure 10.33) indicates abscess formation. While the MRI finding of an ill-defined heterogeneous but predominantly lower signal intensity area within the testis has been described as specific for orchitis, allowing the differentiation between an inflammatory process and tumor,[17] the number of cases reported at present is small, and because of the paramount importance of not missing or delaying the diagnosis of tumor, caution should be exercised.

MRI in relation to other imaging modalities

If the clinical diagnosis of epididymitis needs reinforcement because the history and physical examination are limited, or if the response to antibiotic therapy is inadequate, imaging can be used as an adjunct to the physical examination. In those instances, ultrasound is the initial study of choice. Although the sonographic diagnosis of epididymitis is highly accurate, orchitis cannot be differentiated from testicular tumor based on imaging findings alone. MRI studies are reserved for cases in which ultrasound is limited or additional information is required. MRI, however, based on imaging findings only, will not differentiate benign from the malignant disease.

Testicular tumors

Benign tumors of the testes are rare representing 3 to 4 per cent of all primary testicular tumors. They are mostly (90 per cent) nongerminal tumors arising from the interstitial Leydig cells, Sertoli cells, or the connective tissue stroma.[38,39] Benign epidermoid cysts can also occur.[38,39]

Most testicular tumors are malignant.[39,40] Although cancer of the testes accounts for only 1 per cent of all cancers in the male, its socioeconomic impact is accentuated by its high prevalence in the young adult.[40] In males aged 15–34 years, testicular cancer is the most common cancer, and it accounts for 8.8 per cent of all cancer deaths.[39,40] Furthermore, incidence of testicular cancer is steadily increasing.[40] In the United States the incidence of testicular cancer in white males has nearly doubled in the past 40 years.[41] In the vast majority of cases (over 90 per cent), testicular cancers are malignant germinal cell tumors with one of four histologic patterns: (1) seminoma (37.8 per cent); (2) embryonal carcinoma (31.6 per cent); (3) teratoma (26.5 per cent); or (4) choriocarcinoma (1.8 per cent).[39,42] Clinical examination—palpation of a testis mass—may be suggestive as to the type of cancer.[39] Seminoma tend to expand and infiltrate the entire testicular substance while embryonal carcinoma and terotoma each demonstrate a discrete nodular mass.[39] Malignant testicular tumors of nongerminal origin are most commonly lymphoma, which may cause localized or diffuse involvement of the testis. Testicular lymphoma constitutes only 5 per cent of all testicular neoplasms, but they are the most common tumor of the testes in patients over 50 years of age.[42] The testes may also be involved in acute lymphocytic leukemia. Clinical involvement occurs in only 8–16 per cent of cases. Autopsy studies, however, demonstrate an occurrence rate ranging from 70–92 per cent. Metastatic disease of the testis can occur from melanomas, carcinoma of the prostate, the lungs, the gastrointestinal tract, and the kidney.[42]

Testicular tumors most commonly present with painless enlargement of the testis or the incidental finding of a testicular nodule. Approximately 40 per cent of patients complain of a dull ache or heavy sensation in the scrotum, inguinal area or lower abdomen.[39] Occasionally, a testis tumor may present with acute pain, in which case it must be differentiated from testicular torsion. Since testicular tumors are more commonly associated with dull pain and discomfort, epididymitis is a more important differential diagnosis. It has been reported that as many as 55 per cent of patients with testicular tumor were initially treated for presumed epididymitis resulting in a delay of cancer treatment ranging from several weeks to nine months or longer.[39] In approximately 10 per cent of patients the initial clinical presentation is related to the metastatic disease. Initial treatment of primary testicular carcinoma, regardless of their histologic type, is orchiectomy, and is usually performed through an inguinal approach. When tumor invades the wall of the scrotum, hemiscrotectomy is required. Serial histologic analysis is essential as different types of cancer can be present concomitantly. Furthermore, the local staging of the disease is based on pathology (Table 10.1). At present, the detection of nodal metastasis (N staging) relies primarily on the CT findings, and for some tumor types, on serum markers. In seminoma, elevated

Table 10.1   Classification and MR imaging criteria for local staging of primary testicular tumors

Stage	TNM criteria	MR criteria
T0	No evidence of primary tumor	No evidence of primary tumor
T1	Confined to testis	Normal testicular tissue surrounding the tumor and/or tunica albuginea intact
T2	Extends beyond tunica albuginea	Localized interruption of tunica albuginea on T2-predominant images; mass extending beyond tunica
T3	Involves rete testis or epididymis	Obliteration of low signal intensity mediastinum on T2-predominant images or direct tumor extension to the epididymis
T4a	Invades spermatic cord	Obliteration of fat on T1-predominant images; enlargement of the spermatic cord and low signal intensity on T2-predominant images
T4b	Invades scrotal wall	Invasion of scrotal wall

Carotid Triplex Exam Protocol

Proximal and Distal Disease

Lesions which occur proximal (innominate) or distal (carotid siphon) to the carotid can be detected with duplex evaluation of the neck vessels.

Intracranial Disease

Doppler changes have been found to occur in the common carotid artery when a stenosis of 75 percent or greater is present in the intracranial internal carotid artery.

The Doppler findings which indicate intracranial disease are:

1. The ipsilateral common carotid artery will exhibit a dampened waveform (i.e. blunted systolic profile and absent or decreased diastolic component).

2. The contralateral common carotid artery will exhibit normal or slightly increased flow with a normal waveform profile.

3. The external carotid arteries will remain normal bilaterally.

4. The ipsilateral internal carotid artery will exhibit overall decreased flow.

Diasonics

human chorionic gonadotropin (HCG) is seen in only 10 per cent of the patients, but in nonseminomatous tumors, alpha-fetoprotein (AFP) and HCG tumor markers are helpful in the search for metastatic disease. If nodal metastasis is suspected in patients with seminoma (nodes are not bulky and there are fewer than five nodes present), the patients are customarily treated with radiation therapy, while patients with any trace of nonseminomatous tumors undergo retroperitoneal dissection. Multidrug chemotherapy is the primary treatment for bulky nodal disease or presence of metastasis.

MRI appearance

MRI appearance of solid benign tumors of the testis is similar to their malignant counterpart. They often demonstrate homogeneous medium signal intensity (similar to normal testicular tissue) on T1-weighted images and show marked decrease in signal intensity on T2-weighted images, as shown in Figure 10.34. While benign solid tumors cannot be differentiated from malignant ones, testicular cysts have a characteristic MRI appearance. As illustrated in Figure 10.35, testicular cysts are sharply outlined and they demonstrate homogeneous low signal intensity on T1-weighted images and increase in signal intensity on T2-weighted images. When such a signal intensity pattern is seen, the imaging can suggest the benign nature of the lesion, and can influence the surgical approaches. However, if the fluid content within the cyst is more proteinaceous, the imaging diagnosis of benign lesion is no longer feasible.

Malignant testicular neoplasm can manifest a spectrum of findings on either T1- or T2-weighted images. On T1-weighted images, as shown in Figure 10.36, most testicular cancers have a signal intensity similar to the adjacent normal testicular tissue.[9,11–15] The homogeneous or heterogeneous high signal intensity of the tumors, however, can be seen. On T2-weighted images, the majority of testicular tumors (Figure 10.36) are characterized by decrease in signal intensity as compared with adjacent normal testicular tissue.[9,11–15] However, tumors demonstrating heterogeneous signal intensity, or signal intensity similar to normal testicular tissue, have been reported. It has been suggested that MRI can be used to diagnose specific tumor type based on signal intensity and heterogeneity of the lesion. Seminomatous tumors are reported to be isointense with testicular tissue on T1-weighted images and hypointense and homogeneous on T2-weighted images. While this is correct for some of the tumors, exceptions often exist. As shown in Figure 10.37, seminoma can demonstrate signal intensity higher than expected on T1-weighted images. Tumor which demonstrates medium signal intensity on the T1-weighted image and heterogeneous high signal intensity on the T2-weighted image is shown in Figure 10.38. Figure 10.39 demonstrates seminoma with high signal intensity on the T1-weighted image and heterogeneous signal intensity with numerous septations on the T2-weighted image. Figure 10.40 illustrates heterogeneous high signal intensity of the seminoma on the T1- and T2-weighted images which correlated with acute bleeding. A nonseminomatous tumor (Figure 10.41) usually demonstrates heterogeneous signal intensity and often shows a dark margin towards the normal testicular tissue. The latter correlates with a fibrous tumor capsule on histologic examination.

A secondary tumor of the testis similar to a primary lesion in a majority of cases causes decrease in signal intensity on T2-weighted images (Figure 10.42). While MRI is very sensitive in depicting the pathology, the specificity as to the tumor type is very rarely possible.

Local staging of testicular tumors has been attempted by MRI.[9] Because MRI consistently demonstrates low signal intensity of the tunica albuginea, it was expected that extension beyond the tunica would be easily depicted.[12] However, as the low signal intensity tumor extends to the proximity of the tunica, any disruption of the tunica is difficult to assess. Similarly, false positive results of the tumor extension to the spermatic cord have been encountered.[9] The inflammatory changes in the cord, obliterating the fat planes and mimicking tumor extension, are shown in Figure 10.43. Therefore, while the initial expectations for the MRI accuracy of local tumor staging were optimistic,[12] as more experience was gained, the 64 per cent staging accuracy of MRI was disappointing.[9]

MRI in relation to other imaging modalities

Ultrasound is considered the primary imaging modality in the evaluation of testicular tumors.[1,2,43] In the presence of localized testicular lesions, the accuracy of ultrasound is similar to that of MRI and no advantages over MRI have been shown.[9] However, if ultrasound is technically suboptimal, MRI studies are the next procedure of choice. MRI studies are also warranted when there is a discrepancy between ultrasound and clinical findings. In diffusely infiltrative disease, or in disease extending into both testicles (Figure 10.44), the limitations of ultrasound are well documented and MRI should be the procedure of choice in these patients. Similarly, if sonography suggests a benign epidermoid cyst, the cystic nature of the lesion can be confirmed with MRI.

Although the detection of testicular tumor is highly accurate with MRI, MRI is not tissue specific and cannot be used to determine the tumor's histologic characteristics. In addition, local tumor staging with MRI is no more accurate than with ultrasound. In fact, CT is the recommended modality for the staging of testicular cancer since the detection of lymph node metastasis is essential. MRI is preferred for follow-up investigation of lymph nodes in patients with previous lymph node dissection, because surgical clips do not distort MRI image quality.

References

1 HRICAK H, FILLY RA, Sonography of the scrotum, *Invest Radiol* (1983) **18**:112–21.

2 BENSON CB, DOUBILET PM, RICHIE JP, Sonography of the male genital tract. Review Article, *AJR* (1989) **153**:705–13.

3 SUBRAMANYAM BR, HORII SC, HILTON S, Diffuse testicular disease: sonographic features and significance, *AJR* (1985) **145**:1221–4.

4 SCHWERK WB, SCHWERK WN, RODECK G, Testicular tumors: prospective analysis of real-time US patterns and abdominal staging, *Radiology* (1987) **164**:369–74.

5 HUSBAND JE, HAWKES DJ, PECKHAM MJ, CT estimations of mean attenuation values and volume in testicular tumors: a comparison with surgical and histologic findings, *Radiology* (1982) **144**:553–8.

6 MARINCEK B, BRUTSCHIN P, TRILLER J et al, Lymphography and computed tomography in staging nonseminomatous testicular cancer: limited detection of early stage metastatic disease, *Urol Radiol* (1983) **5**:243–6.

7 COALSAET BLRA, Varicocele syndrome, venography determining the optimal level for surgical management, *Radiology* (1981) **140**:266.

8 HOLDER LE, MELLOUL M, CHEN DCP, Current status of radionuclide scrotal imaging, *Semin Nucl Med* (1981) **11**:232–49.

9 THURNHER S, HRICAK H, POBIEL R et al, Imaging the testis: comparison between MR imaging and US, *Radiology* (1988) **167**:631–6.

10 BAKER LL, HAJEK PC, BURKHARD TK et al, MR imaging of the scrotum: normal anatomy, *Radiology* (1987) **163**:89–92.

11 RHOLL KS, LEE JKT, LING D et al, MR imaging of the scrotum with a high-resolution surface coil, *Radiology* (1987) **163**:99–103.

12 BAKER LL, HAJEK PC, BURKHARD TK et al, MR imaging of the scrotum: pathologic conditions, *Radiology* (1987) **163**:93–8.

13 THOMSEN C, JENSEN KE, GIWERCMAN A et al, Magnetic resonance: in vivo tissue characterization of the testes in patients with carcinoma-in-situ of the testis and healthy subjects, *Int J Androl* (1987) **10**:191–8.

14 SEIDENWURM D, SMATHERS TL, LO RK et al, Testes and scrotum: MR imaging at 1.5 T, *Radiology* (1987) **164**:393–8.

15 JOHNSON JO, MATTREY RF, PHILLIPSON J, Differentiation of seminomatous from nonseminomatous testicular tumors with MR imaging, *AJR* (1990) **154**:539–43.

16 FRITZSCHE PJ, HRICAK H, KOGAN BA et al, Undescended testis: value of MR imaging, *Radiology* (1987) **164**:169–73.

17 TRAMBERT MA, MATTREY RF, LEVINE D et al, Subacute scrotal pain: evaluation of torsion versus epididymitis with MR imaging, *Radiology* (1990) **175**:53–6.

18 HRICAK H, Testicular MRI, *Contemporary Urology* (In press).

19 BAKER LL, HAJEK PC, BURKHARD TK et al, Polyorchidism: evaluation by MR. Case Report. *AJR* (1987) **148**:305–6.

20 TZIKA AA, MOSELEY ME, HRICAK H et al, Comparison of MR imaging and P-31 MR spectroscopy in a rat model of testicular torsion. Presented at the 75th Scientific Assembly and Annual Meeting of the *Radiological Society of North America*, Chicago, 1989.

21 BRETAN PN JR, VIGNERON DB, HRICAK H et al, Assessment of testicular metabolic integrity with P-31 MR spectroscopy, *Radiology* (1987) **162**:867–71.

22 CHEW W, HRICAK H, MCCLURE RD, The assessment of human testicular function by ^{31}P MRS. Presented at the 73rd Scientific Assembly of the Radiologic Society of North America, Nov 29–Dec 4, 1987, *Radiology* (in press).

23 CHEW W, HRICAK H, CARROLL P, Clinical utility of P-31 MR spectroscopy in the evaluation of human testicular abnormalities. For presentation at the 75th Scientific Assembly and Annual Meeting of the *Radiological Society of North America*, November, 1989.

24 LIERSE W, Testis. In: *Applied Anatomy of the Pelvis*, (Springer Verlag: Berlin 1984) 188–98.

25 ROUVIERE H, Anatomy of the human lymphatic system. Compendium. Tobias MJ (translator). (Edwards Brothers: Ann Arbor, Michigan 1983).

26 SEMELKA R, ANDERSON M, HRICAK H, Prosthetic testicle: appearance at MR imaging, *Radiology* (1989) **173(2)**:561–2.

27 GLASS AR, Identical twins discordant for the 'rudimentary testes' syndrome, *J Urol* (1982) **127**:140–1.

28 HANCOCK RA, HODGINS TE, Polyorchidism, *Urology* (1984) **24**:303–7.

29 RAJFER G, WALSH PC, Testicular descent: normal and abnormal, *Urol Clin North Am* (1978) **5**:223–5.

30 WYNDHAM NR, A morphological study of testicular descent, *J Anat* (1943) **77**:179.

31 KOGAN SJ, Cryptorchidism. In: Kelalis King B ed. *Clinical Pediatric Urology*, 2nd edn. (WB Saunders, Philadelphia 1985) 864–87.

32 FALLON B, WELTON M, HAWTREY C, Congenital anomalies associated with cryptorchidism, *J Urol* (1982) **127**:91–3.

33 KOGAN SJ, Cryptorchidism and infertility: an overview, *Dial Pediatr Urol* (1981) **4**:2–3.

34 ROSENFELD AT, BLAIR DN, MCCARTHY S, The pars infravaginalis gubernaculi and associated structures. An imaging pitfall in the identification of undescended testis, *AJR* (1989) **153(4)**:775–8.

35 WEISS RM, CARTER AR, ROSENFIELD AR, High resolution real-time ultrasonography in the localization of the undescended testis, *J Urol* (1986) **135**:936–8.

36 BUNCE PL, Scrotal abnormalities. In: Glenn JF, ed. *Urologic Surgery*, (Harper and Row: New York 1975) 232.

37 GONDA RL, KARO JJ, FONTE RA et al, Diagnosis of subclinical varicocele in infertility, *AJR* (1987) **148**:71–5.

38 MOSTOFI FK, Testicular tumors, epidemiologic, etiologic and pathologic features, *Cancer* (1973) **32**:1186.

39 EINHORN LH, CRAWFORD ED, SHIPLEY WU et al, Cancer of the testes. In: DeVita VT Jr, Hellman S, Rosenberg SA, eds. *Cancer Principles and Practice of Oncology*, Vol 1, Ch 35, 3rd edn. (JB Lippincott: Philadelphia 1989) 1071–98.

40 SILVERBERG E, Cancer in young adults (ages 15 to 34). *CA* (1982) **32**:32.

41 SCHOTTENFELD D, WARSHAUER ME, SHERLOCK S et al, The epidemiology of testicular cancer in young adults, *Am J Epidemiol* (1980) **112**:232.

42 MOSTOFI FK, PRICE EP JR, Tumors of the male genital system: In: Firminger HI, Haslan I, eds. *Atlas of Tumor Pathology.*

(1973) Fascicle 8, Series 2, Washington, D.C., Armed Forces Institute of Pathology.

43 BENSON CB, The role of ultrasound in diagnosis and staging of testicular cancer, *Semin Urol* (1988) **6**:189–202.

Figure 10.1

Diagrammatic section
demonstrating the testis and its
fascia.

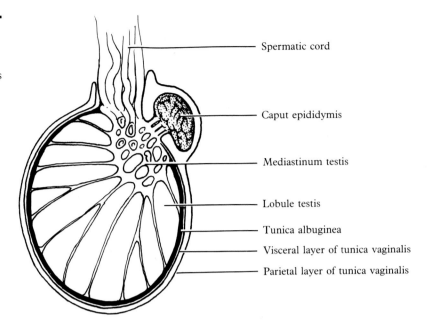

Spermatic cord

Caput epididymis

Mediastinum testis

Lobule testis

Tunica albuginea

Visceral layer of tunica vaginalis

Parietal layer of tunica vaginalis

Figure 10.2

Schematic drawing of the
spermatic cord and the inguinal
canal. (**a**) Window to
demonstrate the layers of the
inguinal canal, (**b**)
demonstration of the cord
structures with fascia removed
and (**c**) course of the ductus
deferens.

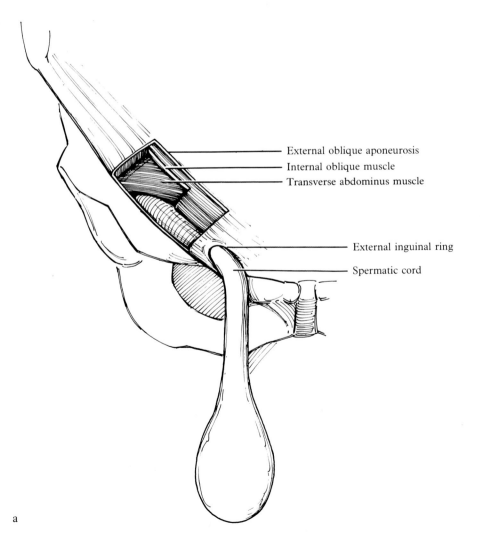

External oblique aponeurosis
Internal oblique muscle
Transverse abdominus muscle

External inguinal ring
Spermatic cord

a

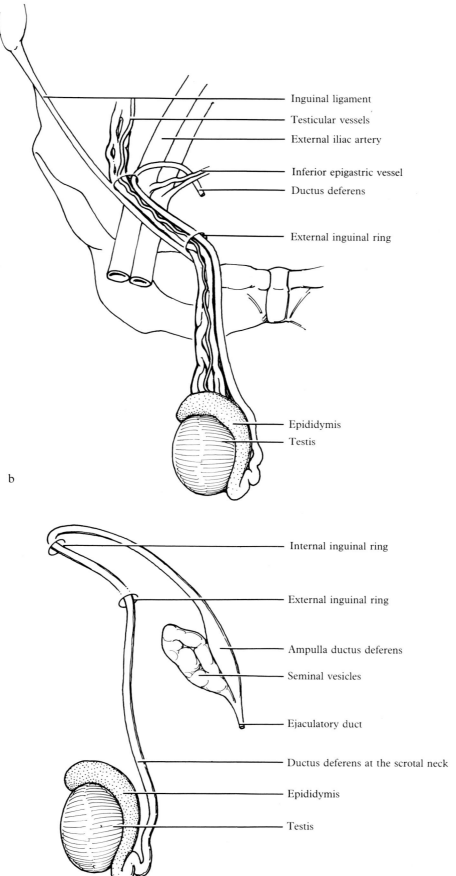

Inguinal ligament

Testicular vessels

External iliac artery

Inferior epigastric vessel

Ductus deferens

External inguinal ring

Epididymis

Testis

b

Internal inguinal ring

External inguinal ring

Ampulla ductus deferens

Seminal vesicles

Ejaculatory duct

Ductus deferens at the scrotal neck

Epididymis

Testis

c

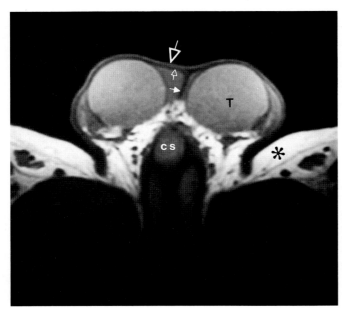

a

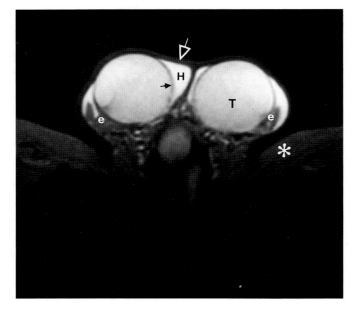

b

Figure 10.3

Normal testis, transaxial plane of imaging. (**a**) T1-weighted and (**b**) T2-weighted images. On the T1-weighted image, the testis (T) images with homogeneous medium signal intensity (the signal intensity of the testis (T) is similar to that of the corpus spongiosum (CS) and is lower than the signal intensity of the subcutaneous fat (asterisk)). The testis (T) signal intensity increases on a T2-weighted image and is higher than adipose tissue (asterisk). The signal intensity of the epididymis and hydrocele are similar on the T1-weighted image, but on the T2-weighted image the epididymis (e) decreases in signal intensity while the fluid of the hydrocele (H) increases in signal intensity, making the differentiation between the two easy. The tunica albuginea is visible on the T2-weighted image (solid black arrow). On the T1-weighted image, within the scrotal skin, the inner low signal intensity stripe (small open white arrow) corresponding to the dartos muscle and fascial layers can be separated from higher signal intensity scrotal skin (large open arrow). The septum (solid white arrow), however, demonstrates low signal intensity. On the T2-weighted image layers of the scrotal wall cannot be separated, and they demonstrate low signal intensity.

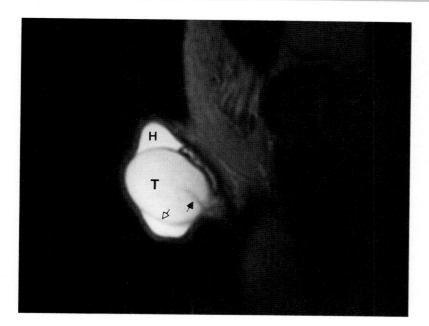

Figure 10.4

Mediastinum testis on the sagittal T2-weighted image. The mediastinum testis (small black arrow) is of low signal intensity and it is seen invaginating within the higher signal intensity testicular tissue (T). (Open black arrow)-tunica albuginea; (H)-hydrocele.

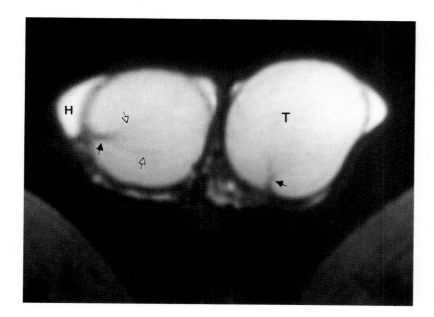

Figure 10.5

The intratesticular septulae, transaxial T2-weighted image. From the mediastinum testis (small black arrows) emanate fine low signal intensity stripes (open black arrows), probably representing slighter thickened septulae between the lobules. (T)-testis; (H)-hydrocele.

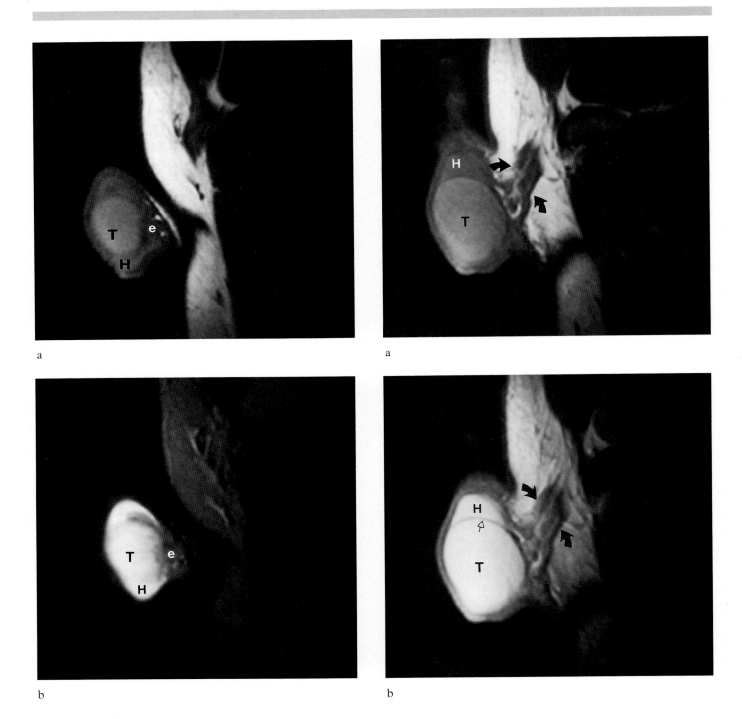

a

b

a

b

Figure 10.6

The epididymis shown in the sagittal plane of imaging. (**a**) T1-weighted, and (**b**) T2-weighted images. The epididymis (e) and the hydrocele (H) are of medium signal intensity on the T1-weighted image. However, on the T2-weighted image, the hydrocele (H) increases in signal intensity while the epididymis (e) decreases in signal intensity rendering excellent contrast between the two. (T)-testis.

Figure 10.7

Spermatic cord at the level of the scrotal neck. Sagittal (**a**) T1- and (**b**) T2-weighted images. (Curved arrows)-level of the spermatic cord at the scrotal neck; (T)-testis; (small open black arrow)-tunica albuginea; (H)-hydrocele.

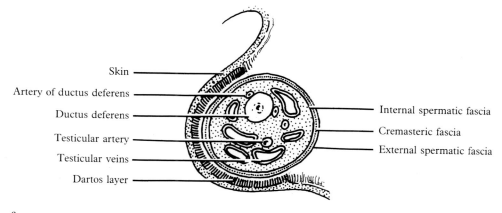

Skin

Artery of ductus deferens

Ductus deferens

Testicular artery

Testicular veins

Dartos layer

Internal spermatic fascia

Cremasteric fascia

External spermatic fascia

a

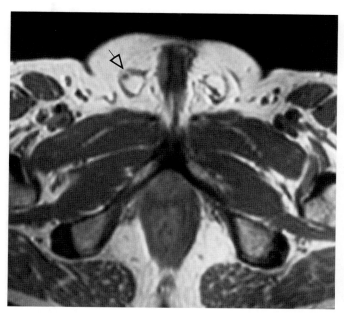

b

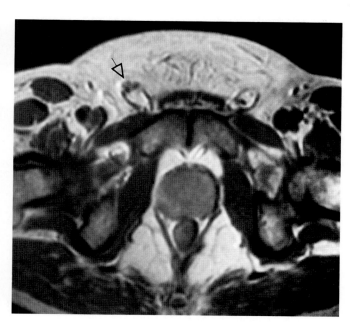

c

Figure 10.8

Contents of the spermatic cord. (a) Schematic drawing at the level of the scrotal neck, (b) transaxial proton density image at the level of the scrotal neck, and (c) transaxial proton density image section at the upper border of the symphysis pubis.

On the MRI image at the level of the scrotal neck, the low intensity ring of the spermatic cord is contrasted to the surrounding adipose tissue. Within the cord, there are fat and low signal intensity structures, the largest of which should be the ductus deferens. Separate identification of each individual component of the spermatic cord is not possible. (Open arrows)-spermatic cord.

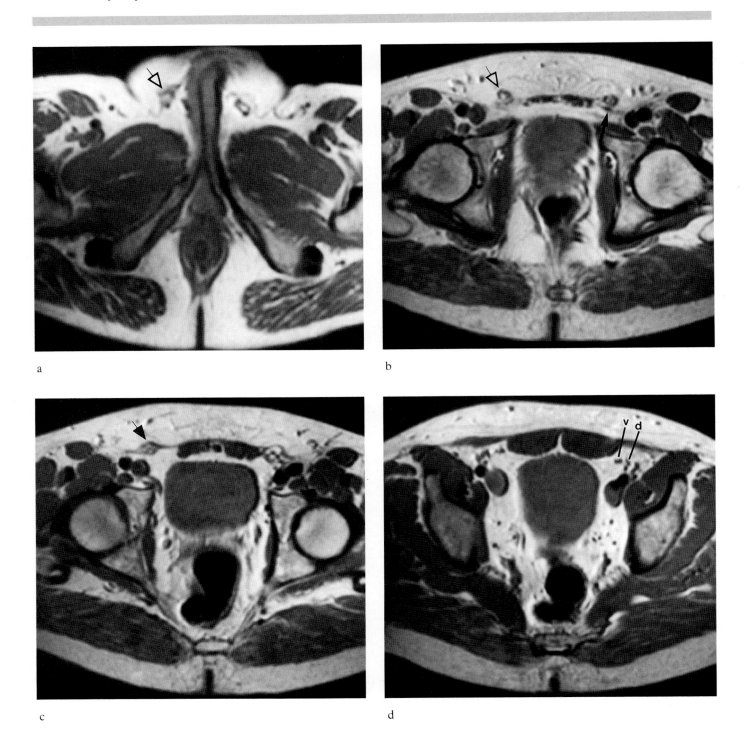

a

b

c

d

Figure 10.9

Anatomical landmarks of the spermatic cord and the inguinal canal as seen on a serial transaxial proton density image. (**a**) Spermatic cord (open arrow) at the level of the scrotal neck, (**b**) spermatic cord just outside the external ring. The spermatic cord is seen anterior to the external oblique muscles (long black arrow), (**c**) at the level of the external inguinal ring (black arrow). The aponeuroses of the oblique muscles are seen on either side of the spermatic cord, (**d**) located just outside the inguinal canal, proximal to the internal inguinal ring. The ductus deferens (d) is seen lateral to the inferior epigastric vessels (v).

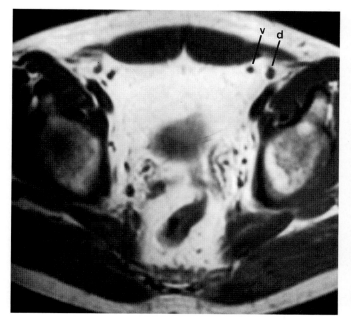

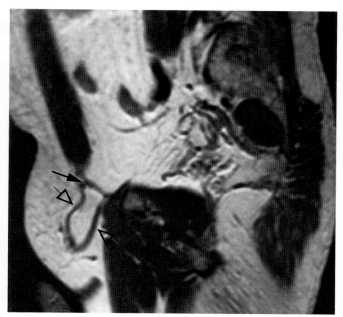

a

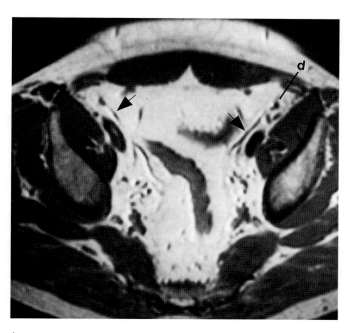

b

Figure 10.11

The spermatic cord in the sagittal plane, proton density image. Fat within the spermatic cord emphasizes the low signal intensity wall (open arrows). The course of the spermatic cord to the external ring (long black arrow) is well seen in the sagittal image.

Figure 10.10

Course of the ductus deferens. (**a**) Outside the level of the internal inguinal ring, where the ductus deferens (d) and surrounding vessels are seen lateral to the inferior epigastric vessels (V). (**b**) The ductus deferens (d) is seen passing downwards towards the seminal vesicles. The straight portion of the ductus deferens before looping can be seen (black arrows).

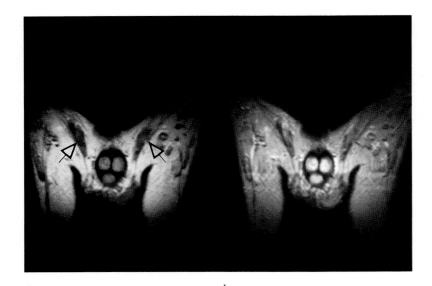

a   b

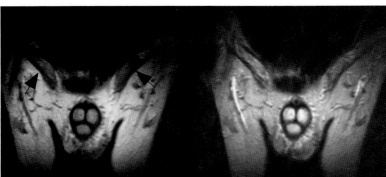

c   d

Figure 10.12

The spermatic cord (open arrowheads) and the inguinal canal (solid arrowhead) in the coronal plane of imaging. (**a**) and (**b**) are proton density and T2-weighted images of the spermatic cord, and (**c**) and (**d**) demonstrate the inguinal canal (solid black arrows).

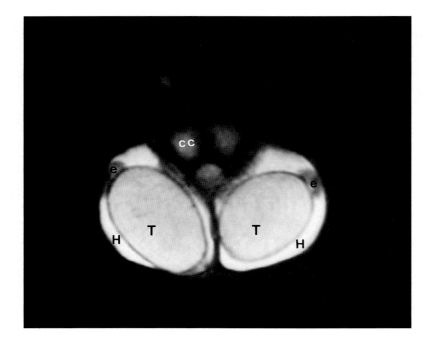

Figure 10.13

Normal testis as seen in a T2-weighted coronal image. The coronal plane of imaging allows comparison between the signal intensity of the right and left testis (T). (H)-hydrocele; (e)-epididymis. Note that in this patient the signal intensity of the testicular tissue is much higher than that of the corpora cavernosa (cc).

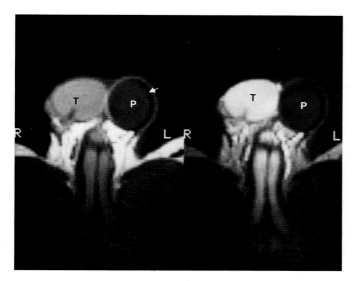

a   b

Figure 10.14

Testicular prosthesis, transaxial
(**a**) T1- and (**b**) T2-weighted
images. The right testis (T) is
normal. On the left side the
testicular prosthesis (P)
demonstrates low signal
intensity on both T1- and T2-
weighted images. The
chemical-shift artifact (arrow) is
pronounced around the
prosthesis but not seen around
the testis.

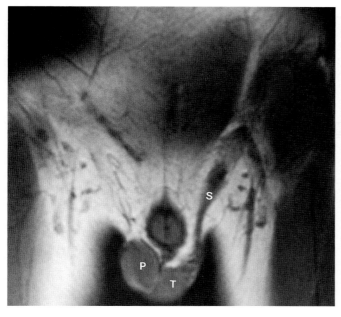

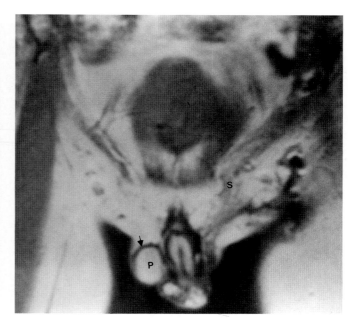

a   b

Figure 10.15

Testicular prosthesis (made of
solid elastomer). Coronal (**a**)
T1- and (**b**) T2-weighted
images. The prosthesis (P)
demonstrates signal intensity
similar to the normal testis (T)
on the T1-weighted image. It
increases on the T2-weighted
image, and the only
identification of the prosthesis
(P) is by the demonstration of
the chemical-shift artifact
(black arrow) and lack of the
spermatic cord on the right
side. (S)-left spermatic cord.

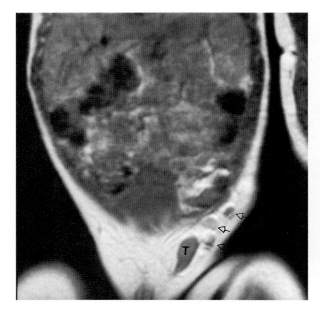

a

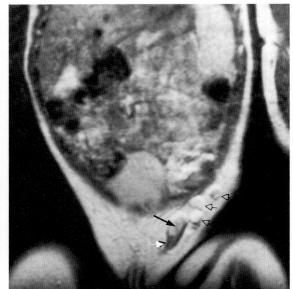

b

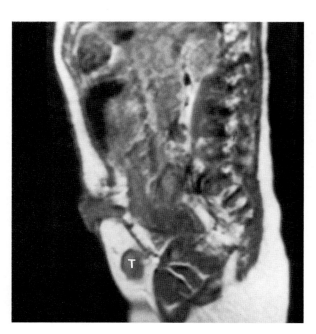

c

Figure 10.16

Undescended testis located 2 cm beyond the external inguinal ring (high scrotal position). Coronal (**a**) proton density image, (**b**) T2-weighted image, and (**c**) sagittal proton density image. The undescended testis (T) is of normal signal intensity on the T1- and T2-weighted images. The mediastinum testis (long black arrow) is visible and the gubernaculum testis (solid white arrow) demonstrates low signal intensity on the T2-weighted image. (Open black arrows)-inguinal lymph nodes.

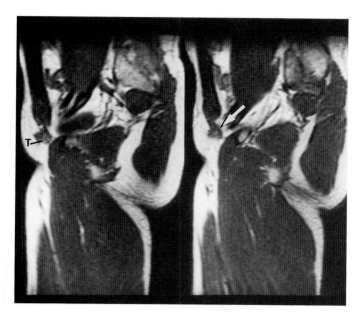

a   b

Figure 10.17

Undescended testis located just outside the external inguinal ring. Sagittal T2-weighted image, (**a**) and (**b**) are two consecutive sections. The undescended testis (T) is seen just outside the aponeurosis of the oblique muscle (white arrow). The testis (T) is small and of lower than normal signal intensity indicating fibrosis.

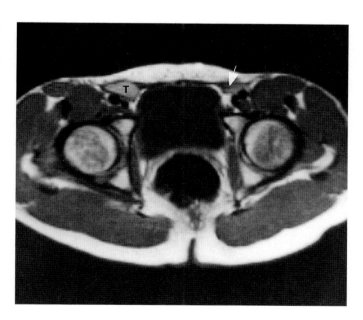

Figure 10.18

The undescended testis intra-abdominal in location. Transaxial T1-weighted image. The orientation of the right undescended testis (T) is horizontal, indicating that the testis is no longer within the inguinal canal. At surgery, it was located just outside the internal inguinal ring. The left testis (white arrow) was also undescended, and was located at the level of the internal inguinal ring.

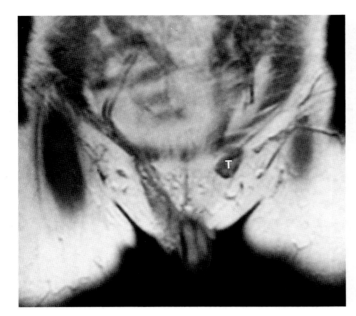

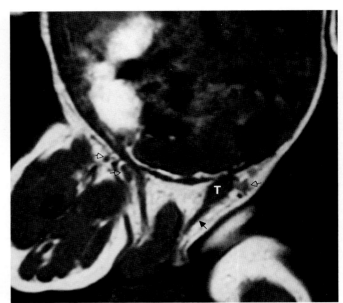

a

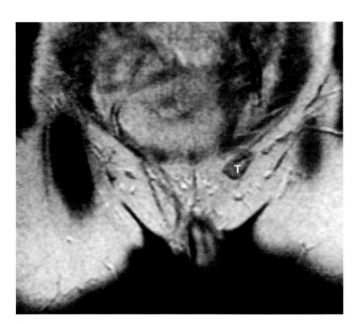

b

Figure 10.19

Atrophic undescended testis.
Coronal plane (**a**) proton
density, and (**b**) T2-weighted
images. The left undescended
testis (T) is located beyond the
external inguinal canal. The
testis, however, is of low signal
intensity on the T2-weighted
image indicating atrophy.

Figure 10.20

Retractile (migratory) testis.
Coronal T1-weighted image.
The testis (T) in the left
spermatic cord is in high scrotal
position. The cord, distal to the
testis (black arrow), is well
developed. The right testis was
in a normal scrotal position.
(Open arrows)-inguinal nodes.

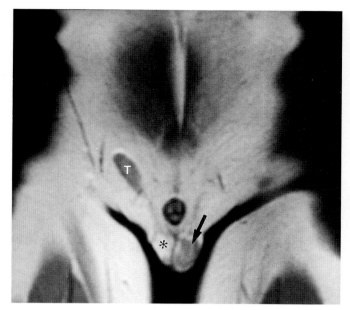

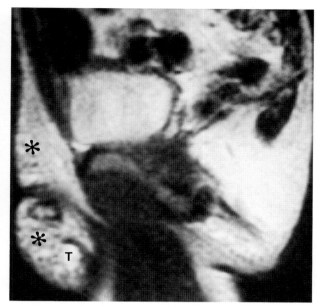

a

b

Figure 10.22

Six-month-old boy with extensive lymphedema of the scrotum and the anterior abdominal wall limiting the clinical and ultrasound evaluation. The sagittal T2-weighted image demonstrates the testis (T) and the extension of lymphedema (asterisks).

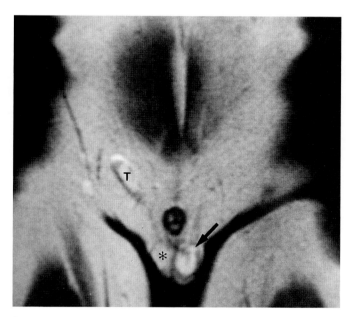

Figure 10.21

Undescended testis. Coronal plane, (**a**) proton density and (**b**) T2-weighted images. The undescended testis (T) in the right high scrotal position is of similar size and signal intensity to the contralateral normal testis (black arrow). (Asterisk)-empty right scrotal sac.

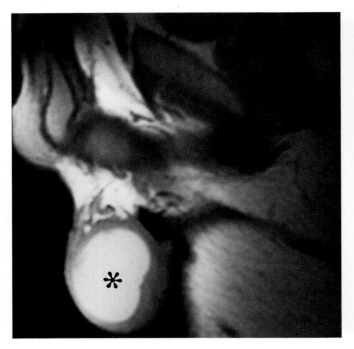

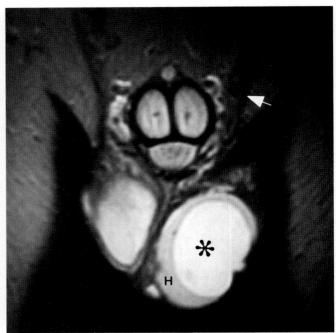

a   b

___

Figure 10.23

Intermittent testicular torsion, (**a**) sagittal T1-weighted image and (**b**) coronal T2-weighted image. The left testis (asterisk) is enlarged and is of high signal intensity on both the T1- and T2-weighted images. Diffuse testicular hemorrhage is suggested from the imaging findings. The surrounding hydrocele can be seen (H). The spermatic cord on the left is enlarged (arrow). In combination with the findings on ^{31}P MR spectroscopy, the diagnosis of intermittent torsion was made and subsequently proven at surgery.

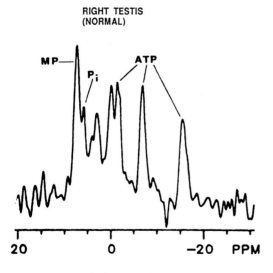

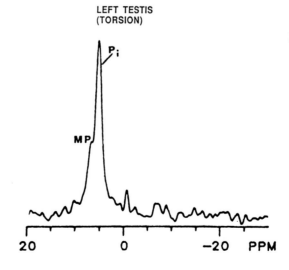

___

Figure 10.24

^{31}P MR spectra in a patient with acute torsion of the left testis. The right testis is normal. The left testis demonstrates loss of ATP peaks and marked decrease of PM (phosphomonoester) levels. The P_i (inorganic phosphate) peak is markedly increased.

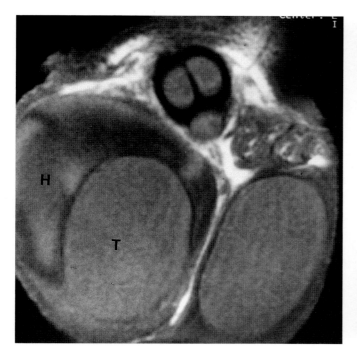

a

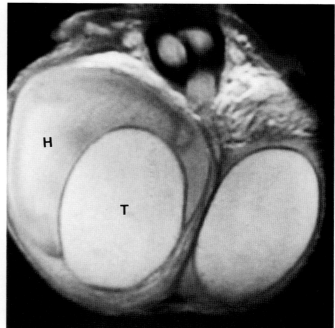

b

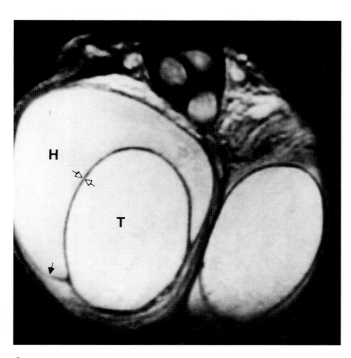

c

Figure 10.25

Hydrocele. (**a**) T1-weighted image, (**b**) proton density image, and (**c**) T2-weighted image. The fluid collection (H) around the right testis (T) is of lower signal intensity than the testis on the T1-weighted image, and of higher intensity than the testis on the T2-weighted image. The hydrocele is the fluid accommodation between the visceral and parietal layers of the tunica vaginalis. This permits visualization of the parietal layer of the tunica vaginalis (black arrow). The tunica albuginea cannot be differentiated from the visceral layer of the tunica vaginalis (open arrows).

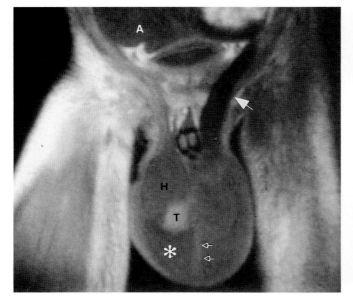

a

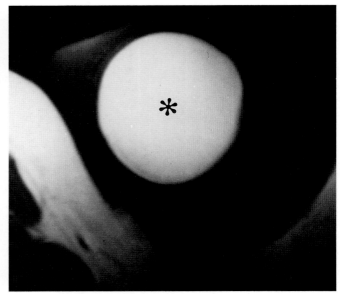

a

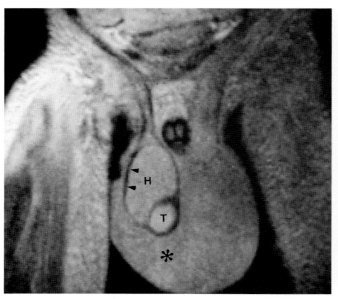

b

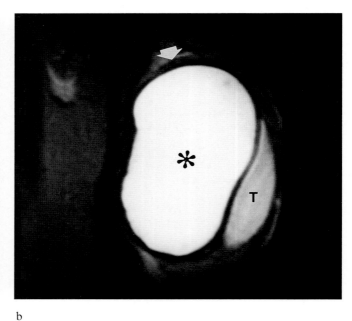

b

Figure 10.26

Scrotal lymphedema and bilateral hydrocele. Coronal plane (**a**) T1-weighted image and (**b**) T2-weighted image. The hydrocele (H) is imaged with medium signal intensity on the T1-weighted image and increases in signal intensity on the T2-weighted image. (T)-testis. The tissue outside the parietal layer of the tunica vaginalis (black arrowheads) is edematous scrotal skin (asterisk). The scrotal septum can be seen (open arrows). There is a communicating hydrocele on the left side, as the fluid (solid white arrow) is present within the left spermatic cord. (A)-ascites.

Figure 10.27

Chronic hematocele, (**a**) transaxial T1-weighted image, and (**b**) coronal T2-weighted image. Hematocele (asterisk) is imaged with high signal intensity on both the T1- and T2-weighted images. A thick capsule around the hematocele (white arrow) is seen. The left testis (T) is compressed.

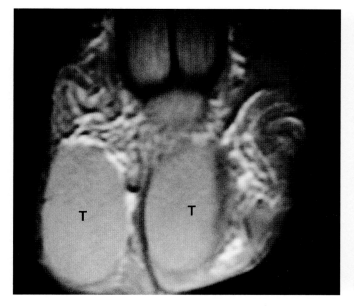

a

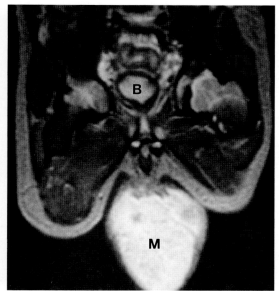

a

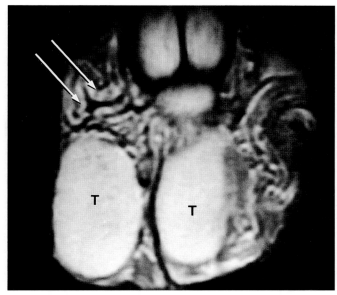

b

b

Figure 10.28

Bilateral varicoceles, coronal plane (**a**) proton density image, (first echo) and (**b**) T2-weighted image (second echo). Numerous serpiginous tubular structures are seen superior to the testis (T). They exhibit medium signal intensity on the first echo, but on the second echo image, some are of high signal intensity and some remain of medium signal intensity depending on flow velocity. The dilated veins of the pampiniform plexus—varicoceles—are visible on the T2-weighted image (long white arrows).

Figure 10.29

Meconium within the scrotal sac presenting as a large scrotal mass in a newborn. T2-weighted images, (**a**) coronal and (**b**) sagittal. The scrotum is markedly enlarged, and a large mass (M) is of heterogeneous, predominantly high signal intensity. A punctate low signal intensity area (arrows) corresponded to calcifications seen on the plain film. (B)-urinary bladder.

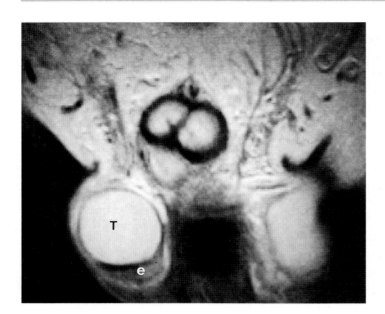

Figure 10.30

Epididymitis. Coronal T2-weighted image. The right testis (T) is normal. The epididymis (e) is enlarged, but remains of low signal intensity.

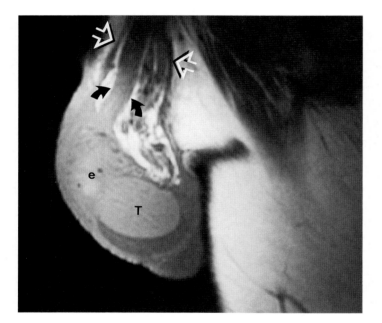

Figure 10.31

Epididymitis with extension along the ductus deferens. Sagittal T1-weighted image. (T)-testis. The epididymis (e) is enlarged and there is enlargement of the ductus deferens (curved arrows) within the spermatic cord (open arrows).

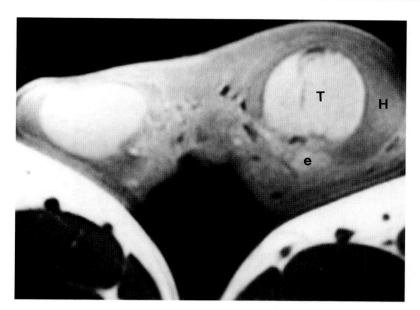

a

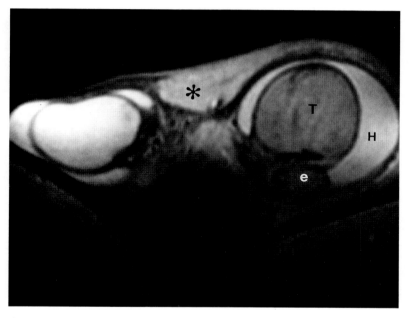

b

Figure 10.32

Epididymitis and orchitis, transaxial (**a**) proton density and (**b**) T2-weighted images. The left epididymis (e) is enlarged and is of low signal intensity on the T2-weighted image. The left testis (T) is also enlarged. On the T2-weighted image, the testis is of homogeneous low signal intensity as compared to the normal high signal intensity right testis. (H)-hydrocele. The scrotal skin (asterisk) on the left is also swollen and is of high signal intensity on the T2-weighted image.

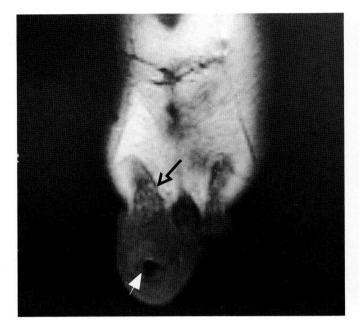

a

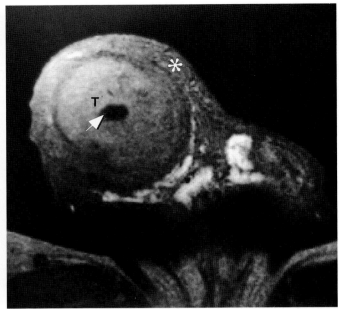

b

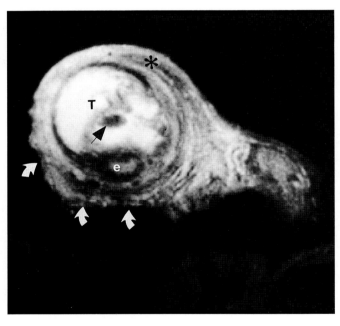

c

Figure 10.33

Abscess of the right scrotum,
(**a**) coronal T1-weighted image,
transaxial (**b**) T1-weighted
image and (**c**) T2-weighted
image. The right scrotum is
markedly enlarged. The
epididymis (e) is enlarged.
Within the testis (T) there is an
air collection (solid arrow). The
scrotal skin (asterisk) is
thickened and of
inhomogeneous signal intensity
with marked irregularity and
ulcerations along its inferior
aspect (white curved arrows).
The infection ascends along the
spermatic cord (open arrow).

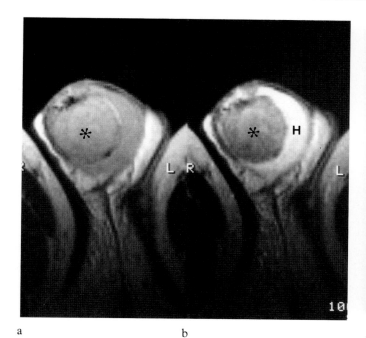

a   b

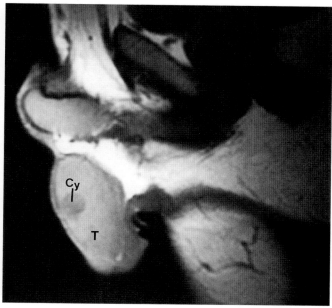

a

Figure 10.34

Leydig cell tumor of the right testis, transaxial (**a**) proton density and (**b**) T2-weighted images. On the proton density image, the tumor (asterisk) has similar signal intensity to the adjacent hydrocele. On the T2-weighted image, the hydrocele (H) markedly increases in signal intensity while the tumor (asterisk) demonstrates homogeneous decrease in signal intensity. Tumor infiltrates the entire testis.

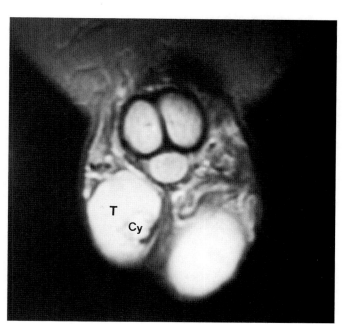

b

Figure 10.35

Testicular cyst, right testis. (**a**) T1-weighted and (**b**) T2-weighted images, coronal plane. Within the right testis (T) there is a sharply outlined cystic (Cy) mass of low signal intensity on the T1-weighted image and of high signal intensity on the T2-weighted image. These findings are characteristic of testicular cysts.

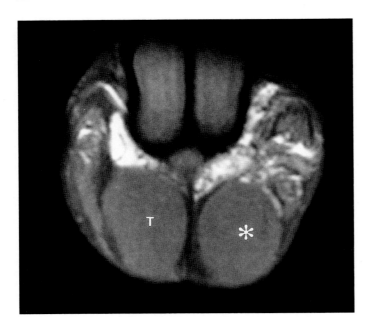

a

Figure 10.36

Seminoma of the left testis.
Coronal (**a**) T1-weighted and
(**b**) T2-weighted images. On the
T1-weighted image, the signal
intensity of the left testis
(asterisk) is homogeneous and
is similar to that of the normal
contralateral right testis (T). On
the T2-weighted image, the
testicular tumor (asterisk)
demonstrates low signal
intensity contrasted to the high
signal intensity of the right
testis.

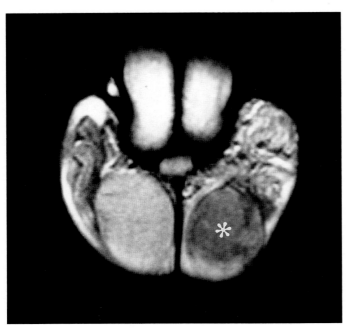

b

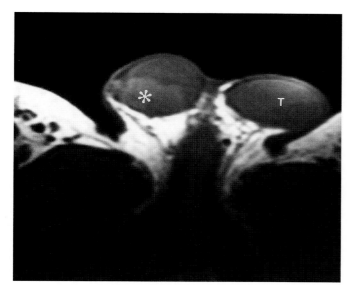

a

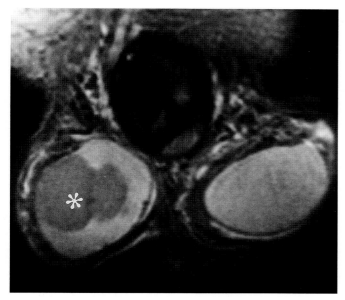

b

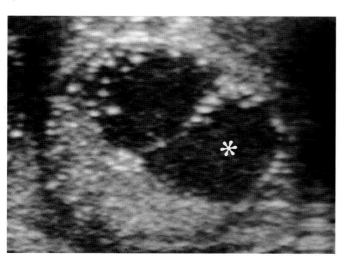

c

Figure 10.37

Seminoma of the right testis. (**a**) Transaxial T1-weighted image, (**b**) coronal T2-weighted image and (**c**) comparison ultrasonogram. In this patient, the testicular tumor (asterisk) demonstrates signal intensity which is homogeneous but higher than the adjacent normal testicular tissue or the contralateral normal left testis (T) on the T1-weighted image. On the T2-weighted image, the tumor (asterisk) demonstrates homogeneous lower signal intensity. The bilobe tumor configuration corresponds to the hypoechoic mass (asterisk) seen on the ultrasonogram.

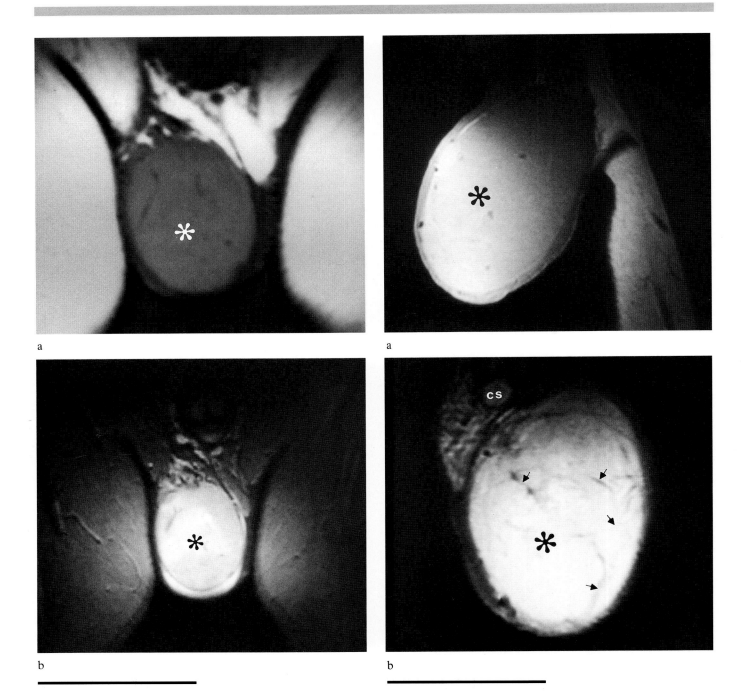

a

a

b

b

Figure 10.38

Seminoma of the right testis.
Coronal (**a**) T1-weighted and
(**b**) T2-weighted images. In this
patient, the entire right testis is
infiltrated by tumor (asterisk).
It is enlarged, and on the T1-
weighted image, it is of
unremarkable medium signal
intensity. However, on the T2-
weighted image, the entire
testis exhibits heterogeneous
but high signal intensity. The
signal intensity of the testicular
tumor is higher than that of the
adjacent adipose tissue.

Figure 10.39

Large seminoma of the left
testis (asterisk). (**a**) Sagittal T1-
weighted and (**b**) coronal T2-
weighted images. On the T1-
weighted image, the testis is
markedly enlarged and is of
higher signal intensity than the
adjacent scrotal skin or the
adipose tissue. On the T2-
weighted image, the testis
demonstrates high signal
intensity (higher than the
corpus spongiosum (cs)) with
many septa (arrows).

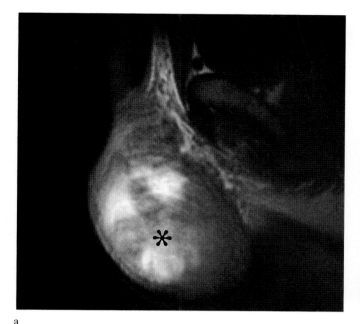

a

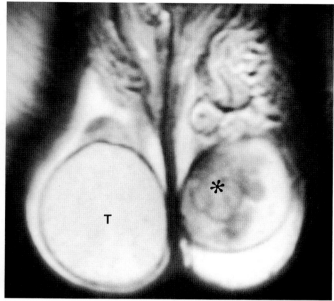

Figure 10.41

Embryonal cell carcinoma, coronal T2-weighted image. The tumor (asterisk) demonstrates heterogeneous signal intensity and is lobulated and septated. (T)-normal right testis.

b

Figure 10.40

Seminoma (asterisk) of the left testis. (**a**) Sagittal T1-weighted image and (**b**) coronal T2-weighted image. On the T1-weighted image, the left testis is of heterogeneous signal intensity with areas of high signal intensity which subsequently corresponded to hemorrhage. On the T2-weighted image, the testis is of heterogeneous low and high signal intensity. The right compressed testis (T) can be seen. The patient presented with acute pain and a diagnosis of epididymitis and orchitis was entertained for three weeks. Following the MRI study supplemented with MRS spectroscopy, surgery was performed revealing seminoma. The acute pain was due to hemorrhage.

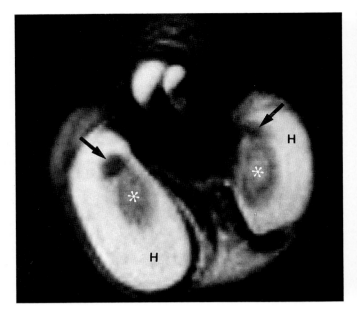

a

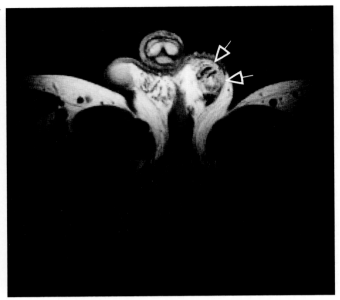

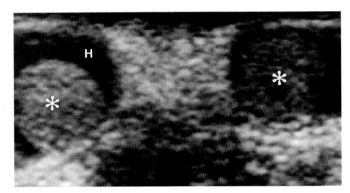

b

Figure 10.43

Enlargement of the left spermatic cord. Transaxial T1-weighted image. The left spermatic cord (arrows) is enlarged and of medium signal intensity. Tumor extension was suspected from imaging but only edema was found at surgery.

Figure 10.42

Lymphocytic leukemia involving both testicles. (**a**) Coronal T2-weighted image and (**b**) ultrasound scan. On ultrasound, both the right and left testis (asterisks) are normal in size and echogenicity. (H)-hydrocele. On the T2-weighted MR image, both testicles (asterisks) are of abnormally low signal intensity. (Long black arrow)-head of the epididymis; (H)-hydrocele.

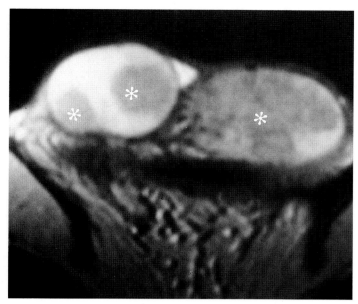

a

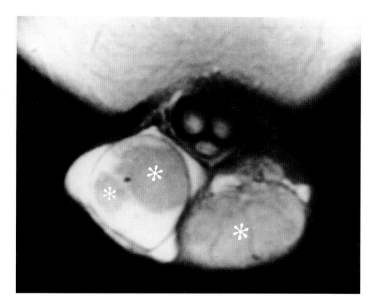

b

Figure 10.44

Bilateral seminomas, T2-weighted images, (**a**) transaxial and (**b**) coronal. Multifocal low signal intensity lesions are seen in the right testis (asterisks) and a large, almost completely infiltrating, lesion is present in the left testis. On ultrasound, the lesion within the right testis was detected but the diffusely infiltrative lesion in the left testis was overlooked.

11

The Penis and Male Urethra

Hedvig Hricak

Clinical indications for radiologic evaluation of the penis are increasing, and it has become evident, especially with the introduction of cross-sectional imaging, that radiology has a significant contribution to make in the management of a variety of disorders affecting the penis. Although the corpora cavernosogram has been available for many years, the technique has recently been perfected and applied to the evaluation of congenital anomalies, trauma, and erectile dysfunction.[1] The indications for penile imaging have been further expanded with the introduction of CT, and even more so with high resolution real-time ultrasonography.[2-4] MR imaging brings unique advantages to radiologic evaluation of the penis. MRI is especially useful in the demonstration of penile anatomy, penile and urethral trauma, and in the staging of proximal penile carcinoma.[5] The large field-of-view, operator independence, and the ease with which the examination is performed contribute to the usefulness of MRI. Indications for the use of MRI are rapidly expanding, and it is likely that MRI will become a valuable tool in the evaluation of penile pathology.

Normal anatomy of the penis and urethra

Penis

The male phallus develops from the **genital tubercle**, a surface elevation which appears at the cranial end of the cloacal membrane and lengthens to form the phallus. The phallus then enlarges to form the penis, and its apex become the glans. The genital folds fuse and enclose the phallic part of the urogenital sinus, forming the urethral bulb posteriorly and the greater part of the spongious urethra anteriorly. The glans and shaft of the penis are recognizable by the third month.[6]

In the adult, the penis consists of three erectile bodies—the two lateral **corpora cavernosa** and the ventral and medial **corpus spongiosum**. The penis, with its corporeal portions, can be divided into the radix (root) of the penis, located in the perineum, and the corpus of the penis, the free pendulous portion.[7]

In the **radix penis** the posterior portions of the corpora cavernosa are called the **crura**. As illustrated in Figure 11.1, the diverging crura are firmly attached to the ischiopubic ramus, and their medial aspect is covered by the **ischiocavernosus muscle**. The **transversus perinei superficialis muscle** can be seen at the posterior end of each crus. The posterior end of the corpus spongiosum is expanded in the radix penis and is called the **bulb of the penis.** It is attached to the perineal membrane (**urogenital diaphragm**). Just inferior to the bulb of the penis is the **bulbospongiosus muscle**, which also attaches to the transversus perinei superficialis muscle.[7-9]

The major portions of the two corpora cavernosa and the corpus spongiosum are found in the free pendulous part of the penis. At its distal end, the corpus spongiosum expands to form the **glans penis.** The corpora cavernosa and the corpus spongiosum are intimately attached structures. As shown in Figure 11.2, all three corpora are covered by the **tunica albuginea.** The tunica albuginea is composed of a collagen fiber network which is interspersed with a coarse mesh of elastic fibers. The tunica around the corpora cavernosa is thicker (approximately 3 mm in the flaccid state thinning to 0.5–1 mm in the erect state) than the tunica surrounding the corpus spongiosum (approximately 0.3–0.5 mm) (Figure 11.2). The portion of the tunica albuginea that is interposed between the paired corpora cavernosa forms an incomplete septum, allowing free communication between them.[7,9] However, there is no communication between the corpora cavernosa and corpus spongiosum in the normal patient. As depicted in Figure 11.3, the layer next to the tunica albuginea is the deep fascia of the penis (**Buck's fascia**). Buck's fascia is a fibrous tube-like envelope that surrounds the tunica albuginea and separates the penis into its dorsal (corpora cavernosa) and ventral (corpus spongiosum) compartments. The suspensory ligament of the penis blends with the Buck's fascia, and as a paired structure it extends from the fascia of the penis to the front of the symphysis pubis.

Vascular supply

The corpora cavernosa and the corpus spongiosum are erectile tissues, and their arteries open directly into the cavernous spaces without any intervening capillaries.

The portion of the **internal pudendal artery** after it gives off its perineal branch is called the **penile artery**.[9] The penile artery passes through the urogenital diaphragm, and continues along the medial margin of the inferior ramus of the pubis. It divides into its terminal branches—the **bulbourethral**, **cavernous** and **dorsal arteries**—near the urethral bulb. The bulbourethral artery, relatively short and of large caliber, passes through the urogenital diaphragm to enter the bulb of the penis. The cavernous (deep) artery travels along the dorsomedial surface of the corpus cavernosum and enters the hilum of the corpora cavernosa adjacent to the junction of both cavernous bodies. It continues distally in the center of the corpora cavernosa almost to their tips (Figure 11.3). Along its intracavernous course, it gives off multiple terminal branches to the cavernous spaces (the **helicine arteries**). The dorsal artery passes anterior to the crura and courses distally along the dorsum of the penis between the deep dorsal vein medially and the dorsal nerve of the penis laterally. Along its course, the dorsal artery gives off several circumflex branches that accompany the circumflex vein around the lateral surface of the corpora cavernosa. The dorsal artery primarily supplies the glans penis, although the circumflex arteries may also provide blood to the cavernous bodies.

Our understanding of the venous drainage of the penis has changed markedly in the last few years.[9] The venous drainage of the corpora cavernosa has long been a matter of controversy.[9] Until recently, most investigators believed that the corpora cavernosa were drained mainly by the deep dorsal vein. It is now known that the main venous drainage of the corpora cavernosa is via the **cavernous veins**, with additional drainage through the circumflex, deep dorsal, and

crural veins. The cavernous veins, in turn, drain into the internal pudendal vein. The **deep dorsal vein** provides the main venous drainage for the glans penis, the corpus spongiosum, and the distal two-thirds of the corpora cavernosa. The dorsal vein of the penis drains into the periprostatic plexus.

Lymphatic drainage

The lymphatic vessels of the penis follow the geographic distribution of the blood vessels. The glans of the penis drains into the **superficial inguinal nodes**, and the proximal part of the penis, including the penile urethra, drains into the **deep inguinal nodes.** Direct drainage into the **internal iliac nodes** along the course of the internal pudendal artery is also possible.[7]

Male urethra

From its origin in the bladder to its termination at the end of the penis, the male urethra is approximately 18–20 cm long.[10,7] Its circumference varies from 10–15 mm in the proximal prostatic part, where it is widest, to 7–8 mm at the external urethral meatus, where it is most narrow.

The urethra is divided into three regional parts—the prostatic part, the membranous part, and the penile (spongy) part. The latter is further divided into the bulbar and the anterior penile urethra. The prostatic urethra (approximately 3–4 cm in length) is the most proximal segment, is surrounded by the prostate and is briefly described in Chapter 8. The membranous urethra measures about 1 cm in length. Passing through the urogenital diaphragm, it extends from the apex of the prostate gland to the roof of the bulb of the penis. The levator ani muscle (its pubococcygeal part) lies in close proximity to the membranous urethra, but is anatomically separate from the urethral wall. Embedded in the adventitia of the membranous urethra, on its posterior aspect, are the two bulbourethral glands (Cowper's glands). The wall of the membranous urethra consists of a muscle coat which has an inner layer of smooth muscle bundles and a prominent outer layer of circularly orientated striated muscle fibers. The latter forms the so-called 'external urethral sphincter'. The sphincter is thickest around the membranous urethra but it also extends into the wall of the distal part of the prostatic urethra. The penile urethra is about 15 cm long. The urethra, after piercing the roof of the bulb, dilates to form the intrabulbar fossa and curves downwards and forwards to take a central position within the corpus spongiosum. The ducts of the bulbourethral glands accompany this portion of the urethra for 1–2 cm before opening obliquely through the urethral floor. From the bulbar fossa, the penile urethra narrows before it dilates again within the glans penis to form the fossa navicularis. For the most part, the penile urethra does not have a definitive muscle coat except for the circularly arranged bundles of smooth muscle cells in its inner aspect.

Histologically, the urethra is made up of mucous membrane (which is continuous internally with that of the bladder and externally with the skin covering the glans penis) and is supported by submucosa which connects it to the tissues it passes through. The epithelium lining of the urethra changes in its respective regions. In the proximal prostatic urethra, the epithelium is of the transitional type. Below the openings of the ejaculatory duct, this epithelium changes to a pseudostratified or stratified columnar variety which also lines the membranous urethra and the major part of the penile urethra. Towards the distal end of the penile urethra, the epithelium once again changes, becoming stratified squamous in character. This type of epithelium lines the fossa navicularis and becomes keratinized at the external meatus.

Vascular supply

Like the artery supplying the bulb of the penis, the **urethral artery** passes through the urogenital diaphragm to enter the corpus spongiosum. It travels through the corpus spongiosum to reach the glans penis, supplying the urethra and surrounding erectile tissue.

Lymphatic drainage

Lymphatics from the membranous part of the urethra follow the internal pudendal artery and pass mainly to the **internal iliac nodes**, although a few may end in the **external iliac nodes.** Lymphatics from the spongious urethra accompany those of the glans penis, terminating primarily in the **deep inguinal nodes.** Some may drain to the **superficial inguinal nodes**, and others may reach the **external iliac nodes** via the inguinal canal.

MRI appearance

Penis

On T1-weighted images, as shown in Figure 11.4, the erectile tissue (the corpora cavernosa and the corpus spongiosum) of the penis demonstrates medium signal intensity lower than that of the adjacent adipose tissue

and higher than that of striated muscle, eg, ischiocavernosus muscle. The corpora cavernosa and the corpus spongiosum can only be differentiated by the knowledge of their respective anatomic positions.[5,11] On T1-weighted images, the tunica albuginea images with lower signal intensity than the adjacent corporeal bodies. Sometimes, as shown in Figure 11.5, the tunica albuginea and the Buck's fascia can be separated on either the T1-weighted or the proton density image.

On T2-weighted images, both the corpora cavernosa and corpus spongiosum demonstrate increased signal intensity (Figure 11.4). The normal corpus spongiosum demonstrates a homogeneous increase in signal intensity, interrupted only by the low signal intensity urethra or septum located posteriorly at its base (Figure 11.4b). The signal intensity of the corpora cavernosa, however, can vary widely and may be lower than, similar to, or higher than that of the adjacent fat. Furthermore, the signal intensity of the corpora cavernosa can be homogeneous or heterogeneous. These wide variations in signal intensity reflect changes in penile blood flow and cavernosal blood volume. Changes in signal intensity of the corpora cavernosa may even be seen during the course of a single examination.[5] At the beginning of the study, the corpora cavernosa may demonstrate lower signal intensity towards the periphery, and by the end of the study, they may demonstrate uniform high signal intensity. The cavernous artery demonstrating low signal intensity is seen in the center of the corpora cavernosa (Figure 11.6).

The tunica albuginea demonstrates low signal intensity on T2-weighted images, providing good contrast with the high signal intensity of the corpora. The T2-weighted sequences offer the best contrast for separating the tunica albuginea and corpora cavernosa (Figure 11.4). Buck's fascia, however, also demonstrates low signal intensity on T2-weighted images, and the two fascias blend together and can no longer be differentiated. The deep dorsal vein can be seen between the tunica albuginea and Buck's fascia, and sometimes the superficial dorsal vein outside the Buck's fascia can also be identified.

Following gadolinium-DTPA injection, there is marked increase in the signal intensity of the corpora cavernosa and corpus spongiosum, as demonstrated in Figure 11.7. Use of gadolinium-DTPA allows identification of the penile anatomy similar to that achieved on the T2-weighted image. The tunica albuginea does not enhance, thus providing excellent contrast between the fascia and the corporeal tissue. Similarly, there is minimal muscle enhancement so that the difference between the ischiocavernosus muscle and the crura of the corpora cavernosa is clearly visualized. When gadolinium-DTPA is combined with the fat saturation technique, the anatomy is even more clearly displayed (Figure 11.7b).

At present, most of the available knowledge has been acquired using a conventional spin-echo technique. However, fat suppression images can be utilized as well. On T1-weighted fat suppression images, as shown in Figure 11.8, the signal intensity of either the corpora cavernosa or the corpus spongiosum appears higher as compared to the conventional spin-echo images using the same imaging parameters. The latter is due to the signal suppression from the fat and therefore automatic computer-adjusted gray scale resulting in higher signal intensity of the corpora. As a result, the differentiation between the corpora and the adjacent tunica albuginea is of higher contrast as compared to the conventional spin-echo image.

The anatomy of the penis is well displayed in all three orthogonal planes. The bulb of the penis consisting of corpus spongiosum, adjacent fascia and muscles, is well visualized in all of the planes. In the transaxial plane, the corpus spongiosum in the bulb of the penis with its surrounding tunica albuginea (Figure 11.4) is well displayed. In the posterior part of the bulb of the penis, the invaginating septum of varying length (Figure 11.4b) can also be identified. This normal septum should not be mistaken for a congenital anomaly. The surrounding muscle of the corpus spongiosum (known as either the bulbospongiosus or the bulbocavernosus muscle—the term is used interchangeably) is seen in either the sagittal or the coronal plane of section. As demonstrated in Figure 11.9, on sagittal plane images the bulbospongiosus muscle can be seen as a low signal intensity stripe inferior to the corpus spongiosum. The relation between the bulb of the penis and the transversus perinei superficialis muscle is best seen on the transverse plane of imaging (Figures 11.4 and 11.7), where it can be seen dividing the posteriorly located anal canal from the anteriorly located bulb of the penis. However, as shown in Figure 11.10, the transversus perinei superficialis muscle can be identified if serial sagittal planes of section are viewed.

The corpora cavernosa can be visualized on any of the orthogonal planes of imaging. The crura of the corpora cavernosa are well displayed in a transaxial (Figures 11.4 and 11.7) or coronal plane of section. The corpora cavernosa distal to the symphysis pubis are, however, best displayed in the coronal plane (Figure 11.11). The attachment of the crura to the ischium and the demonstration of the ischiocavernosus muscle which covers the medial aspect of the crura can be visualized on either the transaxial (Figure 11.4) or the coronal (Figure 11.10) plane of imaging. Similarly, the septum between the two corpora cavernosa can also be demonstrated on either transaxial (Figure 11.4) or coronal (Figure 11.6) sections. The cavernous artery is best displayed in the coronal plane of section (Figure 11.6), although sometimes the level of the hilum of the corpora cavernosa (entrance of the cavernous artery)

can be seen in the transaxial plane as well. The dorsal vein can sometimes be seen between Buck's fascia and the tunica albuginea of the corpora cavernosa. The suspensory ligament of the penis is demonstrated on sagittal section (Figure 11.9), and on T2-weighted images it demonstrates low signal intensity. Distally, the corpora cavernosa terminate in the glans, and on transaxial images the distal aspect of the intercavernous septum (Buck's fascia) is seen as a dark line separating the conical ends of the corpora cavernosa from the glans. The signal intensity of the glans does not differ from that of more proximal corpora cavernosa on either T1- or T2-weighted images.

The anatomy of the penis, with differentiation of the corporeal bodies and their surrounding muscle and fascia, is well demonstrated regardless of the patient's age. At birth, the penis is fully developed, and as shown in Figure 11.12, the anatomy can be appreciated. Any change in the anatomic position in patients with congenital anomalies, trauma or following surgery, such as abdominoperineal resection (Figure 11.13), can also be seen.

Changes in erection

MRI can assess the morphologic changes in the penis during erection. The findings include change in the size of the corpora cavernosa, change in the corporeal signal intensity, and change in the thickness of the tunica albuginea. In the flaccid state, the musculature of the terminal arterioles and sinusoidal spaces within the corpora cavernosa is in a contracted state, resulting in marked resistance to arterial inflow.[12] Only a small amount of blood enters for nutritional and metabolic purposes. This muscular tone is dynamic, being mediated by elements of the neurovascular system. Decrease in the corporeal blood volume results in homogeneous or inhomogeneous decrease in signal intensity of the corpora cavernosa on the T2-weighted image. In normal patients, the low signal intensity of the corpora cavernosa has been reported to be present in as many as 20 per cent of patients studied.[5] During erection, the smooth muscles of the sinusoids and arterioles relax. As a result of this relaxation, sinusoidal compliance increases and peripheral resistance decreases. Tumescence results from increased arterial flow, dilatation of the arterial tree, and distension of the sinusoids.[12] The increased arterial flow and consequent increase in cavernosal blood flow exhibits increase in signal intensity on the T2-weighted image. With the enlargement of the corpora cavernosa, the tunica albuginea stretches and thins, and this finding can be demonstrated on an MRI image. The difference in the appearance of the penis between the flaccid state and the erect state is shown in Figure 11.14. As illustrated in Figures 11.14 and 11.15, MRI can also demonstrate the known physiologic difference between the erection induced by prostaglandin injection (the injection which produces results similar to those occurring in a natural erection, ie, increased arterial flow, sinusoidal relaxation, and increased venous resistance), and the erection achieved by the vacuum constriction device (which passively pulls blood into the penis, presumably through expansion of the venous sinusoids, analogous to lung expansion resulting from negative intrathoracic pressure).[13] In erection induced by intracorporeal prostaglandin injection, very little change occurs in the corpora spongiosa (this is similar to normal physiologic erection), while with the vacuum constriction device, all three corporeal bodies enlarge.

When the fibrosis within the corpora cavernosa prevents its expansion, the finding can also be documented on MRI (Figure 11.16).

Penile prosthesis

The MRI appearance of penile prostheses varies, depending on the type of prosthesis. As depicted in Figure 11.17, a semirigid silicone prosthesis images as a signal void, regardless of the imaging sequence. Inflatable prostheses, however, often image with medium signal intensity on T1-weighted images and increase in signal intensity on T2-weighted images. As illustrated in Figure 11.18, the signal intensity at the edge of the prosthesis remains persistently low.

MRI is particularly useful in evaluating the placement of a prosthesis within the corpora cavernosa and the relation between the distal end of the prosthesis and the crura of the corpora cavernosa (Figure 11.17). Complications associated with the placement of a prosthesis, including injury and hematoma or infection, are easily and clearly displayed on MRI scans.

Male urethra

The MRI appearance of the prostatic urethra and the differentiation between the MRI features of the proximal and distal prostatic urethra are described in Chapter 8. The membranous urethra can be visualized in the transverse plane of section. On T1-weighted images, the signal intensity of the urethra is similar to the adjacent tissue. However, because the wall of the membranous urethra contains thick striated muscles (external sphincter), on T2-weighted images the urethra demonstrates a low signal intensity ring surrounding the higher signal intensity epithelial surface (Figure 11.19). On the sagittal plane T2-weighted image the membranous urethra can be seen as a low signal intensity stripe. As shown in Figure 11.20, the zonal anatomy is not seen, but the normal relation between the apex of the prostate gland,

membranous urethra and the bulb of the penis is well displayed. In either a transaxial or coronal plane of section, the muscle of the periurethral levator ani can be separated from muscle fibers of the external sphincter (Figure 11.19). The location of the bulbar urethra as it pierces the roof of the penis can be seen on either the sagittal or the coronal plane of section (Figure 11.20).

Within the bulb of the penis, the urethra can sometimes be visualized in the transaxial plane (Figure 11.4), but it is consistently visualized in the coronal plane of section. Regardless of the plane of imaging, the urethra demonstrates a ring-like appearance on T2-weighted images, and its anterior position at the level of the symphysis pubis (Figure 11.21) is demonstrated.

While the wall of the urethra can be seen, the lumen of the urethra cannot be identified unless the indwelling catheter is placed as shown in Figure 11.22. The anterior penile urethra—the part of the urethra within the penile shaft—is very rarely visualized on the MRI image, and MRI is not applicable for the evaluation of any anomaly in that location.

Recommended imaging sequences

Both T1- and T2-weighted images are necessary to evaluate the penis and urethra accurately. T1-weighted images emphasize the contrast between the corporeal bodies and the surrounding fat. T2-weighted images illustrate the difference between the corporeal bodies and the adjacent tunica albuginea, demonstrate the location of the urethra and the cavernous artery and are helpful in demonstrating intrapenile anatomy and pathology.

Although the penis can be seen on all three planes of imaging, each has limitations and advantages. The transaxial plane of section allows demonstration of the radix penis including the bulb of the penis and the crura of the corpora cavernosa. It is also best for displaying the relation between the bulb and the transversus perinei superficialis muscle. The sagittal plane allows evaluation of the bulb of the penis and its relation to the urogenital diaphragm as well as the bulbospongiosus muscle. Although the corpora cavernosa can be seen in the transaxial or sagittal planes, coronal images provide the best views of the anatomy and any pathology affecting the corpora cavernosa. Evaluation of the membranous urethra is facilitated on the transverse plane of imaging. The relation between the membranous and the bulbar urethra, such as in the case of trauma, is best appreciated in either the coronal or the sagittal plane of imaging. The evaluation of the penile urethra is not applicable by MRI.

Pathology of the penis and urethra

Congenital anomalies

Although the penis and urethra are the site of a variety of forms of congenital anomalies, many have little clinical significance or are readily apparent on inspection. Anomalies which are more serious, and may require radiologic assessment, include anomalies in number, such as penis diphallus, and malformations of the urethral groove, such as hypospadias and epispadias.

Penis diphallus

Penis diphallus is a rare anomaly in which there are various combinations of duplication ranging from four completely developed corpora cavernosa and two corpora spongiosa, to any combination of number of corporeal bodies.[14,15] In addition, there are often two urethras.

MRI appearance.   Each of the corporeal bodies can be clearly demonstrated on MR images. The signal intensity of the corpora cavernosa is unremarkable (normal) on both T1- and T2-weighted images.[5] The thickness of the tunica albuginea can be seen to vary in the different parts of the penis diphallus. This disorder is frequently associated with other perineal anomalies, such as a short perineum or asymmetrical development of the ischiocavernosus muscles. As illustrated in Figure 11.23, all the associated anatomic variations can be displayed on MRI. When two glans penis are present (Figure 11.24), the anomaly is demonstrated, but the extent of the associated urethral duplication cannot be assessed.

Epispadias

Epispadias is a rare congenital anomaly almost always associated with bladder exstrophy (see Chapter 12).[16] When it occurs alone it is considered a milder form of the exstrophy complex. In this anomaly the roof of the distal urethra is absent, and the proximal urethra may open anywhere from the base to the glans of the penis. There is also widening of the symphysis pubis, and the separated pubic bones are joined by fibrous bands. The attachment of the corpora cavernosa follows the bony anomaly. The urethra is usually short and incompletely developed, and instead of pointing downwards towards the perineum it points upwards as the corpus spongiosum becomes more anterior in location.

MRI appearance.   MRI allows unique evaluation of the epispadias complex.[5] Since the corpora cavernosa are attached to the ischium, and the orientation of the ischial bone is changed, the direction of the corpora cavernosa is changed as well. As illustrated in Figure 11.25, the corpora cavernosa are spread apart, and the corpus spongiosum, which is normally the most inferior structure at the level of the symphysis pubis, becomes located superiorly. Because the bulbar urethra is an anterior cephalad structure within the corpus spongiosum, the urethra in this anomaly opens onto the dorsal part of the penis (Figure 11.26).

MRI in relation to other imaging modalities

Both US and corpora cavernosography have been recommended in the evaluation of congenital penile anomalies. Because of the superiority of MRI in displaying penile anatomy, MRI is likely to have a significant role in defining all aspects of penis diphallus and associated structural anomalies, which require complex plastic reconstruction.

The use of MRI in epispadias is especially useful in the assessment of the development of the corpora cavernosa and in the understanding of this complex anomaly in order to design the optimal surgical correction.

Inflammatory disorders

Peyronie's disease

Peyronie's disease, an inflammatory disease of unknown etiology, affects the tunica albuginea of the penis and extends to varying degrees into the corpora cavernosa.[17] It occurs most commonly in middle-aged men, and is characterized by a firm plaque or band usually situated in the dorsum of the penis. Plaques, which are caused by replacement of the normally elastic connective tissue with a hyalinized or fibrous scar, may range in size from a few millimeters to a broad sheet occupying a large segment of the penile shaft.[17] Pain on erection is a common complaint. Physical examination is often sufficient for the diagnosis of Peyronie's disease. However, imaging may be performed if additional information about the size and thickness of the plaque is needed or if there is the possibility of compromise of cavernous arteries.

MRI appearance.   The only abnormality identified on T1-weighted images is asymmetrical thickening of what appears to be tunica albuginea. On T2-weighted scans, however, the Peyronie's plaque can be differentiated from the normal tunica albuginea.[5] As illustrated in Figure 11.27, the plaque images with lower signal intensity than the adjacent tunica albuginea, and the distance between the plaque and the deep artery of the corpora cavernosa is consistently demonstrated. The finding of asymmetrical low signal intensity contiguous with the tunica albuginea is diagnostic for Peyronie's disease. Surgical treatment for Peyronie's disease is changing, and laser therapy is becoming more popular. As it becomes more commonly used, identification of the precise location and extent of the plaque by MRI may become more important.

MRI in relation to other imaging modalities. Ultrasound using a high frequency transducer has been advocated as an adjunct to physical examination in the diagnostic evaluation of Peyronie's disease.[3,18] The plaque appears as a localized thickening of the tunica albuginea with an echo pattern that varies with the age of the plaque, raising the possibility of differentiating mature calcified plaques from more recent ones. Such a differentiation would be helpful in determining the mode of medical or surgical treatment.[3] The use of ultrasound in measuring the distance between the plaque and cavernous artery has also been reported.[3,11] At present, the differentiation between the mature calcified plaque and the recent plaque has not been performed on MRI. However, MRI offers a larger field-of-view and is devoid of operator dependence in identifying the lesion and measuring the distance between artery and plaque, the finding utilized in planning the extent of the surgical excision.

Fibrosis of the penis

Penile fibrosis is a known complication of prolonged priapism and collagen vascular disease such as lupus erythematosus. It is also a recently recognized complication of intracavernous injection of vasoactive agents. Biopsy is often required for the diagnosis of this disorder, and MRI offers a sensitive, noninvasive alternative.

MRI appearance. On T1-weighted images, the signal intensity in an area of fibrosis varies and it may be similar to or lower than the adjacent corpora cavernosa. As illustrated in Figure 11.28, on T2-weighted images a fibrotic area is identified as a low signal intensity focus within an otherwise higher signal intensity corpora cavernosa. The margin between the fibrosis and the adjacent corpora is sharp, and the underlying tunica albuginea is usually normal (Figure 11.29). Fibrosis can be distinguished from hematoma which, in the subacute phase, usually images with high signal intensity. Fibrosis of any etiology, as seen in Figure 11.30, has a similar MRI appearance.

MRI in relation to other imaging modalities. Corpora cavernosograms can also be used in the assessment of intracorporeal fibrosis (Figure 11.29), but the technique is invasive and may, as shown in Figure 11.29, overestimate the extent of the disease. Anecdotal reports on the ultrasound appearance of penile fibrosis can be found, but a large study comparing the sensitivity of ultrasound and penile biopsy validating the use of this modality is not available.[19] Similarly, a large series assessing the ability of MRI in identifying intracorporeal fibrosis has not been carried out. However, on the basis of the excellent performance of MRI in the identification of fibrosis within the tissue elsewhere in the body, it can be suspected that MRI will be a valuable modality in diagnosing, as well as evaluating, the extent of intracorporeal fibrosis.

Trauma

Urethral and penile trauma can be divided into penile rupture, which may or may not be associated with injury to the male urethra,[20] and complex injuries of the urethra, corpus spongiosum and corpora cavernosa as a consequence of blunt or bony injury to the pelvis.

Penile trauma

Traumatic rupture of the corpus cavernosum or fracture of the penis is uncommon. All reported injuries have occurred to the erect penis as a result of direct blunt trauma that bends the organ.[20] During erection, the tunica albuginea of the corpora cavernosa is thinned and relatively inelastic. This makes it susceptible to injury, usually a tear in a transverse orientation. This type of injury usually occurs during coitus, but it may also be caused by abnormal bending of the penis, by attempting to place the erect penis into the pants, or from other trauma such as rolling over in bed or bumping into furniture. The injury can occur anywhere along the shaft, but it is common at the base where the corpora cavernosa are somewhat fixed by the penile suspensory ligament. Usually only one corporeal body is injured, but both corpora can be affected depending on the nature and severity of the trauma.[20] Physical findings are often sufficient to make the diagnosis.

MRI appearance. Coronal plane images obtained with a surface coil are essential for the demonstration of a penile fracture. As illustrated in Figure 11.31, on T2-weighted images the torn tunica is seen as an interruption of the normal low signal intensity ring of the tunica albuginea. Peripenile hematoma can also be identified and, because the patient is usually seen in the acute phase of injury, the hematoma demonstrates medium signal intensity on T1-weighted images and increased signal intensity on T2-weighted images. In addition, hematoma can be differentiated from fibrosis, which demonstrates low signal intensity on T2-weighted images.

MRI in relation to other imaging modalities. Corpora cavernosography has been advocated for the evaluation of penile trauma, mainly for the demonstration of the tear of the tunica albuginea and extravasation of the contrast media into pericorporeal tissue. However, a number of false-negative corpora cavernosograms can be accounted for. It is difficult to perform corpora cavernosography in an already injured penis, and in addition associated severe vasoconstriction and tamponade caused by the adjacent hematoma result in false-negative studies as they may be the cause for lack of demonstration. The demonstration of peripenile hematoma consequent to acute rupture of the penis appearing as an echo-poor mass adjacent to the corpora cavernosa has been reported on an ultrasound study.[4] However, due to the small field-of-view and often the location of the injury at the level of the symphysis pubis, ultrasound can be technically difficult to perform and a small rupture of the tunica may be overlooked. MRI is not operator dependent, allows a large field-of-view, is noninvasive, and by the combination of thin sections and coronal T1- and T2-weighted images, offers a very accurate and elegant way of identifying rupture of the tunica albuginea and presence of adjacent peripenile hematoma.

Urethral trauma (traumatic posterior urethral rupture)

Injury to the membranous urethra is usually associated with complex injury to the pelvis, often including numerous pelvic fractures, hemorrhage, and multi-organ injury.[21] In incomplete rupture voiding may be possible, and hematuria is inevitable. Blood expressed from the urethral meatus also indicates urethral trauma. If the rupture is complete, extravasation causes a suprapubic mass. Repair, if possible, may be accomplished by primary anastomosis or urethrostomy.

MRI appearance. MRI is applicable only for the demonstration of the associated soft tissue injury and for the documentation of urethral dislocation. The type of the urethral injury or the assessment of the urethra requires contrast studies. In the evaluation of the pelvic floor trauma, thin sections in all three imaging planes are essential. On T1-weighted images, major organ displacement such as posterior dislocation of the prostate gland (Figure 11.32) can be seen. Also

identified is soft tissue injury such as the presence of hematoma and bony fractures. It is the T2-weighted image, however, which is essential for the demonstration of the membranous urethra, and the assessment of any lateral displacement. The T2-weighted image will also allow the evaluation of the associated corporeal injury as well as muscular hematomas. The findings on MRI that can contribute to the design of the optimal surgical approach include: (1) dislocation of the urethra; (2) extension of the fibrosis and soft tissue injury; and (3) associated fracture of the penis. The dislocation between the apex of the prostate gland, membranous urethra and the bulb of the penis, can occur in the anterior-posterior direction, as seen in Figure 11.32. Posterior dislocation of the prostatic apex and the length of the urethral injury are best determined on a combination of midline, parasagittal and coronal plane images. The lateral displacement of the urethra can also occur. The lateral displacement of the prostate or urethra is best evaluated on the coronal plane of imaging. As demonstrated in Figure 11.33, the misalignment between the apex of the prostate gland and the bulbar urethra may be minor, or as illustrated in Figure 11.34, the misalignment-dislocation may be as much as 1.5 cm. With urethral dislocation, associated hematoma and fibrosis will be present, and these can also be demonstrated on MRI. Fibrosis and/or organized hematoma will demonstrate low signal intensity on the T2-weighted image. With extensive pelvic injury, displaced fracture and avulsion of the corpora cavernosa can be seen as well. Fracture of the corpora cavernosa without their displacement is shown in Figure 11.35. These fractures are always associated with fracture of the ischium, and an adjacent hematoma which will be of high signal intensity on T2-weighted images can be identified. Fracture of the corpora cavernosa can, however, be associated with avulsion of the corpora cavernosa, as seen in Figure 11.36. MRI is also a sensitive modality for the associated bony fractures which are sometimes difficult to define on the plain conventional radiographs. The patient in Figure 11.37 had an unsuspected fracture of the ischium and avulsion of the corpora cavernosa. Impotence is a common sequel of avulsion of the corpora cavernosa, and therefore MRI findings are very valuable in patient counselling.

MRI in relation to other imaging modalities. As part of a complex pelvic injury, urethral trauma is a difficult clinical problem and selection of the best surgical approach for repair often represents a dilemma. Traditionally, retrograde urethrography and cystography have been used to characterize the defects that develop after traumatic rupture of the membranous urethra. The length of the urethral injury and the associated soft tissue injuries are, however, difficult to evaluate with these modalities. Furthermore, it is difficult to obtain precise information about prostatic and urethral dislocation, necessary in deciding whether to use a transperineal or suprapubic approach for repair.

MRI can be used to complement conventional cystourethography as an accurate and useful imaging study before repair of a post-traumatic membranous urethral defect. By defining the pelvic anatomy accurately, it provides information essential in planning the appropriate surgical approach.

Tumors of the penis and urethra

Penile carcinoma

Carcinoma of the penis is an uncommon disease (incidence 2–5 per cent of all urogenital cancers; 1 per cent of all cancer in males).[22,23] While the disease can be present in young men, it usually occurs in the fifth and sixth decades of life.[22,23] The etiology is uncertain, but the disease is rarely seen in circumcised men and is strongly correlated with the presence of a foreskin and the irritant effects of smegma combined with the products of poor hygiene within the preputial sac.[23] The most common presenting symptom is a mass or persistent sore or ulcer of the glans or foreskin. Occasionally the initial symptoms are related to inguinal lymphadenopathy.[23] Since most lesions are painless, many patients delay up to a year before seeking treatment, by which time the cancer has infiltrated and deeper structures are involved.

Diagnosis is made by biopsy, which reveals squamous cell carcinoma in over 95 per cent of cases. Different staging systems have been proposed among which the Jackson classification was the most popular (Table 11.1). The Jackson classification, however, does not subcategorize the inguinal node involvement, and at present, staging by the TNM system is widely accepted[23] (Table 11.2). Treatment depends on the structures involved and may include partial penile amputation (at least 2 cm proximal to the lesion but leaving enough of the penis for adequate direction of the urinary stream) or total penectomy with the formation of a perineal urethrostomy. The lymphatic drainage of penile tumors tends to result in metastasis to superficial or deep inguinal nodes. Palpable nodes are often removed surgically, since radiation therapy has not been as effective.

Urethral carcinoma

Carcinoma of the male urethra is extremely rare, only approximately 600 cases have been reported in the world literature.[23] Although significant etiologic factors have not been identified, chronic inflammation may play a role since many patients give a history of prior venereal disease, urethritis, or urethral stricture. An increased incidence has also been reported with smoking or occupational exposure to known carcinogens. Symptoms, such as urethral bleeding and a weak urinary stream, are nonspecific and are often attributed to benign stricture disease rather than to malignancy. As a result there is often delay, five months on average, before the diagnosis is made.

Transurethral or needle biopsy is required for definitive diagnosis. In the majority of cases (78 per cent) the cancer is a squamous cell carcinoma. Other

Table 11.1   Jackson classification for penile carcinoma

Stage	Criteria
I	Tumor confined to glans or prepuce
II	Invasion into shaft or corpora; no nodal or distant metastases
III	Tumor confined to penis; inguinal metastases that are operable
IV	Tumor involves adjacent structures; inoperable and/or distant metastases

Table 11.2   TNM classification for penile carcinoma

T-Primary Tumor	
T1	Tumor not more than 1 cm in largest dimension and clearly superficial
T2	Tumor 1 cm in any dimension and clearly superficial
T3	Tumor of any size invading underlying tissues
T4	Tumor invading adjacent structures, that is, corpus, urethra, symphysis, perineum

N-Regional Lymph Nodes	
N0	No evidence of involvement of regional lymph nodes
N1	Involvement of single regional node
N2	Involvement of single bilateral inguinal nodes or multiple unilateral nodes
N3	Fixation of regional nodes or ulceration of skin over involved regional nodes

M-Metastases	
M0	No evidence of distant metastases
M1	Distant metastases present

types include transitional cell carcinoma (15 per cent), adenocarcinoma (6 per cent), and undifferentiated carcinomas (1 per cent). Initial spread is by direct extension to adjacent structures via the vascular spaces of the corpus spongiosum and the periurethral tissue. Carcinoma of the bulbomembranous urethra often extends to the urogenital diaphragm. Hematogenous spread is uncommon except in advanced cases.

Metastases to regional lymph nodes occur by lymphatic embolization. The lymph node chain involved is dictated by the location of the carcinoma. As discussed earlier, lymphatics from the anterior urethra drain into the superficial and deep inguinal nodes and occasionally to the external iliac nodes. Lymphatics from the posterior urethra, however, drain into the external iliac, obturator and internal iliac nodes.

When the disease involves the distal part of the penis, the extent of local involvement can be determined by careful inspection and by bimanual examination. Cancer in the bulbomembranous urethra, however, requires radiologic evaluation. Carcinoma of the prostatic urethra is rare. The approach to staging is based on the location of the carcinoma, as is the treatment. Carcinoma of the distal urethra can be treated by resection, partial penectomy, or total penectomy, depending on the extent of disease. Lesions in the bulbar urethra or more proximal lesions require extensive surgical resection (possibly including *en bloc* removal of the penis, urethra, prostate, bladder with overlying pubis, and pelvic lymph nodes) and an ileal diversion. Unfortunately, there are no reports of survival figures for all forms of surgical treatment.

Metastatic tumor

Metastatic tumors to the penis are very rare with approximately only 200 cases reported in the literature. The metastatic penile lesions originate most commonly from the genitourinary tract with carcinoma of the prostate, urinary bladder and testis being the most common primary sites. The most likely routes of spread are retrograde venous and lymphatic transport or arterial embolism. Direct extension can occur as well, in which case carcinoma of the rectum is included among the primary sites. Leukemic or lymphomatous infiltrate can be present as well. As the metastatic tumors are often infiltrative, their most frequent clinical presentation is priapism. In those cases, the clinical evaluation is very difficult, and because the priapism in over 90 per cent of cases is idiopathic, the possibility of the metastatic cause is often overlooked and the patient undergoes prolonged treatment for priapism missing the underlying disease. Biopsy is essential to determine the diagnosis, and treatment consists of the local control only. For leukemic or lymphomatous infiltrate, treatment of systemic disorders is required.

MRI appearance

Although penile and urethral carcinomas are clinically separable entities in their early stages, once the lesions have infiltrated and deeper structures become involved, their MRI appearance is the same. On T1-weighted images, urethral or penile carcinoma demonstrates a signal intensity similar to or lower than that of the surrounding corporeal body. On T2-weighted images, as seen in Figure 11.38, tumors have a low signal intensity regardless of their histologic type. Urethral tumors, especially when located in the glans penis, will be associated with extensive inflammatory reaction and often abscess formation. In those instances, underlying inflammatory changes will influence the signal intensity of the involved region. Often on T1-weighted images, they may demonstrate medium or low signal intensity, and marked increase in signal intensity on T2-weighted images (Figure 11.39). In this way the extent of the disease can accurately be evaluated. MRI has a limited role in the evaluation of the disease extent of the carcinoma located in the glans penis. However, when the tumor extends into the radix penis, clinical examination becomes limited and the value of MRI increases. The tumor extension is identified by the demonstration of the low signal intensity tumor within corporeal tissue. On the T2-weighted image (Figure 11.40) involvement and tumor extension into the septum of the corpora cavernosa or tunica albuginea can be demonstrated. Tumor extension into the bulb of the penis and extension across the urogenital diaphragm is an important feature in the therapy decision—radiation versus surgery. The tumor staging can follow the TNM classification. In stage T1 when tumor invades only the subepithelial connective tissue, the role of MRI is limited, and the differentiation between the inflammatory changes and small tumor cannot be made. As the tumor increases in size, so does the value of MRI. Tumor invasion of the corpus spongiosum or cavernosum (stage T2) can be demonstrated. The sagittal plane of section facilitates the evaluation of tumor cranial extension, across the urogenital diaphragm (stage T3). Evaluation of the tumor extension to the adjacent structures is facilitated by the excellent soft tissue contrast of MRI and its capacity for direct multiplanar imaging. Early reports indicate that MRI may be useful in the staging of the disease and in planning surgical approach, but its usefulness is limited to the carcinomas located at the root of the penis.

MRI can also be applied to the evaluation of the metastatic disease of the penis. A metastatic tumor causes decreased signal intensity on T2-weighted images. The tumor margins are usually ill-defined, and while the abnormality is detected, the differentiation between primary and metastatic lesion cannot be made. Tumor extension and invasion of the tunica albuginea can be seen by the interruption of the low signal intensity tunica on T2-weighted images. When complicated with priapism, as seen in Figure 11.41, clinical diagnosis and physical examination are very limited. The use of MRI in those cases can be helpful.

MRI in relation to other imaging modalities

The role of radiology in the evaluation of penile carcinoma has been confined to the assessment of lymphadenopathy for which lymphangiography or CT were most commonly used. The evaluation of possible distant metastatic disease has utilized a number of radiologic modalities including CXR, CT, and liver and bone scans. Local staging of the disease, however, was not attempted before the introduction of MRI. The ability of MRI to assess the local tumor extent may impact on the design of the therapeutic approach. MRI is applicable, however, only to larger lesions and especially lesions located in the radix penis where clinical examination is limited. However, although local tumor extension can be accurately determined from MR images, it should be emphasized that MR imaging is not specific for tumor diagnosis, nor is it yet known whether urethral carcinoma can be differentiated from diffuse fibrous, inflammatory or postsurgical changes.

References

1 LUE TF, HRICAK H, SCHMIDT RA et al, Functional evaluation of penile veins by cavernosography in papaverine-induced erection, *J Urol* (1986) **135**:479–82.

2 LUE TF, HRICAK H, MARICH KW et al, Vasculogenic impotence evaluated by high-resolution ultrasonography and pulsed Doppler spectrum analysis, *Radiology* (1985) **155**:777–81.

3 BALCONI G, ANGELI E, NESSI R et al, Ultrasonographic evaluation of Peyronie's disease, *Urol Radiol* (1988) **10**:85.

4 OESTERLING JE, BROMBERG WD, ALBERTSON PC, Xeroradiography and ultrasonography in the evaluation of a penile injury, *J Urol* (1986) **135**:791–3.

5 HRICAK H, MAROTTI M, GILBERT TJ et al, Normal penile anatomy and abnormal penile conditions: evaluation with MR imaging, *Radiology* (1988)- **169**:683–90.

6 FELIX W, The development of the urogenital organs. In: Keibel F, Mall FP, eds. *Manual of Human Embryology*, Volume III (JB Lippincott: Philadelphia 1912) 881–975.

7 LIERSE W, Penis. In: *Applied Anatomy of the Pelvis* (Springer-Verlag: Berlin 1984) 139–48.

8 THOREK P, *Anatomy in Surgery*, 3rd edn. (Springer-Verlag: New York 1985).

9 BREZA J, ABOSEIF SR, ORVIS BR, Detailed anatomy of penile neurovascular structures: surgical significance, *J Urol* (1989) **141**:437–43.

10 GOSLING JA, DIXON JS, HUMPHERSON JR, Gross and microscopic anatomy of the urethra I: male urethra. In: *Functional Anatomy of the Urinary Tract* (Gower Medical Publishing: London 1982) 4.2–4.22.

11 LUE TF, HRICAK H, Ultrasound of the penis. In: Resnick MI, Rifkin MD, eds. *Ultrasound of the Urinary System*, 3rd edn. (Williams & Wilkins: Baltimore 1988).

12 WAGNER G, Erection physiology and endocrinology. In: Wagner G, Green R, eds. *Impotence: Physiological, Psychological–Surgical Diagnosis and Treatment*, (Plenum Press: New York 1981) 25–36.

13 ANDERSON MW, BRODERICK G, HRICAK H, Penile imaging at 1.5 T: the effect of blood flow. Presented at the 74th Scientific Assembly and Annual Meeting of the Radiological Society of North America, Chicago, 1988.

14 JOHNSON CF, CARLTON CE, POWELL NB, Duplication of penis, *Urology* (1974) **4**:722.

15 REMZI D, Diphallia, *Urology* (1973) **1**:462.

16 MUECKE EC, Exstrophy, epispadias, and other anomalies of the · bladder. In: Walsh PC, Gittes RF, Perlmutter AD et al, eds. *Campbell's Urology*, 5th edn. (WB Saunders Company: Philadelphia 1986) 1856–80.

17 VORSTMAN B, LOCKHART J, Peyronie's disease, *Problems in Urology* (1987) **1**:507–17.

18 HAMM B, FRIEDRICH M, KELAMI A, Ultrasound imaging in Peyronie's disease, *Urology* (1986) **28**:540–45.

19 HAMM B, FRIEDRICH M, KELAMI A, Ultrasound imaging of the corpora cavernosa after priapism, *Eur Urol* (1985) **11**:210–11.

20 MERRILL DC, PALMER JM, Male genital trauma. In: *Trauma Management* (1985) **2**:97–107.

21 PALMER JK, BENSON GS, CORRIERE JN Jr, Diagnosis and initial management of urological injuries associated with 200 consecutive pelvic fractures, *J Urol* (1983) **130**:712–14.

22 MELICOW MM, ROBERTS TW, Pathology and natural history of urethral tumors in males, *Urology* (1978) **11**:83–9.

23 FAIR WR, PEREZ CA, ANDERSON T, Cancer of the penis. In: DeVita VT, Hellman S, Rosenberg SA, eds. *Cancer Principles & Practice of Oncology*, Vol 1, 3rd edn. (JB Lippincott: Philadelphia 1989) 1063–70.

Figure 11.1

Normal anatomy of the radix penis. Schematic drawing.

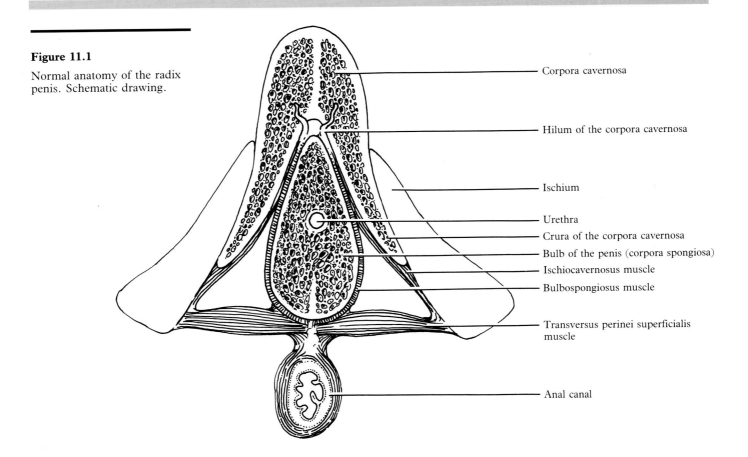

— Corpora cavernosa

— Hilum of the corpora cavernosa

— Ischium

— Urethra
— Crura of the corpora cavernosa
— Bulb of the penis (corpora spongiosa)
— Ischiocavernosus muscle
— Bulbospongiosus muscle

— Transversus perinei superficialis muscle

— Anal canal

Figure 11.2

Thick histologic section through the body of the penis. The corpora cavernosa (CC) and the deep artery of the corpora cavernosa (small black arrow) are both visible. Note that the tunica albuginea of the corpora cavernosa (asterisk) is thicker than the tunica albuginea of the corpus spongiosum (curved black arrow). The tunica albuginea (septum) between the two corpora cavernosa shows multiple interruptions (open arrows). (CS)-corpus spongiosum; (U)-urethra; (large open arrow)-Buck's fascia between the tunica albuginea of the corpora cavernosa and the corpus spongiosum.

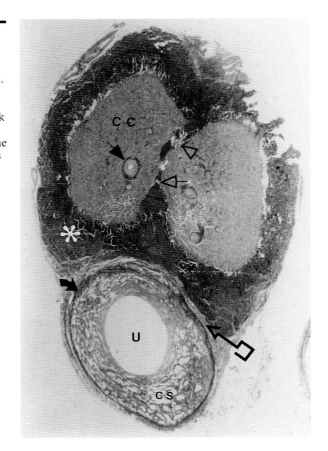

Figure 11.3

Normal anatomy of the penis. Schematic drawing showing corpora of the penis with their fascias and blood vessels.

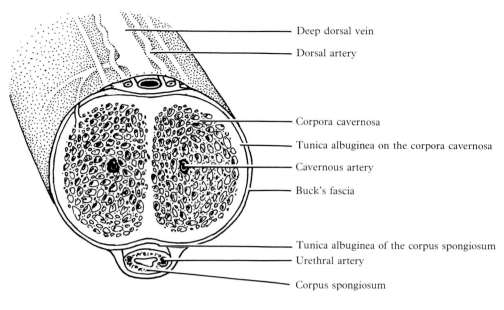

Deep dorsal vein

Dorsal artery

Corpora cavernosa

Tunica albuginea on the corpora cavernosa

Cavernous artery

Buck's fascia

Tunica albuginea of the corpus spongiosum

Urethral artery

Corpus spongiosum

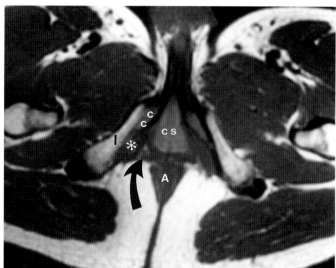

a

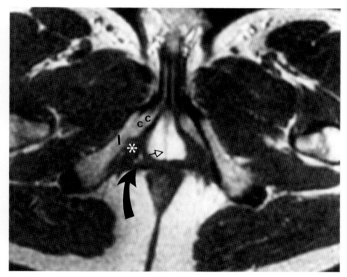

b

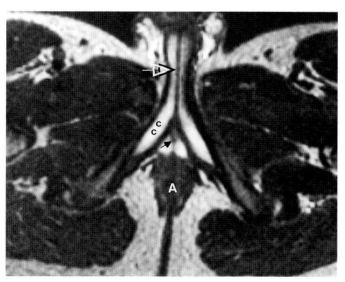

c

Figure 11.4

Normal anatomy of the radix penis in the transaxial plane. (**a**) T1-weighted, (**b**) T2-weighted images, and (**c**) T2-weighted section obtained 1 cm cranially to the section depicted in (**b**). The corpora cavernosa (CC) and corpus spongiosum (CS) are of medium signal intensity on the T1-weighted image and of high signal intensity on the T2-weighted image. (A)-anal canal; (I)-ischium; (curved arrow)-transversus perinei superficialis muscle; (asterisk)-ischiocavernosus muscle. The urethra (small solid black arrow) and the septum between the corpora cavernosa (large open arrow) can be seen on (**c**). The septum of the corpus spongiosum (small open arrow) is visible on (**b**).

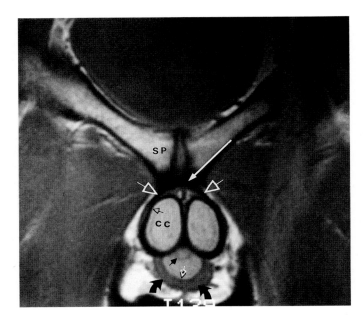

Figure 11.5

Normal anatomy of the fascia of the penis. Proton density coronal image at the level of the symphysis pubis. (SP)-symphysis pubis; (long arrow)-suspensory ligament; (large open white arrows)-Buck's fascia; (small open black arrow)-tunica albuginea of the corpora cavernosa; (CC)-corpora cavernosa; (small black arrow)-urethra within corpus spongiosum; (small open black and white arrow)-tunica albuginea of the corpus spongiosum (note that this fascia is thinner than the tunica albuginea of the corpora cavernosa); (curved arrows)-bulbospongiosus muscle.

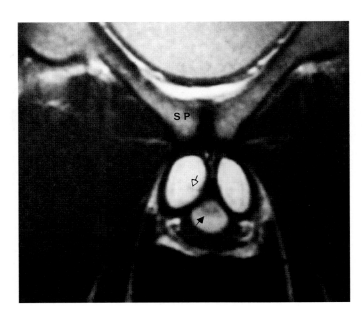

Figure 11.6

Normal anatomy at the level of the hila of the corpora cavernosa showing the oblique course of the artery of the corpora cavernosa. Coronal T2-weighted image. (SP)-symphysis pubis; (small open arrow)-deep cavernous artery; (small black arrow)-urethra within the corpus spongiosum.

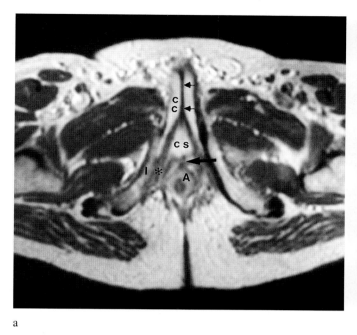

a

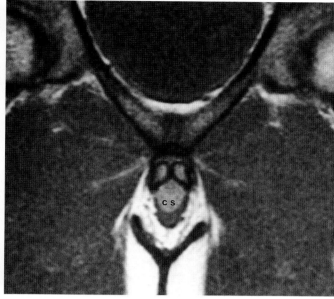

a

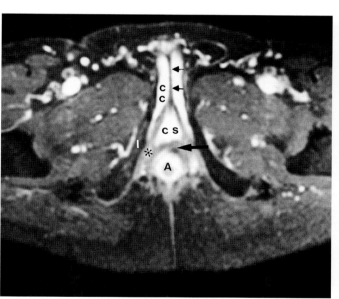

b

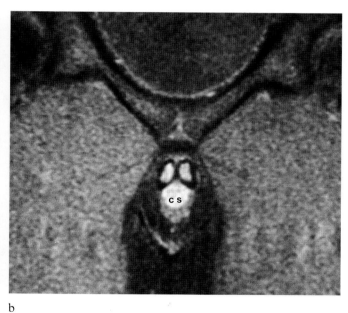

b

Figure 11.7

Normal anatomy of the penis. Transaxial Gd-DTPA-enhanced T1-weighted image at the level of the radix penis. (**a**) Conventional spin-echo image, and (**b**) fat-saturation image. (CC)-corpora cavernosa; (small black arrows)-septum of corpora cavernosa; (CS)-corpus spongiosum; (asterisk)-ischiocavernosus muscle; (I)-ischium; (A)-anal canal showing zonal anatomy; (large solid arrow)-transversus perinei superficialis muscle.

Figure 11.8

Normal anatomy of the penis on a T1-weighted image, coronal plane (**a**) conventional spin-echo and (**b**) fat-saturation images. Although all of the imaging instrument parameters are the same, the signal intensity of the corpora cavernosa and corpus spongiosum (CS) appears higher on the fat-saturation image as compared to the conventional study.

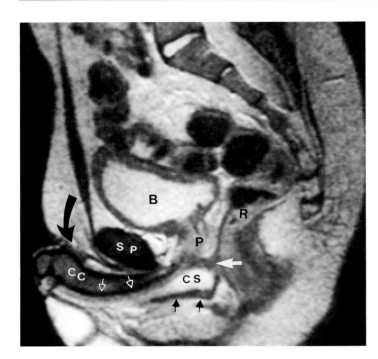

Figure 11.9

Sagittal T2-weighted midline section showing the normal anatomy of the penis and its suspensory ligament. (B)-urinary bladder; (P)-prostate; (white closed arrow)-urogenital diaphragm; (SP)-symphysis pubis; (large curved black arrow)-suspensory ligament; (CC)-corpora cavernosa; (open arrows)-tunica albuginea of corpora cavernosa; (CS)-corpus spongiosum; (small black arrows)-bulbospongiosus muscle; (R)-rectum.

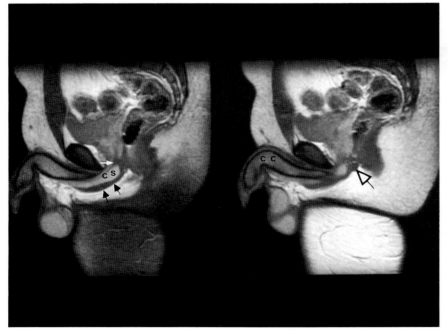

a   b

Figure 11.10

Normal penile anatomy and the demonstration of the transversus perinei superficialis muscle in the sagittal plane. Two consecutive proton density sagittal sections. (**a**) Midline, and (**b**) 1 cm lateral section, showing the relationship between the corpus spongiosum (CS) of the bulb of the penis, the membranous urethra (white arrow) and the apex of the prostate gland in the midline parasagittal plane. (CS)-corpus spongiosum; (CC)-corpora cavernosa; (black arrow)-bulbospongiosus muscle; (open arrow)-transversus perinei superficialis muscle.

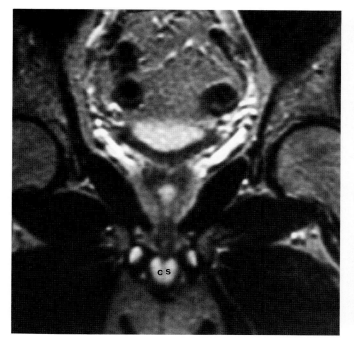

a

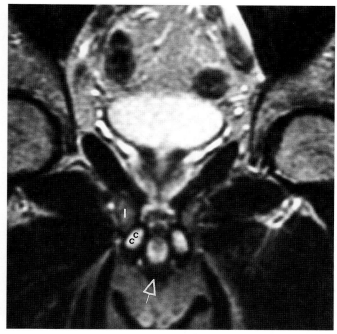

b

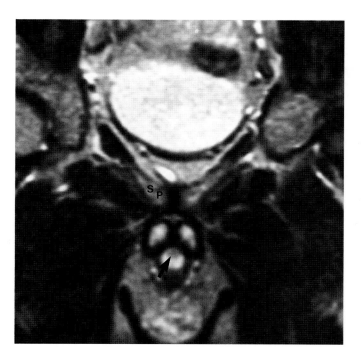

c

Figure 11.11

Normal anatomy of the penis in the coronal plane. Serial T2-weighted images at the level of (**a**) the penile bulb, (**b**) the crura of the corpora cavernosa, and (**c**) the symphysis pubis. (CS)-corpus spongiosum; (CC)-corpora cavernosa; (I)-ischium; (open arrow)-bulbospongiosus muscle; (SP)-symphysis pubis; (black arrow)-urethra.

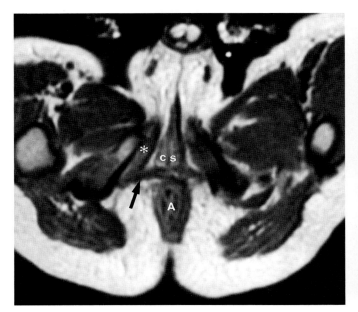

a

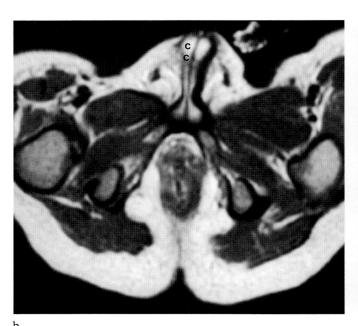

b

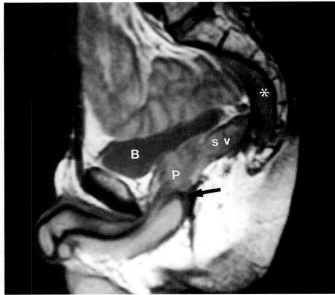

a

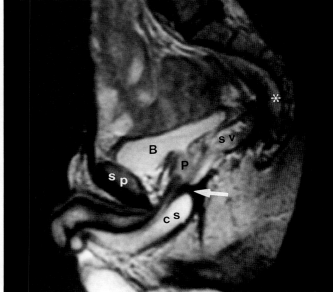

b

Figure 11.12

Normal anatomy of the penis. One-month-old infant. Axial proton density images, (**a**) at the level of the base of the corpus spongiosum (CS) and (**b**) through the corpora cavernosa (CC). (Asterisk)-ischiocavernosus muscle; (arrow)-transversus perinei superficialis muscle; (A)-anal canal. The normal penile anatomy is clearly displayed regardless of the patient's age.

Figure 11.13

Altered anatomic relations following abdominoperineal resection for carcinoma of the rectum. Sagittal plane (**a**) proton density and (**b**) T2-weighted images. (Asterisk)-scar tissue in the presacral region; (SV)-seminal vesicles; (B)-urinary bladder; (P)-prostate; (SP)-symphysis pubis; (CS)-corpus spongiosum. There is upward and dorsal retraction of the bulb of the penis (arrow). The roof of the bulb of the penis (arrow) is retracted 2 cm cranially from the inferior pubic ramis which is its normal position.

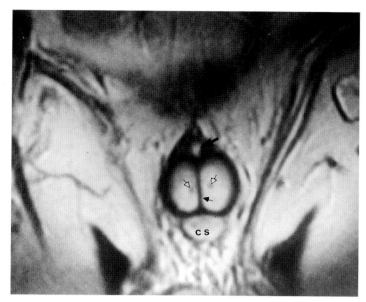

a

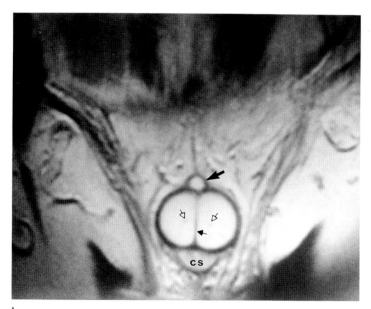

b

Figure 11.14

Signal intensity of the corpora cavernosa as a function of cavernosal blood volume. T2-weighted images, coronal plane. Penis in (**a**) flaccid and (**b**) erection states. The erection was achieved with intracorporeal 10 µg prostaglandin E1 injection. When the penis is in the flaccid state, the corpora cavernosa image with inhomogeneous signal intensity, lower at the periphery. During erection, besides enlargement of the corpora cavernosa, the signal intensity is uniformly high and the septum–tunica albuginea (small black arrow) thins and stretches. The corpus spongiosum (CS) does not enlarge following corporeal injection of prostaglandin. (Large black arrow)-dorsal vein of penis; (open arrows)-cavernous artery.

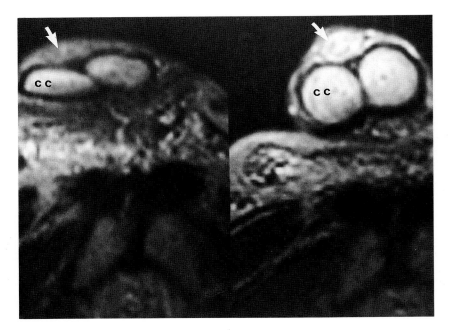

a   b

Figure 11.15

Appearance of the penis (**a**) before and (**b**) during erection produced by a vacuum constriction device. Notice that with this mode of inducing erection, the corpus spongiosum (white arrow) shares the enlargement with the corpora cavernosa (CC).

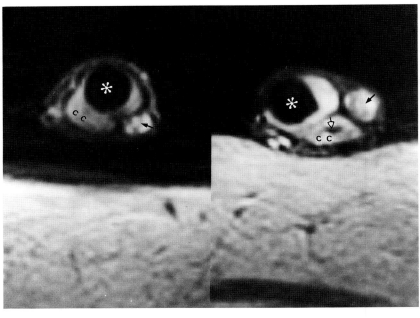

a   b

Figure 11.16

Silicone prosthesis placed in only one corpus cavernosum, T2-weighted images: (**a**) penis in flaccid state, (**b**) vacuum constriction device induced erection. The corpus cavernosum around the prosthesis (asterisk) enlarges and increases in signal intensity during erection. The contralateral corpus cavernosum (CC) demonstrates a scar (small open arrow) and fails to enlarge. Notice the enlargement of the corpus spongiosum. (Small black arrow)-the urethra within the corpus spongiosum.

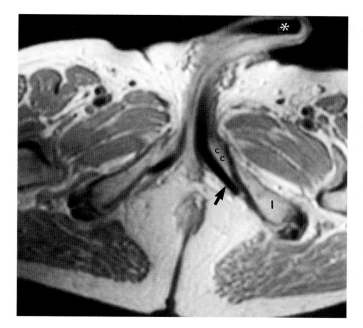

a

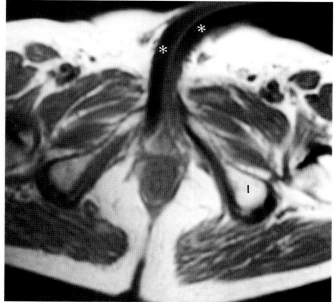

b

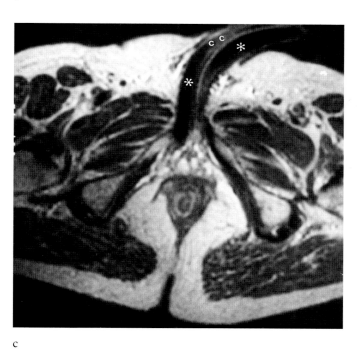

c

Figure 11.17

Silicone penile prosthesis. (**a**) Proton density image at the proximal crura of the corpora cavernosa, (**b**) proton density image through the shaft of the penis and (**c**) T2-weighted image at the same level as (**b**). The penile silicone prosthesis images with signal void on both the proton density and T2-weighted scans. (Asterisk)-prosthesis; (CC)-corpora cavernosa; (I)-ischium. As the prosthesis is placed blindly its proximal end (arrow) is often incorrectly positioned.

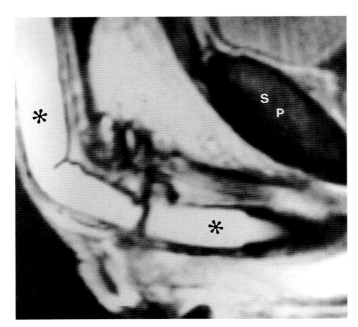

Figure 11.18

Inflatable penile prosthesis (asterisks) showing high signal intensity with a low intensity border on this T2-weighted image. (SP)-symphysis pubis.

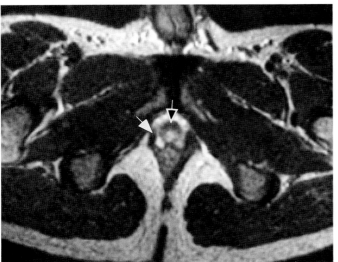

Figure 11.19

Membranous urethra in the transaxial plane of section, T2-weighted image. The urethral wall (black and white arrow) images as a low signal intensity ring surrounding the higher signal intensity epithelial surface. The levator ani muscle (white arrow) is clearly separated from the urethra.

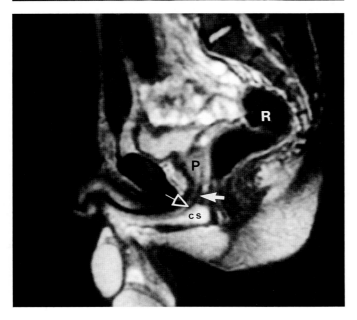

Figure 11.20

Distal prostatic, membranous and proximal bulbar urethra seen on a sagittal T2-weighted image. The urethra images as a low signal intensity stripe and its zonal anatomy is not seen. However, the relationship between the urethra in the distal prostate gland (P), the membranous urethra (white arrow), and the bulbar urethra (open arrow) as it pierces the roof of the corpus spongiosum (CS) is demonstrated. (R)-rectum.

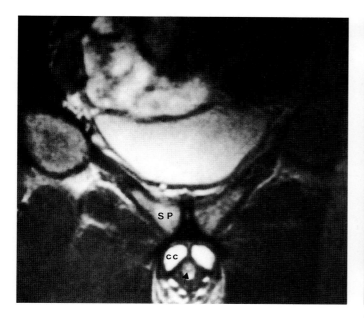

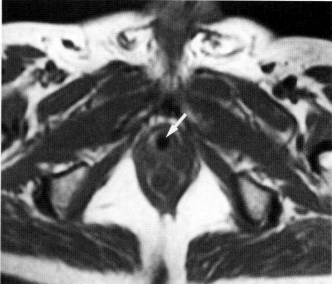

a

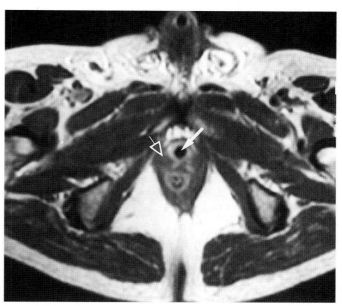

b

Figure 11.21

Anatomy of the penis showing the relationship between the corpora cavernosa (CC) and the corpus spongiosum with a cephalad location of the urethra (arrow) at the level of the symphysis pubis (SP). Coronal plane T2-weighted image.

Figure 11.22

Indwelling catheter (solid white arrow) in the membranous urethra. (**a**) Noncontrast, and (**b**) gadolinium-enhanced T1-weighted images. The identification of the lumen of the urethra is facilitated by the placement of the indwelling catheter. Following gadolinium injection, the wall of the urethra shows enhancement indicating an inflammatory component. The wall of the urethra can be separated from the levator ani muscle (open arrow).

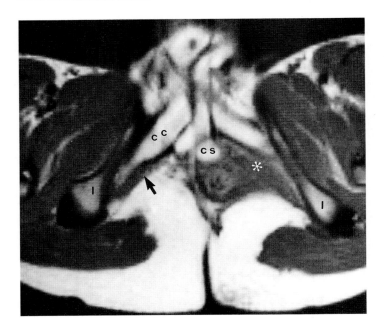

Figure 11.23

Penis diphallus. T2-weighted image showing asymmetrical development of the right (CC) and left corpora cavernosa. The corpus spongiosum (CS) is duplicated. The ischiocavernosus muscles are seen to be asymmetrically developed. (Arrow)-right ischiocavernosus muscle; (asterisk)-left ischiocavernosus muscle. The ischium (I) is malrotated.

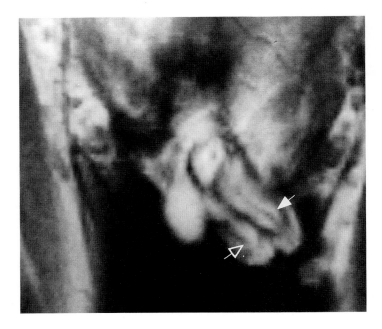

Figure 11.24

Penis diphallus. Proton density image showing two glans penis (open and solid arrows).

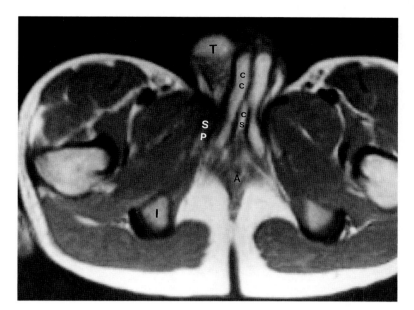

Figure 11.25

Epispadias. Proton density image. The corpora cavernosa (CC) are separated, as is the symphysis pubis (SP). The perineum is shortened, and the anal canal is displaced anteriorly. (CS)-corpus spongiosum; (T)-testicle; (A)-anal canal; (I)-ischium. (0.35T.)

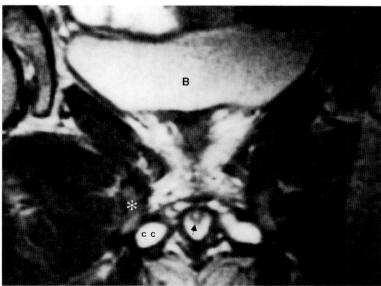

Figure 11.26

Epispadias. T2-weighted image in the coronal plane. The symphysis pubis (asterisk) is separated, and the corpora cavernosa (CC) are spread apart. The corpus spongiosum is displaced upwards and located between the corpora cavernosa. The urethra (arrow) therefore is the most cephalic in location.

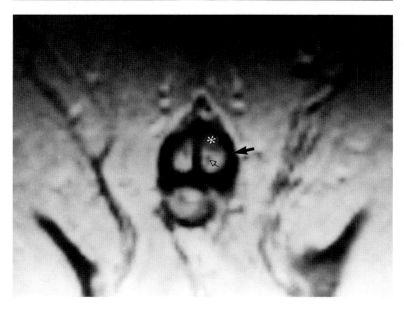

Figure 11.27

Peyronie's disease. T2-weighted coronal image showing the thick low signal intensity tunica albuginea (black arrow). The fibrous plaque (asterisk) has also imaged with low signal intensity, lower than the corpora cavernosa but higher than the tunica albuginea. The distance between the plaque and the deep artery of the corpora cavernosa (small open arrow) can be appreciated.

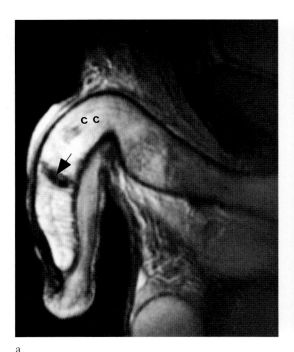

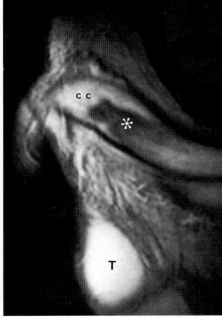

a

Figure 11.29

Idiopathic penile fibrosis. (**a**) T2-weighted sagittal image and (**b**) corpora cavernosogram. The large irregularly shaped area of low signal intensity (asterisk) in the corpora cavernosa (CC) is sharply outlined. It is seen on the corpora cavernosogram as a large filling defect. (T)-testicle. The dorsal vein of the penis (white arrow) is draining into the preprostatic vein (veins of Santorini) (open arrows), draining in turn into the vesicoprostatic plexus (large open arrow with box).

a

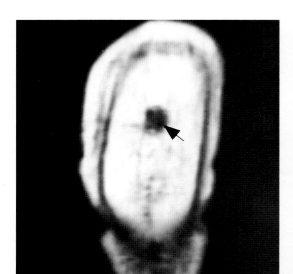

b

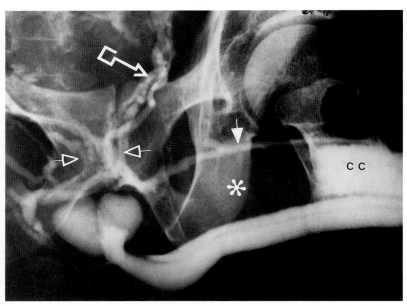

b

Figure 11.28

Self-inflicted corporeal penile fibrosis due to repeated intracorporeal prostaglandin E1 injections. T2-weighted images, (**a**) sagittal, (**b**) coronal planes. The corpora cavernosa (CC) are of inhomogeneous signal intensity with the localized area of low signal intensity (arrow) at the site of injections indicating fibrosis.

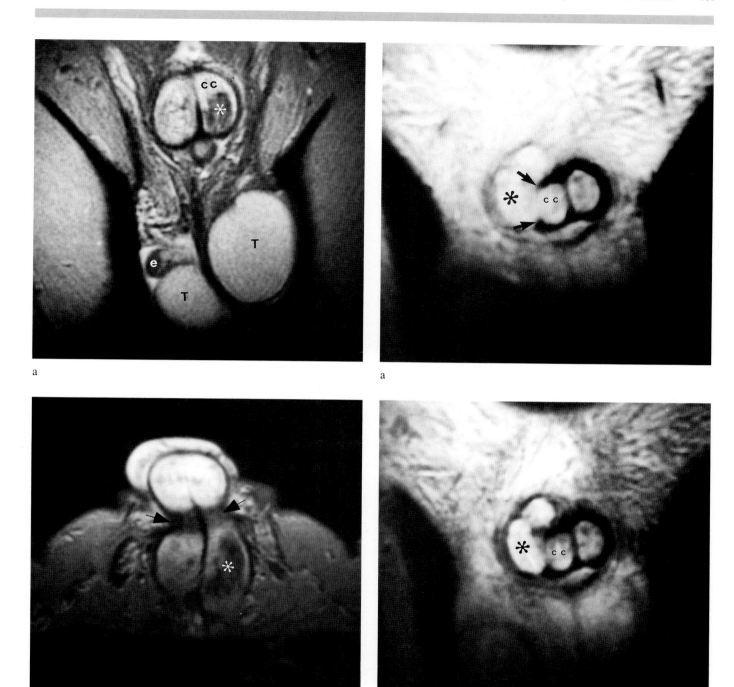

a

b

a

b

Figure 11.30

Fibrosis of the corpora cavernosa (asterisk) probably due to lupus erythematosus and fibrosis at the site of a patient applied constriction ring, placed in order to prolong erection (arrows). (**a**) Coronal and (**b**) transaxial T2-weighted images. (CC)-corpora cavernosa; (E)-head of epididymis; (T)-testicles.

Figure 11.31

Acute fracture of the penis, coronal plane (**a**) proton density, and (**b**) T2-weighted images. There is a break in the continuity of the tunica albuginea (arrows) with formation of a pericorporeal hematoma (asterisk). The corpora cavernosa (CC) are of inhomogeneous signal intensity on the T2-weighted image.

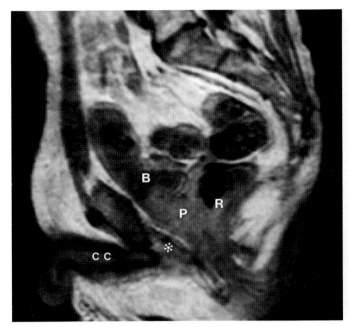

a

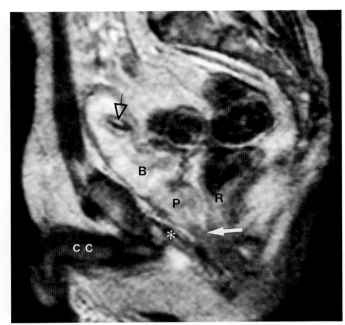

b

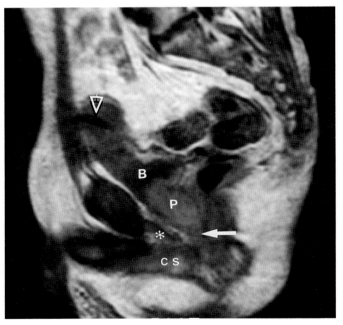

c

Figure 11.32

Pelvic trauma with fracture of the membranous urethra. Sagittal (**a**) proton density, and (**b**) T2-weighted images in the midline and (**c**) proton density image 1 cm to the left. The bulb of the penis (CS) is not in the same midline plane as the apex of the prostate (P) due to fracture at the level of the membranous urethra. (Open arrow)-suprapubic catheter; (B)-urinary bladder; (P)-prostate; (white solid arrow)-apex of the prostate; (R)-rectum; (asterisk)-organized hematoma; (CC)-corpora cavernosa.

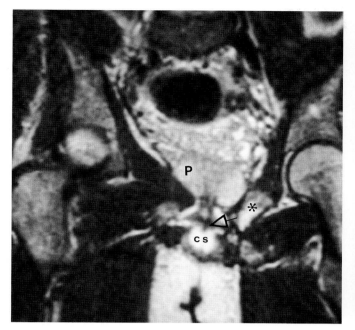

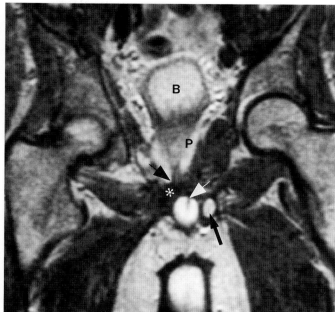

a

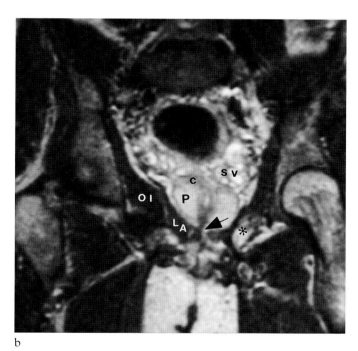

b

Figure 11.34

Severe dislocation of the bulbar urethra (white arrow) which is displaced to the left, while the apex of the prostate (short black arrow) is displaced to the right of the midline (1.5 cm lateral misalignment). Coronal T2-weighted image. There is fibrosis in the region of the membranous urethra (asterisk). The penis is also fractured and only one corpus cavernosum (long black arrow) is visualized in this plane.

Figure 11.33

Minor misalignment of the apex of the prostate (solid arrow) with the bulbar urethra (open arrow). Two consecutive coronal T2-weighted images (**a**) and (**b**). (SV)-seminal vesicles; (C)-central zone of the prostate; (P)-peripheral zone; (LA)-levator ani muscle; (OI)-obturator internus muscle; (asterisk)-chronic hematoma; (CS)-corpus spongiosum.

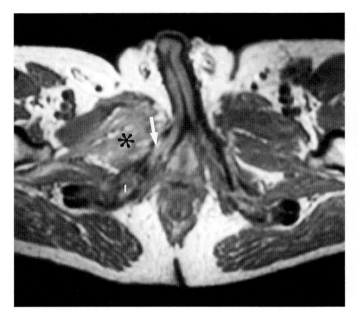

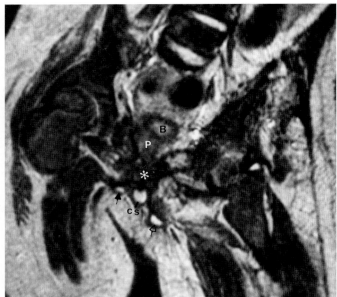

a

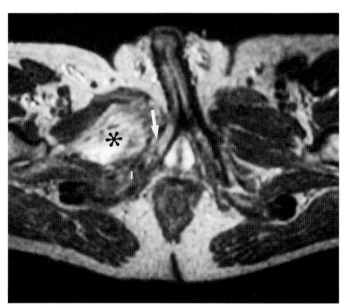

b

Figure 11.36

Separation of the corporeal bodies due to severe pelvic trauma. Coronal T2-weighted image. The right (solid arrow) and the left (open arrow) corpora cavernosa are separated from the corpus spongiosum (CS). (P)-prostate gland; (B)-urinary bladder; (asterisk)-extensive fibrosis in the membranous urethra. The distance between the bulbar urethra and the apex of the gland is 2 cm.

Figure 11.35

Undisplaced fracture of both corpora cavernosa and compound fractures of the ischial bones. Transverse (a) proton density and (b) T2-weighted images. (I)-fractured right ischium; (asterisk)-hematoma; (arrow)-undisplaced fracture of the right corpus cavernosum.

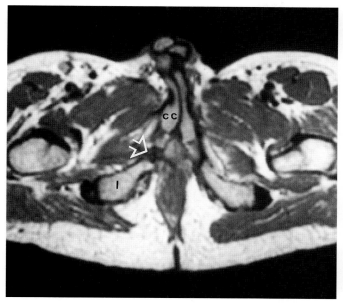

a

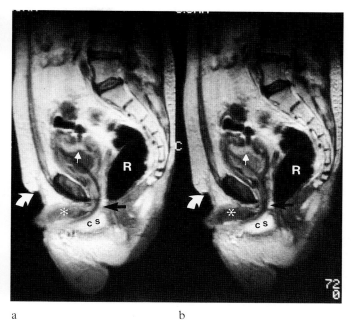

a   b

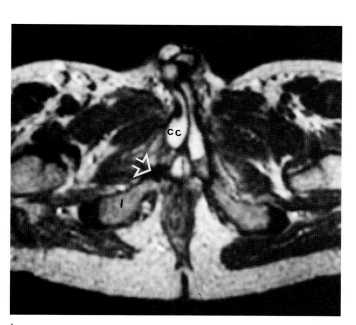

b

Figure 11.38

Penile carcinoma, stage T2. Sagittal (**a**) proton density and (**b**) T2-weighted images. Advanced penile carcinoma with skin ulceration (curved arrow), and autoamputation of the penile shaft are visible. Carcinoma has invaded the corpora cavernosa (asterisks) and demonstrates low signal intensity on the T2-weighted image. The corpus spongiosum (CS) is not invaded. The tumor did not spread beyond the urogenital diaphragm (black straight arrow). The bladder wall is thickened and the mucosa (white arrow) is of high signal intensity. The findings indicate catheter induced cystitis. (R)-rectum. (0.35T.)

Figure 11.37

Fractured corpora cavernosa with the separation (open arrow) between the right corpus cavernosum (CC) and the ischium (I). Transaxial (**a**) proton density and (**b**) T2-weighted images.

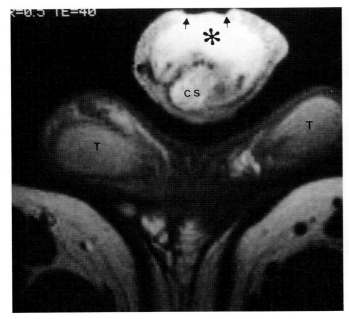

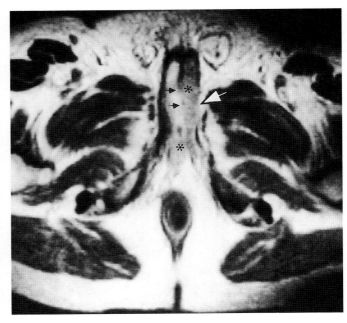

a

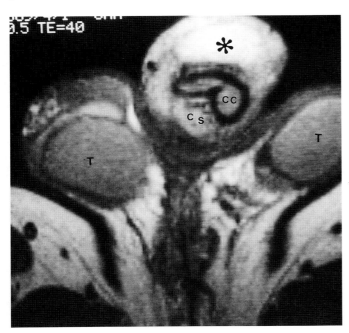

b

Figure 11.40

Urethral carcinoma, transitional cell carcinoma at the base of the penis with invasion of the bulb of the penis. (Asterisks)-corpora cavernosa; (black arrows)-septum of the corpora cavernosa and tunica albuginea (white arrow) along its left side, stage T3. T2-weighted image. (0.35 T.)

Figure 11.39

Penile carcinoma (squamous cell carcinoma), stage T2, in the glans penis with large abscess formation (asterisk), skin ulceration (small arrows) and invasion of the corpora spongiosum (CS) in the glans, but not the corpora cavernosa (CC). Transaxial proton density image at the level of (**a**) the glans penis and (**b**) 1 cm proximally. (T)-testis. (0.35 T.)

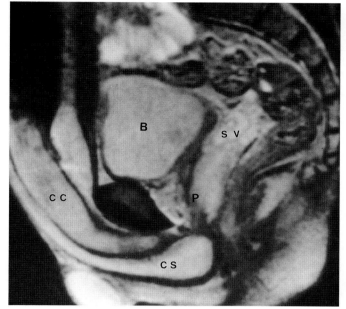

a

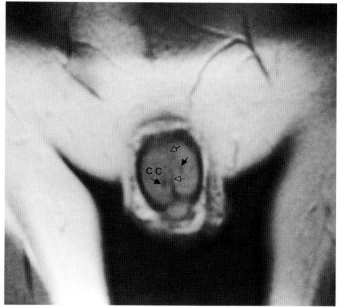

b

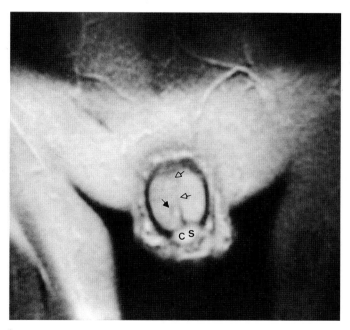

c

Figure 11.41

Infiltrative metastases from testicular cancer, primary carcinoma of the testis causing priapism. (**a**) T2-weighted sagittal image, (**b**) proton density and (**c**) T2-weighted coronal images. The penis is erect, the corpora cavernosa are of inhomogeneous signal intensity and the septum (open arrows) is disrupted. (Black arrows)-cavernous artery; (CS)-corpus spongiosum; (B)-urinary bladder; (SV)-seminal vesicles; (CC)-corpora cavernosa; (P)-prostate.

12
The Bladder and Female Urethra

Hedvig Hricak

For many years radiologic evaluation of the urinary bladder and urethra was limited to intravenous urography (IVU) and retrograde and voiding cystourethrography. The development of cross-sectional imaging modalities such as ultrasound (US), computed tomography (CT) and magnetic resonance imaging (MRI), however, has changed the diagnostic approach to the urinary bladder and urethra, and has markedly improved the preoperative assessment of congenital anomalies, the evaluation of the extent of trauma, and the staging accuracy of bladder and urethral tumors.

Normal anatomy of the bladder and urethra

Urinary bladder

The urinary bladder is a muscular organ located extraperitoneally in the pelvis beneath the peritoneum and behind the symphysis pubis.[1,2] In the male, the inferolateral aspect of the base of the bladder is adjacent to the seminal vesicles. Medial to each seminal vesicle, the bladder base is in contact with the ampulla ductus deferens. The bladder neck is in close contact with the base of the prostate gland. In the female, the posterior bladder base is loosely attached to the anterior wall of the cervix and vagina (the **uterovesical space**), and the bladder neck is in close contact with the periurethral muscles and urethra. In infants, the bladder lies higher than it does in adults; and the internal sphincter of the bladder neck often lies well above the symphysis pubis. In adult males, the vesical neck lies either just below the upper border of the symphysis or, in females, opposite the lower third of the pubic bone.

The size of the bladder varies. In children, the upper border of the full bladder should not rise above the level of the first sacral vertebra. In an adult, the bladder should not reach above the second or third sacral segment.

The shape of the normal bladder is influenced by the degree of filling and by pressure from adjacent organs. In the male, the bladder base may be indented by the prostate gland (even when the prostate is not enlarged), and the levator ani muscle may produce an impression on the bladder floor in either sex.

Embryologically, the bladder develops in two stages.[3] Initially it develops from the cloaca, but the trigone differentiates later, from the primitive urogenital sinus. The belief that the cloaca separates into two structures—the rectum and the primitive urogenital sinus—is controversial, and today most theories suggest that the hind gut starts above the cloaca, and that the rectum forms largely from the hind gut.[3]

Histologically, the wall of the urinary bladder consists of three layers: an advential layer of connective tissue, a smooth muscle coat, and an inner layer of mucous membrane.[4] The mucosal lining, with the exception of the trigone which is always smooth, is rugose in the undistended organ and becomes smoother as filling proceeds. When the bladder is fully distended, the wall should not be more than 5 mm thick. The bladder fundus has a serosal covering of peritoneum.

Vascular supply

The bladder receives its principal blood supply from the superior and inferior **vesical arteries**, which are derived from the internal iliac artery.[1,2] Branches from the **obturator** and **inferior gluteal arteries** also supply

417

the bladder, as do branches of the **uterine** and **vaginal arteries** in the female. Venous drainage is via a complicated plexus on the inferolateral surface (vesico-prostatic plexus in the male), which ultimately drains into the internal iliac veins.

Lymphatic drainage

Lymphatics from the trigone, the bladder base, and the superior surface of the bladder nearly all drain to the **external iliac nodes.** Some vesical lymphatics may drain to the **internal** or **common iliac group**.[1]

Female urethra

In the female the urethra is a thin-walled muscular tube, about 4 cm long, which starts at the internal urethral orifice of the bladder (opposite the symphysis pubis) and runs in a craniocaudal direction to its termination (the external urethral orifice) just anterior to the opening of the vagina and behind the clitoris.[1] Only the female urethra will be discussed in this chapter. The male urethra is discussed together with the penis in Chapter 11.

The wall of the urethra is composed of three layers—the mucosa, the submucosa, and the external muscle coat.[4,5] The **mucosa** (the inner mucous layer) extends the entire length of the urethra and contains stratified squamous, pseudostratified columnar, or transitional epithelium, depending upon which area of the urethra is being studied.[5] The **submucosa (lamina propria)** extends through the length of the urethra, and consists of loose connective tissue with blood vessels and elastic fibers as well as a few smooth muscle fibers. Because of the cavernous character of the submucosa, the urethra was sometimes falsely referred to as the corpus spongiosum of the female. The **external striated muscle** layer, continuous with that of the bladder, is thickest at the anterior wall and towards the middle of the urethra.[6]

The urethra is divided into three portions—the upper-, middle-, and lower-thirds—which have differing histologic characteristics. The **upper-third** is composed primarily of the external muscular coat, a continuation of the tissue which forms the bladder neck. At the level of the bladder neck, the middle (circular) layer of the bladder wall is prominent, encircling the lower portion of the bladder and extending downwards to form the upper part of the urethra. The submucosa in the upper-third is composed of fibrous connective tissue, rich in fine elastic fibers with moderate vascularization.

The **middle-third** of the urethra is characterized by an outer layer of circular striated muscle and a submucosa of highly vascularized involuntary muscle bundles.

At the **lower-third** of the urethra the substantia propria becomes extremely thick and the lower-third is composed almost entirely of fibrous tissue. At the external urethral orifice, the paraurethral ducts (which run through the mucosa on each side of the urethra) end in a small aperture.

Vascular supply

The major arterial supply is through the urethral artery which is the branch of the inferior vesical artery. The distal post of the urethra is often supplied by the branches of the internal pudendal artery. The drainage is through the vesical plexus, veins of Santorini or vaginal veins and vulvar venous plexus.

Lymphatic drainage

In the female, lymphatics from the urethra drain primarily to the **internal iliac nodes**, although a few may pass to the **external iliac nodes.** Lymphatics from the membranous part of the urethra follow the path of the internal pudendal artery.

MRI appearance

Urinary bladder

The urinary bladder is clearly demonstrated on MRI, regardless of the degree of bladder distension.[7] Since both urine and muscle have a relatively long T1 relaxation time, both the bladder wall and urine within the bladder image with low signal intensity on T1-weighted images (Figure 12.1a).[7] In contrast, the T2 relaxation times of urine and smooth muscle are markedly different, enhancing differentiation between the two on T2-weighted scans. Urine has a long T2 relaxation time, and as illustrated in Figure 12.1b, images with high signal intensity, whereas the smooth muscle of the bladder wall has a short T2 relaxation time, and it images with low signal intensity on T2-weighted scans.[7]

It is important to differentiate the normal low intensity of the bladder wall from the chemical-shift artifact caused by the different resonant frequencies of the hydrogen nuclei of urine and fat. The chemical-shift artifact (see Chapter 1) depends on the direction (polarity) of the gradient readout. As shown in Figure 12.2, on transverse images it is seen as a dark bend along the lateral wall of one side of the bladder and a bright stripe along the lateral wall of the opposite side.

On sagittal (Figure 12.3) or coronal (Figure 12.4) images, the chemical-shift artifact is seen along the base and dome of the bladder. Knowledge of the appearance of this artifact prevents an erroneous diagnosis of bladder pathology.

On T1-weighted fat-saturation images, the bladder wall (Figure 12.5a) demonstrates signal intensity slightly higher than either urine within the urinary bladder or the perivesical fat. As illustrated in Figure 12.5b, on T2-weighted images, the bladder wall shows decrease in signal intensity but due to saturation of the adjacent perivesical fat the low signal intensity wall is only seen when contrasted to high signal intensity perivesical structures such as the vesicoprostatic venous plexus or seminal vesicles. The fat-saturation images reduce chemical-shift artifact. The value of the fat saturation technique in the study of bladder tumors needs to be further established. At present most of the results are based on the use of conventional spin-echo images. Following gadolinium-DTPA injection on the immediate scan as seen in Figure 12.6, no enhancement of the wall of the urinary bladder is seen. However, on the delayed scan, there is signal enhancement of the bladder wall. The appreciation of the enhancement of the bladder wall is accentuated when the fat-saturation technique is combined with gadolinium-DTPA enhancement as shown in Figure 12.7.

Female urethra

On T1-weighted transaxial images, as depicted in Figure 12.8, the female urethra is of medium signal intensity and differentiation between the urethra and the posteriorly located vagina is not possible.[8] On T2-weighted MR images in the transaxial plane, the characteristic target-like appearance of the urethra can be seen (Figure 12.8). The rings seen on MR scans can be correlated with the histologic layers of the urethral wall.[8] The outer low signal intensity ring most probably corresponds to the outer striated muscle of the urethra. On both histologic and MRI studies this striated muscle ring is found to be most prominent in the mid-urethra and may be complete or incomplete posteriorly. It may also be less prominent in post-menopausal women.[6] The somewhat thicker middle zone of the urethra, which on T2-weighted images demonstrates a higher signal intensity, probably corresponds to the smooth muscle layer, with a contribution from the submucosa which consists of loosely woven connective tissue with an elaborate vascular plexus. The central portion of the urethra images as a low signal intensity dot, and is possibly related to folded stratified epithelium which has compact cells and very little extracellular space.[8] Using the fat-saturation spin-echo technique the zonal anatomy of

the urethra can be seen readily on T1-weighted images, and is accentuated on proton density or T2-weighted images as shown in Figure 12.9. On the fat-saturation images the enhancement of the periurethral and perivaginal vascular areolar tissue is better seen than on conventional spin-echo images (Figure 12.10).

Following administration of gadolinium-DTPA, as illustrated in Figure 12.11 the target-like appearance of the urethra can be seen on T1-weighted images.[8] The outer striated muscle and the central low intensity dot do not enhance, and the middle zone shows marked enhancement, allowing differentiation of the zonal anatomy.

On T2-weighted or Gd-DTPA-enhanced T1-weighted images in the sagittal plane, the urethra is usually visualized with lower signal intensity than the posteriorly located vagina, but the target-like appearance is not demonstrated (Figure 12.12). The urethra may be difficult to find on coronal plane images, even when thin sections are used.

Recommended imaging sequences

Urinary bladder

Both T1- and T2-weighted images are essential for evaluation of the urinary bladder. T1-weighted images often allow detection of intraluminal bladder pathology, but tissue characterization of the bladder wall and staging of bladder carcinoma require T2-weighted images.

Although the normal bladder wall is clearly seen in all planes of imaging, specific regions of the bladder are better seen with particular planes. Therefore, the plane of imaging depends on the location of the pathologic process being evaluated. Transaxial images are helpful in evaluating the lateral walls of the bladder, whereas sagittal images are essential in evaluating the dome or the base of the bladder. Similarly, tumors located at the anterior or posterior wall of the bladder are optimally displayed on the sagittal plane of imaging. Coronal images are complementary in the evaluation of the dome and base of the bladder and are most beneficial in the evaluation of the lateral wall of the bladder.

On the scans taken immediately after gadolinium-DTPA administration, the bladder wall does not enhance. However, there is enhancement of the bladder wall on delayed scans. Therefore, if tumor staging is required early postgadolinium sections are most helpful.

Female urethra

Transaxial images are essential for the evaluation of the female urethra, and both T1- and T2-weighted scans should be obtained. T1-weighted images offer excellent contrast between the medium signal intensity urethra and the high signal intensity anterolateral adipose tissue. T2-weighted images allow identification of the zonal anatomy of the urethra, which can also be seen on T1-weighted images following gadolinium enhancement.

Although images in the transverse plane are required for the demonstration of zonal anatomy, two planes of imaging are recommended in the evaluation of urethral pathology. Transaxial images are needed for the identification of urethral diverticula, but craniocaudal extension is best seen in the sagittal plane. Spread of urethral carcinoma to the urinary bladder is best appreciated on sagittal films, and tumor spread to the vagina requires a combination of transaxial and sagittal scanning.

Pathology of the bladder and urethra

Congenital anomalies

Urinary bladder

The major anomalies of the urinary bladder include agenesis, hypoplasia, duplication, exstrophy and diverticula.[3] **Bladder agenesis** is a rare condition usually associated with absence of the urethra and with other congenital abnormalities incompatible with life. **Bladder hypoplasia (dwarf bladder)** is also extremely rare and is associated with other anomalies of the urinary tract.

Bladder duplication. This extends to different degrees. In a complete bladder duplication there are two separate bladders, each with its own muscle wall and mucosa, separated by a peritoneal fold of varying depth.[9] In addition to two urethras, there are often two penises, or a partially duplicated penis, in males and two vaginas and two uteri in females. In incomplete bladder duplication, there may be two separate fundae, but there is only a single base and one urethra. Incomplete duplication may be caused by sagittal or frontal division. Multiseptated bladders are also known to occur.

MRI appearance. Magnetic resonance plays only a limited role in the evaluation of the congenital anoma-

lies of the urinary bladder. As shown in Figure 12.13, MRI can demonstrate bladder duplication. The septum between the two halves of the bladder exhibits low signal intensity on both T1- and T2-weighted images. The bladder wall in both halves is of similar thickness and signal intensity (Figure 12.13). This finding is best appreciated on transaxial or coronal planes of imaging. Associated duplications of the urethra can also be demonstrated.

Bladder exstrophy. There are many variations in the presentation of bladder exstrophy.[9] The most common is classic exstrophy, which includes epispadias and increased separation of the pubic bones (the distance between the pubic bones should be no more than 10mm at any age). In classic exstrophy the anterior wall of the bladder and the corresponding portion of the anterior abdominal wall fail to fuse during fetal development. In severe cases the inner surface of the posterior bladder wall protrudes into the abdomen. Bladder exstrophy may be associated with bilateral inguinal hernias, undescended testis, and a shortened penis (see Chapter 11).

MRI appearance. MRI does not play a decisive role in the clinical diagnosis of bladder exstrophy, but can contribute the information about associated skeletal, muscular, and perineal anomalies including development and the position of the sex organs. The diagnosis of bladder exstrophy is clinical and the evaluation of the urinary tract is by conventional studies including IVP and/or cystograms. MRI will demonstrate musculoskeletal anomalies, such as anomalous rotation of the pelvic bones and separation of the symphysis pubis. The separation and frequent underdevelopment of the rectus abdominis muscle is illustrated in Figure 12.14. The presence of umbilical hernia is easily documented on MRI images. Because of excellent soft tissue contrast, either the transaxial or sagittal plane of imaging (Figure 12.15) can display the shortening of the perineum and the anterior position of the anus. In males, the prostate gland changes the direction of its long axis (the apex is displaced anteriorly) and subsequently the seminal vesicles lie inferior and anterior or at the level of the bladder base (Figure 12.16). The clinical usefulness of all of these findings at present has not been ascertained, but MRI is helpful in improving the understanding of this complex anomalous syndrome.

Bladder diverticulum. Congenital bladder diverticula are hernias of the bladder mucosa through the detrusor muscle of the bladder. Ninety-eight per cent are seen in males, and most occur in the region of the bladder base. When they are located in the region of the ureteral meatus they are known as Hutch's diverticula, and often cause ureteral obstruction. When Hutch's diverticula enlarge and extend laterally and posteriorly to the ureteral meatus, they may cause urethral obstruction.[3]

MRI appearance. Bladder diverticula are easily displayed on MR images. The diverticulum has a thin wall, in contrast to the native bladder wall which is often thickened as a result of associated bladder outlet obstruction. The thick bladder wall images with low signal intensity on T2-weighted images. The bladder wall, however, may remain of normal thickness in which case, as shown in Figure 12.17, the radiologic differentiation between the large bladder diverticulum and bladder duplication is not possible.

Congenital bladder diverticula, Hutch's diverticula (Figure 12.18), can be identified by their characteristic location in the posterolateral aspect. The optimal plane of imaging depends on the location of the diverticula. For lateral diverticula transverse or coronal images are preferred. For diverticula located posteriorly, sagittal or transaxial images are recommended.

MRI in relation to other imaging modalites. Conventional radiographic studies, IVP and cystogram, coupled with cystoscopy are the primary mode of evaluation for the congenital anomalies of the urinary bladder. The increased popularity of ultrasound has advanced the use of US in many bladder anomalies. The cross-sectional modalities, CT and MRI, are rarely used. Between the two, MRI has better tissue contrast and its capability of direct multiplanar imaging makes it more suitable than CT in the assessment of associated bony and soft tissue anomalies.

Urachal abnormalities

Discussion of congenital anomalies of the urinary bladder includes anomalies of the urachus. The urachus is a patent canal in the fetus which connects the bladder with the allantois. In the first stage of the fetal development of the bladder, a diverticulum grows out of the cloaca in a cranioventral direction, and this diverticulum is called the urachus. At the level of the umbilicus the cranioventral end of the urachus opens into the allantois. Late in embryonic and fetal life, or early in postnatal life, the urachal lumen becomes obliterated. The obliterated urachus, covered by peritoneum, is located in the midline and is known as the **median umbilical fold** (see Chapter 4). In one-third of adults the urachus is not completely obliter-

ated and has microscopic communications with the bladder.

There are four types of congenital urachal anomalies: (1) patent urachus; (2) urachal cyst; (3) urachal sinus; and (4) urachal diverticulum.[10,11] The **patent urachus** is often associated with urethral atresia or obstructed posterior urethral valves. A **urachal cyst** develops if the urachus is obliterated at the level of the umbilicus and bladder, but remains patent between the two areas. An infected urachal cyst can lead to the development of a **urachal sinus**, which may open either into the umbilicus or the urinary bladder. A **urachal diverticulum** forms when the urachus closes at the umbilicus, but not at the bladder. This anomaly is common in the prune-belly syndrome, and is often associated with in utero bladder outlet obstruction.

MRI appearance. Because the median umbilical fold is well seen in the transaxial or sagittal plane of MR imaging, urachal cysts (Figure 12.19) and urachal diverticula can be identified as well.[12] To demonstrate a sinus tract or fistula, however, contrast studies are needed, although lateral sagittal MR scans may also be helpful. Sagittal images are helpful in identifying the anomalies between the dome of the urinary bladder and the umbilicus. It is the morphologic findings that are helpful because the fluid composition of uncomplicated urachal anomalies may overlap.

MRI in relation to other imaging modalities. US is often the initial study in the diagnosis of urachal anomalies. MRI, except for morphologic display, has little to offer in the study of urachal sinuses or tracts. Urachal diverticula and cysts can be seen on both CT and MRI, but the sagittal plane MR images depict with high accuracy the urachal anomalies within the median umbilical fold.

Female urethra

Congenital anomalies of the female urethra represent anomalies in both number (duplication) and form (strictures, polyps, and diverticula). Anomalies are rare, and nearly all cases of congenital urethral polyps occur in males.

Urethral duplications. There are several different types of urethral duplications in the female, including double urethra and double bladder, double urethra and single bladder, and an accessory urethra which opens into the bladder on one side.[3] Although patients usually have no evidence of virilization, related genital anomalies, such as abnormalities of the labia, introital stenosis, absence of the vaginal vestibule, absence of the hymen, and vaginal introitus may be present.

MRI appearance. In an anecdotal report, it appears that MRI is helpful in defining the extent of the anomaly. On T2-weighted transaxial images, the morphologic anomalies of the urethra are well displayed.

Urethral diverticula. Diverticula of the female urethra are difficult to diagnose clinically and may go undetected even following urethroscopy. Although small urethral diverticula may be asymptomatic, when they become infected the symptoms may mimic bladder or urethral infection or tumor.[13]

MRI appearance. Urethral diverticula have a characteristic MRI appearance.[8] On T1-weighted images the urethra is usually of homogeneous medium signal intensity. Occasionally an area of lower signal intensity can be seen. As illustrated in Figure 12.20, on T2-weighted images the fluid content within the submucosal region of a urethral diverticulum demonstrates high signal intensity. The outer, low signal intensity wall is usually intact, although it may be thinned. Craniocaudal extension of the diverticulum can be appreciated on sagittal plane images. Following gadolinium-DTPA administration, the submucosal region is enhanced, but the area of diverticulum is not, permitting confirmation of the diagnosis of urethral diverticulum. The advantage of Gd-DTPA in the demonstration of urethral diverticulum is shown in Figure 12.21.

MRI in relation to other imaging modalities. Double-balloon catheter technique (Figure 12.22)—a conventional urographic study—for many years has been considered a standard diagnostic modality for the demonstration of urethral diverticula.[14] However, the study is sometimes technically difficult (short urethrae are particularly difficult to examine) and it is known that both cystoscopy and a double-balloon catheter study can overlook the urethral diverticula. In the clinical setting when there is suspicion of urethral diverticula and they are not demonstrated during cystoscopy or conventional studies, an MRI study should be obtained. As MRI becomes more widely available, its use in the study of urethral diverticula will probably expand even further.

Inflammatory disease of the urinary bladder (cystitis)

Radiologic studies do not play a major role in the diagnosis of cystitis. The diagnosis depends on history, culture, cystoscopic examinations, and, sometimes, biopsy.[15] Most cases of cystitis occur in adult women, often in combination with urethritis and vaginitis. *Escherichia coli* is the predominant organism. The histologic hallmark of chronic cystitis is irregularity of the bladder wall associated with trabeculation and often a small bladder capacity. The presence of gas within the bladder wall is often associated with emphysematous cystitis and can be seen following instrumentation of the genitourinary tract, in cases of fistula formation between the intestinal and genital tracts, and in diabetes mellitus.

MRI appearance

Inflammation usually causes bladder wall thickening, which can be appreciated on MR images. The thickened wall is usually of medium signal intensity, or as shown in Figure 12.23, of heterogeneous higher signal intensity on T1-weighted images. On T2-weighted images, the inflamed bladder wall demonstrates an increase in signal intensity. Radiation cystitis has a unique MR appearance. Although the bladder wall images with homogeneous signal intensity on T1-weighted images (Figure 12.24), on T2-weighted images an inner lower signal intensity stripe is preserved whereas the larger outer part of the thickened bladder wall exhibits high signal intensity. As depicted in Figure 12.25, bullous edema within the bladder wall can also be demonstrated on MR images.

Following administration of Gd-DTPA, the inflamed bladder wall (Figure 12.26) demonstrates various degrees of enhancement. The enhancement can be homogeneous or heterogeneous in distribution. The use of Gd-DTPA does not add to the specificity of MRI findings.

MRI in relation to other imaging modalities

MRI has a very limited role in the evaluation of bladder inflammation. The only specific findings for MRI is the appearance of the radiation cystitis. However, even for the diagnosis of radiation cystitis, cystoscopy is always required.

Bladder calculi

Bladder calculi can arise as a result of stasis, infection, or foreign bodies, or they may descend from the kidneys. Stasis is probably the most common cause. The stones are usually composed of magnesium, ammonia, or uric acid.[16]

MRI appearance

Bladder calculi exhibit a lack of signal intensity (ie, they are seen as signal voids). They may be difficult to detect on T1-weighted images because they are surrounded by low signal intensity urine. However, on T2-weighted scans (Figure 12.27) urine images with high signal intensity, providing excellent contrast to the lack of signal intensity of the calculi.

MRI in relation to other imaging modalities

Because of their composition, bladder calculi are often not seen on plain films, while conventional contrast radiographic studies such as IVU or cystogram will demonstrate the size and number of calculi. If a noninvasive study is to be performed, ultrasound is not only widely available but it is highly accurate. The finding of bladder stones on MRI is usually incidental and is discernible only when calculi are 0.5 cm or larger.

Bladder tumors

Bladder carcinoma is the most common cancer of the urinary tract. It accounts for approximately 4 per cent of all malignant tumors, and is the fifth leading cause of death among men over 75 years of age.[17] In addition, its incidence appears to be rising, a situation believed to be due to increased exposure to environmental carcinogens such as tobacco, artificial sweeteners, coffee, cyclophosphamides, and various aromatic amines.[18] Bladder cancer is three times more common in men than in women, and although it is most commonly seen in the sixth and seventh decades, it is being found in an increasingly large number of patients aged less than 30 years of age.[18] Bladder carcinoma most frequently arises in the region of the trigone and in the lateral and posterior walls. The tumors may be single or, more often, multicentric.

Primary bladder tumors are usually epithelial in origin and less than 10 per cent arise from nonepithelial sources.[18] Nonepithelial tumors include both benign (eg, **leiomyoma** and **fibroma**) and malignant (eg, **leiomyosarcoma** and **rhabdomyosarcoma**) neoplasms. Other primary tumors of the bladder include **pheochromocytoma**, **hemangioma**, **leukoplakia** and **endometriosis**. The bladder may also be the site of metastatic disease, although this occurrence is rare.

All **epithelial tumors** of the bladder are malignant, and the majority are **transitional cell carcinomas** (up to 90 per cent). **Adenocarcinomas** account for only 2 per cent of bladder cancers, and **squamous cell carcinomas** account for only 5–10 per cent. Although relatively rare compared with transitional cell carcinomas, squamous cell carcinomas are the most prevalent form of neoplasia in patients with chronic inflammatory disease of the bladder.[18]

Recent advances in the understanding of the biology of bladder cancer have helped to establish guidelines for prognosis and therapy. The most important variable in the prognosis of bladder carcinoma is its stage or extent at the time of diagnosis. Other variables include site, number (single versus multiple), degree of differentiation (grade), and pattern of growth (papillary, sessile, or combined papillary and sessile). Although analysis of these features assists in prediction of tumor behavior, there is considerable variability in the clinical course of disease, and appropriate treatment of bladder cancer that has invaded muscle or surrounding tissue (stages T2 to T4) is still controversial. The relative merits of radical radiotherapy, surgery, or a combination of both are the subjects of ongoing studies. Accurate preoperative staging is clearly valuable in making appropriate therapy decisions.

There are two major categories in the staging of bladder tumors: superficial tumors (stages Tis and T1), and invasive tumors (stage T2 and higher). The natural course and prognosis for the two groups are substantially different. In 80 per cent of cases, superficial tumors remain confined to the mucosa and submucosa (stage T1).[18] Occasionally, growth is entirely submucosal, and the mucosa remains intact (carcinoma in situ or stage Tis). Invasive tumors, however, exhibit spread at their initial presentation and are associated with a poor prognosis and propensity to metastasize. Clinical staging, either by the TNM or Jewett–Strong–Marshall system, has a relatively high error rate. In fact, the higher the tumor stage, the lower the clinical accuracy, and errors in as many as 50 per cent of cases have been reported.

MRI appearance

As illustrated in Figure 12.28, MRI can demonstrate benign tumors of the bladder. However, except for the tumor homogeneous appearance and smooth margin, there is no signal intensity pattern that can differentiate benign from malignant bladder lesions.

Bladder cancer on T1-weighted images usually demonstrates medium signal intensity, somewhat higher than the surrounding lower signal intensity urine.[19–25] T1-weighted images are optimal for the evaluation of tumor growth pattern and tumor size.

Table 12.1   Staging bladder carcinoma (see also diagram on opposite page)

TNM	American Urologic System	Histologic description	MRI criteria
Tis	0	Carcinoma in situ	NA
Ta		Noninvasive papillary carcinoma	
T1	A	Superficial limited to mucosa and submucosa	Stages A and B1 or T1 and T2 are diagnosed when the tumor is confined to the bladder wall with the outer bladder wall being of low signal intensity on T2WI
T2	B1	Superficial invasion of muscular wall	
T3a	B2	Deep invasion of muscular wall	Interruption of low signal intensity bladder wall on T2WI
T3b	C1	Perivesical fat invasion	Transmural extension with tumor extension to the perivesical fat on T1WI
T4	C2	Invasion of adjacent organs	Direct invasion of adjacent organs
N1	D1 (pelvic nodes)	Lymph node involvement	> 1.0 cm
M1	D2	Distant metastases	Distant metastases

NA = not applicable, too small for current resolution
T1WI = T1-weighted image
T2WI = T2-weighted image

Papillary tumor growth is illustrated in Figure 12.29. The large tumor protrudes into the urinary bladder and the surface of the tumor is irregular. The infiltrative type of the tumor growth demonstrates asymmetrical bladder wall thickening (Figure 12.30). As depicted in Figure 12.30, the tumor signal intensity is similar to the adjacent bladder wall on the T1-weighted image. However, as shown in Figure 12.31, the tumor demonstrates an increase in signal intensity (tumor signal intensity is higher than the normal bladder wall) on the T2-weighted image. Tumors often demonstrate both papillary and infiltrative tumor growth (Figure 12.32). Although detection of tumors as small as 0.5 cm, as shown in Figure 12.33, is sometimes possible, lesions less than 1 cm are not reliably seen on MR images. On the T2-weighted scans bladder tumors show different degrees of enhancement. Sometimes they image with signal intensity similar to or higher than the surrounding urine, but their signal intensity can vary and can be considerably lower than that of adjacent urine. However, the T2-weighted image is always necessary for tumor staging, as the low signal intensity of the bladder wall is contrasted with the higher signal intensity of the tumor, allowing assessment of the depth of infiltration of the bladder wall.

MRI staging. MRI staging can follow either the TNM or the American Urologic System classifications (Table 12.1). It is difficult to differentiate tumors that are confined to the mucosa and submucosa (stage T1) from superficial invasion of the muscle wall (stage T2). Deep muscle invasion (stage T3a) is diagnosed when there is interruption of the low signal intensity bladder wall. Detection of perivesical fat invasion (stage T3b)

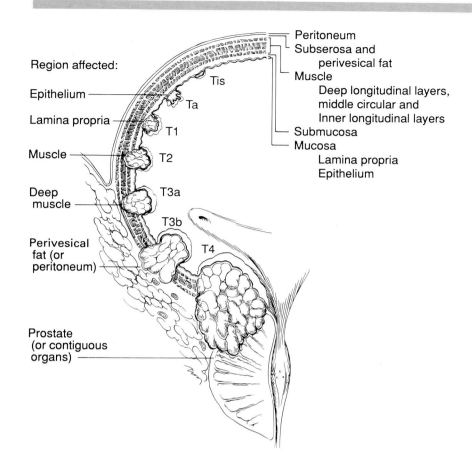

Region affected:

Epithelium

Lamina propria

Muscle

Deep muscle

Perivesical fat (or peritoneum)

Prostate (or contiguous organs)

Tis
Ta
T1
T2
T3a
T3b
T4

Peritoneum
Subserosa and
    perivesical fat
Muscle
    Deep longitudinal layers,
    middle circular and
    Inner longitudinal layers
Submucosa
Mucosa
    Lamina propria
    Epithelium

Diagram

Staging bladder carcinoma.

can be made on MRI scans (Figure 12.34). However, associated inflammatory changes may produce increased signal intensity on T2-weighted images, and false positive results can therefore occur. If the outer low signal intensity muscle layer is intact, no perivesical extension is present. The higher the stage of the tumor, the more accurate the MRI findings.

MRI evaluation of lymph node invasion by bladder carcinoma relies on detection of enlarged nodes (regional nodes larger than 1–1.5 cm are considered abnormal), and malignant nodes cannot be differentiated from hyperplastic ones. MR detection of local invasion, however, should raise the suspicion of lymph node invasion and alert the clinician to the need for lymph node sampling.

Administration of gadolinium-DTPA appears to improve accuracy in tumor detection (via selective enhancement of tumors) (Figure 12.35) and in differ-

entiating stages T2 and T3a from stage T3b. Differentiation between scar tissue and tumor is often, but not always, facilitated because tumor tissue is enhanced after Gd-DTPA administration and scar tissue is usually not. Organ infiltration is also more clearly seen on contrast-enhanced scans. Differentiation between edema and tumor is not facilitated by contrast enhancement. If gadolinium enhancement is used, only early postgadolinium sections should be obtained because the bladder wall enhances on delayed scans.

MRI in relation to other imaging modalities

The diagnosis of bladder cancer is made clinically, based on history (usually including hematuria), cystoscopy, and biopsy. Despite reports of relatively high accuracy rates for tumor detection by radiologic modalities, there is no role for radiologic diagnosis (Figure 12.36) or assessment in the early stages of disease, and radiologic assessment is reserved for the staging of more advanced disease. For staging of superficial disease (stages Tis and T1), biopsy and transurethral bladder resection are usually the only procedures needed. For evaluation of the upper urinary tract, IVU should be performed. For evaluation of suspected stage T2 or more advanced disease, either CT or MRI are recommended.

The overall staging accuracy for MRI, as for CT, varies widely. The accuracy for MRI has been reported to be as high as 90 per cent[23] and as low as 64 per cent.[20] The overall staging accuracy for CT ranges similarly, from 64–92 per cent.[26] CT accuracy in detecting perivesical extension is between 65 per cent and 85 per cent.[27] The use of CT, therefore, renders improved radiation port planning and facilitates the use of computerized dosimetry.[13] CT is also sometimes preferred over MRI because it is more widely available and more physicians are familiar with it. MRI and CT have similar accuracy rates (70–95 per cent) for lymph node detection. On MRI, similar to CT, the differentiation between the hyperplastic and malignant nodes is not possible. The nodal signal intensity change is nonspecific. When the nodes are calcified as illustrated in Figure 12.37, MRI renders lower specificity than CT. However, the advantages of MRI as compared to CT include: (1) better tissue contrast resolution—MRI is therefore better suited for differentiating stage T1–T3a disease from stage T3b or greater; and (2) multiplanar imaging. MRI therefore permits better evaluation of tumors located at the bladder base or dome, whereas CT is limited to direct imaging in the transaxial plane.

Carcinoma of the female urethra

Primary carcinoma of the female urethra is an uncommon lesion (accounting for less than 0.02 per cent of all female malignancies) which usually occurs in women over the age of 40.[28–30] The majority of tumors (40–75 per cent) are squamous cell carcinomas, and the next most common types are transitional cell carcinoma and adenocarcinoma.[28,31,32] Metastatic disease of the urethra also occurs, and melanoma is among the more common primary tumors metastasing to the urethra.[33]

Clinical diagnosis of urethral carcinoma is difficult. Patients often present with symptoms mimicking those of chronic urinary tract infection, and a mass lesion may not be appreciated, even by an experienced clinician. Patients therefore often have advanced disease by the time of diagnosis.[28]

Important prognostic variables include tumor location, size, and stage. Although no statistical correlations have been made between staging and location of urethral tumors, lesions confined to the distal urethra are generally of a lower stage.[34] Once the location is determined, urethral carcinoma may be classified as either anterior (distal)—tumor confined to the distal third of the urethra—or posterior (proximal)—tumor involving the portion of the urethra close to the bladder neck.[29] Some authors classify tumors as 'entire' when any portion of the urethra other than the distal one-third is involved.[29] Tumor size (maximum tumor diameter) is another important factor in patient prognosis.[32] Classification of urethral tumors into those less than 2 cm, those 2–4 cm, and those greater than 4 cm has been suggested.[32]

Spread of urethral carcinoma is usually orderly and in centrifugal fashion, progressing from local extension to lymphatic spread and, finally, to distant metastasis. Local extension is to the periurethral adipose tissue, vagina, and bladder; with more extensive spread to the levator ani muscle, pubic symphysis, and vulva. Sites of lymphatic spread depend on the site of the primary urethral disease. Tumors in the distal third of the urethra spread to the inguinal nodes and then proceed to pelvic nodes. Tumors of the proximal urethra, however, are more likely to initially involve the pelvic nodes, including the obturator and external inguinal nodes. Distant metastases are uncommon at presentation and are reported to occur in 10–15 per cent of patients.[28,34]

MRI appearance

Although carcinoma of the urethra can be detected on MR scans, it is not possible to differentiate among the various malignant tumor types or between malignancy and benign granulation tissue (Figures 12.38 and 12.39).[8] On unenhanced T1-weighted images, as shown in Figure 12.38, the urethral lesions demonstrate low signal intensity and cannot be differentiated from the periurethral muscular layer or from the adjacent low signal intensity anterior wall of the vagina. On T2-weighted images, however, tumors image with increased signal intensity and disrupt the target-like appearance of the normal urethra. Urethral tumors demonstrate signal enhancement following injection of gadolinium-DTPA.

MRI staging. Location, size, and tumor spread can be identified by MRI. Because prognosis for carcinoma of the female urethra depends mainly on the stage of disease rather than on tumor histology, accurate assessment by MRI is clinically useful. MR offers a new and promising imaging approach which can provide information valuable in planning surgical and/or radiation therapy. An MRI tumor classification

Table 12.2 MR staging system modified from Grabstald and associates[29]

	MR stage	MR finding
Q	In situ (limited to mucosa)*	Normal urethra, or on T2WI,
A	Submucosal (not beyond submucosa)	low SI of central urethral dot not seen
B	Muscular (infiltrating periurethral muscle)	On T2WI, the zonal anatomy is distorted and the outer muscular ring is partially or completely of high SI
C	Periurethral	Extension beyond outer muscular ring, with extension to adjacent fat, vagina, bladder, or other tissue
C1	Infiltration of muscular wall of the vagina*	On T2WI, interruption of low signal intensity anterior vaginal wall
C2	Infiltration of vaginal wall and mucosa*	
C3	Spread to other adjacent structures (such as bladder, labia, clitoris)	Extension into bladder or other structures such as labia and clitoris evident by direct tumor invasion and change of SI
D	Metastases	Invasion of the fat best seen on T1WI
D1	Involvement of inguinal lymph nodes	Inguinal nodes > 1.5 cm
D2	Spread to pelvic nodes, below aortic bifurcation	Pelvic nodes > 1 cm bifurcation
D3	Lymph node, above aortic bifurcation	Retroperitoneal nodes > 1 cm
D4	Distant metastasis	

T2WI = T2-weighted image, T1WI = T1-weighted image, SI = signal intensity
*MRI cannot separate stage 0 and stage A and stages C1 and C2.

has been developed from the pathologic staging system proposed by Grabstald (see Table 12.2).[29] When the inner muscular ring is preserved, the tumor does not extend beyond the muscular wall (stage B or less). Early (stage B) disease is sometimes overstaged by MRI because the complete low signal intensity ring of the periurethral muscular layer cannot be detected, and infiltration of the vaginal wall cannot be excluded.

Stage C disease is diagnosed when anterior spread through the periurethral muscular layer (and eventual obliteration of fat posterior to the pubic symphysis) is detected, as shown in Figure 12.40. Tumor spread into periurethral adipose tissue is best seen on T1-weighted images and is always accompanied by complete tumor extension through the periurethral striated muscle, resulting in an increase in the signal intensity of the muscle. Stage C2 disease, infiltration of the vaginal wall and tumor extension into the vagina, can be inferred from loss of the normal low signal intensity wall on T2-weighted images. However, false positive interpretations can result from increased signal intensity due to inflammatory changes. If the vaginal wall retains its low signal intensity, noninvasion can be determined with 100 per cent accuracy. Classification of stage C3 disease is based on direct extension of a proximally located urethral tumor into the urinary bladder. As illustrated in Figure 12.41, bladder invasion is seen as a large tumor bulk extending across the bladder neck with thickening of the bladder wall and increased signal on T2-weighted images. The low signal posterior vaginal wall remains intact. False positive findings of bladder invasion can also result from increased signal related to inflammatory changes.

The identification of stage D (metastatic disease) is based on finding enlarged lymph nodes. Lymphadenopathy is best detected with a combination of T1- and T2-weighted axial images, but the degree of lymphadenopathy may be underestimated.

MRI in relation to other imaging modalities

Present radiologic studies provide rather poor evaluation of urethral carcinoma. Primary lesions may be detected by urethrography, but this method fails to evaluate local spread of disease and does not add to the information gained at cystourethroscopy. CT has been used to evaluate local tumor spread, but the difficulty in differentiating urethra from vagina has been a limitation. CT is further limited in the evaluation of the bladder base, both because the tumor and bladder wall have similar CT density and because the bladder base is difficult to evaluate in the axial plane. Few data are available on ultrasound evaluation for urethral carcinoma, probably because of the difficulty in transabdominal scanning of a structure located just posterior to the pubic symphysis. Endovaginal scanning may circumvent this problem. Evaluation of lymphadenopathy has been attempted by both CT and lymphangiography, but again, limited data are available in the literature.

MRI can play an important role in the evaluation of urethral carcinoma, especially in staging. The value of MRI in detecting urethral tumors is limited because benign granuloma and malignant tumor have similar MRI appearances. Once urethral carcinoma is diagnosed, however, MRI is useful in demonstrating tumor size and location, and in the assessment of tumor spread. The excellent tissue contrast offered by MRI allows signal intensity changes (not just anatomic distortion caused by mass effect) to be used in determining the extent of lesions. Secondly, the ability to image in multiple planes makes MRI particularly useful in evaluating craniocaudal or anteroposterior tumor spread.

MR is highly accurate (90 per cent) in the evaluation of direct tumor extension, with a positive predictive value of 80 per cent and a negative predictive value of 83 per cent in the detection of tumor spread into periurethral adipose tissue. In the evaluation of vaginal wall invasion MRI accuracy is 73 per cent, with a positive predictive value of only 25 per cent. Negative predictive value is 100 per cent. The negative predictive value for bladder invasion is also 100 per cent, and the positive predictive value is 75 per cent.[8]

In summary, MRI evaluation of tumor extent has excellent negative predictive values, but overestimation of tumor extent and lower positive predictive values result from the inability to differentiate among tumor, edema, and inflammation.[8]

Recurrent bladder carcinoma

The management of bladder cancer depends primarily on the stage of the disease and also on tumor growth pattern, degree of differentiation, and whether the lesion is single or multiple. In situ bladder tumors are frequently treated with transurethral resection or fulguration. When papillary, many of the lesions can be controlled locally with conservative therapy in more than 80 per cent of cases. However, when the lesions are more infiltrative and are less differentiated, a recurrence rate of more than 50 per cent has been reported. If the carcinoma in situ is multifocal and diffuse, a combination of adjunct chemo- or radiation therapy is advised. The role of radiology in all of these patients is minimal and patient follow-up is usually by cystoscopy. Partial cystectomy is an attractive alternative for carefully selected patients with a small yet invasive solitary tumor. Following selection criteria, segmental resection is appropriate for only 5 per cent of patients with bladder cancer. Surgical seeding at the time of a partial cystectomy is a consideration and preoperative radiotherapy (in the form of a minimum dose of 1000–2000 rads) is recommended. Patient follow-up is by cystoscopy and flowcytometry, but in selective cases cross-sectional imaging is important. The most aggressive surgical treatment for invasive lesions that have penetrated into the muscularis is radical cystoprostatectomy in men or anterior exenteration in women. When properly selected, failures of radical cystectomy are usually due to distant metastases, in fewer than 10 per cent of patients do local recurrences occur. Radiation therapy and chemotherapy alone or as a combination regimen are today gaining in popularity. Although surgical extirpation has been the mainstay of treatment, therapy combining radiation and chemotherapeutic agents may help to reduce overall mortality from distant metastases and result in an improved long-term disease-free survival rate.

MRI appearance

Following partial cystectomy, localized bladder wall thickening can be seen. On T1-weighted images, asymmetrical bladder wall thickening is detected and that region usually exhibits low signal intensity on the T2-weighted image (Figure 12.42). However, various signal intensities have been reported and because these patients are usually seen after cystoscopy followed by biopsy, it is sometimes difficult to differentiate postbiopsy changes from a small residual tumor. As seen in Figure 12.43, the biopsy site may sometimes bleed, and MRI is not able to differentiate a blood clot at the site of biopsy from a blood clot in the residual underlying tumor, MRI is, however, helpful when surgical seeding following partial cystectomy is present. As seen in Figure 12.44, the recurrent tumor is seen at the bladder base and its anterior wall. There is a soft tissue mass in the anterior abdominal wall at the site of surgical incision. The mass exhibits high signal intensity while the scar tissue is of low signal intensity. As seen in Figure 12.45, following transurethral bladder tumor resection the recurrent tumor is at the base of the bladder and shows full depth anterior bladder wall invasion. Following chemotherapy, MRI can be used to follow the change in tumor response, mainly by following its size (Figure 12.46). The value of MRI following radiation therapy is discussed in Chapter 14.

MRI in relation to other imaging modalities

The exact role of magnetic resonance in the study of recurrent bladder tumors and the relation of MRI to other modalities, mainly CT, remains to be established. CT will detect the recurrent tumor when the tumor projects as a tumor mass, but has difficulties in differentiating asymmetrical bladder wall thickening from a recurrent lesion. Furthermore, when the recurrence occurs at the dome or the base of the bladder, CT limitations in the transverse plane of imaging present a drawback. CT is, however, helpful in following the response to chemotherapy. The advantages of MRI in the study of recurrent bladder tumors are similar to those in the assessment of primary lesions and consist of excellent soft tissue contrast combined with multiplanar imaging and, therefore, the ability to display lesions at the dome or the base of the bladder. As far as tissue specificity is concerned MRI, like CT, is accurate in the diagnosis of recurrence when the tumor projects as an intraluminal mass, but in infiltrative or very small lesions, the tumor recurrence can mimic postsurgical and postbiopsy changes.

References

1 LIERSE W, Chapter IV, Urinary bladder. In: *Applied Anatomy of the Pelvis*, (Springer-Verlag: Berlin 1987) 146–59.

2 WILLIAMS PL, WARWICK R, DYSON M et al, eds. *Gray's Anatomy*, (Churchill Livingstone: New York 1989) 1416–21.

3 FRIEDLAND GW, DE VRIES PA, NINO-MURCIA M et al, Congenital anomalies of the urinary tract. In: Pollack HM, *Clinical Urography*, (WB Saunders: Philadelphia 1990) 559–77.

4 MAXIMOW AH, BLOOM W, *A Textbook of Histology*, 4th edn. (WB Saunders: Philadelphia 1946).

5 KRANTZ K, The anatomy of the urethra and anterior vaginal wall, *Am J Obstet Gynecol* (1951) **62**:374–86.

6 CARLILE A, DAVIES I, RIGBY A et al, Age changes in the human female urethra: a morphometric study, *J Urol* (1988) **139**:532–5.

7 FISHER MR, HRICAK H, CROOKS LE, Urinary bladder MR imaging, *Radiology* (1985) **157**:467–70.

8 HRICAK H, SECAF E, BUCKLEY D et al, MRI in female urethra, *Radiology* (1990) (in press).

9 RETICK AB, BAUER SB, Bladder and urachus. In: Kalalis PP, King LR, eds. *Clinical Pediatric Urology*, (WB Saunders: Philadelphia 1976) 557–64.

10 BLICHERT-TOFT M, KOCH F, NIELSEN DV, Anatomic variants of the urachus related to clinical appearance and surgical treatment of urachal lesions, *Surg Gynecol Obstet* (1973) **137**:51–4.

11 BERMAN SM, TOLIA BM, LAOR E et al, Urachal remnants in adults, *Urology* (1988) **31**:17–21.

12 ROSEN L, HODDICK WK, HRICAK H et al, Urachal carcinoma, *Urol Radiol* (1985) **7**:174–7.

13 WALSH PC, GITTES RF, PERLMUTTER AD et al, *Campbell's Urology*, 5th edn. (WB Saunders: Philadelphia 1986) 1444.

14 GREENBERG M, STONE D, COCHRON ST et al, Female urethral diverticula: double-balloon catheter study, *AJR* (1981) **136**:259–64.

15 FOWLER JE JR, PULASKI ET, Excretory urography, cystography and cystoscopy in the evaluation of women with urinary tract infections, *New Engl J Med* (1981) **304**:462.

16 OTNES B, Correlation between causes and composition of urinary stones, *Scand J Urol Nephrol* (1983) **17**:93.

17 SILVERBERG E, LUBERA J, Cancer statistics, 1989, *CA* (1989) **39**:3–20.

18 RAGHAVAN D, SHIPLEY WU, GARNICK MB et al, Biology and management of bladder cancer, *New Engl J Med* (1990) **322**:1129–38.

19 FISHER MR, HRICAK H, TANAGHO EA, Urinary bladder MR imaging. II. Neoplasm, *Radiology* (1985) **157**:471–7.

20 AMENDOLA MA, GLAZER GM, GROSSMAN HB et al, Staging of bladder carcinoma: MRI-CT-surgical correlation, *AJR* (1986) **146**:1179–83.

21 RHOLL KS, LEE JKT, HEIKEN JP et al, Primary bladder carcinoma: evaluation with MR imaging, *Radiology* (1987) **163**:117–21.

22 BARENTSZ JO, LEMMENSS JAM, RUIJSS SHJ et al, Carcinoma of the urinary bladder: MR imaging with a double surface coil, *AJR* (1988) **151**:107–12.

23 KOELBEL G, SCHMIEDL U, GRIEGEL J et al, MR imaging of urinary bladder neoplasms, *J Comput Assist Tomogr* (1988) **12**:98–103.

24 BUY J-N, MOSS AA, GUINET C et al, MR staging of bladder carcinoma: correlation with pathologic findings, *Radiology* (1988) **169**:695–700.

25 TAVARES N, DEMAS BE, HRICAK H, MR imaging of bladder neoplasm, *Urol Radiol* (1990) **12**:27–33.

26 HODSON NJ, HUSBAND JE, MACDONALD JS, The role of computed tomography in the staging of bladder cancer, *Clin Radiol* (1979) **30**:389–95.

27 SAGER EM, TALLE K, FOSSA S et al, The role of CT in demonstrating perivesical tumor growth in the preoperative staging of carcinoma of the urinary bladder, *Radiology* (1983) **146**:443–6.

28 BRACKEN R, JOHNSON E, MILLER C et al, Primary carcinoma of the female urethra, *J Urol* (1976) **116**:118–92.

29 GRABSTALD H, HILARIS B, HENSCHKE U et al, Cancer of the female urethra, *JAMA* (1966) **197**:835–42.

30 HUISMAN AB, Aspects of the anatomy of the female urethra with special relation to urinary continence, *Contrib Gynec Obstet* (1983) **10**:1

31 PETERSON D, DOCKERTY M, UTZ D et al, The peril of primary carcinoma of the urethra in women, *J Urol* (1973) **110**:72–5.

32 JOHNSON D, O'CONNELL J, Primary carcinoma of the female urethra, *Urology* (1983) **21**:42–5.

33 NISSENKOM I, SERVADIO C, AVIDOR I et al, Malignant melanomas of female urethra, *Urology* (1987) **29**:562–5.

34 BENSON R, TUNCA J, BUCHLER D et al, Primary carcinoma of the female urethra, *Gynecol Oncol* (1982) **14**:313–8.

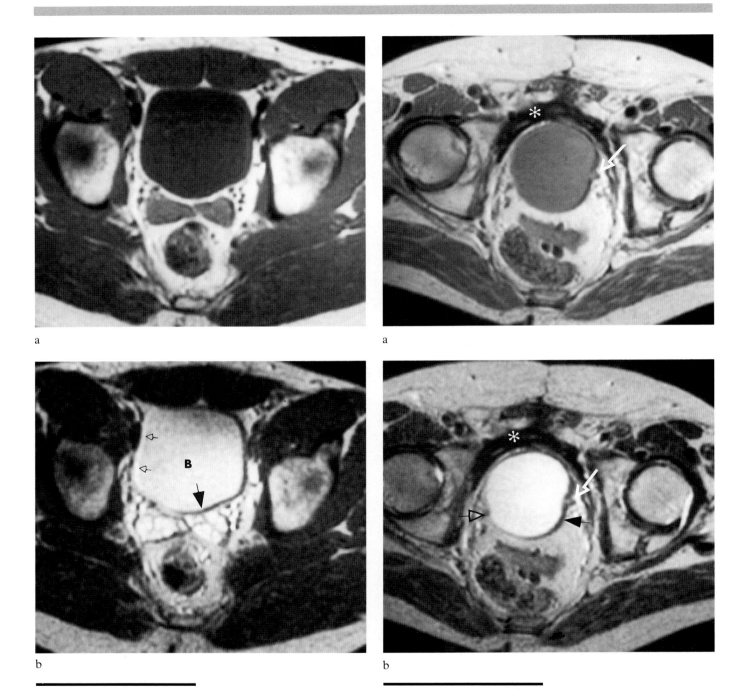

a

b

a

b

Figure 12.1

Normal urinary bladder, transaxial image. (**a**) T1-weighted and (**b**) T2-weighted images. On the T1-weighted scan, both the bladder wall and urine within the bladder image with low signal intensity. On the T2-weighted image, the contrast between the low signal intensity bladder wall (arrow) and high signal intensity urine (B) is enhanced. Chemical-shift artifact accentuates or decreases (open arrows) the bladder wall thickness.

Figure 12.2

Chemical-shift artifact on the transaxial image. (**a**) Proton density and (**b**) T2-weighted images. The polarity of the gradient readout results in a low signal intensity band along the left lateral wall (solid arrow) and a high signal intensity stripe along the right lateral wall (open black arrow) of the bladder. (Open white arrow)-small bladder diverticulum; (asterisk)-postsurgical fibrosis.

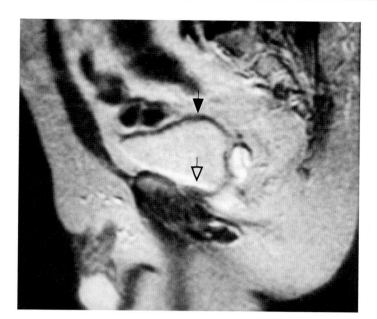

Figure 12.3

Chemical-shift artifact in the sagittal plane. The chemical-shift artifact causes low signal intensity along the dome of the bladder (solid arrow) and high signal intensity along its base (open arrow).

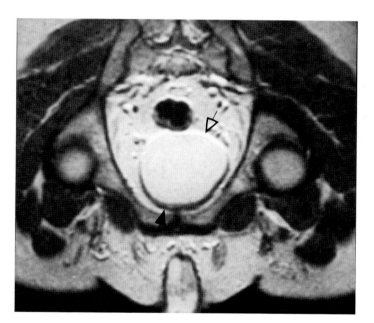

Figure 12.4

Chemical-shift artifact in an oblique coronal plane. Low intensity band (solid arrow) at the base of the bladder and high signal intensity band (open arrow) along its dome.

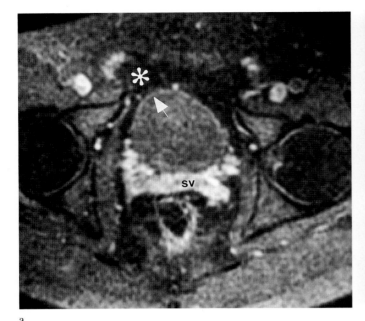

a

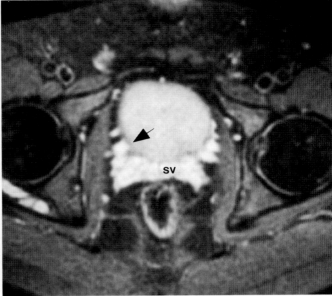

b

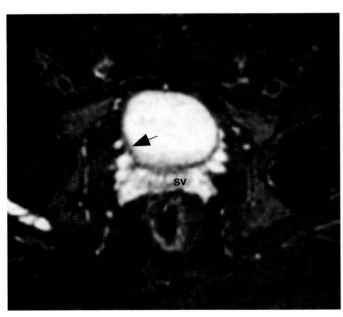

c

Figure 12.5

Normal urinary bladder on fat-saturation images. (**a**) T1-weighted, (**b**) proton density and (**c**) T2-weighted images. On the T1-weighted image, the wall of the urinary bladder (solid white arrow) is of slightly higher signal intensity than the adjacent lower intensity urine or adipose tissue (asterisk). On the proton density and the T2-weighted images, the bladder wall (solid arrow) images with low signal intensity and is well seen when contrasted to the outer high signal intensity of vesicoprostatic plexus or seminal vesicles (SV). Note that the fat-saturation technique diminishes the chemical-shift artifact.

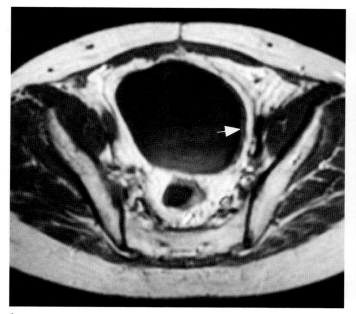

a

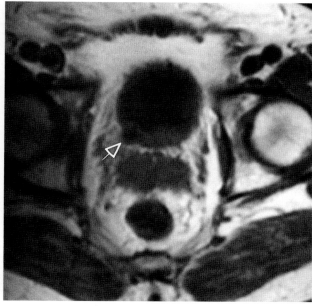

a

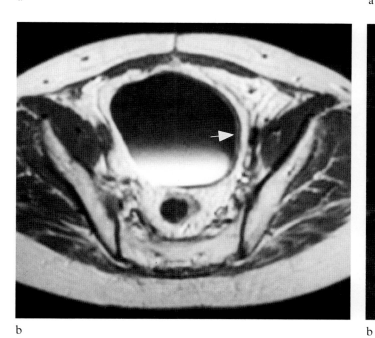

b

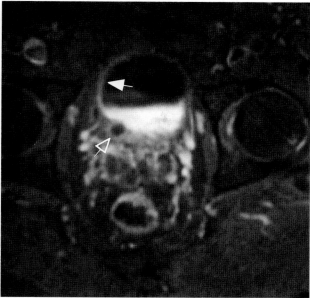

b

Figure 12.6

Appearance of the normal urinary bladder following Gd-DTPA injection. (**a**) Immediate and (**b**) delayed postcontrast T1-weighted images. The wall of the urinary bladder (solid arrow) is of medium signal intensity on the immediate postcontrast scan, but enhancement of the bladder wall (solid arrow) is seen on the delayed postcontrast scan.

Figure 12.7

Appearance of the urinary bladder on combined gadolinium-DTPA-enhanced and fat-saturation image. (**a**) Conventional T1-weighted spin-echo image, (**b**) gadolinium-DTPA-enhanced fat-saturation image demonstrating enhancement of the wall (solid arrow) of the urinary bladder. The wall of the dilated right distal ureter (open arrow) shows enhancement as well.

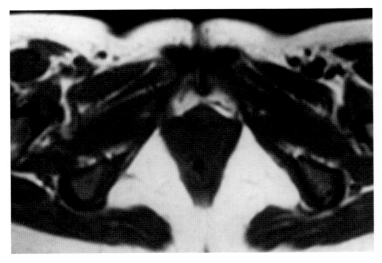

a

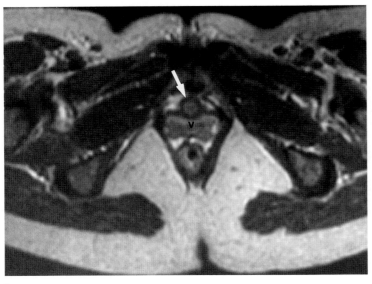

b

Figure 12.8

Normal female urethra transaxial (**a**) T1- and (**b**) T2-weighted images. On the T1-weighted image, the zonal anatomy of the urethra is not seen but on the T2-weighted image the zonal anatomy of the urethra with the lower signal intensity outer ring (long arrow), higher signal intensity submucosa and low signal intensity central dot is well appreciated. Also seen is clear separation between the urethra and the anterior wall of the vagina (V).

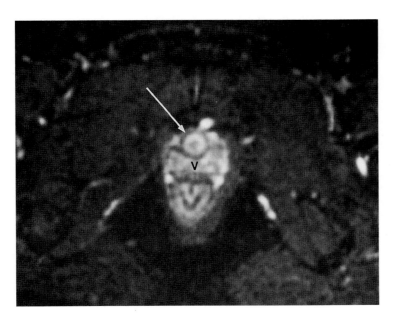

Figure 12.9

Normal urethra. Transaxial plane fat-saturation T2-weighted image. The zonal anatomy of the urethra with differentiation between the low signal intensity outer ring (long white arrow) and the high signal intensity submucosa is clearly visualized, as is the separation between the urethra and the vagina (V).

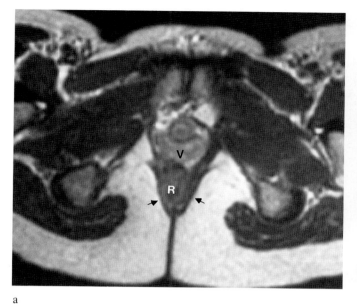

a

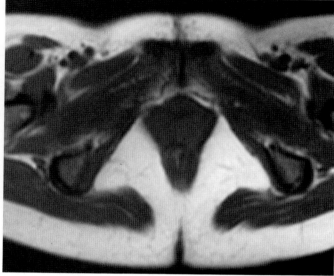

a

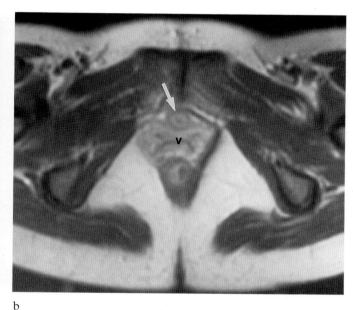

b

b

Figure 12.10

Comparison in appearance of the urethra between two T2-weighted images: (**a**) conventional spin-echo image and (**b**) fat-saturation image. All the instrument parameters (TR = 2000, TE = 70) are identical between the two images. The zonal anatomy of the urethra, vagina (V), and rectum (R) is well seen. On the fat-saturation image, marked enhancement of the periurethral and perivaginal areolar tissue and veins of Santorini (open white arrow) is seen. Also note that the thickness of the levator ani muscle (small arrows) on the fat-saturation image is of identical width on the right and left side while on the regular spin-echo image, due to the chemical-shift artifact, an uneven artificially produced thickness is seen.

Figure 12.11

Normal urethra following gadolinium-DTPA injection. (**a**) T1-weighted nonenhanced image and (**b**) T1-weighted gadolinium-enhanced image. The zonal anatomy of the urethra is seen following gadolinium injection. (Long arrow)- outer low signal intensity ring; (V)-vagina.

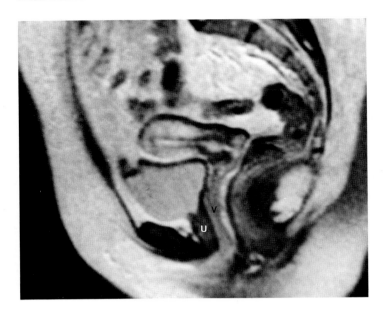

Figure 12.12

Sagittal T2-weighted image. The urethra (U) images with a lower signal intensity than the posteriorly located vagina (V). While the length of the urethra is well seen, the zonal anatomy is not appreciated.

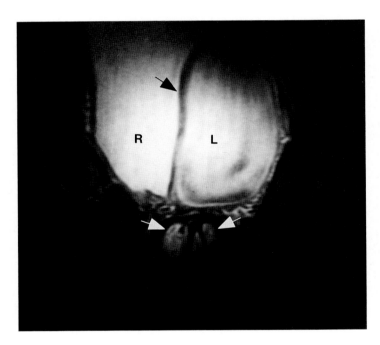

Figure 12.13

Bladder duplication, coronal T2-weighted image. The wall of the urinary bladder on the right (R) is similar in signal intensity and thickness to the wall of the urinary bladder on the left (L). The septum (arrow) between the two halves of the bladder is also of low signal intensity, and it demonstrates greater thickness, as in this patient the septum consisted of two layers of the bladder wall. The patient had two urethras and duplication of the penis (white arrows).

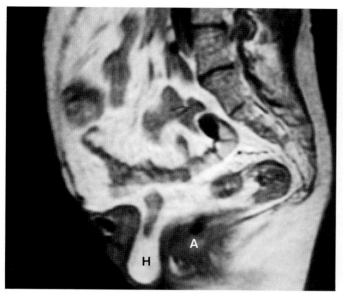

a

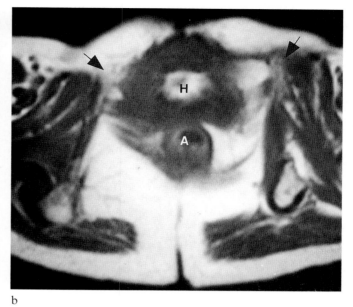

b

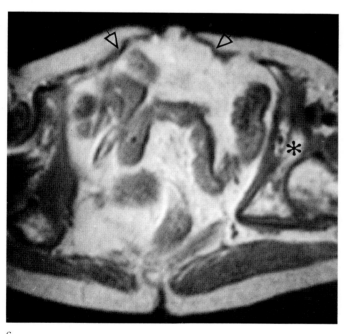

c

Figure 12.14

Bladder exstrophy. Proton density (**a**) sagittal, (**b**) and (**c**) transaxial scans; (**b**) at the level of the symphysis pubis and (**c**) 2 cm cranially. Status postcystectomy. (H)- postoperative hernia. The short perineum in the anal canal (A) postioned anteriorly can be seen. Also visible is the widening of the symphysis pubis (black arrows) and malrotation of the pelvic bones (asterisk). The rectus abdominis muscles (open arrows) are underdeveloped and separated.

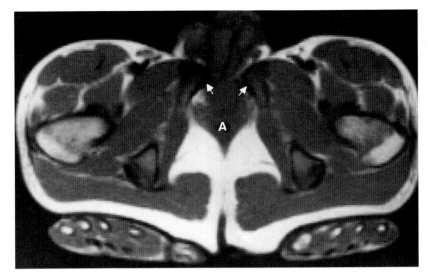

a

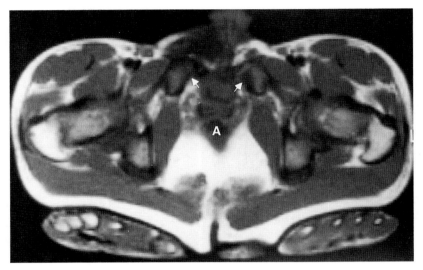

b

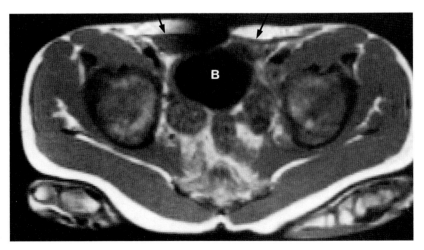

c

Figure 12.15

Bladder exstrophy, serial transaxial T1-weighted images. (**a**) At the level of the bulb of the penis, (**b**) at the level of the prostate gland, and (**c**) through the urinary bladder. There is a separation of the pubic bones (white arrows). The perineum is short and the anus (A) is displaced anteriorly. In this patient the bladder (B) was reconstructed. Note the asymmetrical development of the rectus abdominis muscle (black arrows).

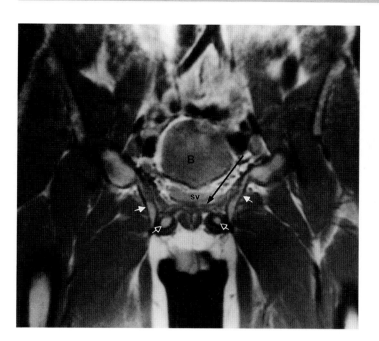

Figure 12.16

Classic bladder exstrophy with epispadias and increased separation of the pubic bones. Coronal proton density image. The urinary bladder (B) was reconstructed. The pubic bones (solid white arrows) are separated and there is separation of the corpora cavernosa (open arrows). Chordee (long black arrow), a classic finding in epispadias complex, is also seen. The seminal vesicles (SV) lie inferior and anterior to the bladder base.

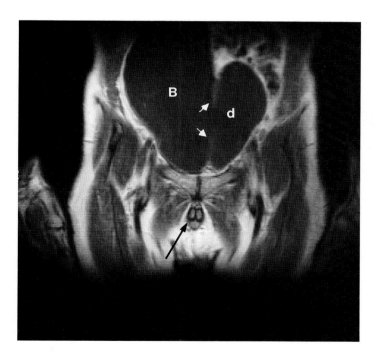

Figure 12.17

Bladder diverticulum. T1-weighted image, coronal plane of section. In this patient the thickness of the wall of the bladder (B) and the diverticulum (d) was similar and on imaging findings alone the differentiation between bladder duplication and the diverticulum is not possible. No urethral anomalies of the urethra or penis (long arrow) are identified. The site of the communication between the bladder and diverticulum (small white arrows) is also seen. (0.35T.)

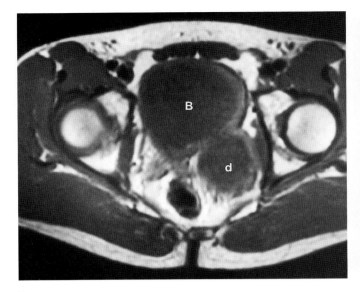

a

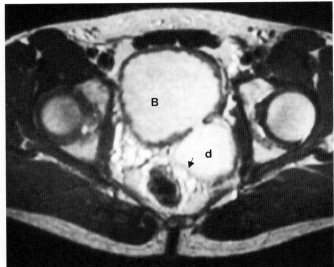

b

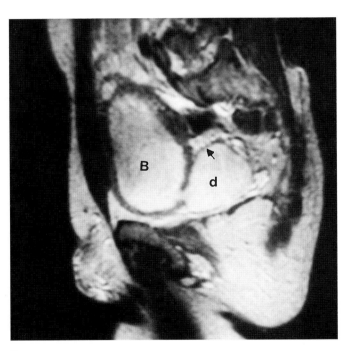

c

Figure 12.18

Hutch's diverticulum.
Transaxial (**a**) T1-weighted and
(**b**) T2-weighted images. (**c**)
Sagittal T2-weighted image.
The urinary bladder (B) has a
thick wall which is of low signal
intensity on the T2-weighted
image. The inner surface of the
bladder wall shows marked
irregularity. The diverticulum
(d) has a thin low signal
intensity wall (black arrow).
The lateral and posterior
location of this diverticulum is
the cause of the bladder outlet
obstruction.

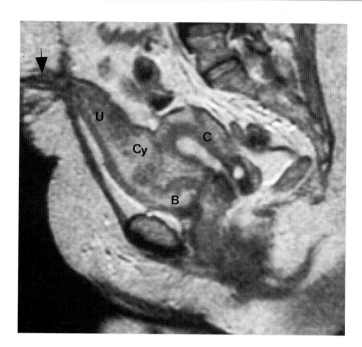

Figure 12.19

Urachal cyst which communicated to the umbilicus, causing a urachal sinus. Sagittal plane, T2-weighted image. The urachal cyst (Cy) is seen at the dome of the urinary bladder (B). (C)-corpus uteri. The urachal tissue (U) above the cyst extends to the umbilical drainage catheter.

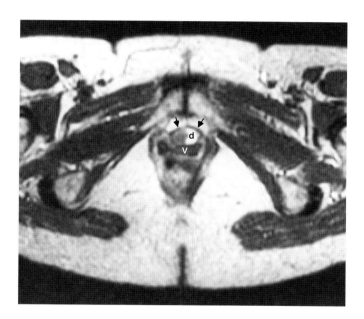

Figure 12.20

Urethral diverticulum as seen on the transaxial T2-weighted image. Urethral diverticulum (d) is seen as a high signal intensity fluid collection within the submucosal region of the urethra. The outer muscular wall of the urethra (arrows) remains of low signal intensity. (V)-vagina.

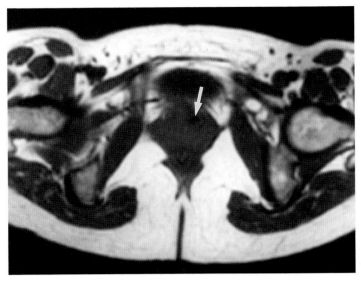

a

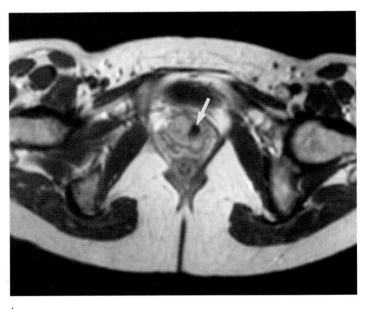

b

Figure 12.21

Appearance of a urethral diverticulum following gadolinium injection. Transaxial (**a**) T1-weighted nonenhanced and (**b**) T1-weighted gadolinium-DTPA enhanced images. On the nonenhanced image, a low signal intensity diverticulum (arrow) within the urethra is identified. Following gadolinium injection, the urethra enhances in signal intensity while the diverticulum (arrow) remains of low signal intensity, confirming the diagnosis of urethral diverticulum.

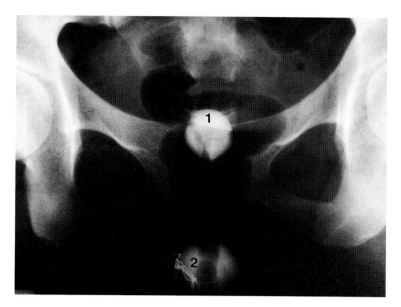

a

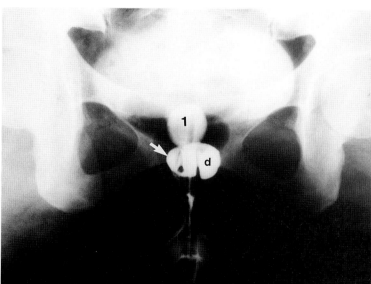

b

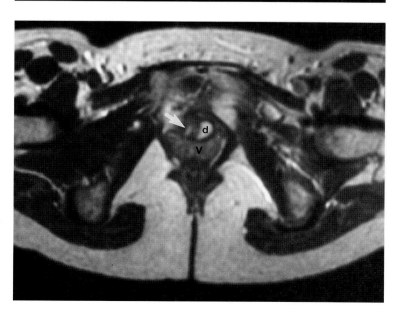

c

Figure 12.22

Bilateral urethral diverticula demonstrated by the double-balloon catheter technique and transaxial T2-weighted imaging. (**a**) The double-balloon catheter in place, (**b**) administration of the contrast media with double-balloon catheter in place, and (**c**) transaxial T2-weighted MR image. Urethral diverticula to the left (d) and to the right (arrow) are seen on each side of the urethral lumen. (V)-vagina; (1)-balloon inflated at the bladder base; (2)-balloon inflated at the urethral meatus.

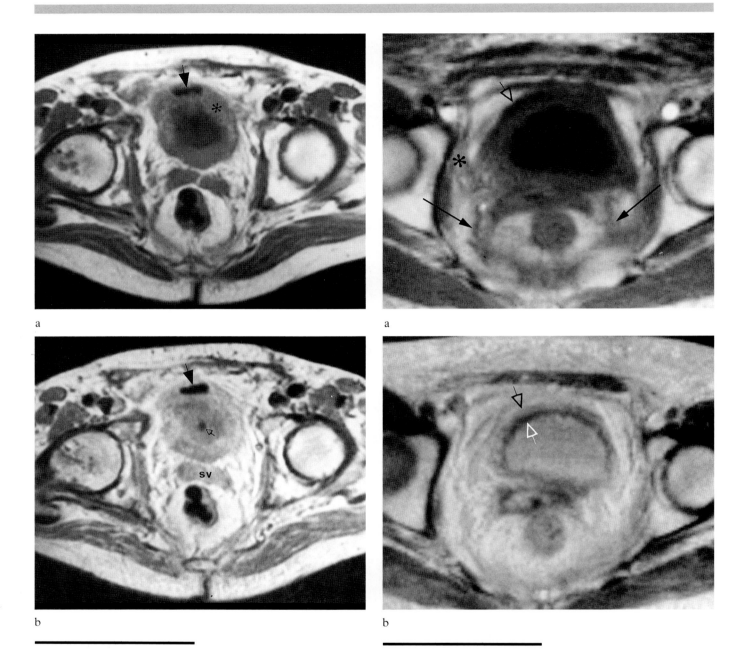

a

b

a

b

Figure 12.23

Emphysematous cystitis, transaxial (**a**) T1-weighted and (**b**) T2-weighted images. On the T1-weighted image, the bladder wall (asterisk) is thick and it is of heterogeneous but somewhat high signal intensity. The air (black arrow) within the bladder wall can be seen. On the T2-weighted image the inflamed bladder wall demonstrates a heterogeneous increase in signal intensity. (Small open arrow)-Foley catheter; (SV)-seminal vesicles.

Figure 12.24

Radiation cystitis. Transaxial (**a**) T1-weighted and (**b**) T2-weighted images. Extensive radiation changes in the subcutaneous fat (asterisk), thickening of the pelvic fascia (long arrows) and infiltration of the presacral fat are visualized. The bladder wall (black open arrow) is thickened. On the T2-weighted image, the outer bladder wall thickening increases in signal intensity while the low signal intensity stripe is seen in its inner surface (white open arrow). The findings are characteristic for radiation cystitis. (0.35T.)

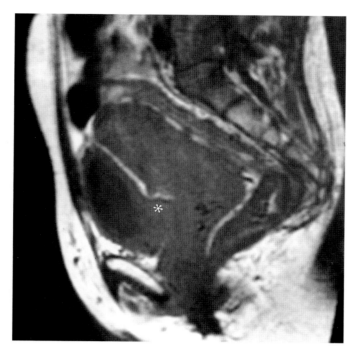

a

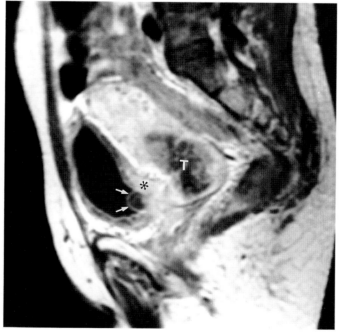

b

Figure 12.25

Radiation cystitis with formation of bullae. Sagittal (**a**) T1-weighted image, (**b**) gadolinium-enhanced T1-weighted image. The bladder wall (asterisk) is thickened and demonstrates enhancement following Gd-DTPA injection. Bullous formation (arrows), especially on the gadolinium-enhanced image, is well demonstrated. (T)-large necrotic carcinoma of the cervix.

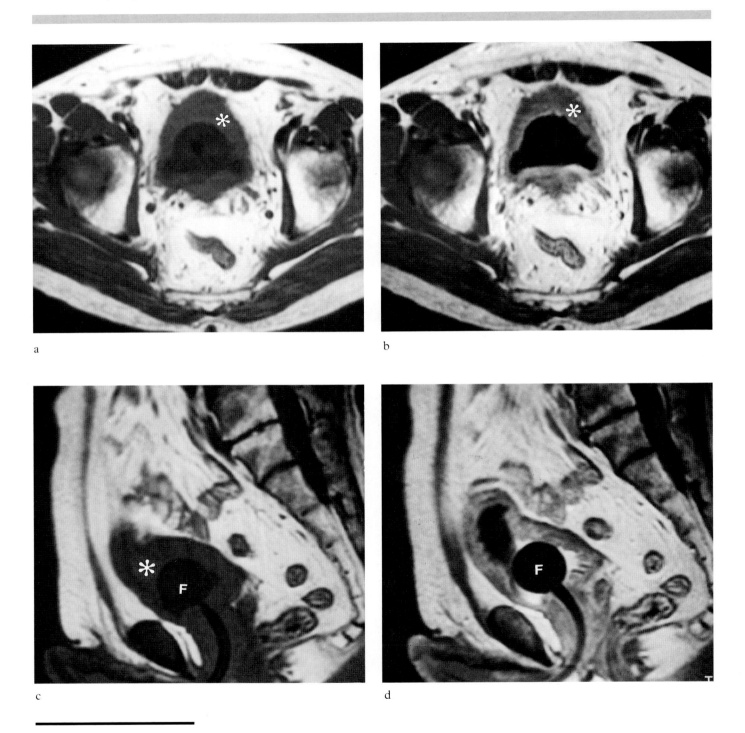

a   b   c   d

Figure 12.26

Bladder inflammation due to a longstanding indwelling urethral catheter. Transaxial (**a**) T1-weighted and (**b**) gadolinium-enhanced T1-weighted images; sagittal (**c**) T1-weighted and (**d**) gadolinium-enhanced T1-weighted images. The bladder wall (asterisk) is thickened with irregularity of its inner surface. Following gadolinium injection, the bladder wall shows heterogeneous signal enhancement. (F)-Foley catheter balloon.

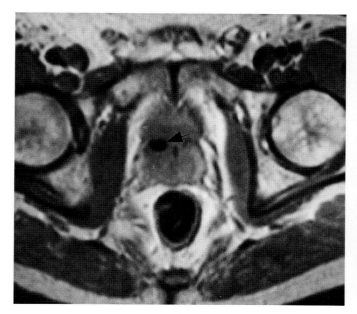

a

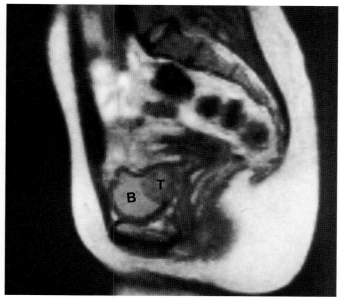

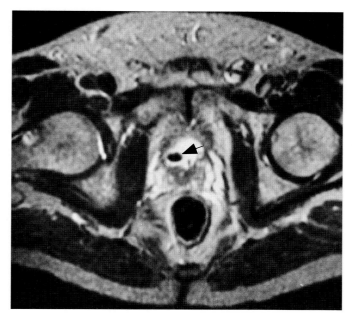

b

Figure 12.28

Benign leiomyoma of the urinary bladder, sagittal T2-weighted image. A smoothly marginated papillary tumor (T) is seen protruding within the lumen of the urinary bladder (B). The tumor is of homogeneous signal intensity. (0.35T.)

Figure 12.27

Bladder calculus located at the base of the bladder. Transaxial (**a**) proton density and (**b**) T2-weighted images. The area of the signal void within the urinary bladder (black arrow) is identified on both the proton density and the T2-weighted images. In correlation with plain X-ray films, this represents a bladder calculus. The signal void on MRI, however, could also be due to air, although the air would be in a more anterior position as opposed to the calculus which is in a dependent location due to gravity.

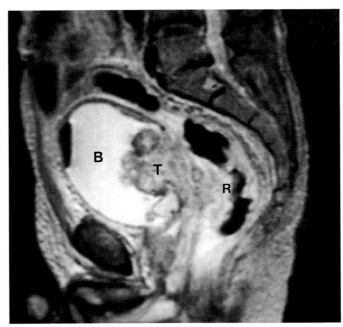

a

Figure 12.29

Sarcoma—papillary tumor growth. (**a**) Sagittal T2-weighted, (**b**) transaxial T1-weighted and (**c**) transaxial T2-weighted images. The tumor (T) in the urinary bladder (B) has a large intraluminal papillary component with irregular margins. There is deep mural invasion of the bladder wall and the tumor also involves the seminal vesicles (SV). Therefore, this is a stage T4 transitional cell carcinoma. High signal intensity of the obturator internus muscle (asterisks) and the wall of the rectum (R) are due to severe acute radiation injury (see Chapter 14).

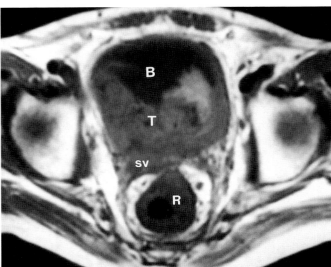

b

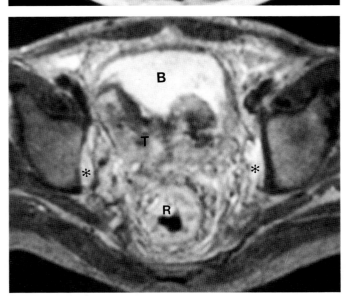

c

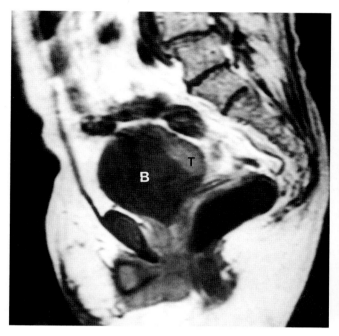

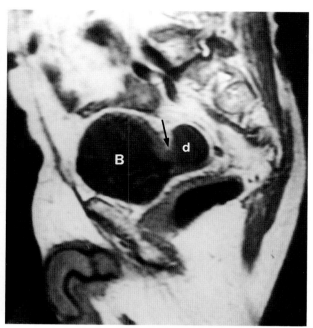

a

b

Figure 12.30

Infiltrative growth pattern of a transitional cell carcinoma. T1-weighted sagittal images (**a**) midline and (**b**) to the left of the midline. Asymmetrical bladder wall thickening indicates presence of an infiltrative tumor (T). The tumor extends (arrow) into the diverticulum (d). (B)-urinary bladder.

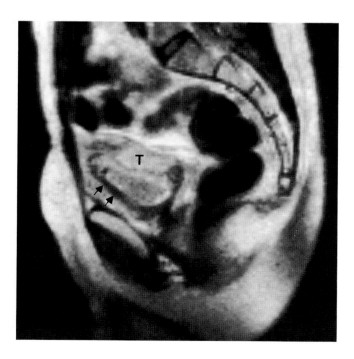

Figure 12.31

Infiltrative type of tumor growth as seen on a T2-weighted image. There is asymmetrical bladder wall thickening along the dome and the posterior wall of the bladder. The large tumor (T) demonstrates high signal intensity on the T2-weighted image in contrast to the low signal intensity of the normal bladder wall (arrows). (0.35T.)

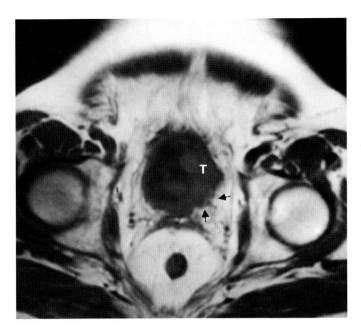

a

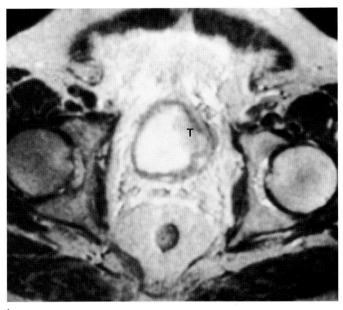

b

Figure 12.32

Papillary and infiltrative tumor growth in a transitional cell carcinoma, stage T3b. (**a**) T1-weighted image, (**b**) T2-weighted image. The tumor (T) along the left lateral wall of the bladder shows both papillary (intraluminal) as well as infiltrative tumor growth. The perivesical fat (small black arrows) is infiltrated, indicating deep muscular invasion and tumor extension into the perivesical region. On the T2-weighted image (**b**) irregular interruption of the normal low signal intensity bladder wall is seen.

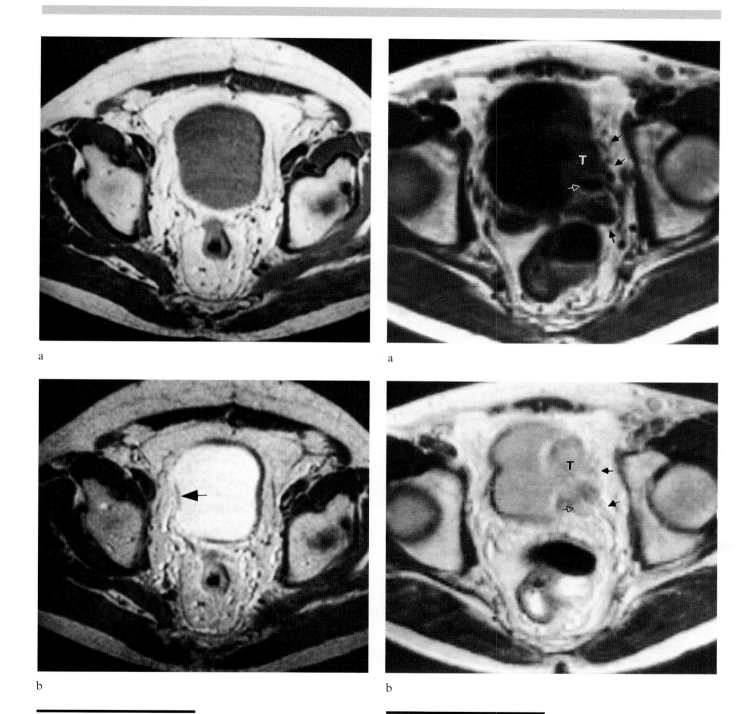

a

b

a

b

Figure 12.33

Small (less than 5 mm in width) infiltrative tumor along the right lateral bladder wall. Transaxial (**a**) proton density and (**b**) T2-weighted images. On the proton density image, no abnormality can be identified. On the T2-weighted image, a localized area of low signal intensity along the right lateral bladder wall (arrow) corresponded to the infiltrative tumor type seen at cystoscopy. No perivesicular spread has occurred, indicating the tumor to be stage T3a or less. The tumor was stage T2 only, no deep invasion of the muscular wall was present. Because of the chemical-shift artifact, the assessment of muscle invasion along the right lateral side is difficult in this transaxial plane of imaging.

Figure 12.34

Stage T3b bladder carcinoma. (**a**) T1-weighted and (**b**) T2-weighted images. A large tumor (T) is seen along the left lateral aspect of the bladder. The tumor exhibits full bladder wall invasion and there is also infiltration of the perivesical fat (small solid arrows). The left ureter is dilated (open arrows). The distal part of the ureter was invaded.

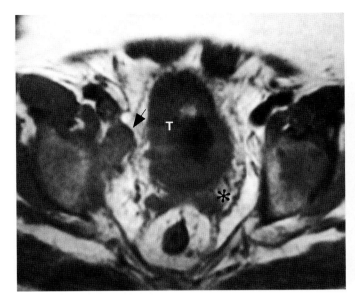

a

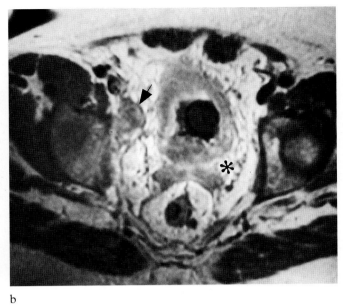

b

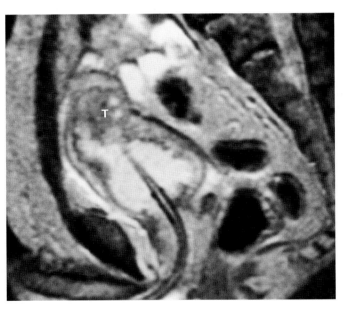

c

Figure 12.35

Transitional cell carcinoma, stage T3a N1. Infiltrative type tumor (T) growth. Transaxial (**a**) T1-weighted image, (**b**) gadolinium-enhanced T1-weighted image, and (**c**) sagittal T2-weighted image. The bladder wall is thickened and shows a heterogeneous increase in signal intensity on the T2-weighted image and enhancement following gadolinium injection. The perivesicular fat (asterisk) is infiltrated and shows enhancement following gadolinium injection. However, only inflammatory reaction was present at histology. (Black arrows)-enlarged nodes of the posterior external iliac chain.

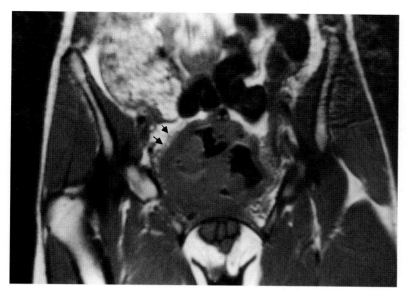

a

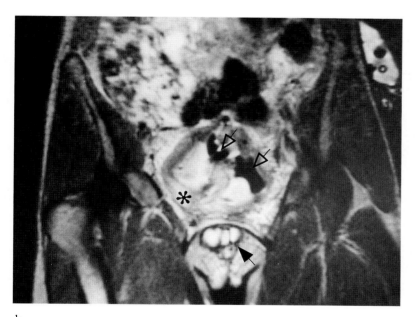

b

Figure 12.36

Extensive postsurgical inflammatory reaction, mimicking tumor on the MRI study. Coronal (**a**) proton density and (**b**) T2-weighted images. In this patient with penile duplication (large black arrow) and congenital duplication of the bladder, bladder unification was performed. Four days after surgery, the patient was in acute retention due to blood clots. The MRI image shows a markedly thickened bladder wall, which on the T2-weighted image demonstrates increased signal intensity (asterisk). The urine is highly proteinaceous–bloody, and images with medium signal intensity on the T1- and high signal intensity on the T2-weighted image. There is air within the bladder (open arrows). Based on the MR imaging findings, the differentiation between the inflammatory region and tumor is not possible. Furthermore, there is perivesical infiltration (small black arrows) with increased signal intensity on the T2-weighted image.

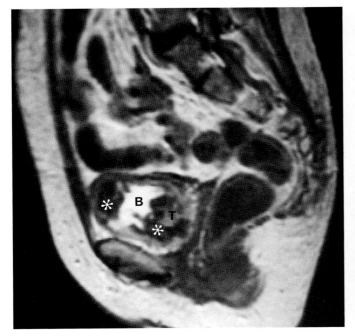

a

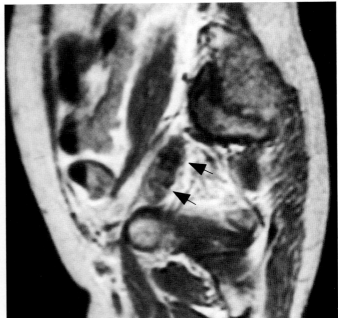

b

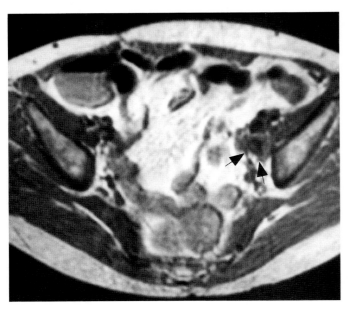

c

Figure 12.37

Primary osteogenic sarcoma of the urinary bladder with lymph node metastasis. Sagittal Gd-DTPA-enhanced images (**a**) at the level of the urinary bladder and (**b**) at the level of the external iliac vessels on the left; (**c**) transaxial T1-weighted image. Dilute Gd-DTPA in the urinary bladder (B) is visible. A heterogeneous low (asterisks) and medium signal intensity tumor (T) is seen. Enlarged nodes of the posterior external iliac chain nodes (arrows) also demonstrate low signal intensity foci. At surgery, the low signal intensity in the bladder and the nodes were found to be calcifications.

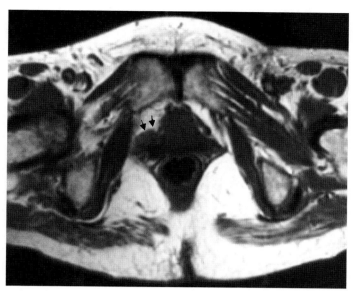

a

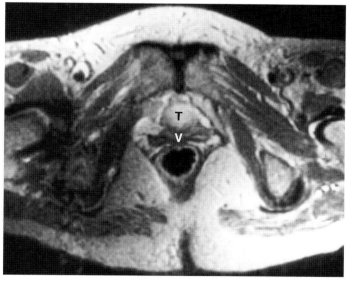

b

Figure 12.38

Urethral tumor–melanoma. Transaxial (**a**) T1-weighted and (**b**) T2-weighted images. The urethra is expanding and on the T2-weighted image, the zonal anatomy is not visualized. The urethral tumor (T) exhibits high signal intensity. There is also perivaginal (arrows) tumor extension. (V)-vagina.

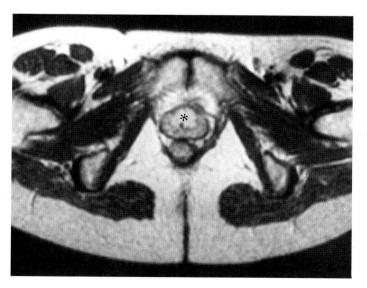

Figure 12.39

Chronic inflammation–granulation involving the urethra. Transaxial T2-weighted image. The urethra is enlarged, the zonal anatomy is not seen and the high signal intensity area (asterisk) mimics tumor. The anterior wall of the vagina is not seen and it was expected that the tumor is invading the anterior wall of the vagina. Only benign granulation tissue was seen following multiple biopsies.

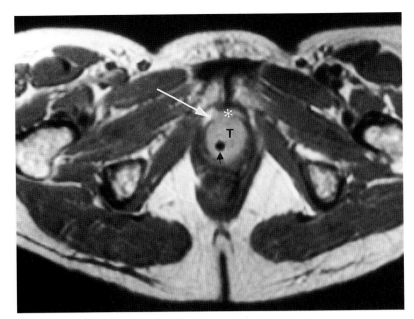

a

Figure 12.40

Stage C carcinoma of the urethra. Transaxial (**a**) proton density and (**b**) T2-weighted images. The urethra is expanded by tumor (T) which demonstrates heterogeneous high signal intensity on the T2-weighted image. The tumor extends beyond the muscular wall of the urethra anteriorly (arrow) and is seen infiltrating the retropubic fat (asterisk). (Black arrow)-Foley catheter.

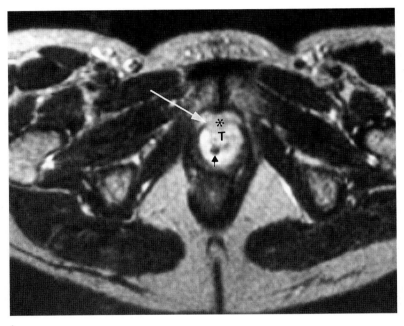

b

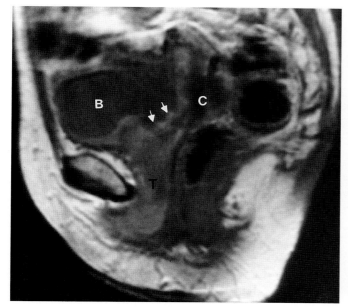

a

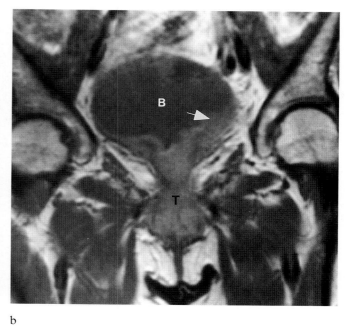

b

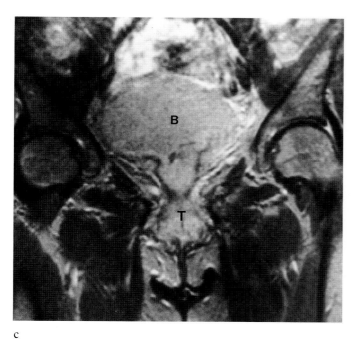

c

Figure 12.41

Urethral tumor with extension into the urinary bladder. (**a**) Sagittal proton density image, (**b**) coronal proton density image, and (**c**) coronal T2-weighted image. The urethra is expanded by a large tumor (T), extending along the entire length of the urethra. (B)-urinary bladder; (C)-uterine cervix. The tumor extends through the bladder base, along the posterior bladder wall (small white arrows) and predominantly along the left lateral wall (large white arrow). On the T2-weighted image, the complete invasion of the bladder wall along the left side is visualized.

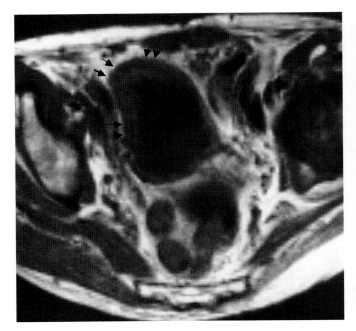

a

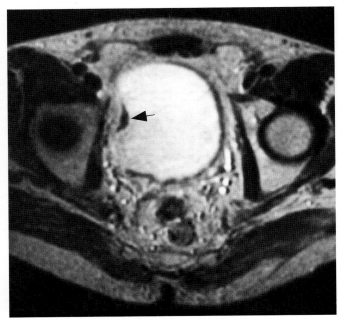

Figure 12.43

Status postpartial cystectomy, and recent cystoscopy with biopsy. Transaxial T2-weighted image. There is a localized low signal intensity area at the right lateral aspect of the bladder (arrow). This may represent a blood clot secondary to recent biopsy, but underlying tumor cannot be excluded.

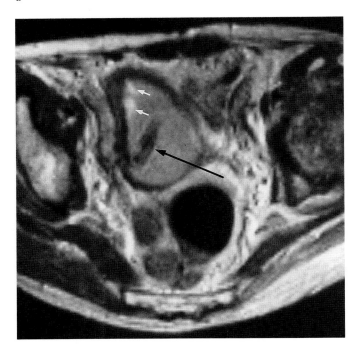

b

Figure 12.42

Bladder following partial cystectomy. (**a**) T1-weighted and (**b**) T2-weighted images. There is an asymmetrical localized bladder wall thickening (black arrows) demonstrating decreased signal intensity on the T2-weighted image. However, at the mucosal surface, there are high signal intensity areas (white arrows), and based on the MRI findings, differentiation between recurrent tumor and postbiopsy edema cannot be made. The patient had cystoscopy with biopsy two days before the MRI study. (Arrow)-Foley catheter.

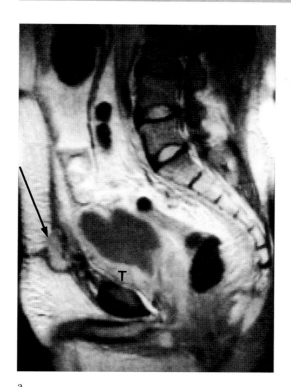

a

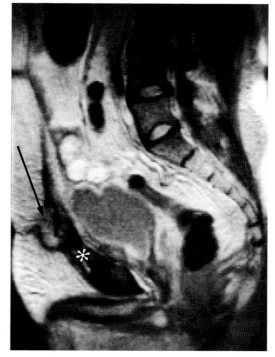

b

Figure 12.44

Recurrent bladder cancer following partial cystectomy with seeding along the surgical tract. Sagittal (**a**) proton density and (**b**) T2-weighted images. The bladder tumor (T) demonstrates irregular asymmetrical bladder wall thickening on the T1-weighted image, but the tumor exhibits relatively low signal intensity on the T2-weighted image. The tumor (long arrow) in the anterior abdominal wall is of high signal intensity on the T2-weighted image. Seeding is suggested from the MRI study. The postsurgical scar (asterisk) is of low signal intensity. (0.35T.)

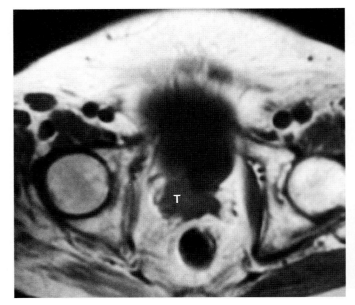

a

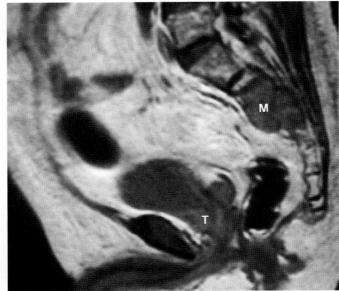

b

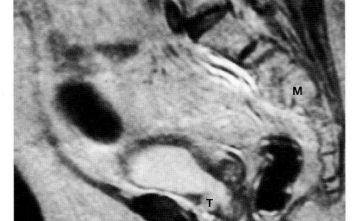

c

Figure 12.45

Recurrent bladder carcinoma following transurethral bladder resection. (**a**) Transaxial T1-weighted, (**b**) sagittal T1-weighted and (**c**) sagittal T2-weighted images. The patient also received radiation therapy. There is a tumor mass (T) at the right bladder base. The tumor exhibits high signal intensity on the T2-weighted image and demonstrates full thickness anterior bladder wall invasion. Also seen are radiation changes in the sacrum as well as bony metastases (M). Changes in the right obturator internus muscle are probably due to irradiation (see Chapter 14).

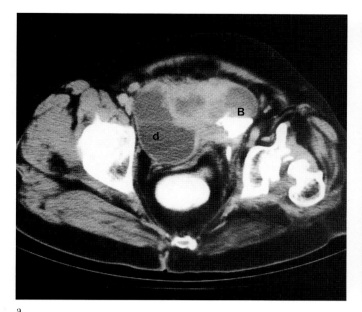

a

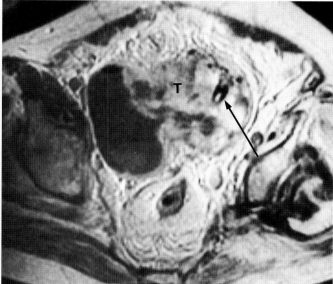

b

Figure 12.46

Transitional cell carcinoma.
Sequential scans following
chemotherapy. (**a**) CT scan, (**b**)
gadolinium-enhanced MRI
image at the time of diagnosis;
(**c**) coronal gadolinium-
enhanced T1-weighted image,
two weeks following
chemotherapy; and (**d**)
transaxial T2-weighted image
three months following
chemotherapy. A large tumor
in the urinary bladder enhances
on the CT scan as well as on the
MRI study. (Long arrow)-
Foley catheter; (d)-bladder
diverticulum; (B)-urinary
bladder. The tumor (T) is
decreasing in size following
therapy. The left kidney (K) is
obstructed and dilute
gadolinium is seen within the
renal pelvis (P). Three months
following therapy, the tumor
has markedly diminished in
size and only a small residual
tumor (T) at the junction
between the urinary bladder
(B) and the diverticulum (d) is
seen. The bladder has a thick
wall but is mostly of low signal
intensity.

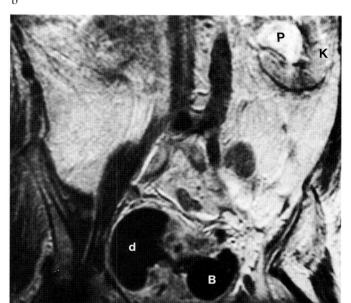

c

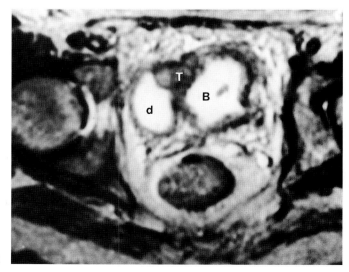

d

13
The Rectum and Sigmoid Colon

Hedvig Hricak

Barium sulfate enema and/or flexible sigmoidoscopy are the primary examinations used in the evaluation of the rectum and sigmoid colon.[1] Both are excellent modalities, showing the mucosal surface with exquisite detail. Sigmoidoscopy has the additional advantage of allowing biopsy of any suspicious lesions. The bowel wall cannot be evaluated with either of these techniques, however, and intra- or extramural pathologic changes are not depicted unless they are large enough to impinge upon the lumen.

With cross-sectional imaging modalities—endorectal ultrasound (ERUS),[1] computed tomography (CT), and magnetic resonance imaging (MRI)—intramural and extramural processes can be demonstrated.[2] With ERUS the individual layers of the bowel wall can be differentiated,[3,4] and this technique is currently being evaluated in many centers for its usefulness in staging rectal carcinoma. The wide field-of-view obtained with CT makes it superior for the demonstration of the bowel wall and the perirectal and perisigmoid tissue. Although the morphologic display with CT is excellent, CT does not offer tissue specificity[5] and lacks the contrast resolution needed to differentiate layers of the bowel wall. Its use in the staging of early cancer of the rectum is therefore limited. The variety of imaging sequences available with MRI provides excellent tissue contrast and allows detailed demonstration of the bowel wall.[6] In addition, multiplanar imaging is advantageous in the evaluation of congenital anomalies and in the assessment of the spread of inflammatory and neoplastic disease. With the use of intravascular and intraluminal gastrointestinal contrast media, MRI for examination of the sigmoid colon and rectum will become even more versatile.[7,8]

Normal anatomy of the rectum and sigmoid colon

The sigmoid colon and rectum are derived from the hind gut, except for the distal portion of the anal canal, which is derived from ectoderm.[9,10] The **sigmoid (pelvic mesenteric) colon** begins at the inlet of the lesser pelvis, where it is continuous with the descending colon, and terminates at approximately the level of the third segment of the sacrum, where it is contiguous with the rectum.[9] The sigmoid colon is an intraperitoneal structure which retains its mesentery. The sigmoid colon generally lies in the true pelvic cavity. When redundant, however, it may extend towards the umbilicus. This position is commonly found in infants. There are wide variations in the length of the sigmoid colon which is, on average, approximately 40 cm long. A redundant sigmoid colon predisposes to volvulus.

The point where the sigmoid colon joins the rectum (the **rectosigmoid junction**) forms an acute angle of varying degrees. Not only is this the narrowest portion of the colon, but it is fixed by the mesentery, and is therefore a frequent site of perforation from overinflation of unduly highly placed rectal balloons.[9]

The **rectum** is formed from the terminal portion of the colon. It begins at the level of the third segment of the sacrum and ends at the anus, as shown in Figure 13.1. Anatomically it is divided into two sections, the rectum proper (10–12 cm in length) and the anal canal (2.5–3 cm in length).[9] The rectum proper contains transverse folds, called the **valves of Houston.** Most frequently there are three of these valves, and the lowest one is usually located on the left side (Figure

13.2).[9] For surgical treatment purposes, the adult rectum is divided into three segments, each approximately 5 cm long, reflecting their arterial supply and lymphatic drainage.[1]

The rectum has no mesentery. The upper portion is totally surrounded by peritoneum. The dorsal part of the rectum, about 12.5 cm from the anus, is not covered by peritoneum. On the anterior and the lateral aspects of the rectum proper, the peritoneum extends to the fifth sacral or first coccygeal vertebra. The peritoneum reflects anteriorly to create the **rectovesical fossa** in the male and the **rectouterine fossa (pouch of Douglas)** in the female. The fascia of the rectum and prostate make up the **rectovesical fascia of Denonvillier** in the male and its equivalent, the **vaginal rectal fascia**, in the female. The lateral peritoneal recesses form the **pararectal spaces**, the right side of which descends lower than the left. The **ischiorectal fossae** are located laterally and form a cone shaped space with its apex pointing cephalad (Figure 13.2). Its lateral boundary consists of the obturator internus muscle and the medial border of the levator ani muscle.

The **anal canal** (the second portion of the rectum) as illustrated in Figure 13.3 is an extraperitoneal structure terminating at the anus, the external aperture of the colon. Descriptions of the anal canal vary, depending on whether the anatomic or surgical designation is being used. The upper margin of the surgical anal canal, reported to be 5–8 cm long, is the anorectal line. However, the upper margin of the anatomic anal canal, reported to be 2–3.5 cm long, is the linea pectinata, believed to be remnant of the proctodermal membrane.[9] The different upper margins account for the differences in reported length. The **levator ani muscle**, as shown in Figure 13.3 attaches laterally to the anal canal, and acts both as an important surgical landmark and as an accessory sphincter. It consists of three parts: the **iliococcygeus muscle**; the **pubococcygeus muscle**; and the **puborectalis muscle.** The iliococcygeus muscle has no relationship to fecal continence. Posteriorly it inserts into the anococcygeal raphe, into the lowest two sacral vertebrae, and into the coccyx. The pubococcygeus muscle is divided into two sections–the medial portion, which attaches to the longitudinal fibers of the rectum, and the lateral portion, which is continuous with the sacrum. The puborectalis muscle is also known as the sphincter muscle of the rectum. Unlike the iliococcygeus and pubococcygeus muscles, it forms a sling which encircles the upper portion of the rectum at the level of the anorectal line and pulls the rectum anteriorly. The puborectalis sling, therefore, demarcates the upper landmark of the surgical anal canal. The perirectal fascia begins at an angle between the levator ani and the internal sphincter muscle and ascends (cranially) cephalad to encircle the extraperitoneal part of the rectum, becoming gradually thinner as it merges with the subserosal connective tissue of the ampulla rectum. At its thickest portion it never exceeds 3 mm.[9]

Two sphincters surround the anal canal. The **internal anal sphincter** is a 2–3 mm thick ring, formed by the thickening of the circular fibers of the muscularis propria. The **external anal sphincter** is elliptical in shape with three concentric layers of striated muscle fibers; deep, superficial, and subcutaneous parts (Figure 13.3).[9]

Histologically, the sigmoid colon, like the rest of the colon, consists of the mucosa, the lamina propria, the muscularis mucosae, the submucosa, the muscularis propria, and, when present, the visceral peritoneum (serosa).[1] Adipose tissue, the subserosa, lies between the muscularis propria and serosa. The mucosa is composed of columnar epithelium and has many goblet cells, both on the surface and in the glands of Lieberkühn. The muscularis mucosae is a thin, smooth muscle layer. The submucosa contains many small vessels and is similar to the submucosa in the rest of the alimentary tube. The muscularis propria has a circular layer, and the longitudinal smooth muscle fibers are arranged in three bands called the **taeniae coli**.[9]

The histologic features of the rectum differ from those of the sigmoid colon. The serosa covers only the upper part of the rectum, and the longitudinal fibers of the muscularis form a continuous layer which is thicker anteriorly and laterally.[1,9] In the anal canal, the longitudinal muscle of the rectum lies adjacent to the internal sphincter and caudally thins out and diverges. The smooth circular muscle layer, as previously described, thickens to form the internal sphincter.

Vascular supply

The sigmoid colon is supplied by the sigmoid artery, a branch of the inferior mesenteric artery. The rectum has a dual blood supply from the inferior mesenteric and internal iliac arteries. The superior rectal (hemorrhoidal) artery, a branch of the inferior mesenteric artery, supplies the upper-third of the rectum. The middle and inferior rectal arteries, derived from the internal iliac artery, supply the middle- and lower-thirds of the rectum. In addition, blood is supplied to the anus and lower rectum via pudendal branches of the internal iliac artery. There are multiple anastomoses between the rectal arteries and in the distal 5 cm of the rectum. This rich arterial network of anastomotic vessels facilitates low rectal resection without the risk of vascular insult.

Venous drainage of the rectum parallels the arterial supply. The sigmoid veins and superior rectal veins drain via the inferior mesenteric vein into the portal circulation. The middle and inferior rectal veins drain via the internal iliac veins directly into the inferior vena cava. The distal portion of the rectum (5–7 cm), therefore, has a dual drainage (the superior rectal veins draining to the portal circulation and middle and inferior rectal veins draining to the pelvic veins). Therefore, distal rectal cancers can produce isolated pulmonary metastases.

Lymphatic drainage

Understanding the pathways of lymphatic drainage is essential in designing appropriate imaging approaches for staging cancer. The lymphatics of the colon are divided into intra- and extramural systems. The intramural lymphatics begin as a plexus in the submucosa where they follow blood capillaries proceeding through the muscularis propria and form a chain of lymph nodes along major blood vessels. Nodal groups along the sigmoid colon are called paracolic, and along the rectum they are known as pararectal nodes.[1] The lymphatics from the sigmoid colon and the upper-two segments of the rectum follow the inferior mesenteric artery to the **lumbar paraaortic lymph nodes.**[1,9,11,12] Lymphatics from the lower part of the rectum (approximately 7–8 cm above the anal verge) drain into the **obturator, internal,** and **common iliac nodes.**[1,9,11,12]

The regional nodes of the anus are the **superficial inguinal nodes.**[1,9,11,12]

MRI appearance

On T1-weighted images the bowel wall is of medium signal intensity. On T2-weighted images the appearance of the colon varies depending on its histologic features. When the sigmoid colon is distended, and the bowel wall thin, it images with medium signal intensity and the separate layers of the wall cannot be seen. As shown on Figure 13.4, the layers of the wall cannot be discerned in the distended rectal ampulla. However, the bowel wall is thicker in the lower rectum and the anal canal, and in these structures separation of the layers of the bowel wall is possible.

As illustrated in Figure 13.5, on T2-weighted images four separate layers of the bowel wall can be seen in the region of the anal canal.[6] The outside low signal intensity ring corresponds to the outer muscular layer (the muscularis propria). The next layer is an area of higher signal intensity, probably corresponding

to the submucosal region. Third is a low signal intensity inner ring, probably representing the muscularis mucosae and lamina propria; and fourth is a central area of high signal intensity, representing the mucosa with its goblet cells.

As shown in Figure 13.5, the bowel wall layers are also seen on Gd-DTPA contrast-enhanced T1-weighted images. Following Gd-DTPA injection, the muscularis propria and muscularis mucosae do not enhance, but the submucosa and inner mucosa do, allowing differentiation between the layers. The thick muscle of the external sphincter demonstrates low signal intensity on T2-weighted images or Gd-DTPA-enhanced T1-weighted images. Visualization of the bowel wall anatomy is further highlighted with fat suppression SE sequences. Using fat suppression technique, zonal anatomy of the anal canal (Figure 13.6) can be seen on nonenhanced proton density and T2-weighted images or, as shown in Figure 13.7, on Gd-DTPA-enhanced T1-weighted images.

The thickness of the bowel wall should be measured only when the bowel is distended. In the sigmoid colon and the rectal ampulla, it should not exceed 5 mm. In the anal canal the wall should not measure more than 10 mm.[9]

The anatomic relations among the rectum proper, the anal canal, the anus, and the surrounding muscular structures can be demonstrated on MR images. As shown in Figure 13.1, the rectum proper extends from S3 to the insertion of the levator ani muscle. The location of the levator sling is easily seen in the sagittal and coronal planes of imaging (Figure 13.1), but in the transaxial plane (Figure 13.8) sequential images need to be reviewed in order to identify the levator ani insertion. The anal canal is surrounded circumferentially by the internal (part of the wall) and external sphincters. Below the level of the transversus perinei superficialis muscle, the wall of the anal canal is surrounded by the subcutaneous portion of the external sphincter (Figure 13.8a). At the level of the transversus perinei superficialis muscle, the superficial part of the external sphincter is present (Figure 13.8b). The superficial part of the external sphincter is thick and it encircles the anal canal (Figure 13.8c). The deep part of the external sphincter becomes thinner cranially (Figure 13.8d). The puborectalis muscle can be seen just superior (cephalad) to the two sphincters, where it forms a sling posteriorly and laterally. The puborectalis muscle does not extend to the ventral portion of the rectal wall, another helpful landmark in locating it. The insertion of the pubococcygeal part of the levator ani is just cephalad to the puborectalis sling, and the muscle fibers (Figure 13.8f) are extending to the coccyx. The perirectal fascia, as illustrated in Figure 13.9, can be seen superior to the level of the levator ani. It is seen as a thin stripe of low signal intensity on both T1- and T2-weighted images.

Recommended imaging sequences

Whenever possible, the rectum and sigmoid should be cleansed with enemas before MRI examination.[13,14] As illustrated in Figure 13.10, retained fecal material cannot be differentiated from tumor. Preparation of the entire alimentary tube, however, is not necessary. Motion, either respiratory or bowel contractions, will degrade the image quality. The routine use of respiratory compensation, even when imaging the rectum, is advised (see Chapter 1). To minimize the motion artifact produced by bowel contractions, glucagon or similar antiperistaltic medications are recommended.[15] Antiperistaltic agents should be administered intramuscularly, in order to prolong their action.[15] In addition to decreased contractility, the antiperistaltic drugs also produce relaxation of the smooth muscle resulting in bowel distension. Air distension of the rectum has been suggested to further improve the evaluation of the bowel wall. As seen in Figure 13.4, the air insufflation in the rectum will distend the rectal ampulla but may induce motion artifacts and therefore degrade the image quality. For lesions in the anal canal however, air insufflation is not only unnecessary, but should not be used as it may hide the lesion. Imaging in the prone position has been suggested but is not essential.

Regardless of field strength, T1- and T2-weighted spin-echo sequences are recommended as the basic technique. T1-weighted images provide an excellent outline of the bowel wall, show intraluminal masses, and demonstrate changes affecting the extravisceral fat. T2-weighted images show tissue changes in the bowel wall (neoplastic and inflammatory), as well as showing better characterization of extracolonic masses.

Although indications for the use of intravenous Gd-DTPA (0.1 mmol/kg intravenously) are still being defined, the use of Gd-DTPA provides anatomic detail on T1-weighted images, and demonstrates enhancement of inflammatory changes and tumors. Because the use of Gd-DTPA allows excellent morphologic detail in shorter imaging time (as compared to T2-weighted images) it is recommended in sick patients or patients who will not tolerate long imaging time. The use of fat suppression techniques, with or without Gd-DTPA administration, is also still being investigated but is promising in improving signal-to-noise ratios and enhancing detail in imaging intra- and extramural pathology.

In addition to the development of intravascular contrast media, a number of intraluminal gastrointestinal contrast media are currently being tested. Two approaches are developing, 'positive' (high signal intensity on T1-weighted images) and 'negative' (low signal intensity on T1-weighted images) contrast agents, the merits of which are still debated.[7,8]

Imaging in the transaxial plane is essential and should always be performed. Imaging in the sagittal plane provides information on the anterior and posterior relationships of the rectum and sigmoid colon and allows measurement of pathological changes in the craniocaudal extension. Coronal plane images demonstrate the relationship of the levator ani muscle to the rectum, as well as changes in the perirectal fat. Oblique dorsal to ventral sections can be used to obtain a better cross-sectional view of the rectum and to simultaneously unfold the sigmoid loop. As shown in Figure 13.11, 35 degree oblique coronal views demonstrate exquisitely the anatomy of the anal canal, rectum and rectosigmoid region with display of surrounding muscles and fascias.

Pathology of the rectum and sigmoid colon

Congenital anomalies

Duplication

Eighty per cent of patients with colonic duplications have associated anomalies, most notably genital and bladder duplications. Duplications may involve the entire colon, from rectum to cecum, or only portions. There may even be two anal openings.[16]

MRI appearance.   The value of MRI in the evaluation of congenital duplications has not been documented. As illustrated in Figure 13.12, anomalies of the extraperitoneal (fixed) portion of the bowel can be delineated on noncontrast MR images. Anomalies of the intraperitoneal colon, however, are difficult to assess without the use of gastrointestinal contrast agents. The diagnosis of duplication of the rectum and adjacent bowel is made by demonstration of two lumens in the extraperitoneal location. Multiplanar imaging and the use of both T1- and T2-weighted images are helpful in identifying rectal pathology.

Stenosis and atresia of the rectum

The severity of anorectal malformations varies widely. Rectal stenosis occurs with varying degrees of severity. The level and the extent of the atresia also varies. It may be relatively mild, for example, a normal rectum with only a cutaneous septum occluding the anus, or quite severe, for example, obliteration of much or all of the rectum and a colon which ends in a blind pouch at varying distances above the anus. An atretic rectum may also be separated from an open, normally placed but hypoplastic anus.

It is the level of the atresia which governs the surgical approach to correction of anorectal anomalies. Historically, three types of atresia were described. Recently, however, the classification was simplified and the atresia were categorized into **supralevator** (high) and **translevator** (low) type.[18] Correction of supralevator atresia requires an initial colostomy followed by definitive repair in later infancy. Accurate identification of the level of the high atretic lesion is important since it will ensure the optimal placement of the colostomy (left iliac placement for intermediate lesions and transverse colostomy for very high lesions).[19] Correction of low, translevator atresia is accomplished by perineal anoplasty in the neonatal period. Approximately 50 per cent of all patients with anorectal anomalies have associated congenital anomalies including, but not restricted to, genitourinary anomalies, vertebral defects, esophageal atresia, and congenital heart disease.[19] In general, associated congenital anomalies are more commonly found with supralevator atresia. The fistulous tracts to the lower genitourinary tract or perineum are, however, rare with supralevator atresia but are found in 50–70 per cent of cases of low translevator atresia. The presence of the fistula is therefore often used as a reliable clinical sign of low atresia.[17–19]

In addition to the location of the atresia, another important factor affecting successful primary repair of an anorectal malformation is the degree of development of the sphincter and musculature available for reconstruction.[17] Although the inferior portion of the puborectalis muscle and the superior portion of the external anal sphincter are contiguous and inseparable on MRI scans, it is possible to locate these structures and evaluate their degree of development.

MRI appearance. The diagnosis of rectal atresia can be made with MRI, and the distance between the atretic rectal pouch and the anal dimple can be assessed.[20–25] As shown in Figures 13.13 and 13.14, the differentiation between translevator (Figure 13.13) and supralevator (Figure 13.14) types of atresia can be diagnosed. In the newborn, the presence of retained meconium (which images with medium signal intensity on T1-weighted scans and increases in signal intensity with T2-weighting) within the atretic section is a helpful anatomical landmark, as shown on Figure 13.14. The wall of the blind pouch is usually thick and images with low signal intensity on T2-weighted scans, allowing precise localization of the atretic stump. As illustrated in Figure 13.15, imaging in the sagittal plane provides the optimal measurement of the distance between the levator ani muscle and the distal end of the rectal pouch. Imaging in the coronal plane further aids in demonstrating the relations between the levator ani sling and the blind rectal end.

In the child in whom an initial colostomy has been performed, the presence of bowel content may present difficulties in the identification of the blind ending, and the use of gastrointestinal contrast such as corn oil, instilled through the colostomy to facilitate delineation of the distal end of the rectal pouch has been recommended.[20] As seen in Figure 13.15, imaging in both the coronal and sagittal plane provides sufficient information and this maneuver is often not necessary. The external sphincter and levator sling are well visualized on T2-weighted MR images and their measurements can be obtained on a combination of transaxial and coronal scans. Figure 13.16 illustrates the normal anal sphincter and puborectal strip in a 12-month-old boy, while Figures 13.15 and 13.17 demonstrate hypoplastic levator sling in an age matched 12-month-old boy.

MRI in relation to other imaging modalities

For many years lateral plain films with the infant inverted (feet held up) were advocated for evaluation of rectal atresia and stenosis. In this position air rises to the end of the blind rectum facilitating its visualization. However, meconium deposited at the bottom of the atretic rectum may falsely increase the distance from the blind end to the anal dimple marker. MRI provides considerably more information in the evaluation of these patients, and it has been advocated as an accurate tool in the assessment of these anomalies. Meconium, rather than leading to a misinterpretation of the extent of the lesion, is clearly visualized and can be used as a landmark. In addition, fistulas communicating with the urogenital tract may be identified with the use of contrast media and accompanying vertebral anomalies can be assessed with sagittal and coronal views. With the combined use of intracavitary contrast injection, which provides excellent tissue contrast, and direct multiplanar imaging, MRI may provide the optimal diagnostic approach. Its superiority over CT examination, especially with respect to the evaluation of the puborectalis muscle, has been reported.[22]

Inflammatory disease

The colon and rectum have a limited spectrum of tissue reactions to a host of noxious agents. These reactions range from the least severe consisting of submucosal edema with thicking of the wall, to more severe yet superficial ulcerations in addition to edema and wall thickening. Deeper ulcers produce localized areas of wall thickening and deep ulcerations, sinus tracts, fistulae and perirectal and pericolonic inflammatory masses and abscesses. The most severe reaction consists of toxic megacolon. The bowel is dilated, the wall is thickened and the mucosa is ulcerated or destroyed over large areas.

The radiologic evaluation can demonstrate these changes. The specific diagnosis, however, requires bacteriologic studies with stool cultures and serum antibody tests, detailed clinical history and often even biopsy obtained at endoscopy.

Chronic ulcerative colitis

Although ulcerative colitis is relatively common in the Western world, its cause is not known and the diagnosis is made on the basis of the exclusion of specific infectious organisms as causative factors. The disease process often begins in the rectum, and spreads to usually involve the entire left colon. Crypt abscesses are the histologic hallmark of early disease. As the abscesses enlarge, they erode the mucosal margins producing small ulcers. With extension of disease into the submucosa, the ulcers coalesce causing denudation of mucosa. Over time, thickening and fibrosis of the bowel wall are encountered. Since by definition the disease is superficial, fistulas and sinuses are not usually seen. These changes are nonspecific and are encountered in a host of infectious processes as well as in ischemic colitis. Malignancy, which is an infrequent complication of long standing disease, has been reported in left sided colitis, but is three to four times less frequent than in pancolitis.[26]

MRI appearance. In sporadic reports the MRI appearance of ulcerative colitis has been described as thickening of the bowel wall without evidence of pericolonic infiltration.[14] The signal intensity of the involved bowel wall on T2-weighted images varies depending on the acuteness of the disease. In acute colitis, the signal intensity increases. Following Gd-DTPA injection, the thickened bowel wall in the acute phase demonstrates enhancement (Figure 13.18). These MRI findings are, however, nonspecific and can be seen in a variety of inflammatory diseases.

MRI in relation to other imaging modalities. The double contrast barium enema, which shows ulcerations as well as the superficial granularity of the mucosa, is the examination of choice in ulcerative colitis. Any form of enema, including the double contrast, however, is **contraindicated** if clinical information and plain films of the abdomen suggest toxic megacolon.

CT and MRI do not contribute significantly to the diagnosis of this disease, nor are they useful in differentiating chronic ulcerative colitis from infectious forms of colitis. They may, however, be helpful in differentiating chronic ulcerative colitis from Crohn's disease.[27]

Crohn's disease (granulomatous colitis)

Crohn's disease, also of unknown etiology, usually, but not exclusively, affects individuals in the second to fourth decade of life. It is a systemic disease affecting multiple organs. The small bowel and colon are most often involved, but the entire gastrointestinal (GI) tract may be affected. Rectal involvement is less common than in chronic ulcerative colitis, but is more severe when it does occur. Up to 10 per cent of patients have anal and rectal fissures or sinuses, or fistulae to the perineum.[28]

By definition, the inflammatory process in Crohn's disease of the intestine (including the colon) is transmural, and deep ulcers proceed to the formation of sinuses and fistulas. Early in the course of the disease, however, there are small granulomatous and shallow aphthous ulcers. With more advanced disease, areas of severe involvement may alternate with areas of normal bowel. Abscesses are frequent, and the involved mesentery or mesocolon becomes thickened and permeated with fat as well as inflammatory tissue.[28]

MRI appearance. The value of MRI in Crohn's disease appears to be in the demonstration of the pericolonic extent of disease.[29] T1-weighted images allow delineation of the extension of the fistulas relative to adjacent organs and show fatty infiltration and inflammatory changes in the tissue surrounding the colon, as shown in Figure 13.19. T2-weighted images show increased signal intensity of the bowel wall, fluid collections within the fistulas, invasion of adjacent organs, and inflammatory muscle changes. Sinus tracts and the perirectal spread of fistulas with respect to the levator ani muscle can also be demonstrated.[29] Gd-DTPA contrast enhancement adds to the usefulness of MRI in the assessment of Crohn's disease. As illustrated in Figure 13.19, after Gd-DTPA administration acute inflammatory tissue is enhanced, increased vascularity of the region is demonstrated, and pericolonic fat infiltration is clearly visualized.

MRI in relation to other imaging modalities. The rectal and sigmoid changes of Crohn's disease are best identified with the double contrast barium enema.[30] Aphthous ulcers, sinuses, and fistulas are also clearly demonstrated by this approach.

CT is excellent for demonstrating sinus tracts, fistulas, and abscesses, particularly when water soluble iodine contrast media enemas are administered.[30] Nonenhanced or Gd-DTPA-enhanced MRI can be used to evaluate pericolonic extension of disease and, as seen in Figure 13.20, to demonstrate sinus tracts and abscesses. Infiltration of fat is clearly seen on T1-weighted images; and fat suppression sequences, supplemented by Gd-DTPA-enhanced MRI, may show the bowel wall changes to better advantage. MRI studies should be used as a complement to, not a substitute for, the barium enema.

Other types of colitis

In addition to chronic ulcerative colitis and Crohn's disease of the colon, numerous infectious and noninfectious inflammatory conditions may present with the same spectrum of pathologic and radiographic changes.

Ischemic colitis involves the rectum only infrequently and the sigmoid colon more often. When present the changes from ischemia may vary from only edema to deep ulcerations, sinus tracts and even to necrosis.

Infectious colitis can be caused by many different viruses, bacteria, fungi, protozoas such as amebae, cryptosporidium, helminths, etc. The changes show a spectrum of findings, from Campylobacter causing the least severe tissue reaction to gonococci, *Entamoeba histolytica* or *Mycobacterium tuberculosis*, capable of causing reactions as severe as those of Crohn's disease with sinuses, fistulae and abscesses. Opportunistic infections in immunosuppressed patients can duplicate the entire range of changes encountered in inflammatory diseases of the rectum and sigmoid colon.

MRI appearance. Following the range of histologic changes, the spectrum of findings seen with MRI extends from thickening of the bowel wall due to edema to pericolic infiltration, sinus tracts and fistula formation. MRI demonstration of thickening of the bowel wall in ischemic colitis has been reported.[14] While MRI has a very limited role in the diagnosis of colitis it can be used in evaluating the severity of the disease by showing associated complications. Perirectal spread of the disease with infiltration of the perirectal fat and thickening of the perirectal fascia are well demonstrated on the T1-weighted image (Figure 13.21). On the T2-weighted image (Figure 13.22) the infiltrative fat demonstrates decrease in signal intensity. Extension of the inflammatory changes to the levator ani muscle, as shown in Figure 13.23, can also be detected, as can spread of the infection into the presacral region with widespread disease (similar to pelvic inflammatory disease in females) (Figure 13.24). Following Gd-DTPA injection, the inflamma-

tory tissue shows various degrees in signal enhancement depending on the acuteness of disease (Figures 13.25, 13.26). The greatest value of MRI is in demonstration of sinus tracts and perirectal abscess, as shown in Figure 13.27. While excellent in the morphologic demonstration of the disease, MRI findings are nonspecific. The type of colitis cannot be diagnosed and furthermore, differentiation between inflammatory and neoplastic disease cannot be made with certainty.

MRI in relation to other imaging modalities. Radiographic evaluation for suspected infectious inflammatory colon disease is requested only when the bacteriologic studies are negative or inconclusive, when patients do not respond to medical therapy, or when pericolonic disease extent or other complications are suspected. Plain films should be the initial study in severe disease to rule out toxic megacolon. Double contrast barium enema is the examination of choice for the evaluation of the mucosa. CT is used when the evaluation of the wall is needed or when pericolonic involvement is suspected. While the role of MRI in the evaluation of nonspecific inflammatory bowel disease is promising, especially in the evaluation of pericolonic disease (Figure 13.27), further assessment is still needed.

Diverticulosis and diverticulitis

Diverticular disease is a phenomenon of the Western world and the 20th century. The occurrence of diverticula seems to be inversely proportional to the amount of roughage in the diet and is associated with localized hypertrophy of the circular layer of the muscularis propria. It is estimated that in Western countries diverticula can be found in more than 50 per cent of individuals over 60 years of age. Diverticula are usually found in the sigmoid colon, but the entire colon may be involved.[31]

Inflammation of diverticula (diverticulitis) may be uncomplicated (requiring only medical therapy) or complicated (needing surgical intervention).[32] Complicated diverticulitis (abscess, colovesical fistula or both) is caused by microperforations, which are known to lead to intramural and subserosal abscesses. The majority of abscesses are pericolonic, but they may track into the gluteal region. Fistulas, although uncommon, may also occur. Open perforations, however, are rare.

MRI appearance

In diverticulosis, the bowel wall is of normal thickness. As shown in Figure 13.28, numerous air-filled outpouchings are seen traversing the wall outside. In **uncomplicated diverticulitis** (Figure 13.29) T1-weighted images demonstrate diverticula and a thickened bowel wall. On Gd-DTPA-enhanced T1-weighted images, the bowel wall shows enhancement. On T2-weighted scans, the thickened bowel wall demonstrates medium signal intensity. Adjacent extravisceral fatty tissue is normal on both T1- and T2-weighted images. In **complicated diverticulitis**, in addition to segmental thickening of the bowel wall and the presence of diverticula (Figure 13.30) there is also evidence of extravisceral inflammatory extension. Infiltration of the pericolonic fat is best seen on T1-weighted images, and as illustrated in Figure 13.31, air or fluid within the pericolonic inflammatory tissue can also be demonstrated. Following Gd-DTPA injection, both the bowel wall and the pericolonic disease show enhancement. On T2-weighted scans, the pericolonic tissue shows an increase in signal intensity.[14] Inflammatory extension into adjacent organs such as the bladder (Figure 13.32) is clearly demonstrated. Imaging in the sagittal plane facilitates visualization of the anteroposterior extension of disease.

MRI in relation to other imaging modalities

Contrast enemas are often diagnostic in diverticulitis. If clinical symptoms suggest frank perforation, water soluble iodine contrast enemas are recommended, as barium is known to produce adhesions and fibrosis in the peritoneum. Tracts leading to abscesses, masses impinging on the lumen with narrowing, and diverticula are the hallmarks of this condition. CT is an excellent complement to the barium enema.[32] When water soluble contrast material is used, CT demonstrates thickening of the wall, sinuses and abscesses, and mesenteric masses.[32] MRI can be helpful in evaluating the extracolonic extent of the disease. However, as illustrated in Figure 13.33, sometimes neither contrast enema, CT, nor MRI can differentiate diverticulitis from carcinoma, and this often presents a difficult clinical problem.

Carcinoma of the sigmoid colon and rectum

In the United States, the incidence of colorectal cancer is second only to carcinoma of the lung. In 1989 there were approximately 151 000 new cases of carcinoma of the colon, 44 000 of which originated in the rectum. Colon cancer is responsible for approximately 60 000 deaths per year, about 8000 of which are due to carcinoma of the rectum.[33] Risk factors include a personal or family history of colon and rectal cancer, polyps, and long standing inflammatory disease.

Although the etiology of colorectal cancer is unknown, an increased incidence of the disease has been associated with diets low in roughage and high in fat. The incidence also increases with age, but a significant proportion of cases are seen in younger individuals. Certain conditions, such as multiple polyposis, Gardner's syndrome, or even Peutz-Jehger's syndrome, carry a genetic predisposition to cancer of the colon.[1,33] The major histologic type of sigmoid and rectum cancer is adenocarcinoma (90–95 per cent of all large bowel tumors). The degree of tumor histologic differentiation, an important prognostic variable, applies only to adenocarcinoma tumor type.

Three tests are valuable in the detection of colorectal cancer—digital rectal examination, the detection of fecal occult blood, and flexible proctosigmoidoscopy.[33] If any of these tests are positive, colonoscopy and/or barium enema should be performed.[1] Lesion biopsy is essential to establish the diagnosis. In cases where the tumor extends no deeper than the submucosa, and the biopsy tissue margin is free of tumor, the 5-year survival rate following surgery is reported to approach 100 per cent.[1,34] Overall, the 5-year survival rate for carcinoma of the rectum is 79 per cent when the tumor is localized, but decreases to 31 per cent when the tumor has spread.[1] There are several tumor morphologic features that constitute prognostic variables and can be assessed radiologically. They include tumor size, configuration, location, and stage including local extent and lymph node metastasis.[1,34]

Tumor size at the time of initial diagnosis impacts on long-term survival. Colon tumors which are 6–10 cm in size are associated with better survival rates than those larger than 11 cm. The relationship between the size of the tumor and survival, however, does not hold true for rectal cancers. Configuration of the primary tumor (growth pattern) has also been reported to have influence on patient prognosis. Survival rates are better in patients with polypoid tumors (ie, tumors projecting into the lumen) than in patients whose tumors have a sessile infiltrative pattern.[1] The pathologic features of local tumor spread found to be of importance include the degree of transmural invasion and adjacent organ involvement.[1] Considerable interest has been expressed in the prognostic value of the local inflammatory reaction (considered to be a favorable prognostic factor) at the primary tumor site.[1]

Involvement of lymphatics and lymph nodes has an important bearing on the prognosis of cancer of the rectum. Both the number of lymph nodes involved, and the level at which they are invaded, are significant.[1] The pathways of lymph node spread depend on the location of the primary lesion. A carcinoma in the anal canal (low-lying rectal cancer) may metastasize along three pathways: (1) via the ischiorectal fossa and perianal lymphatics to the

Table 13.1 1987 AJCC/UICC Staging classification of colorectal cancer[39]

Primary Tumor (T)

Tis	Carcinoma in situ
T1	Invades submucosa
T2	Invades into muscularis propria
T3/T4	Depends on whether serosa is present

Serosa present:
  T3 Invades through muscularis propria into
        Subserosa
        Serosa (but not through)
        Pericolic fat within the leaves of the mesentery
  T4 Invades through serosa into free peritoneal cavity,
        or through serosa into contiguous organ
        Subserosa
        Serosa (but not through)
        Pericolic fat within the leaves of the mesentery
No serosa (distal two-thirds rectum, posterior left of right colon):
  T3 Invades through muscularis propria
  T4 Invades other organs (vagina, prostate, ureter, kidney)

Regional Lymph Nodes (N)

NX	Nodes cannot be assessed (eg local excision only)
N0	No regional node metastases
N1	1–3 positive nodes
N2	4 or more positive nodes
(N3	central nodes positive)

Distant Metastases (M)

MX	Presence of distant metastases cannot be assessed
M0	No distant metastases
M1	Distant metastases present

Dukes' staging system correlated with TNM

Dukes' A = T1N0M0
              T2N0M0
Dukes' B = T3N0M0
              T4N0M0
Dukes' C = T(any)N0M0,T(any)N2M0
Dukes' D = T(any)N(any)M1

AJCC = American Joint Commitee on Cancer
UICC = Union International Contre le Cancer

superficial inguinal lymph nodes; (2) laterally, either above or below the levator ani muscle, to the internal iliac nodes; and (3) upwards along the superior rectal artery to the left colic and inferior and superior mesenteric lymph nodes.[1] Tumors arising in the ampulla of the rectum metastasize laterally to the internal iliac lymph nodes and upwards to the left colic and inferior and superior mesenteric nodes. A tumor located more than 10 cm above the anus metastasizes almost exclusively upwards, to the left colic and inferior mesenteric lymph nodes.[1]

Tumor staging was for many years based on Dukes' classification which divides rectal tumors into stage A (penetration into but not through the bowel wall), stage B (penetration through the bowel wall) and stage C (involvement of lymph nodes). As the knowledge of prognostic factors expanded, the Dukes' classification underwent many modifications. Most of the additional prognostic factors have been incorporated in the new AJCC/UICC staging classification of colorectal cancer (Table 13.1).[35]

The primary treatment strategies for potentially

curable sigmoid and rectal cancer is surgery. Postoperative chemotherapy may improve the disease-free survival rate in large lesions. Adjuvant radiation therapy is directed toward maximizing local control. En-bloc surgical resection is therefore the primary treatment approach. Successful surgical treatment of colon cancer requires excision of an adequate amount of normal colon, proximal and distal to the tumor. Pathologic studies indicate that tumor rarely spreads more than 1.2 cm longitudinally beyond the area of gross involvement, and, therefore, a 5 cm margin is considered adequate. The type of surgery (colectomy, anterior resection or abdominoperineal resection) depends on the location of the tumor and its extent, especially the relation of the tumor to the insertion of the levator ani muscles and the distance of the tumor from the anus. On cross-sectional imaging, if feasible, the following features should be assessed and reported: tumor size; configuration; location with respect to anal canal and levator ani muscle insertion; tumor spread including depth of wall invasion; size; number and location of lymph nodes.

MRI appearance

On T1-weighted spin-echo images the tumor blends with the rectal wall and the two cannot be separated. As illustrated in Figure 13.34, the tumor diagnosis is based on the detection of an asymmetrical wall thickening and/or presence of an intraluminal mass. Tumor extension beyond the bowel wall is clearly seen on these sequences because the low signal intensity tumor strands are contrasted with high signal intensity perirectal fat.[13,36–39]

On T2-weighted spin-echo sequences, the tumor images with high signal intensity and can be differentiated from the lower signal intensity bowel wall muscle. As shown in Figure 13.35, the T2-weighted sequence allows evaluation of the depth of mural invasion. The T2-weighted sequence is also helpful in the evaluation of adjacent tissue, for example, levator ani muscle (Figure 13.36) and organ invasion.

Following Gd-DTPA injection, the tumor demonstrates enhancement. On Gd-DTPA T1-weighted images (Figure 13.34), the depth of tumor invasion can be evaluated. Gd-DTPA-enhanced T1-weighted sequences provide results similar to T2-weighted sequences but in a shorter scanning time, and the images often have better overall resolution.

In analyzing the morphologic features of sigmoid and rectal carcinoma, the following can be summarized: the size of the lesion is best assessed on T1-weighted and/or proton density images, and this is facilitated by the use of multiple planes (Figure 13.34). The mode of tumor growth being infiltrative (Figure 13.34), circumferential (Figure 13.35), or papillary

(Figure 13.36) is also best demonstrated on the T1- or proton density image. The demonstration of the lesion location, its relation to the levator ani insertion (Figures 13.36, 13.37) and the anal verge require assessment with both T1- and T2-weighted images in the transaxial as well as the coronal and sagittal imaging planes.

MRI staging

MRI staging of colorectal cancer can follow the suggested TNM classification (Table 13.1). MRI is not applicable to the assessment of stage Tis. Tumors staged T1 will demonstrate localized bowel wall thickening with preservation of the low signal intensity of the muscular wall on the T2-weighted image, as shown in Figure 13.38. However, except for the region of the anal canal, the muscularis propria of the wall is not consistently seen. Furthermore, colon cancer is often associated with an inflammatory reaction. The inflammatory process, on the T2-weighted image, causes an increased signal intensity of the bowel wall. It is therefore unlikely that MRI will be consistently helpful in differentiating stage T1 from stage T2 disease (Figure 13.34). In stage T2 disease, the entire bowel wall is thickened and is of high signal intensity on the T2-weighted image. The surrounding pericolonic tissue is normal. As previously described, the limitation to the accuracy in diagnosing stage T2 disease can be due to the fact that inflammatory reaction associated with stage T1 may produce similar changes. MRI is useful, however, in identifying stage T3 and T4 disease. On T1-weighted images pericolonic infiltration can be seen but the evaluation of the adjacent organ invasion requires assessment with T2-weighted images. MRI can also be used for lymph node evaluation. Pararectal nodes of 1 cm or greater in size, as shown in Figures 13.39 and 13.40, can be detected in multiple planes. The number and location of nodes greater than 1 cm should be reported although it should be realized that MRI cannot differentiate large hyperplastic from malignant nodes.

MRI in relation to other imaging modalities

The double contrast barium enema is an integral part of the evaluation of rectal cancer (Figure 13.41). In early stages of the disease, when the depth of mural invasion needs to be assessed, endorectal ultrasound is appropriate for routine preoperative use.[3,4] Endorectal ultrasound may also be used for the detection of low-lying pararectal lymph nodes.

CT is not advocated for routine preoperative staging, and its value rises with more advanced disease. CT has proven helpful in the evaluation of possible nodal and liver metastases. CT can demonstrate enlarged nodes in any location, although the nodes along the inferior mesenteric artery and left colic nodes are difficult to detect unless there is abundant mesenteric fat.

The soft tissue contrast resolution obtained with MRI is superb, allowing differentiation of the layers of the rectal wall on T2-weighted images. In addition, the capability for direct multiplanar imaging enhances the determination of tumor extent, as illustrated in Figure 13.41. The value of MRI in the assessment of colorectal cancer, however, needs further assessment with large patient series. Although early reports indicated that the potential of MRI exceeds that of CT,[13] this early promise needs to be substantiated. Technical advances, such as the development of endorectal surface coils and intraluminal contrast media, may increase the value of MRI in the study of this disease. In the detection of pararectal and pelvic nodes, the accuracy of MRI is similar to that of CT (65–90 per cent). Although it is possible to detect enlarged nodes and assess their size with cross-sectional imaging modalities, it is not possible to differentiate hyperplastic from malignant nodes.

Comparison of ultrasound, MRI, and CT in some studies[2–4] indicates that ultrasound is superior to MRI and CT in determining the depth of mural invasion and in detecting small lymph nodes. MRI, however, as shown in Figure 13.39, is an excellent modality for detecting infiltration of other organs and for demonstrating tumor location providing information helpful in choosing the optimal type of therapy or tumor resection. The staging accuracy of MRI for primary tumors is reported to be 74 per cent, compared to 68 per cent for CT.[38] MRI is especially useful in evaluating perirectal extension, with a sensitivity of over 75 per cent, a specificity of 100 per cent, and staging accuracy following TNM criteria of 79 per cent. MRI is, therefore, particularly useful in selecting patients who are appropriate candidates for local excision.

Metastasis

Metastases to the colon are more often found at autopsy than are recognized clinically or radiographically.[40] Tumors that most commonly metastasize to the colon include stomach, breast, pancreas and gynecologic pelvic malignancies.[40] There are different pathways for metastatic involvement of the colon. The colon can be involved secondarily by direct invasion from contiguous neoplasm, by spread of tumor along lymphatic channels, from intraperitoneal recesses, or by the embolic hematogenous route (the latter is particularly common for metastatic spread of melanoma).

MRI appearance

The metastatic lesion characteristically produces localized thickening of the bowel wall (Figure 13.42). The mucosal folds may be thickened but uninvaded. Such an example is shown in Figure 13.42 (metastasis from carcinoma of the cervix) where there is a localized thickening of the bowel wall with intact muscosa. The intact mucosa shows signal enhancement (greater than that of the tumor) following gadolinium-DTPA injection explaining why in this patient the colonoscopy was negative. As the metastatic lesion enlarges, changes in the colon will be more obvious. Imaging findings with the exception of localized thickening of the colon wall with intact mucosa are nonspecific, and primary and metastatic lesions cannot be distinguished.

MRI in relation to other imaging modalities

Invasion of the colon by metastatic disease can follow multiple routes as described. Metastatic involvement by the lymphatic or hematogenous routes can be detected by the double contrast barium enema which demonstrates characteristic spread and distortion of otherwise preserved mucosal folds. CT and MRI will demonstrate localized bowel wall thickening with a smooth intraluminal surface. When the mucosa is invaded, mucosal irregularities and ulcerations are present. When the involvement is by direct invasion, MRI appears to be superior to CT due to its multiplanar and multiple sequence capabilities. CT, however, has the advantage of better spatial resolution and, at present, has widely available gastrointestinal contrast media.

Recurrent colorectal cancer

The surgical, or pathologic, stage is the most important variable affecting the recurrence of colorectal cancer. The major risk of recurrence is disseminated disease.[1] The liver is involved in as many as two-thirds of patients who die of colon cancer.

Patterns of recurrence include local recurrence at the suture line, regional recurrence in the node-bearing tissue, and peritoneal seeding. The incidence of local recurrence is related to the extent of transmural penetration, to the number of lymph node metastases, and to the involvement of adjacent organs.[1] The local recurrence rate is approximately 30 per cent in disease with transmural extension only. It approaches 50 per cent if five or more lymph nodes are positive at the time of surgery, and it increases to 69 per cent if the tumor has adhered to or invaded adjacent structures. The incidence of local cure failure also depends on the location of the primary tumor, and tumors which cause posterior penetration in the portion of the rectum devoid of serosa are associated with an increased recurrence rate.

Another reason for the failure rate in the cure of colorectal cancer is the incidence of peritoneal seeding. Peritoneal seeding has been reported in 36 per cent of patients who die of colon cancer, and of these, as many as 58 per cent do not demonstrate local or regional recurrence. Ovarian metastases develop in up to 7 per cent of women with colon cancer, although it is still controversial whether the route of spread is direct intraperitoneal or hematogenous. Pelvic recurrence can be secondary to surgical seeding (implanted tumor cells), and tumor implants at the abdominal surgical scar, perineal scar, or even the mucocutaneous margin of the colostomy, have been reported. Peritoneal seeding may also be caused by retained involved lymph nodes and by intralymphatic tumor spread.

MRI appearance

Following anterior resection of carcinoma of the rectosigmoid colon as shown in Figure 13.43, a surgical clip can be seen at the site of anastomosis. The appearance of the bowel wall at the anastomotic site depends on the time interval between surgery and imaging. In the immediate postoperative period, localized inflammatory reaction will cause bowel wall thickening and increase signal intensity on the T2-weighted image. While no data are presently available describing the time course of changes at the postoperative site, usually six months following surgery and thereafter, the inflammatory reaction will have subsided and the bowel at the site of anastomosis will be of normal thickness and signal intensity (Figure 13.43). Local tumor recurrence at the suture line will be most commonly a round or irregular shaped tumor mass. Unlike the primary tumor which has a tendency to grow circumferentially, tumor recurrence as seen in Figure 13.44 has an exophytic growth tendency, and additional tumor masses as shown in Figure 13.45 can be seen adjacent to the recurrent lesion. Tumor recurrence in the presacral region (Figure 13.46) is easily demonstrated with MR multiplanar imaging. Similarly, tumor extension into adjacent organs such as seminal vesicles in the male (Figure 13.46) or the urinary bladder (Figure 13.47) can also be assessed. While the morphologic features of tumor recurrence are very well displayed on MRI, the tumor signal intensity varies. When the tumor recurrence exhibits high signal intensity on the T2-weighted image, its diagnosis is not difficult. In some instances, however, tumor recurrence will be of low signal intensity on the T2-weighted image as shown in Figure 13.48. In those cases, it is the morphologic finding of asymmetrical

tumor mass that raises the suspicion of tumor recurrence and warrants biopsy. In advanced cases, tumor recurrence will extend posteriorly and involve the sacrum. Sacral involvement is best seen on T1-weighted images, and again a combination of multiplanar imaging facilitates its evaluation (Figure 13.49). Tumor recurrence can be diffuse and, as seen in Figure 13.50, can invade the adjacent muscle. Following abdominoperineal (AP) resection, there is distortion of the normal anatomy. Direct multiplanar orthogonal imaging supplemented with T1 and T2 sequences allows correct anatomical display. A thick low intensity postsurgical scar, as shown in Figure 13.51, can be seen. The postsurgical scar, however, can also present heterogeneous low to medium signal intensity. In most instances, the reactive scar tissue follows the internal pelvic surface. Foci of tumor, often growing in thin sheaths within the scar tissue, cannot be detected by MRI. There are, however, many advantages to MRI, which is often a helpful modality in the evaluation of tumor recurrence. Scar tissue can be of heterogeneous signal intensity on T2-weighted images as late as 1 to 1½ years after surgery or subsequent radiation therapy. When the scar tissue as seen in Figure 13.51 is of homogeneous low signal intensity and follows the internal pelvic surface, the findings usually indicate benign process. In patients in whom thin sheaths grow within the scar, tumor recurrence cannot be diagnosed. Follow-up examinations are helpful, as seen in Figure 13.52. In the initial study, the small focus of high signal intensity within the scar tissue was thought to be nonspecific but six months later the tumor showed interval growth.

Metastases from colorectal cancer can be found in the ovary. In these cases, the metastasis may be cystic (Figure 13.53). Only anecdotal reports describing peritoneal seeding in conjunction with rectal carcinoma are available. An example of such peritoneal seeding is seen in Figure 13.53.

MRI in relation to other modalities

CT is helpful in the detection of locally recurrent colorectal cancer. The accuracy of CT in the evaluation of suspected recurrence is significantly better than for preoperative staging. A CT accuracy of 87 per cent with a sensitivity of 91 per cent and specificity of 72 per cent[41] has been reported. The CT examination is accurate in detecting local recurrence and lymph node metastasis. Difficulties are, however, frequently encountered in distinguishing recurrence from fibrosis and in assessing tumor spread into neighboring viscera.

Following AP resection the normal anatomic landmarks are disturbed, and the limited tissue contrast resolution of CT coupled with limitations of direct imaging in the transverse plane only limit the value of CT.

The value of MRI in the evaluation of recurrent rectal cancer has received much publicity and remains a controversial topic.[41-46] Reports describing the excellence of MRI[44] can be found in the literature along with those emphasizing the MRI tissue nonspecificity.[44] In general, it is felt that MR imaging can be useful in determining the extent of suspected recurrent tumor, but that changes in signal intensity on T2-weighted images do not permit a histologic diagnosis. Increases in signal intensity may indicate neoplastic changes (benign or malignant), inflammation, or edema. An area of low signal intensity may correspond to scar tissue, but tumor desmoplastic reaction has a similar appearance. MRI does, however, offer multiplanar imaging and better tissue characterization than CT, and when the MR finding of a mass is combined with an increase in signal intensity on T2-weighted images, the diagnosis of recurrence can be made with confidence. Demonstration of invasion of adjacent organs will further substantiate the diagnosis.

In spite of all technical advances and developments in imaging, it is still difficult to differentiate small locally recurrent tumors from postoperative or radiation fibrosis, and biopsy is often essential.

References

1 COHEN AM, SHANK B, FRIEDMAN MA, Colorectal cancer. In: DeVita VT, Hellman S, Rosenberg SA, eds. *Cancer: Principles and Practice of Oncology*, 3rd edn. (JB Lippincott: Philadelphia 1989) 895–964.

2 INOUE I, NAKAYAMA H, ODA N et al, Studies of diagnosis of rectal cancer using MRI, CT and intrarectal ultrasonography, *Rinsho Hoshasen* (1989) **34(5)**:573–81.

3 BEYON J, FOY DMA, ROE AM et al, Endoluminal ultrasound in the assessment of local invasion in rectal cancer, *Br J Surg* (1986) **73**:474.

4 HILDEBRANDT U, FEIFEL G, Preoperative staging of rectal cancer by intrarectal ultrasound, *Dis Colon Rectum* (1985) **28**:42–6.

5 MOSS AA, MARGULIS AR, SCHNYDER P, A uniform CT-based staging system for malignant neoplasms of the alimentary tube, *AJR* (1981) **136**:1051.

6 SUGIMURA K, CARRINGTON BM, QUIVEY JM et al, Postirradiation changes in the pelvis: assessment with MR imaging, *Radiology* (1990) **175**:805–13.

7 LANAIDO M, KORNMESSER W, HAMM B et al, MR imaging of the gastrointestinal tract: value of Gd-DTPA, *AJR* (1988) **150**:817–21.

8 HAHN PF, STARK DD, LEWIS JM et al, First clinical trial of a new super-paramagnetic iron oxide for use as an oral gastrointestinal contrast agent in MR imaging, *Radiology* (1990) **175**:695–710.

9 LIERSE W, *Applied Anatomy of the Pelvis*, (Springer-Verlag: Berlin 1984) 218–65.

10 MONIE IW, Embryology. In: Margulis AR, Bucherul HJ, eds. *Alimentary Tract Radiology*, 4th edn. (CV Merly: St Louis 1989) 215–30.

11 SPIESSEL B, BEAHRS OH, HERMANEK P et al, eds. *TNM Atlas: Illustrated Guide to the TNM/pTNM-Classification of Malignant Tumours*, 3rd edn. (Springer-Verlag: Berlin 1989).

12 ROEVIERE H, Anatomy of the human lymphatic system. Compendium. Tobias MJ (translator). (Edwards Brothers: Ann Arbor, Michigan 1938).

13 BUTCH RJ, STRAK DD, WITTENBERG J et al, Staging rectal cancer by MR and CT, *AJR* (1986) **146**:1155–60.

14 GOLDBERG HI, THOENI RF, MRI of the gastrointestinal tract, *Radiol Clin of North Am* (1989) **27(4)**:805–12.

15 WINKLER MR, HRICAK H, Pelvis imaging with MR: technique for improvement, *Radiology* (1986) **158**:848–9.

16 CAFFEY J, *Pediatric X-Ray Diagnosis*, 5th edn. (Year Book Medical Publishers, Inc: Chicago 1967) 579–686.

17 SMITH ED, The bath water needs changing but don't throw out the baby: an overview of anorectal anomalies, *J Pediatr Surg* (1987) **22**:335–48.

18 DE VRIES PA, COX KL, Surgery of anorectal anomalies, *Surg Clin North Am* (1985) **65**:1139–69.

19 STEPHENS FD, SMITH ED, *Ano-rectal malformations in children*, (Year Book Medical: Chicago 1971).

20 SATO Y, PRINGLE KC, BERGMAN RA et al, Congenital anorectal anomalies: MR imaging, *Radiology* (1988) **168(1)**:157–62.

21 PANUEL M, GUYS JM, DEVRED P et al, Magnetic resonance imaging of high anorectal malformations. A preliminary study apropos of 15 cases, *Chir Pediatr* (1988) **29(5)**:243–6.

22 VADE A, REYES H, WILBUR A et al, The anorectal sphincter after rectal pull-through surgery for anorectal anomalies: MRI evaluation, *Pediatr Radiol* (1989) **19(3)**:179–83.

23 POMERANZ SJ, ALTMAN N, SHELDON JJ et al, Magnetic resonance of congenital anorectal malformations, *Magn Reson Imaging* (1986) **4**:69–72.

24 MEZZACAPPA PM, PRICE AP, HALLER JO et al, MR and CT demonstration of levator sling in congenital anorectal anomalies, *J Comput Assist Tomogr* (1987) **11**:273–5.

25 PRINGLE KC, SATO Y, SOPER RT, Magnetic resonance imaging as an adjunct to planning an anorectal pull-through, *J Pediatr Surg* (1987) **22**:571–4.

26 LOCKHART-LEAMMERY HE, MORSON BC, Crohn's disease: regional enteritis and its distinction from ulcerative colitis, *Gut* (1960) **1**:87.

27 GORE RM, MARN CS, KIRBY DF et al, CT findings in ulcerative, granularistous and indeterminate colitis, *AJR* (1984) **143**:279.

28 FARMER RG, HAWK WA, TURNBULL RB, Clinical patterns in Crohn's disease: a statistical study of 615 patients. *Gastroenterology* (1975) **6**:627.

29 KOELBEL G, SCHMIEDL U, MAJER MC et al, Diagnosis of fistulae and sinus tracts in patients with Crohn's disease: value of MR imaging, *AJR* (1989) **152(5)**:999–1003.

30 THOENI RF, MARGULIS AR, Colon: inflammatory diseases. In: Margulis AR, Burhenne HJ, eds. *Alimentary Tract Radiology*, 4th edn. (CV Merly: St Louis 1989) 963–1016.

31 PAINTER NS, BURKITT DP, Diverticular disease of the colon: a deficiency disease of Western civilization, *Br Med J* (1971) **2**:450.

32 LABS JD, SARR MG, FISHMAN EK et al, Complications of acute diverticulitis of the colon: improved early diagnosis with computerized tomography, *AJR* (1988) **155(2)**:331–6.

33 *Cancer Facts & Figures-1989* (American Cancer Society: Atlanta 1989).

34 ENKER WE, Cancer of the rectum: operative management and adjuvant therapy. In: Fazio VW, ed. *Current Therapy in Colon and Rectal Surgery* (BC Decker: Toronto 1990) 120–30.

35 1987 AJCC/UICC staging classification of colorectal cancer. In: (modified) *American Joint Committee on Cancer: Manual for Staging of Cancer*, 3rd edn. (JP Lippincott: Philadelphia 1987) and *Union Internationale Contre le Cancer: TNM Classification of Malignant Tumors*, 4th edn. (UICC: Geneva 1987).

36 HODGMAN CG, MACCARTY RL, WOLFF BG et al, Preoperative staging of rectal carcinoma by computed tomography and 0.15 T magnetic resonance imaging, *Dis Colon Rectum* (1986) **29**:446–50.

37 GUINET C, BUY JN, SEZEUR A et al, Preoperative assessment of the extension of rectal carcinoma: correlation of MR, surgical, and histopathologic findings, *J Comput Assist Tomogr* (1988) **12(2)**:209–14.

38 BUTLER H, BRYAN PJ, Magnetic resonance imaging of rectal carcinoma, *J Natl Med Assoc* (1989) **81(1)**:87–90.

39 GUINET C, BUY JN, GHOSSAIN MA, Comparison of magnetic resonance imaging and computed tomography in the preoperative staging of rectal cancer, *Arch Surg* (1990) **125(3)**:385–8.

40 MEYERS MA, MCSWEENEY J, Secondary neoplasms of the bowel, *Radiology* (1972) **105**:1.

41 THOMPSON WM, HALVORSEN RA Jr, Computed tomographic staging of gastrointestinal malignancies. Part II: The small bowel, colon and rectum, *Invest Radiol* (1987) **22**:96–105.

42 RAFTO SE, AMENDOLA MA, GEFTER WB, MR imaging of recurrent colorectal carcinoma versus fibrosis, *J Comput Assist Tomogr* (1988) **12(3)**:521–3.

43 DE LANGE EE, FECHNER RE, WANEBO HJ, Suspected recurrent rectosigmoid carcinoma after abdominoperineal resection: MR imaging and histopathologic findings, *Radiology* (1989) **170(2)**:323–8.

44 KRESTIN GP, STEINBRICH W, FRIEDMANN G, Recurrent rectal cancer: diagnosis with MR versus CT, *Radiology* (1988) **168(2)**:307–11.

45 KRESTIN GP, STEINBRICH W, FRIEDMANN G, Diagnosis of recurrent rectal cancer: comparison of CT and MRI, *ROFO* (1988) **141(1)**:28–33.

46 GOMBERG JS, FRIEDMAN AC, RADECKI PD et al, MRI differentiation of recurrent colorectal carcinoma from postoperative fibrosis, *Gastrointest Radiol* (1986) **11**:361–3.

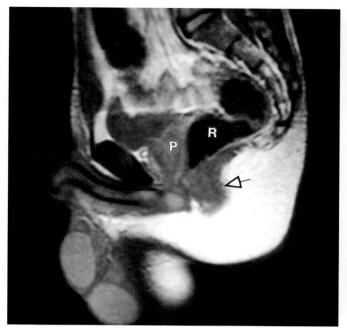

a

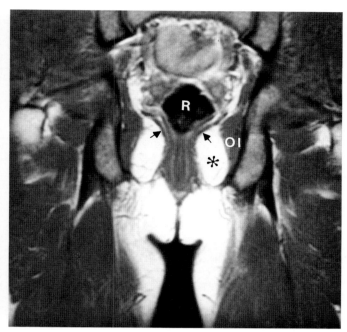

b

Figure 13.1

Anatomy of rectum and anal canal, proton density images, (**a**) sagittal plane and (**b**) coronal plane. The rectum (R) as seen in the sagittal plane extends from the level of the third sacral vertebrae to the anus (open arrow). On the coronal image, the insertion of the levator ani muscle (black arrows) demarcating the surgical anorectal junction is seen. The ischiorectal fossa (asterisk) is bounded laterally by the obturator internus muscle (OI). (P)-prostate.

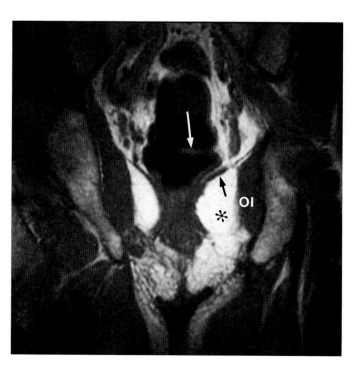

Figure 13.2

Valve of Houston (white arrow), T1-weighted image, coronal plane. (Asterisk)-ischiorectal fossa; (black arrow)-levator ani muscle; (OI)-obturator internus muscle.

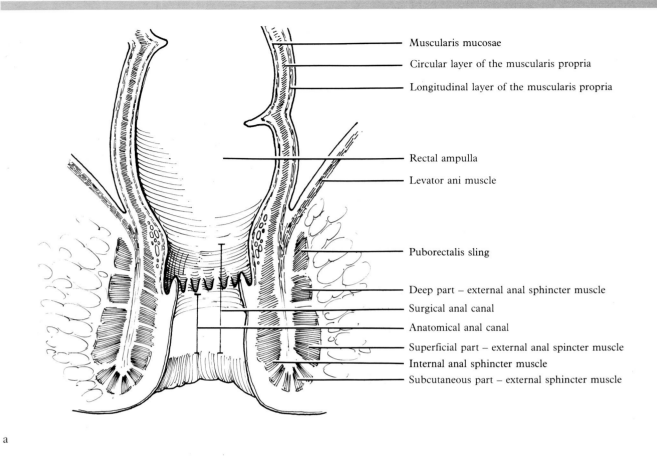

Muscularis mucosae
Circular layer of the muscularis propria
Longitudinal layer of the muscularis propria

Rectal ampulla
Levator ani muscle

Puborectalis sling

Deep part – external anal sphincter muscle
Surgical anal canal
Anatomical anal canal
Superficial part – external anal spincter muscle
Internal anal sphincter muscle
Subcutaneous part – external sphincter muscle

a

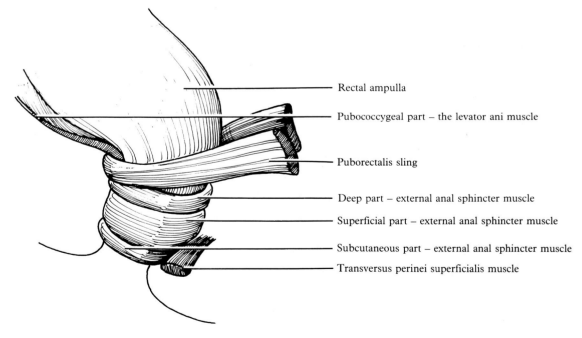

Rectal ampulla

Pubococcygeal part – the levator ani muscle

Puborectalis sling

Deep part – external anal sphincter muscle
Superficial part – external anal sphincter muscle
Subcutaneous part – external anal sphincter muscle
Transversus perinei superficialis muscle

b

Figure 13.3

Schematic drawing of the anal
canal and its surrounding
musculature, (**a**) coronal and
(**b**) sagittal plane.

a

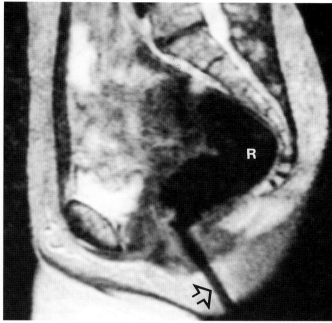

b

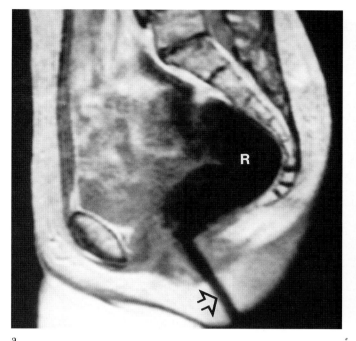

c

Figure 13.4

Anatomy of the rectum proper. Sagittal plane (**a**) proton density image, (**b**) T2-weighted image, and (**c**) transaxial T2-weighted image. The rectum (R) is fully distended by air insufflated through an inserted enema tip (open arrow). The layers of the rectal wall (arrows) cannot be discerned, and the anterior margin of the rectosigmoid junction is not sharp, probably due to induced contractility. (B)-urinary bladder.

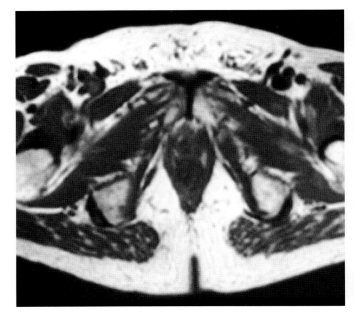

a

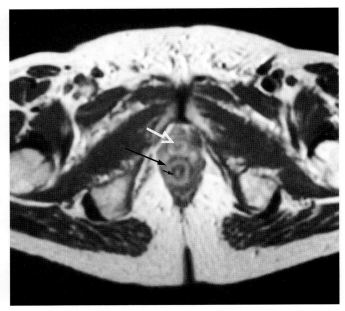

b

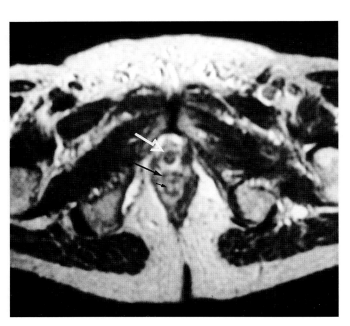

c

Figure 13.5

Anatomy of the anal canal. (**a**) T1-weighted image, (**b**) Gd-DTPA-enhanced T1-weighted image and (**c**) T2-weighted image. On the T1-weighted image, the wall of the anal canal demonstrates homogeneous medium signal intensity. On either the Gd-DTPA-enhanced T1-weighted image or the T2-weighted image, four layers of the bowel wall can be seen. The outside low signal intensity ring (long black arrow) is followed by high intensity submucosa, followed by a third layer—a low intensity ring (muscularis mucosae and lamina propria) (small black arrow) and a fourth central high signal intensity area (mucosa). (Open white arrow)-urethra.

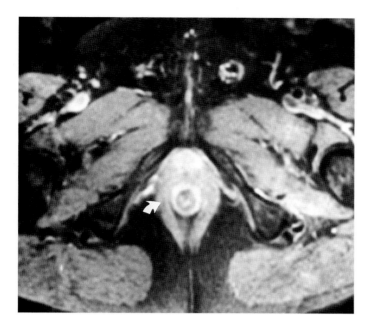

a

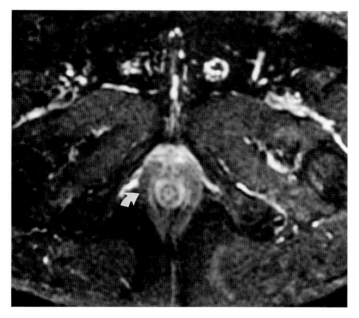

b

Figure 13.6

Anatomy of the anal canal on fat suppression SE sequence. (**a**) Proton density image, (**b**) T2-weighted image. The anal sphincter (curved white arrow) and the zonal anatomy of the bowel wall are both well seen.

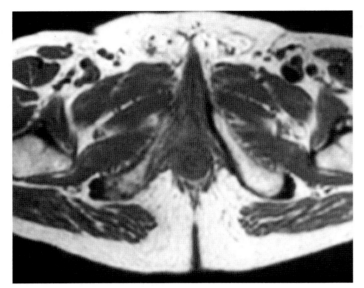

a

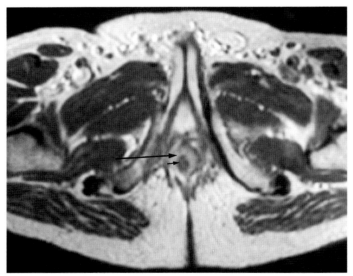

b

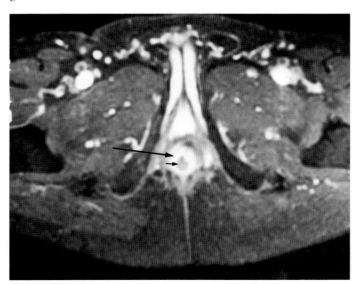

c

Figure 13.7
Zonal anatomy of the anal canal, T1-weighted images. Zonal anatomy with differentiation between high intensity submucosa (long black arrow), lower intensity inner ring (small black arrow), and high signal intensity mucosa (center) can be seen following Gd-DTPA injection. (**a**) SE T1-weighted image, (**b**) SE Gd-DTPA-enhanced T1-weighted image and (**c**) fat suppression SE Gd-DTPA-enhanced T1-weighted image.

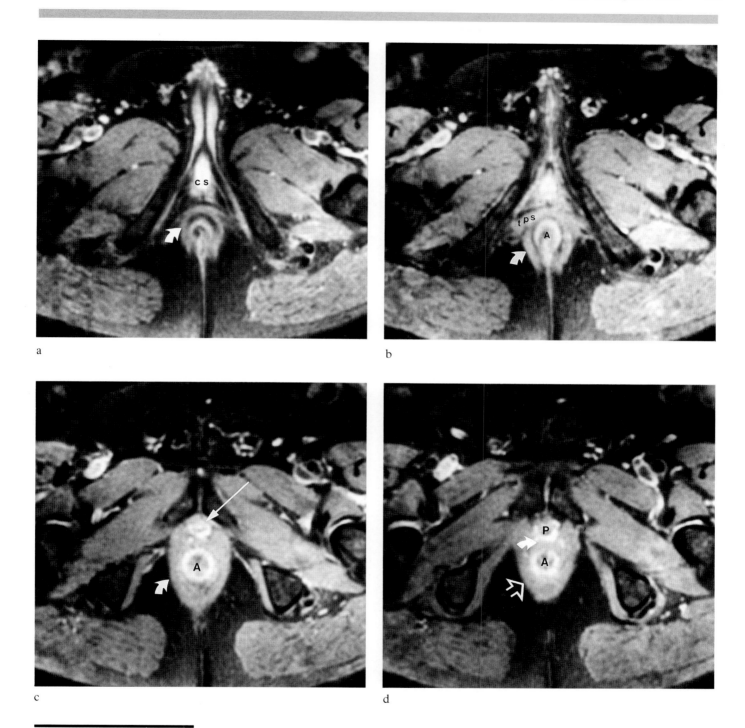

a

b

c

d

Figure 13.8

Anatomy of the anal sphincters. Fat-saturation proton density images. (**a**), (**b**), (**c**), (**d**), and (**e**) are consecutive transaxial sections. (**a**) Below the level of the perineum, the subcutaneous part of the external sphincter (curved arrow) is seen. (CS)-corpus spongiosum. (**b**) At the level of the perineum. Transversus perinei superficialis muscle (tps) is seen anterior to the anal canal (A). Laterally, external and internal muscles surrounding the anal canal cannot be separated (curved white arrow). (**c**) At the level of the membranous urethra (white straight arrow) the sphincter (white curved arrow) completely surrounds the anal canal (A). (**d**) At the apex of the prostate gland (P), the external sphincter (curved white arrow) is seen between the prostate (P) and the anal canal (A). While the sphincter is thinned, the wider muscle portion laterally is due in part to the addition of the puborectalis sling (open white arrow).

continued overleaf

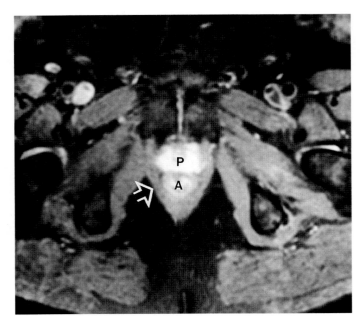

e

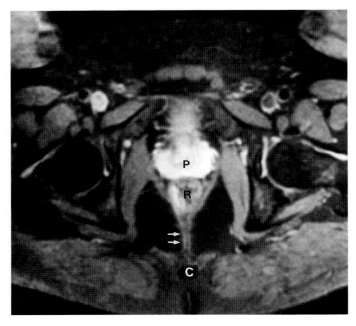

f

Figure 13.8 *continued*

(**e**) Section at the upper margin of the surgical anal canal showing the prostate (P) anteriorly, the anal canal (A) posteriorly, and no muscle between the two. (Open white arrow)-puborectalis sling. (**f**) Superior section demonstrating the pubococcygeal part of the levator ani muscle (arrows) extending from the rectum (R) to the coccyx (C) posteriorly.

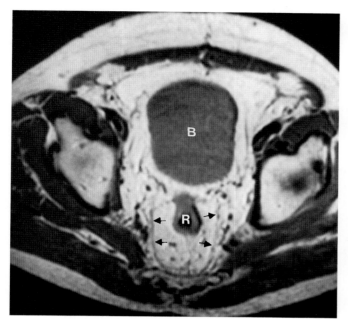

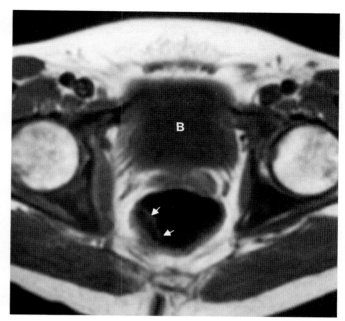

a

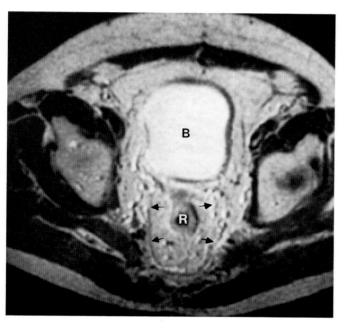

b

Figure 13.10

Retained fecal material within the rectal ampulla, T1-weighted image. Whenever possible, the rectum should be cleansed with an enema. Retained fecal material (white arrows) cannot be distinguished on MR images from neoplasms. (B)-urinary bladder.

Figure 13.9

Perirectal fascia, (**a**) proton density, (**b**) T2-weighted images. (Arrows)-perirectal fascia; (R)-rectum; (B)-urinary bladder.

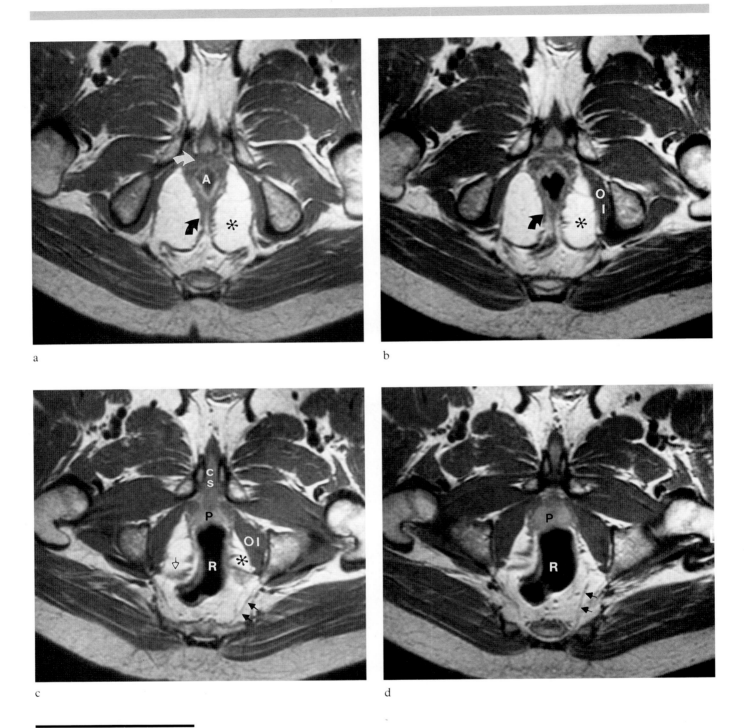

a

b

c

d

Figure 13.11

Anatomy of the anal canal and the rectum as demonstrated on a 35° oblique dorsal to ventral transaxial plane; proton density images. (**a**) to (**d**) sequential scans along the anal canal and rectum showing the anatomy of the anal canal (A) external sphincter (curved white arrow); pubococcygeal part of the levator ani muscle (black curved arrow); the levator ani (open black arrow); the ischiorectal fossa (asterisk); the obturator internus muscle (OI); the perirectal fascia (black arrowheads); unfolded rectosigmoid loop (R); prostate (P); and corpora spongiosa (cs).

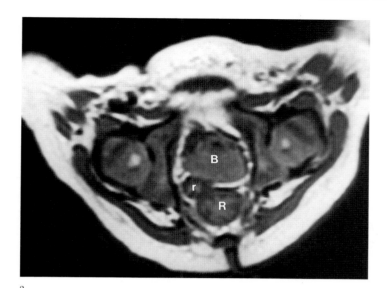

a

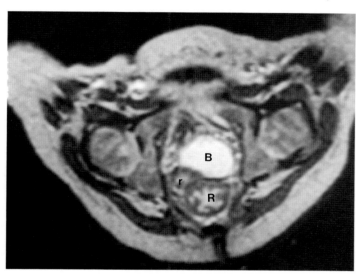

b

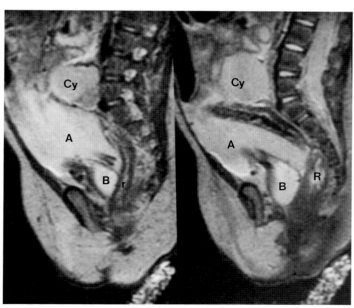

c   d

Figure 13.12

Congenital duplication of
rectum, transaxial plane, (**a**)
proton density, (**b**) T2-
weighted image, (**c**) and (**d**) two
consecutive T2-weighted
sagittal images. Rectal
duplication with the rectum (R)
opening into the anus and the
smaller duplicated portion (r)
seen anteriorly and to the right.
(A)-ascites; (Cy)-mesenteric
cyst; (B)-urinary bladder.

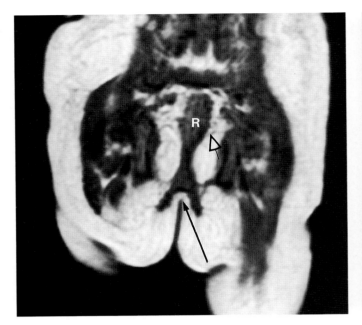

a

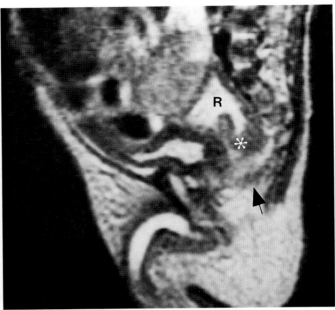

Figure 13.14

Supralevator (high) rectal atresia in a newborn; sagittal T2-weighted image. The rectal pouch (R) is above the levator sling (black arrow). Meconium within the rectal pouch (R) images with high signal intensity on T2-weighted images while the undistended wall of the rectal pouch demonstrates low signal intensity (white asterisk).

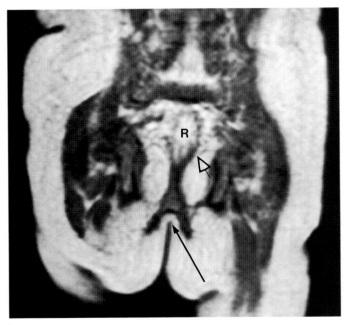

b

Figure 13.13

Translevator (low) anal atresia. Coronal (**a**) proton density and (**b**) T2-weighted image. The atretic rectal stump (R) extends below the level of the levator ani sling (open arrow). Measurement between the anal dimple (long arrow) and the atretic stump can also be made. The puborectalis sling and anal sphincter muscles are well developed. (Compare to Figure 13.15.)

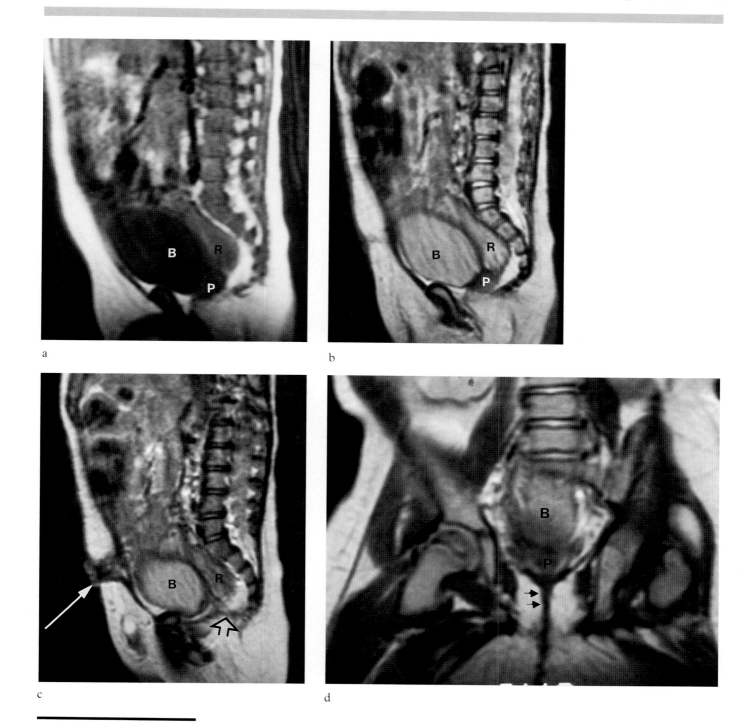

a

b

c

d

Figure 13.15

Supralevator (high) anal atresia in a 12-month-old child with a colostomy (long white arrow). Sagittal (**a**) T1-weighted, (**b**) and (**c**) T2-weighted, and (**d**) coronal T2-weighted images. The demonstration of the blind pouch (R) and the distance between the pouch and the levator ani muscle (open black arrow) are well seen. The levator ani sling and the external sphincter are hypoplastic (small black arrows). (B)-urinary bladder; (P)-prostate.

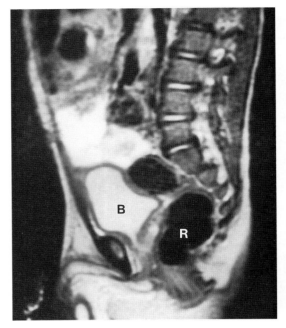

a

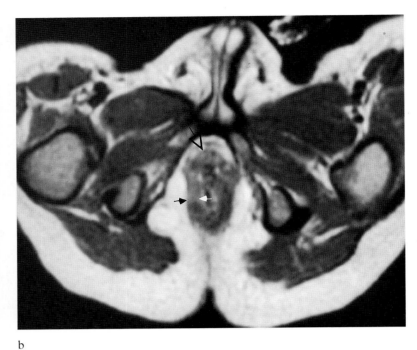

b

Figure 13.16

Normally developed anal
sphincter in a 12-month-old
boy. (**a**) Sagittal T2-weighted
image and (**b**) transaxial T2-
weighted image. (Arrows)-well
developed external sphincter;
(large open arrow)-
membranous urethra; (B)-
urinary bladder; (R)-rectum.

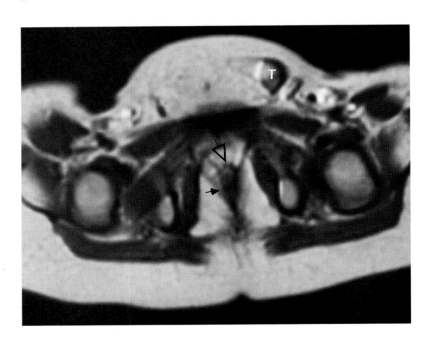

Figure 13.17

Hypoplastic anal sphincter in
12-month-old child with rectal
atresia, transaxial T2-weighted
image. The hypoplastic
external anal sphincter muscle
(black arrow) is seen. (Compare
to Figure 13.16.) The
membranous urethra (open
arrow) is seen anteriorly. (T)-
undescended testes.

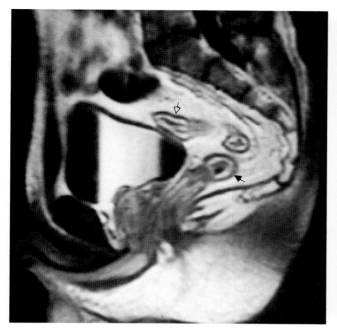

a

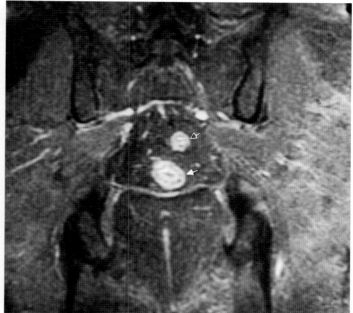

b

Figure 13.18

Ulcerative colitis. (**a**) Gd-DTPA-enhanced T1-weighted image, sagittal plane, (**b**) Gd-DTPA-enhanced fat-saturation image, coronal plane and (**c**) T2-weighted image, coronal plane. The wall of the rectum (solid arrow) and sigmoid colon (open arrow) is thickened; it demonstrates enhancement following Gd-DTPA injection. The pericolonic fat (compared to the Gd-DTPA-enhanced fat-saturation image in Figure 13.19b) is normal (not infiltrated).

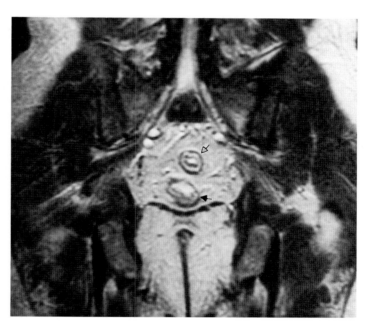

c

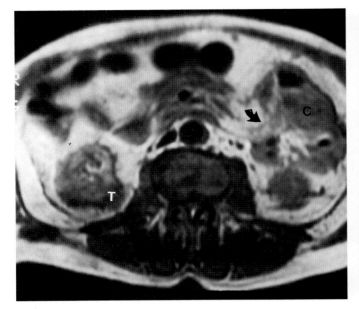

a

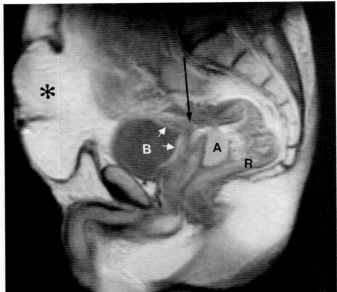

a

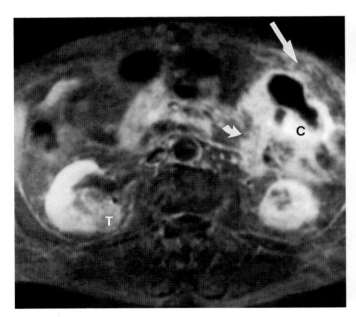

b

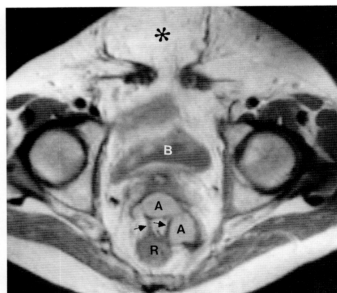

b

Figure 13.19

Crohn's disease with extensive pericolonic inflammatory changes. The patient also has a right-sided renal cell carcinoma (T). (**a**) T1-weighted image and (**b**) Gd-DTPA-enhanced T1-weighted fat-saturation image. On the T1-weighted image, the pericolonic fat infiltration (curved black arrow) demonstrates medium signal intensity shading. (C)-bowel wall. Following the injection of Gd-DTPA the bowel wall (C) enhances and there is also extensive enhancement in its medial (curved white arrow) and lateral (straight arrow) pericolonic tissue. The renal tumor (T) also shows enhancement.

Figure 13.20

Perirectal abscess in a patient with Crohn's disease. (**a**) Proton density sagittal and (**b**) transaxial plane images. There is tethering of a thickened bladder wall (white arrows) with a sigmoid vesical fistula (straight vertical arrow) and a lobulated abscess (A) with low signal intensity sinus tracts (black arrows). (Asterisk)-incisional hernia; (R)-rectum.

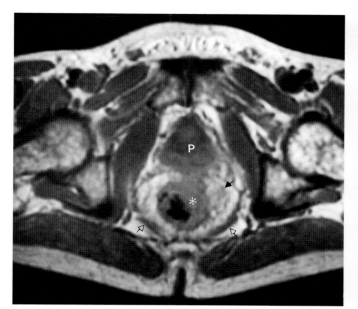

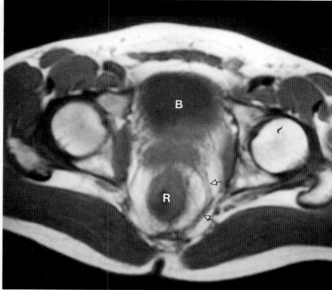

a

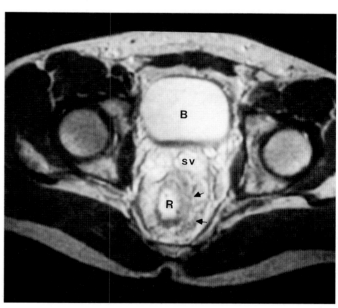

b

Figure 13.21

Nonspecific colitis, T1-weighted image, transaxial plane. The wall of the rectum (asterisk) is irregularly thickened. There is infiltration of the perirectal fat (black arrow). The perirectal fascia is thickened (open arrows). (P)-prostate gland.

Figure 13.22

Nonspecific colitis with involvement of perirectal fat and perirectal fascia. Transaxial (**a**) T1- and (**b**) T2-weighted images. On the T1-weighted image, the wall of the rectum (R) is thickened. There is asymmetrical thickening of the perirectal fascia (open arrows). On the T2-weighted image, the wall of the rectum and the infiltration in the perirectal fat show decrease in signal intensity (black arrows). (SV)-seminal vesicles; (B)-urinary bladder.

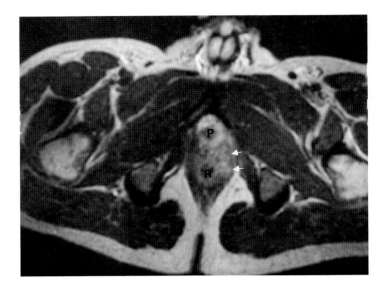

Figure 13.23

Extensive inflammatory bowel disease, extending into the left levator ani muscle; transaxial T2-weighted image. The levator ani muscle on the left (small arrows) is of higher signal intensity compared to the right side, indicating inflammatory disease. In this patient, the inflammatory process was from the bowel disease. (R)-rectum; (P)-prostate gland.

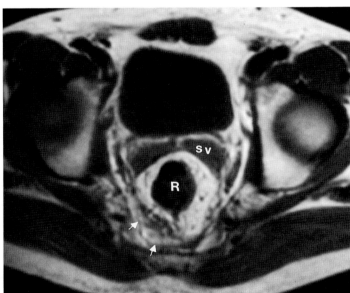

Figure 13.24

Inflammatory bowel disease, extending along the perirectal fascia into the presacral region; transaxial (**a**) T1- and (**b**) T2-weighted images. On the T1-weighted image, there is indistinctness and thickening to the perirectal fascia (small white arrows). On the T2-weighted image, increased signal intensity is seen along the same pathways into the presacral region (small white arrows). (R)-rectum; (SV)-seminal vesicles.

a

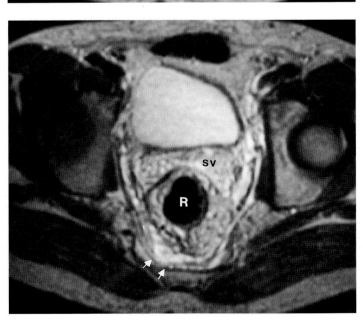

b

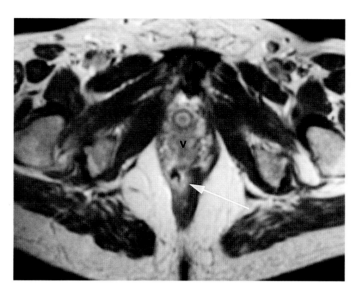

Figure 13.25

Inflammatory changes in the rectum. Contrast-enhanced transaxial T1-weighted image. There is marked enhancement of the rectal mucosa (long white arrow). MRI, however, cannot differentiate between inflammatory and neoplastic changes. (V)-vagina.

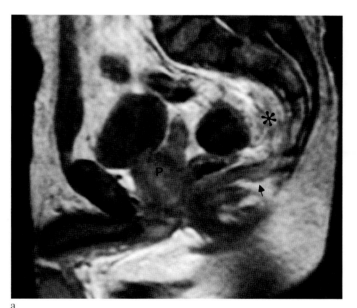

a

Figure 13.26

Pelvic inflammatory disease with extension into the presacral region; sagittal (**a**) T1-weighted image, (**b**) Gd-DTPA-enhanced T1-weighted image, and (**c**) T2-weighted image. Pelvic inflammation originating from the bowel has spread into the presacral region (asterisk) and shows infiltration of the fat on the T1-weighted image and only minor enhancement following gadolinium injection. The inflammation involves the pubococcygeus muscle (black arrow) which is thickened. (P)-prostate. On the T2-weighted image, the presacral area of inflammatory infiltration demonstrates a heterogeneous signal.

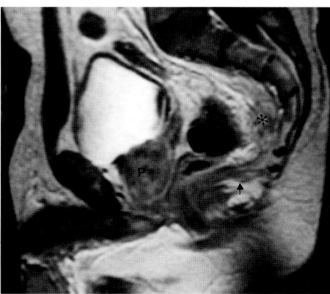

b

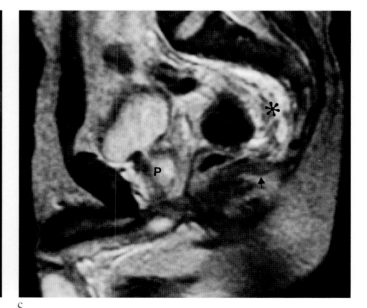

c

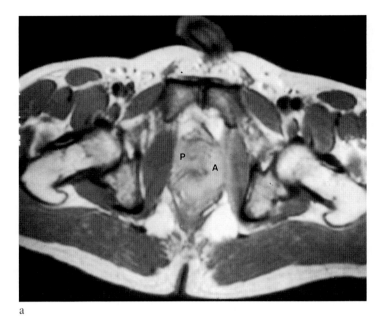

a

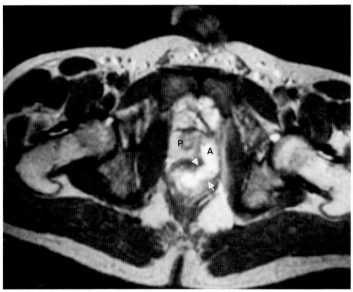

b

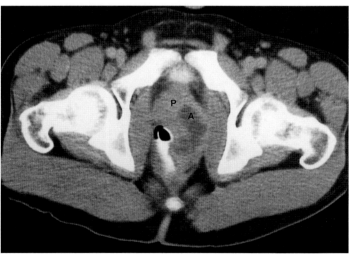

c

Figure 13.27

Periprostatic abscess with sinus tract to the rectum. (**a**) Proton density image, (**b**) T2-weighted image, and (**c**) CT scan. On both the proton density and CT scans, the area of abscess (A) is seen extending between the rectum and the prostate (P). While on both images the abscess formation is highly suspected, the extension of the abscess into the prostate gland cannot be excluded. On the T2-weighted image, however, the sinus tract (small white arrows) with the abscess formation (A) is clearly delineated and the prostate gland (P) is seen to be displaced but not involved.

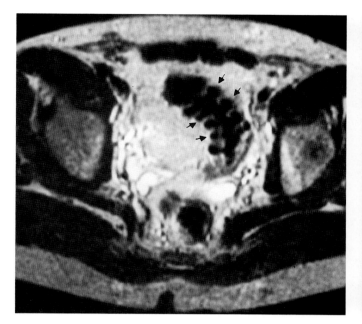

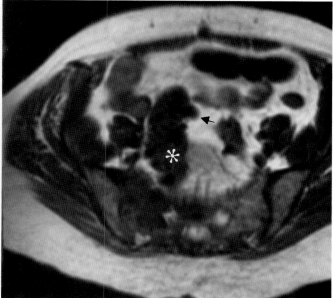

a

Figure 13.28

Diverticulosis of the sigmoid colon; T2-weighted image. Numerous air-filled diverticula (small black arrows) are seen; the bowel wall is of normal thickness.

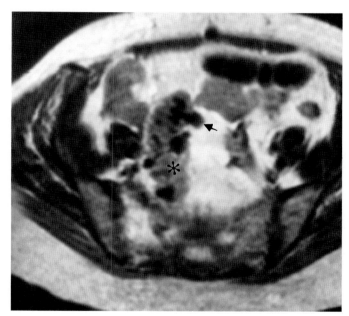

b

Figure 13.29

Uncomplicated diverticulitis; transaxial (**a**) T1-weighted image, and (**b**) Gd-DTPA-enhanced T1-weighted image. Small diverticula (small black arrow) are seen. The bowel wall is thickened (asterisk) and shows enhancement following gadolinium injection. The pericolonic fat tissue is normal.

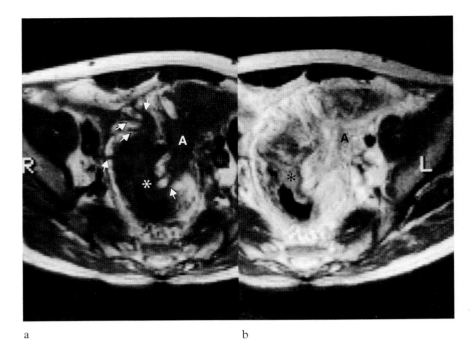

a   b

Figure 13.30

Complicated diverticulitis; (**a**) T1- and (**b**) T2-weighted transaxial images. The bowel wall (asterisk) is thickened, and on the T2-weighted image demonstrates heterogeneous high signal intensity. There is extensive infiltration of the pericolonic fat (small white arrows) and soft tissue mass (A) representing an abscess. Both pericolonic infiltrate and the region of abscess (A) show an increase in signal on the T2-weighted image.

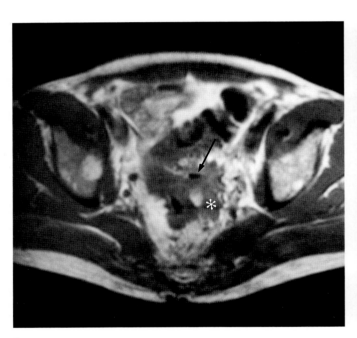
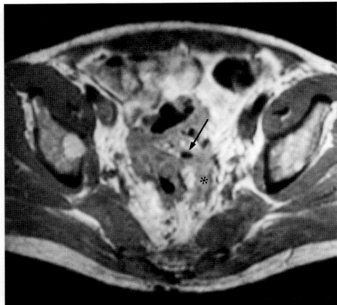

a   b

Figure 13.31

Complicated diverticulitis, with gas within the abscess. (**a**) T1-weighted image, and (**b**) Gd-DTPA-enhanced T1-weighted image. There is extensive infiltration of the pericolonic fat with air (long arrow) seen within the infiltrated tissue. (Asterisk)-abscess. Following gadolinium injection, there is enhancement of inflammatory tissue.

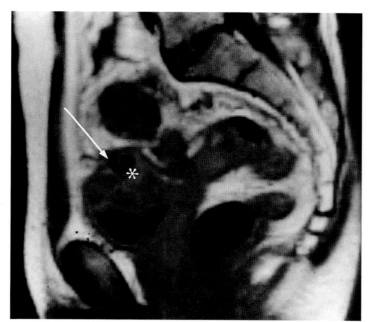

a

Figure 13.32

Acute diverticulitis with extension into the urinary bladder. (**a**) T1- and (**b**) T2-weighted sagittal images. A large inflammatory mass is seen extending to the bladder dome (asterisk). The inflammatory process is extending into the bladder, demonstrating high signal intensity (small black arrows) of the bladder mucosa. There is air within the inflammatory mass (long arrow).

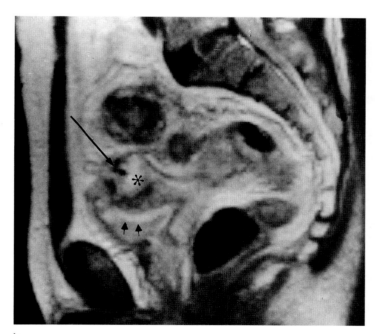

b

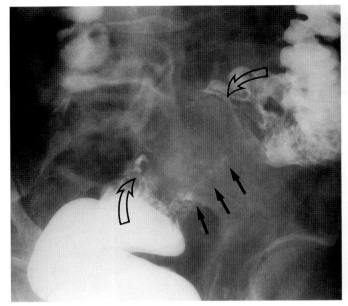

a

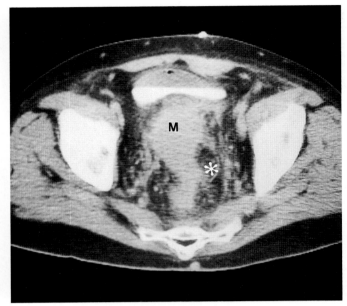

b

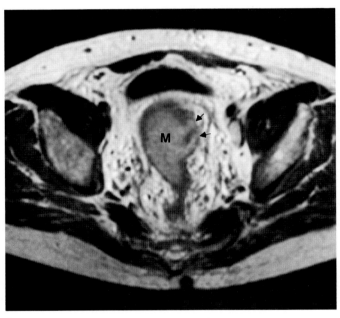

c

Figure 13.33

Extensive diverticulitis, which on multiple studies: (**a**) barium enema; (**b**) CT; or (**c**) to (**g**) MR images could not be differentiated from sigmoid cancer. The MRI studies are as follows: (**c**) transaxial Gd-DTPA-enhanced T1-weighted image, (**d**) sagittal T1- and (**e**) T2-weighted images, (**f**) coronal proton density, and (**g**) coronal T2-weighted images. On the barium enema study, a large irregular filling defect with eccentric lumen (arrows) and overhanging margins (curved open arrows) is seen. On the CT scan, a large tumor mass (M) with extensive pericolonic infiltration (asterisk) is identified. On the transaxial contrast-enhanced MR image, section comparable to CT, the mass (M) demonstrates enhancement, and there is evidence of segmental interruption of the low intensity wall (black arrows) seen on the left side. On the sagittal images, a 15 cm long intraluminal expanding lesion (mass) is seen in the sigmoid colon. Numerous pericolonic nodes are identified (long arrows). In the coronal plane on the proton density image, the large mass (M) is visualized extending into the pericolonic fat (curved arrow), and on the T2-weighted image, there is interruption of the low signal intensity bowel wall (small arrow).

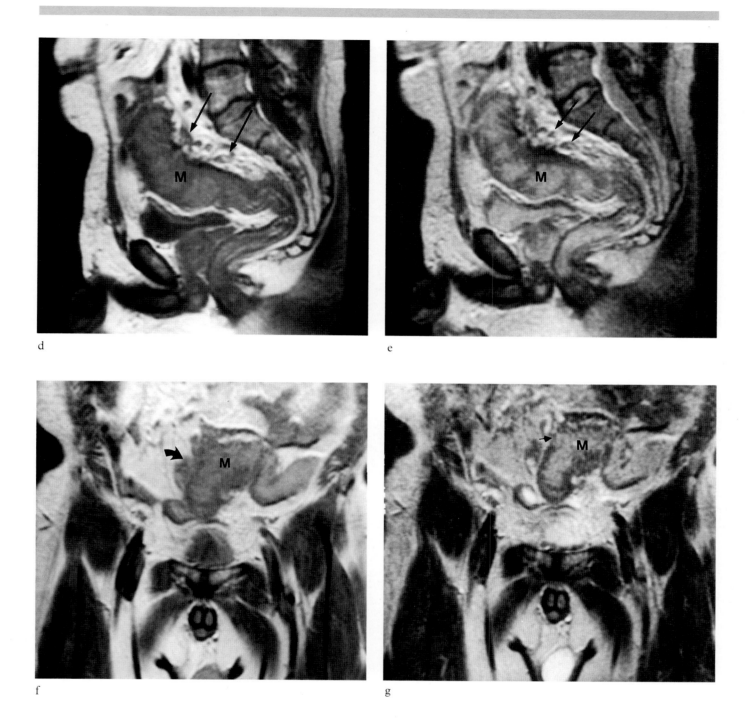

d

e

f

g

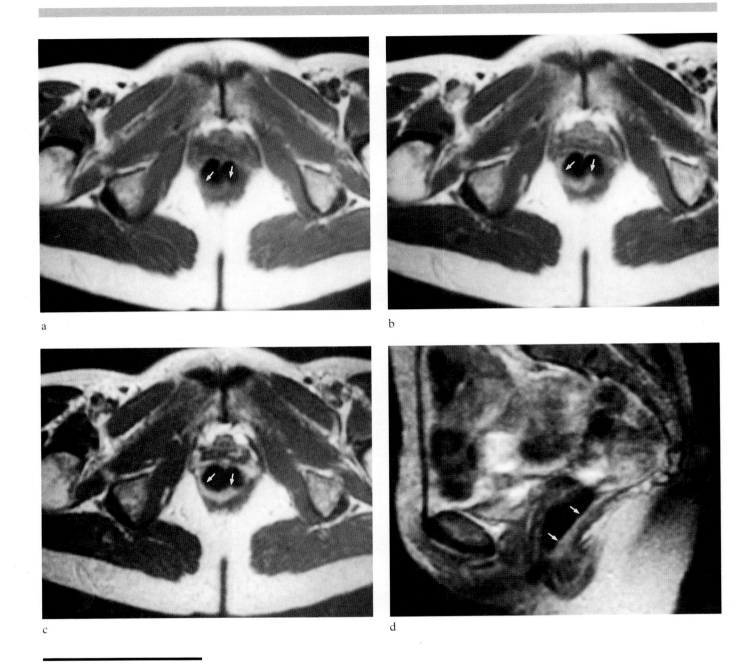

a

b

c

d

Figure 13.34

Carcinoma of the rectum, stage T1N0M0. Transaxial (**a**) T1-weighted image, (**b**) Gd-DTPA-enhanced T1-weighted image, (**c**) T2-weighted image, and (**d**) sagittal T2-weighted image. On the T1-weighted image, the tumor (arrows) blends with the rectal wall and its diagnosis can be suggested only by the demonstration of localized wall thickening. Following injection of Gd-DTPA, the tumor enhances allowing distinction from the adjacent low signal intensity muscle. The T2-weighted image is similar to the Gd-DTPA scan. On the sagittal film, the tumor extension along the posterior wall of the rectum (arrows) is well seen. As the entire thickened wall enhances on MRI, it is impossible to differentiate stage T1 from stage T2 by MRI.

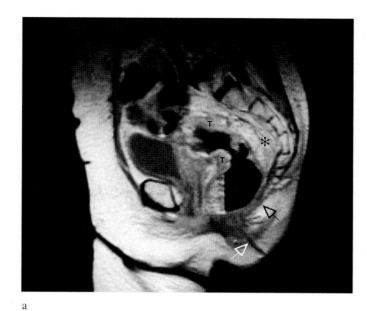

a

Figure 13.35

Stage T3N0M0, carcinoma of the rectum. Sagittal plane (**a**) proton density, (**b**) T1-weighted image, (**c**) T2-weighted image, (**d**) CT scan without contrast injection, and (**e**) CT scan following contrast injection. In the sagittal projection, the circumferential tumor growth (T), tumor length and location with respect to the levator ani muscle (pubococcygeus muscle, open black arrow) and anal canal (enema tip in the anal canal, open white arrow) are well seen. Also seen is tumor infiltration in the presacral region (asterisk). There is no difference between the signal intensity of the tumor and the adjacent wall on the T1-weighted images. The tumor spread along perirectal fascia (small black solid arrows) and the perirectal fat to the presacral region (asterisk) is seen. On the T2-weighted transaxial image, the bowel wall muscle on the left remains of normal low signal intensity, while there is complete mural invasion on the right side (white arrows). These findings cannot be appreciated on CT images either with or without contrast injection. (0.35T.)

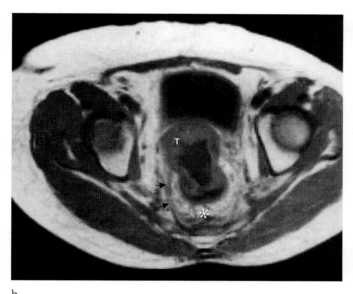

b

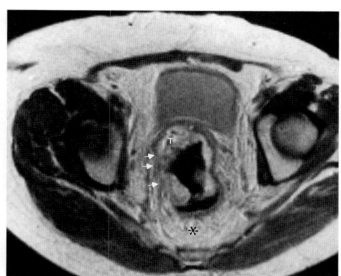

c

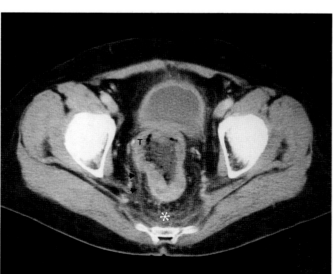

d

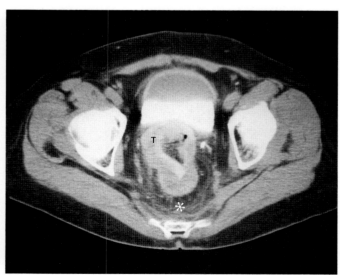

e

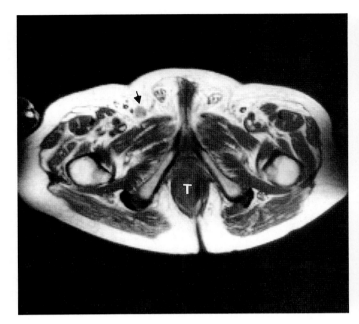

a

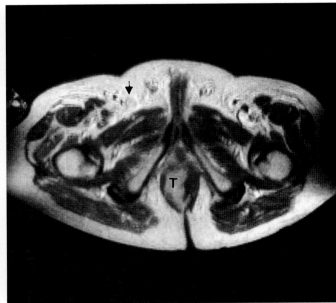

b

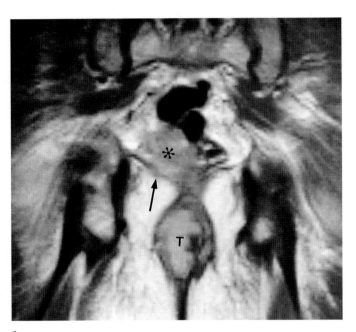

c

Figure 13.36

Carcinoma of the rectum with extension to the anal canal, stage T3N1M0 transaxial (**a**) T1- and (**b**) T2-weighted images. (**c**) Coronal T2-weighted image. On the T1-weighted image, the tumor (T) blends with the adjacent bowel wall, but on the T2-weighted image, the tumor images with high signal intensity contrasted to the low intensity sphincter. In the coronal plane, the tumor (asterisk) invasion of the right levator ani muscle (long arrow) is seen. There is a right inguinal lymph node (small arrow). Presence of inguinal adenopathy indicates the presence of tumor in the anal canal.

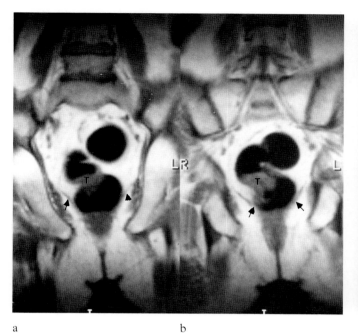

a   b

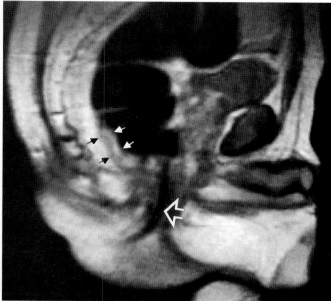

a

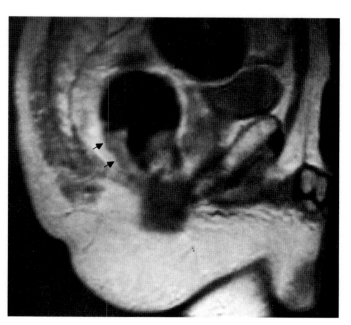

b

Figure 13.37

Carcinoma of the rectum, stage T2N0M0. (**a**) and (**b**) are two consecutive coronal T2-weighted images. The polypoid tumor (T) is seen in the rectal ampulla. The distance between the tumor (T) and the levator ani insertion (small arrow) is well appreciated in the coronal plane.

Figure 13.38

Stage T1N0M0, rectal carcinoma. Sagittal T2-weighted images. (**a**) and (**b**) are two consecutive sections. There is a localized bowel wall thickening (arrows). The outer muscular wall remains of low signal intensity (small black arrows) indicating that the muscularis propria is not invaded, classifying the disease as stage T1. The rectum is distended (enema tip open arrowhead). Imaging was performed with the patient in prone position.

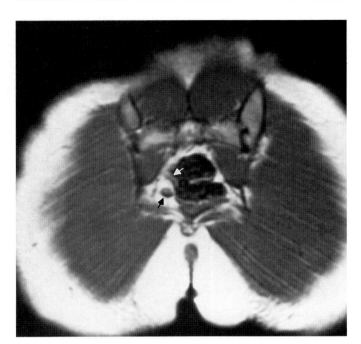

Figure 13.39

Perirectal lymph node, coronal T1-weighted image. In this patient, the primary tumor was very small and was thought to be fully excised by biopsy. There is, however, localized rectal wall thickening (white arrow) which may represent either postbiopsy edema or residual tumor. A small 1 cm pararectal node (black arrow) is present.

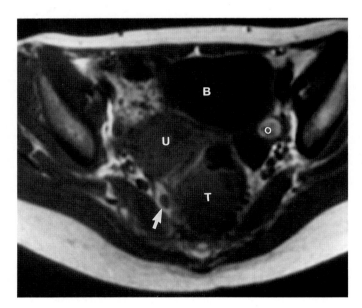

Figure 13.40

Carcinoma of the rectum with pericolonic infiltration and presence of lymph node stage T3N1M0, T1-weighted image. A large tumor (T) shows perirectal infiltration. There is a perirectal lymph node 1 cm in size (short white arrow). (U)-uterus; (O)-ovarian cysts; (B)-urinary bladder.

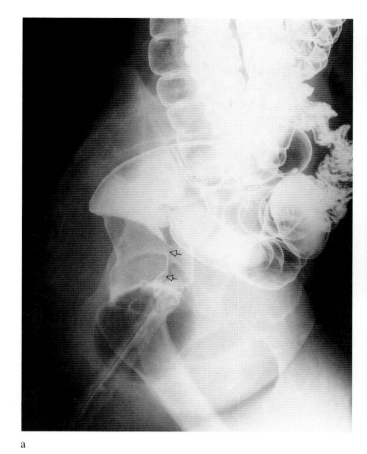

a

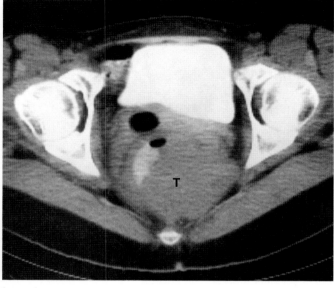

b

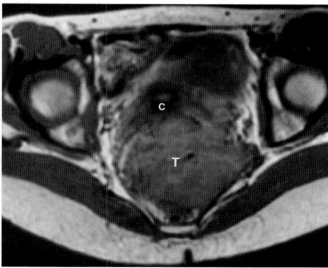

c

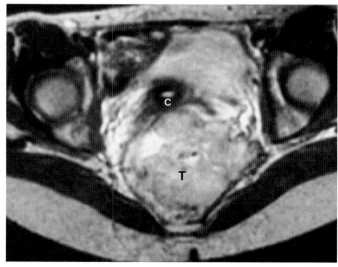

d

Figure 13.41

Cloacogenic carcinoma. (**a**) Barium enema study; (**b**) CT examination; transaxial (**c**) T1-weighted and (**d**) T2-weighted images.

continued overleaf

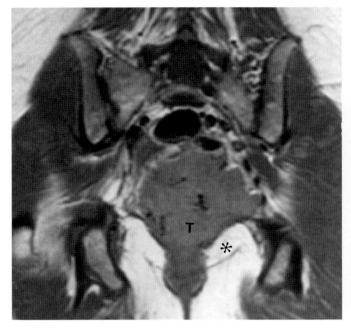

e

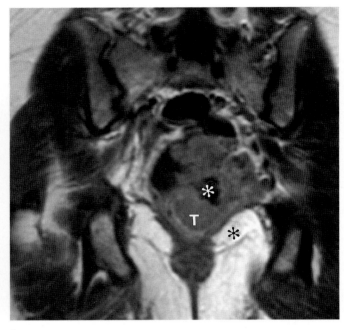

f

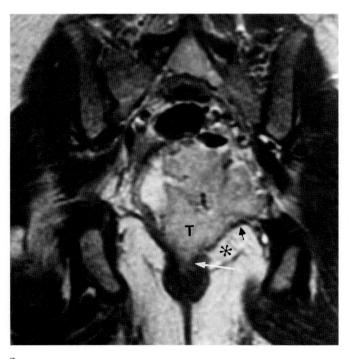

g

Figure 13.41 *continued*

Coronal (**e**) T1-weighted image, (**f**) Gd-DTPA-enhanced T1-weighted image, and (**g**) T2-weighted image. The large cloacogenic carcinoma (T) is seen involving the rectal ampulla and extending into the anal canal [long arrow on (**g**)]. Following gadolinium injection, an area of necrosis within the tumor [white asterisk on (**f**)] can be seen. On the transaxial images, whether CT or MRI, lateral tumor extension cannot be accurately assessed, and it appears that the tumor extends into the ischiorectal fossa and invades the levator ani muscle. (C)-cervix. On the coronal images, however, while the tumor extends towards the left lateral wall, the ischiorectal fossa (black asterisk) is intact and the levator ani muscle (small black arrow) is of normal low signal intensity. The open black arrows on the barium enema study demonstrate an asymmetric impression on the lumen of the rectum.

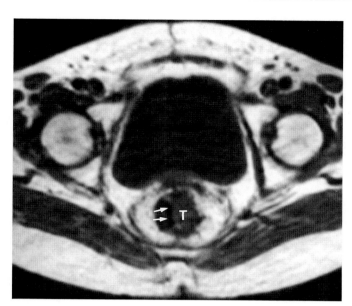

a

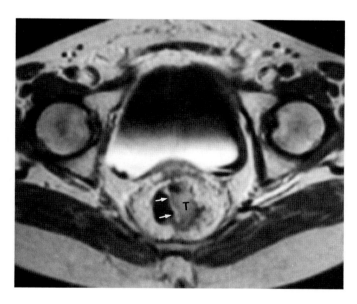

b

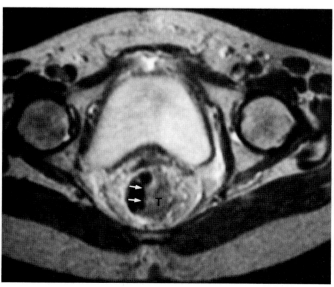

c

Figure 13.42

Metastasis to the rectal wall, primary tumor, carcinoma of the cervix; transaxial plane (**a**) T1-weighted image, (**b**) Gd-DTPA-enhanced T1-weighted image, and (**c**) T2-weighted image. The tumor (T) demonstrates localized bowel wall thickening with narrowing and distortion of the lumen. The mucosal surface (small white arrows) is intact and shows marked enhancement following Gd-DTPA injection.

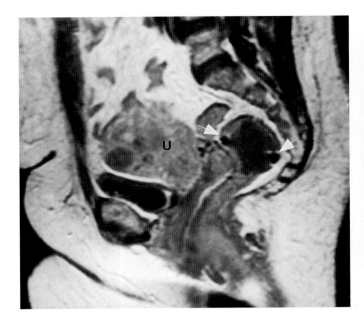

a

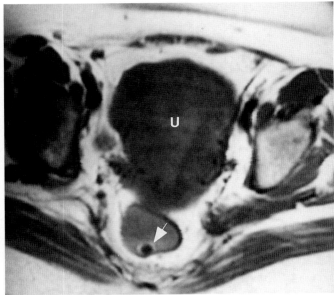

b

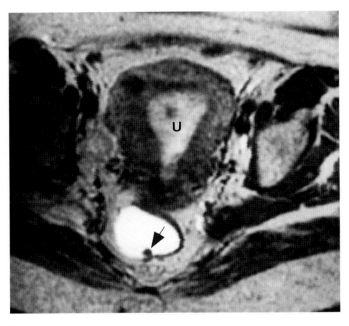

c

Figure 13.43

Normal appearance of the rectum following anterior resection. (**a**) Sagittal Gd-DTPA-enhanced T1-weighted image, (**b**) transaxial T1-weighted image, and (**c**) transaxial T2-weighted image. The surgical clip (solid arrows) (causing metallic artifact) is seen in either plane. The adjacent bowel wall is normal in thickness and signal intensity. (U)-uterus.

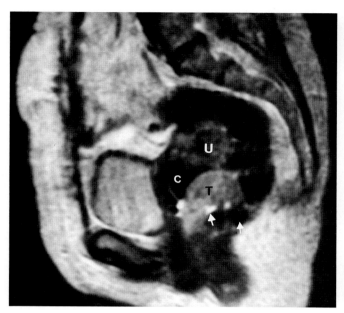

a

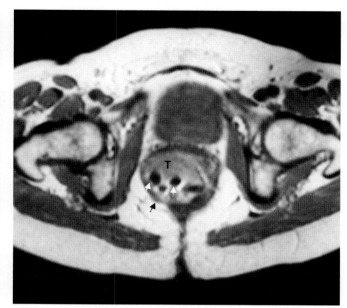

b

Figure 13.44

Recurrent carcinoma of the rectum; sagittal (**a**) T2-weighted image, transaxial (**b**) proton density, and (**c**) T2-weighted images. Tumor (T) recurrence at the site of anastomosis (surgical clips small black and white arrows) demonstrates asymmetrical extraluminal growth pattern, and is displacing but not invading the cervix (c) and corpus uterus (U).

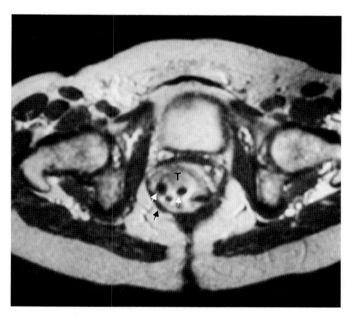

c

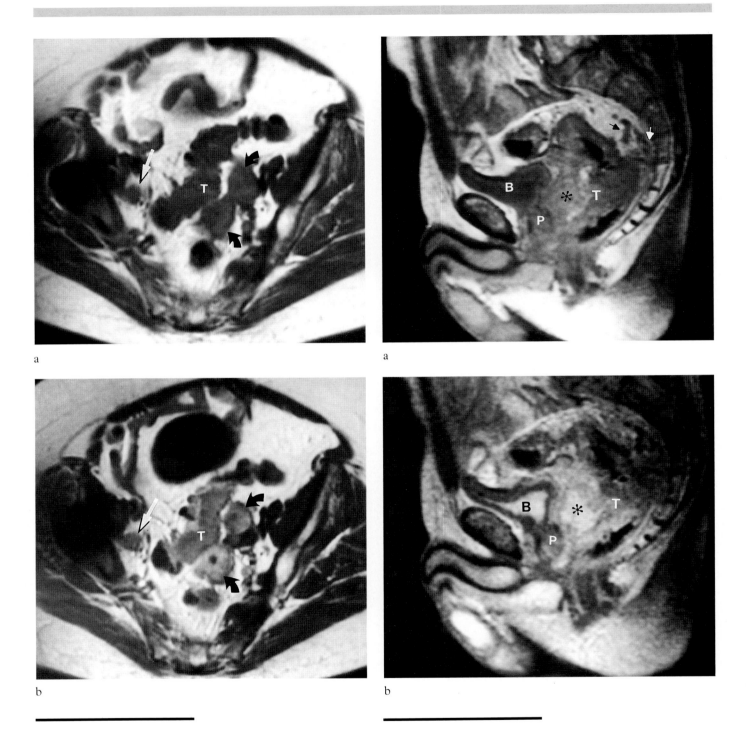

a

b

a

b

Figure 13.45

Recurrent rectosigmoid carcinoma (T) (following anterior resection) with a lobulated extracolonic mass (black curved arrows), and nodal metastasis (arrow); transaxial (**a**) T1-weighted image and (**b**) Gd-DTPA-enhanced T1-weighted image.

A large tumor (T) and a pericolonic mass (curved arrows) increase in signal intensity following Gd-DTPA injection. An enlarged lymph node (small arrow) also shows some enhancement following Gd-DTPA injection.

Figure 13.46

Recurrent carcinoma of the rectum (following low anterior resection) with tumor (T) spread to the presacral region (small arrows), to the cul-de-sac (asterisk), and with tumor invasion of the seminal vesicles. The urinary bladder (B) and prostate gland (P) are not invaded. Sagittal plane (**a**) proton density and (**b**) T2-weighted images. While the tumor size and perirectal tumor invasion are better seen on the proton density image, invasion of seminal vesicles as well as lack of invasion of the urinary bladder and prostate can be assessed only on the T2-weighted image.

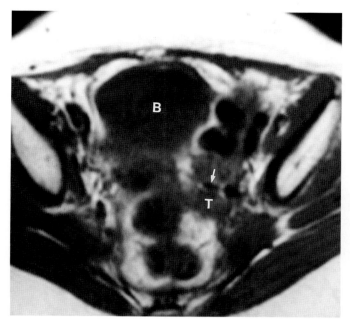

a

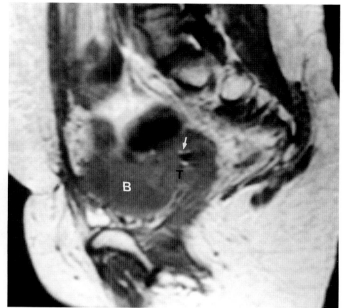

b

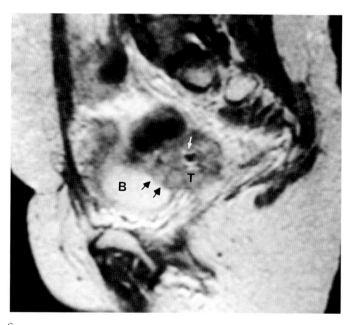

c

Figure 13.47

Recurrence at the suture site (following anterior resection). (**a**) Transaxial T1-weighted image, (**b**) sagittal proton density, and (**c**) sagittal T2-weighted images. At the site of anastomosis which is identified by the clip artifact (arrow), a tumor mass (T) is present. On the T2-weighted image, the tumor mass is seen to have heterogeneous high signal intensity. As seen on the T2-weighted image, the tumor invades (small black arrows) the urinary bladder (B).

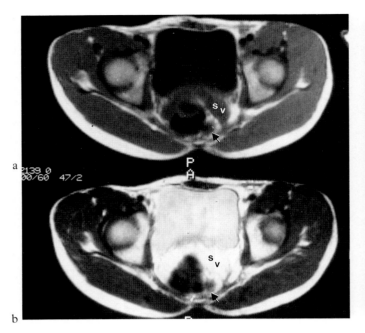

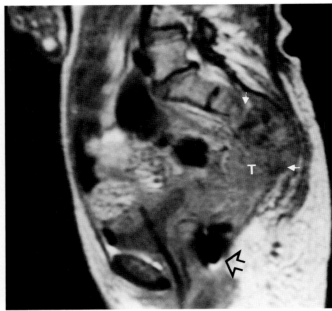

Figure 13.48

Recurrent carcinoma of the rectum following anterior resection demonstrating low signal intensity on the T2-weighted image. (**a**) T1-weighted image and (**b**) T2-weighted image. A small perirectal tumor mass (arrow) demonstrates low signal intensity on the T1- and T2-weighted images. A recurrent tumor was proven at biopsy. (SV)-seminal vesicles. (0.35T.)

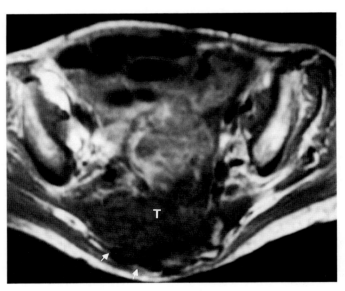

Figure 13.49

Large recurrent rectal carcinoma with extensive bony invasion. (**a**) Sagittal proton density image, and (**b**) transaxial T1-weighted image. A large tumor mass (T) is seen extending from the site of anastomosis (open arrow) and causing extensive bony invasion (white arrows). (Open arrowhead)-surgical clip.

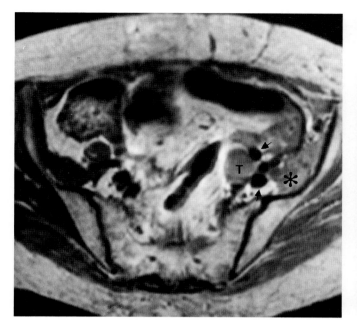

a

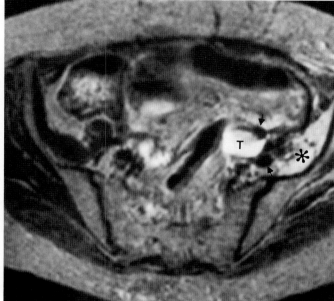

b

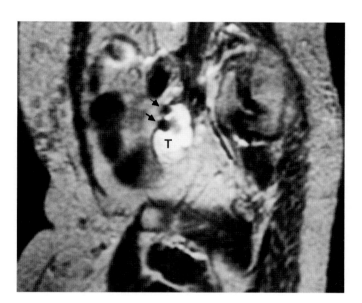

c

Figure 13.50

Recurrent carcinoma of the rectum (T) at the site of surgical intervention (small black arrows) with tumor invading the adjacent psoas and iliacus (asterisk) muscle. Transaxial (**a**) proton density image, (**b**) T2-weighted image, and sagittal (**c**) T2-weighted image. The psoas muscle was exposed during initial surgery, and the present tumor spread may be due to surgical seeding.

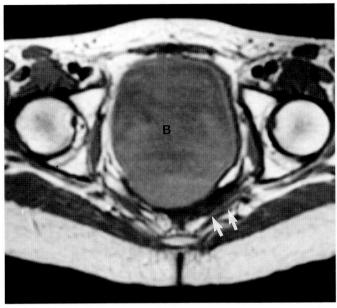

a

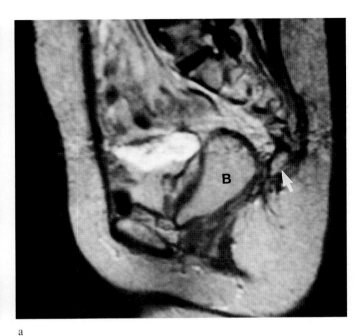

a

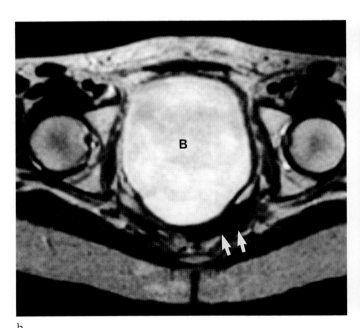

b

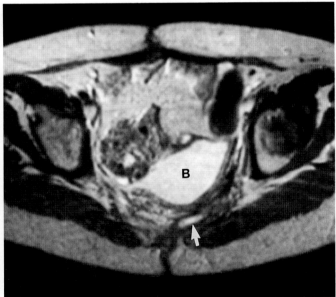

b

Figure 13.51

Appearance of the female pelvis following AP resection. Transaxial (**a**) proton density and (**b**) T2-weighted images. There is extensive postsurgical scarring seen posterior to the urinary bladder (B). The surgical scar is of homogeneous low signal intensity on the T2-weighted image, and the configuration of the scar tissue follows the pelvic boundary (arrows).

Figure 13.52

Recurrent carcinoma of the rectum arising within the postsurgical scar. Figures (**a**) sagittal and (**b**) transaxial T2-weighted images are the initial MRI studies obtained one year after surgery. Within the region of the surgical scar which is of medium high signal intensity, there is a small localized area of high signal intensity (white arrow).

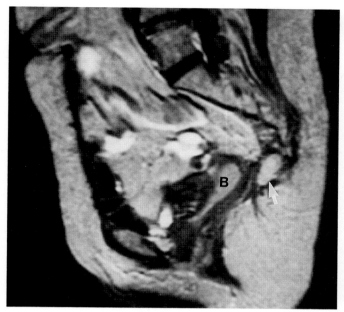

c

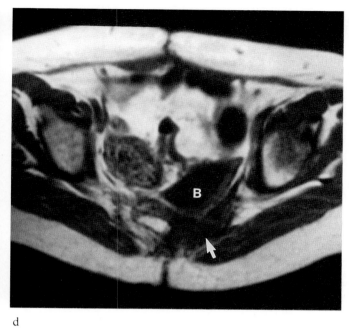

d

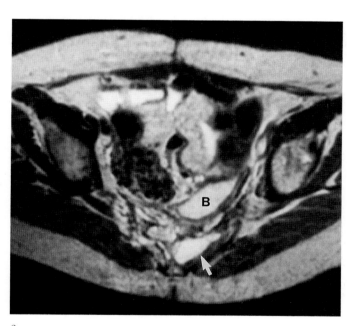

e

Figures (**c**), (**d**) and (**e**) are from an MR study obtained six months later. Figure (**c**) is a sagittal T2-weighted image, (**d**) is a transaxial T1-weighted image, and (**e**) is a transaxial T2-weighted image. In the six-month interval, the presacral soft tissue has increased in size and the region of high signal intensity has now expanded. Interval growth combined with higher signal intensity on the T2-weighted image and mass effect indicate tumor recurrence, which was proven by biopsy. Displacement of the urinary bladder (B) is due to abdominoperineal resection.

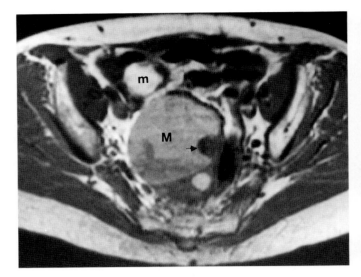

a

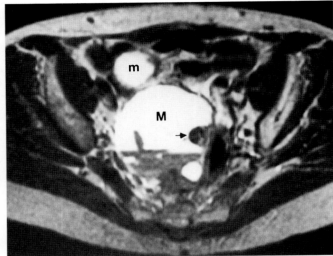

b

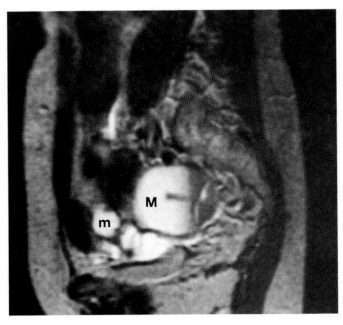

c

Figure 13.53

Cystic ovarian metastasis (M) and peritoneal metastatic seeding (m) from the primary rectal cancer. (**a**) Transaxial proton density, (**b**) transaxial T2-weighted image, and (**c**) sagittal T2-weighted image. A large mass (M) is seen in the region of the right ovary. The lesion is of heterogeneous predominantly high signal intensity on the T2-weighted images with debris level. An intramural nodule (arrow) is present. At surgery, the large lesion represented a cystic metastatic ovarian tumor. An intraperitoneal cystic metastasis was also identified (m).

14
Postoperative and Postradiation Pelvis

Bernadette Carrington

The correct radiologic interpretation of postoperative and postradiotherapy pelvic changes is important in several clinical situations. In the immediate postoperative period the effects of surgery have to be differentiated from residual disease and postsurgical complications. Assessment of treatment efficacy and identification of recurrent disease also necessitate an appreciation of treatment-induced changes. Delineation of pelvic anatomy is also important in selecting the correct surgical approach in patients who require multiple surgical procedures. This is particularly important when different surgical subspecialists may operate independently.

The superior contrast resolution offered by MRI results in the identification of subtle post-treatment tissue changes which may not be visible with other imaging modalities. The facility for multiplanar imaging permits optimal delineation of altered anatomy and, in addition, MRI is capable of differentiating between treatment changes and residual or recurrent disease.

Postoperative appearances

Female pelvis

Uterine surgery

Myomectomy. Myomectomy is performed to remove uterine leiomyomata in patients wishing to achieve pregnancy. If there are only a few submucosal leiomyomata, a hysteroscopic surgical approach may be adopted. However, laparotomy is required for all intramural leiomyomata and for multiple or large lesions.[1,2]

MRI appearance. After myomectomy there may be no identifiable scar and the absence of previously noted leiomyomata may be the only evidence of surgical intervention. Sometimes the uterus may demonstrate localized low signal intensity due to fibrosis at the surgical site.

Total abdominal hysterectomy. Total abdominal hysterectomy involves removal of the body of the uterus, the cervix, and a small cuff of vagina. The uterosacral, uterovesical, round, and broad ligaments are incised, but the cardinal ligaments, which are intimately related to the ureters, are left intact.[3] The proximal vagina is sutured. Subtotal hysterectomy, with the cervix left in situ, used to be an alternative procedure, but it offers no advantage over conventional hysterectomy and the retained cervix poses a potential risk of carcinoma.

MRI appearance. Since the uterus and cervix are absent, the vagina can be seen to end blindly at its proximal origin, as shown in Figure 14.1. The scar tissue of the vaginal vault demonstrates low signal intensity on both T1- and T2-weighted images (Figure 14.2). The opposed vaginal fornices typically form a linear soft tissue density, but some nodularity may be seen at the lateral margins (Figure 14.2) due to postsurgical reactive tissue.

519

Radical hysterectomy.   In a radical hysterectomy, the ureters are dissected free from the paracervical tissues and the bladder is dissected free from the upper one-third of the vagina. The uterosacral ligaments are incised near their point of origin posteriorly, and the cardinal ligaments are severed at the lateral pelvic sidewall. The uterus, the upper-third of the vagina, and the parametrial, paracervical, and upper paravaginal tissues are removed, together with the uterine ligaments.[2] Lymphadenectomy is also performed, and all the pelvic nodes distal to the common iliac vessels are removed. Paraaortic lymphadenectomy may also be performed.

MRI appearance.   In the central pelvis, radical and simple hysterectomies have a similar MRI appearance (Figure 14.2). However, in a radical hysterectomy there may be evidence of lymphadenectomy, with the presence of metallic clips along the pelvic sidewall, and the residual vagina is smaller in length.

Ovarian surgery

Transposition.   Ovarian transposition is performed to move the ovaries out of a pelvic radiation field, in order to preserve their function. The ovary is transplanted by sectioning its attachments to the uterus and the posterior broad ligament and is then transposed, with the ovarian vessels acting as a long pedicle. Typically, the ovary is placed in an intraperitoneal position in the flank, usually in the region of the paracolic gutter.[4,5] Ovarian transposition may be mistaken for recurrent disease.[6]

MRI appearance.   Usually, the ovary is visualized laterally in the flank, and images with medium signal intensity on T1-weighted images and increased signal intensity on T2-weighted images. Sometimes the ovaries may be placed in a retrocecal location.[6]

Vaginal surgery

Neovagina.   Most commonly, a neovagina, or vaginal substitute, is fashioned from a segment of sigmoid colon, which is anastomosed to the perineum. The surgery is performed after an anterior pelvic exenteration. The mucous secretions from the substitute colon act as a lubricant, and sexual intercourse is thereby facilitated. Gracilis muscle flaps have been used to form a neovagina in patients undergoing total pelvic exenteration.

MRI appearance.   A neovagina has a characteristic MRI appearance, as illustrated in Figure 14.3. There is absence of the normal urethra and vagina within the urogenital triangle, and in the corresponding position the neovagina is seen running anteroposteriorly. It is of medium signal intensity on both T1- and T2-weighted images.

Male pelvis

Prostate surgery

Prostate surgery is performed for the resection of benign hypertrophy or prostatic malignancy. In benign disease, three surgical procedures are currently employed: **transurethral resection of the prostate (TURP)**, **suprapubic prostatectomy**, and **retropubic prostatectomy.**[7]

The surgical approach is determined primarily by the size of the prostate gland. When the enlarged prostate weighs less than 50 g—an assessment which can be made clinically, by transrectal ultrasound, or by MRI—the most common method of resection is TURP. TURP involves cystoscopic resection of the hyperplastic transition zone and periurethral tissue from the base of the bladder to the verumontanum. A conical or spinning top widening of the proximal urethra results with regrowth of the urethral epithelium to cover the defect.

If the gland weighs more than 50 g, a suprapubic or retropubic approach is necessary. These approaches are used to avoid the metabolic disturbances which result from systemic absorption of large quantities of cystoscopic irrigation fluid through the raw surface of a TURP defect during protracted surgery. Suprapubic prostatectomy is also performed when treatment for coexistent bladder pathology is required, for example removal of a diverticulum. An extraperitoneal abdominal approach is used in suprapubic prostatectomy, and prostatic tissue is removed after incising the bladder mucosa over the prostate. In retropubic prostatectomy, the approach is via the lower abdomen, and the retropubic space is dissected between the bladder and the pubic bone to remove the hypertrophic tissue via the anterior prostate.

Radical retropubic prostatectomy.   This is the surgical treatment of choice for prostate carcinoma. In this procedure the entire prostate, seminal vesicles, and prostatic urethra are removed.[8] A variable portion of the bladder base is excised, depending on identification of tumor involvement. During the procedure, the vesicoprostatic plexi are ligated, the puboprostatic ligament is transected, and Denonvilliers' fascia is used as the plane of dissection between the prostate and rectum. In addition, the obturator and both internal and external iliac lymph nodes are dissected to the level of the common iliac bifurcation. The residual bladder base is anastomosed to the membranous urethra, and the patient relies on the external sphincter mechanism of the urogenital membrane for continence.

MRI appearance. The MRI appearance after prostate surgery is governed by the surgical approach. After TURP, the proximal prostatic urethra is dilated from the base of the bladder to the verumontanum, as seen in Figure 14.4. No scar tissue is identified in the suprapubic region. After a suprapubic or retropubic prostatectomy, however, in addition to the widened proximal prostatic urethra, scar tissue is identified in the suprapubic region and the bladder wall may demonstrate irregularity in those patients who have had suprapubic surgery. Figures 14.5 and 14.6 are examples of the suprapubic and retropubic approaches.

Figure 14.7 illustrates the pelvic appearance after radical prostatectomy, in which there is no identifiable prostate or seminal vesicles. The bladder base is low, lying beneath the symphysis pubis, due to its anastomosis with the membranous urethra. Metallic surgical clips may produce punctate regions of signal void at the anastomotic site and adjacent to the iliac vessels. Fibrous scarring at the anastomostic site may cause it to image with low signal intensity on both T1- and T2-weighted images.

Bladder surgery

Bladder resection is performed most commonly for primary bladder neoplasms and may be partial or total. Secondary bladder involvement from adjacent pelvic cancers, typically cervical carcinoma, necessitates a **total cystectomy**, either alone or as part of a pelvic exenteration procedure. Occasionally, **partial cystectomy** is performed when there is a solitary tumor which is not related to the bladder neck or trigone, with an otherwise stable bladder uroepithelium.

Radical total cystectomy is performed for malignant bladder lesions, and may be employed as the primary curative treatment after radiotherapy failure or for palliation when patients are incapacitated by severe hematuria.[9] In all patients, the bladder is resected and bilateral pelvic lymphadenectomy and retroperitoneal lymph node dissection is performed. In males the prostatic urethra, seminal vesicles, fat, and overlying pelvic peritoneum are removed. In females the urethra, uterus, ovaries, fallopian tubes and a

segment of the anterior vagina are resected in the same procedure.

After total cystectomy, a urinary diversion is necessary and currently there are three alternatives:[10] (1) a **urinary conduit (ureteroentero–cutaneous diversion)**; (2) a **continent urinary reservoir**; and (3) a **bladder substitute.** A conduit is formed using a non-detubularized bowel loop, usually ileum, which then opens onto the skin surface. Urine is transported by peristalsis within the bowel segment into a collecting bag. A continent urinary reservoir involves detubularizing a small bowel segment and forming a low pressure pouch into which the ureters are anastomosed. A valve mechanism, such as the ileocecal valve, connects the pouch to the exterior abdominal wall. The valve is competent, preventing leakage, and the patient catheterizes the reservoir periodically to drain the urine. In females, continent urinary reservoirs can be pelvic in location, with the valve mechanism connecting to the perineum. For example, cecum can form the reservoir, with the ileocecal valve forming the continence mechanism, and the distal terminal ileum forms a channel to the perineum.

With new surgical techniques it is now possible to construct a bladder substitute in male patients. The substitute is fashioned from cecum, sigmoid colon, or stomach, and is anastomosed to the membranous urethra. The voluntary external urethral sphincter remains intact, preserving continence. This procedure is impossible in females because the urethra is completely resected during the cystectomy procedure.

MRI appearance

A urinary conduit is recognized by its position, typically in the right iliac fossa, where the diverted bowel loop may be visualized traversing the abdominal wall through the rectus abdominis muscle to reach the skin surface. Unless they are hydronephrotic, the ureters are not identified entering the loop. Figure 14.8 shows the MRI appearance of a urinary conduit.

A continent urinary reservoir can also be depicted on MR scans and is illustrated in Figure 14.9. The reservoir is seen adjacent to the anterior abdominal wall, and it has the configuration of bowel with a lobulated outline and identifiable haustra. It contains fluid with the signal characteristics of urine, that is, low signal intensity on T1-weighted images and high signal intensity on T2-weighted images. The valve mechanism connecting the reservoir to the skin surface is also depicted, and in some patients signal void from surgical clips may be identified.

A bladder substitute, illustrated in Figure 14.10, lacks the smooth outline of the normal bladder and is seen as a slightly lobulated, thin-walled, urine-filled structure. The inferior border of the bladder substitute is beneath the level of the symphysis pubis, and the site of anastomosis may be seen in the region of the membranous urethra. Again, signal void from surgical clips may be seen at the urethral anastomosis and along the pelvic lymph node chains.

Rectal surgery

Rectal resection is usually performed for carcinoma and there are two main surgical procedures, either an **anterior resection** or an **abdominoperineal (AP) resection**. Many factors govern the choice of operation, of which the most important is the level of the tumor within the rectum.[11,12] Generally, the distal margin of resection should be approximately 4 cm below the tumor, and an additional 2–3 cm of anal tissue is required to fashion an end-to-end low anterior anastomosis. Therefore, when the inferior tumor resection margin is greater than 8 cm from the anal verge, patients are treated by anterior resection. Those tumors with an inferior resection margin less than 8 cm from the anal verge are treated by AP resection. Other factors which govern the choice of operation include extent of circumferential tumor involvement; fixity of the tumor; degree of differentiation on biopsy; the presence of lymphadenopathy or perirectal spread; and patient factors such as body habitus, age, and other systemic disease.

A low anterior resection consists of complete mobilization of the rectum from the hollow of the sacrum, and division of the lateral ligaments containing the middle rectal arteries. A portion of the rectum is resected, and anastomosis is effected in the residual rectum distal to the visceral peritoneum. The anastomosis is usually achieved with metal staples. Lymph node dissection is performed at the same time.

During AP resection the abdomen is explored for the presence of metastatic disease and the sigmoid colon is used to form a colostomy. The rectum is mobilized, separated from adjacent organs, and the lateral rectal ligaments are divided. Synchronous perineal dissection is performed, and the rectum is pulled through into the perineum and completely removed. The procedure involves dividing and then resuturing the levator ani muscles to reconstitute the pelvic floor. In women, a posterior vaginectomy is simultaneously performed. Hysterectomy is indicated if there is tumor penetration through the rectal wall to involve the uterus.

MRI appearance

After anterior resection, the site of rectal anastomosis can be recognized by the ring of metallic staples, as seen in Figure 14.11. Localized fibrotic tissue is sometimes seen surrounding the anastomosis, and it demonstrates low signal intensity on both T1- and T2-weighted images. The anastomotic site may cause rectal wall irregularity and localized decrease in the diameter of the rectal lumen (Figure 14.11). The residual rectum is reduced in length, and this may cause a decrease in the anterior rectal concavity and an increase in width of the presacral space (greater than 1.5 cm at S4/5 vertebral level).

AP resection is characterized by the complete absence of the rectum and the identification of a sigmoid colostomy, as demonstrated in Figure 14.12. Frequently, there is fibrosis in the presacral space and it demonstrates low signal intensity on all spin-echo sequences. The levator ani muscles show evidence of prior incision and re-anastomosis, as illustrated in Figure 14.13. There is evidence of low signal intensity fibrosis on both T1- and T2-weighted images, in addition to asymmetry of position. On transaxial images at the level of the perineum, the posterior or anal triangle is deficient due to resection of the anal canal (Figure 14.14). Another consequence of AP resection is a redistribution of the residual pelvic contents, with the bladder and seminal vesicles or uterus moving posteriorly in the true pelvis (Figure 14.15).

Pelvic exenteration

Pelvic exenteration is performed for recurrent or persistent pelvic malignancy, most frequently carcinoma of the cervix.[2,13] It may also be indicated in patients who are severely affected by changes caused by pelvic radiation. Total exenteration consists of removal of the bladder, urethra, uterus, vagina, and rectum; together with all the pelvic supporting and connective tissues. Partial exenteration is either anterior, with preservation of the rectum, or posterior, with retention of the bladder and urethra. Most exenterations are supralevator and the pelvic floor musculature is preserved. However, infralevator exenteration is occasionally necessary, and in these cases the pelvic floor muscles and vulva are also resected.

MRI appearance

As shown in Figure 14.16, MRI scans after total exenteration demonstrate complete absence of the normal pelvic organs. The potential space is occupied by small bowel and a variable amount of fibrous tissue. If the patient has had subsequent radiotherapy, there may be a considerable degree of fibrosis. Patients have both a urinary diversion and a colostomy, which may be visualized during the MRI examination.

In patients with anterior pelvic exenteration, there is no identifiable bladder or pelvic genitalia, and the potential space is filled by bowel. As shown in Figure 14.17, in these patients the rectum often occupies a more anterior position. In posterior pelvic exenteration (Figures 14.18 and 14.19) the bladder extends in a posterior direction over the pelvic floor muscles which display a low signal intensity on all sequences due to postsurgical fibrosis.

MRI in relation to other imaging modalities

Postsurgical MRI appearances are usually noted co-incidentally during the course of an examination requested for other clinical reasons. Some postoperative changes can be identified on ultrasound scans, and CT scans may provide additional detailed information. However, MRI is superior to both US and CT in the depiction of surgical changes, and this is of particular relevance in the evaluation of residual or recurrent disease.

MRI appearance of postoperative complications

A variety of pelvic complications may occur in the postoperative patient. The most common are infection and hematoma formation; others include surgically-induced fistulas and sinus tracts, often secondary to protracted or severe infection. In patients who have had lymphadenectomy, there is a small risk of the development of lymphoceles. MRI is capable of detecting all types of postsurgical complications and can be used to accurately delineate the position, size, and extent of the abnormality.

Hematoma

The MRI appearance of blood is complex since its signal intensity depends on the relative amounts of hemoglobin degradation products, which vary with the time from the initial hemorrhage. The site of bleeding is also important. For example, the temporal changes in signal intensity of intracranial hemorrhage are different from those seen in bleeds occurring elsewhere in the body. In the acute phase (up to one week) hemorrhage is of low signal intensity on T1-weighted images and high signal intensity on T2-weighted images. In the subacute phase after hemorrhage, illustrated in Figure 14.20, blood is of high signal intensity on both T1- and T2-weighted images, and thereafter has similar characteristics for a variable period.

Abscess

Infection is a common complication of surgery, especially when bowel has perforated pre-operatively or been incised during the procedure. An abscess is a circumscribed area of infection containing central necrosis. On T1-weighted images it can be seen as a medium signal intensity mass, and it increases in signal intensity on T2-weighted images. In some abscesses multiple foci of necrosis and liquefaction may produce a heterogeneous appearance. Air may form in an abscess, and its presence is indicated by the identification of regions of very low signal intensity on both T1- and T2-weighted images. Figure 14.21 demonstrates extensive pelvic sepsis.

Fistula or sinus tract

A **fistula** is an abnormal communication between two epithelial surfaces and a **sinus** is a blind-ending abnormal tract which communicates with only one epithelial surface. Both occur most frequently as a result of infection, which may be secondary to surgery or to inflammatory gastrointestinal conditions such as Crohn's disease. Fistulas may also be caused by penetrating tumors or radiotherapy. Unless they are large, fistulas are usually not identified on MRI. Indirect evidence, such as air in an abnormal location, as shown in Figure 14.22, usually leads to their identification. Sometimes the site of the fistula is seen, and in cases of long-standing disease it is often fibrotic and demonstrates low signal intensity on all spin-echo sequences (Figure 14.22).

A sinus tract is identified by its orientation, its inflammatory content, the fibrotic nature of its wall, and reactive inflammatory changes in surrounding tissues. Sinuses are linear or tubular structures which run from the pelvis to the skin surface, usually the perineum. A sinus is of medium signal intensity on T1-weighted images and high signal intensity on T2-weighted images due to necrotic debris or fluid discharge. The tract is lined by low signal intensity fibrous tissue as demonstrated in Figure 14.23.

Lymphocele

Lymphoceles represent accumulations of lymph fluid adjacent to the pelvic sidewall, which are contained by the parietal peritoneum. They are relatively uncommon complications of lymphadenectomy, occurring in less than 5 per cent of patients. Lymphoceles may develop either rapidly or more slowly over the course of several months, and there is great variation in size as well as outcome. Some lymphoceles disappear spontaneously, whereas others become symptomatic and require aspiration. As seen in Figure 14.24, which illustrates the MRI appearance of bilateral lymphoceles, lymphoceles are visualized as well circumscribed oval structures which demonstrate medium signal intensity on T1-weighted images and very high signal intensity on T2-weighted images due to their protein content. The configuration and position of a lymphocele, together with its signal characteristics, facilitate recognition on imaging studies, particularly when there is a history of previous lymph node dissection.

MRI in relation to other imaging modalities

MRI is not routinely advocated for the investigation of postsurgical complications since both US and CT can provide equally diagnostic results. However MRI is indicated in those patients in whom US and CT are equivocal, and in the evaluation of residual disease or suspected recurrence where recognition of postsurgical complications helps ensure accurate patient assessment.

Radiation therapy effects

Many pelvic malignancies are treated by radiation therapy with the intention of delivering a uniform tumor dose without injuring normal tissues. However, the adjacent normal organs inevitably receive a small proportion of the total tumor dose and therefore radiation-induced tissues changes may occur. The development of radiation injury is known to be dependent on the total dose received, the volume of tissue irradiated, and additional factors such as the overall treatment time and the size of administered radiation fractions.[14,15] Concurrent surgery or chemotherapy are synergistic with radiation therapy, and patients receiving combined treatment are more likely to suffer from radiation tissue toxicity. However, it is recognized that great individual variation exists both in the occurrence of radiation injury and in the development of clinical symptoms.

The mechanisms by which radiation causes injury remain unclear. We know that absorption of radiation energy causes ionization of intracellular atoms, increasing their reactivity or promoting their breakdown into more reactive or toxic substances. These radiation-induced changes have maximum effect on the intermitotic cells of actively proliferating tissue such as bowel, bladder, and bone marrow.[16] Radiation effects are also seen in small blood vessels, which develop an endarteritis and increased endothelial permeability resulting in the formation of interstitial edema and congestion. Vascular fibroblast activity is stimulated, and produces vessel occlusion and ische-

mia leading to further cell death. Interstitial fibrosis is also promoted by radiation therapy.[16]

Clinically, radiation reactions are divided into acute reactions (those occurring up to three months from the start of therapy), subacute reactions (those occurring three months to one year after treatment), and chronic reactions (those occurring more than one year after institution of therapy).[17,18] Acute reactions are due to parenchymal cell death, and the patient has symptoms relating to the affected organs, for example mucositis, diarrhea, or cystitis. Long-term symptoms result from fibrosis, causing impaired organ function or stricture formation.

It is not possible to identify acute organ changes due to radiotherapy with conventional radiologic imaging modalities, but chronic fibrotic sequelae have been recognized, especially in the gastrointestinal and urinary tracts. Treatment of rectal carcinoma has been reported to cause pelvic postradiation changes identified on CT.[19,20]

With the superior contrast resolution of MRI, radiation effects on every pelvic organ and tissue have been recognized.[21–25] As would be expected, the incidence of tissue change identified on MR examinations is proportional to the total radiation dose and is significantly increased over a threshold dose of 4500cGy.[21] Observed tissue changes appear to be independent of the method of radiotherapy administration, and are seen after both external beam treatment and brachytherapy.[21]

MRI appearance of postradiation changes

Female pelvis

The female genitalia demonstrate a variety of radiation tissue effects. As seen in Figure 14.25, the **uterus** may undergo several changes in women of reproductive age.[22] On T2-weighted images there is a generalized decrease in signal intensity of the myometrium, which may be seen as early as one month after treatment. The uterine zonal anatomy becomes indistinct after approximately three months, and there is a decrease in the thickness and signal intensity of the endometrium, which becomes apparent after about six months. The uterus may also decrease in size after radiotherapy. Two mechanisms account for these changes—a direct radiation effect on the uterine tissues and radiation-induced ovarian hypofunction, which leads to reduced hormonal stimulation of the uterus. No radiation effects on the uterus can be seen on MRI scans in postmenopausal patients. The uterus remains of low signal intensity on T2-weighted images, without discernible zonal anatomy.

The **ovaries** become smaller after radiotherapy, and demonstrate decreased signal intensity on T2-weighted images, reflecting atrophy of the ovarian follicles and increased fibrosis and vascular sclerosis.

The wall of the **vagina** demonstrates increased signal intensity on T2-weighted images after radiation therapy, as demonstrated in Figure 14.26. This change is presumably related to the presence of edema and a hypervascular inflammatory response. Intravenous Gd-DTPA administration causes enhancement of the vaginal tissues (Figure 14.26). In the long term, fibrosis results in low signal intensity of the vagina on all imaging sequences.

Male pelvis

After radiotherapy the **prostate** is decreased in size, and of uniformly low signal intensity on T2-weighted images. There is also loss of the normal prostatic zonal anatomy (see Chapter 8). The **seminal vesicles** decrease in size after radiotherapy, and they display altered signal characteristics, with medium or low signal intensity on T2-weighted images instead of the normal high signal intensity (as shown in Figure 14.27).

Bladder

Postradiation MRI studies of the bladder demonstrate a range of changes which correlates with the severity of histologic findings. The earliest MRI feature is high signal intensity of the bladder mucosa on T2-weighted images with preservation of the normal bladder wall thickness (less than 5 mm). This high signal intensity usually commences at the trigone, as shown in Figure 14.28, but may spread to involve the whole mucosa. With more severe radiation injury, the bladder wall increases in width to more than 5 mm (Figure 14.26) and it demonstrates uniformly high signal intensity on T2-weighted images (Figure 14.29). After Gd-DTPA administration the bladder wall enhances uniformly but there may be increased enhancement of the mucosa (Figure 14.26). In its most extreme form, bladder radiation change includes the formation of a fistula arising from the bladder, in addition to thickening and abnormal signal characteristics of the bladder wall. The grades of bladder radiation injury are not related to the interval from start of therapy, and some of the more minor radiation changes may be identified in asymptomatic patients.

Rectum and perirectal tissues

The earliest sign of radiotherapy change in the rectum (Figure 14.30) is an increase in signal intensity of the submucosa on T2-weighted images. With progression of radiation therapy effects, the rectal wall becomes thickened (greater than 6 mm in the distended state) and demonstrates abnormal high signal intensity in the outer muscular layer on T2-weighted images. Differentiation between the submucosa and muscle layers is lost, as displayed in Figures 14.26, 14.29, 14.31 and 14.32. As seen in Figure 14.33, the rectal tissue enhances after Gd-DTPA administration, but there is no distinction between the component layers. The most severe rectal changes, shown in Figure 14.34, include evidence of a fistula from the rectum. As with bladder radiation injury, all degrees of rectal change are visible irrespective of the time from the start of treatment, and minor rectal MRI findings may be seen in asymptomatic patients.

Changes in the perirectal tissues are seen in Figures 14.26 and 14.27. The perirectal fascia becomes thickened after radiation therapy, measuring greater than 3 mm at the S4/5 vertebral level. Changes are more commonly seen in the subacute phase following treatment. The presacral space, which normally has a maximum diameter of less than 1.5 cm at the S4/5 vertebral level, shows increased width (Figures 14.27 and 14.29), most often in the chronic phase after treatment. The space may be filled with fat (high signal intensity on both T1- and T2-weighted images) or fluid (low signal intensity on T1-weighted images and high signal intensity on T2-weighted images). Alternatively, presacral tissue may demonstrate a low signal intensity on both T1- and T2-weighted images, most likely due to fibrosis.

Pelvic fat

Normal pelvic fat demonstrates homogeneous high signal intensity on T1-weighted images. Radiation therapy changes, shown in Figures 14.29 and 14.32, lead to a heterogeneous decrease in signal intensity on T1-weighted images.

Pelvic sidewall muscles

Normal striated muscle is of medium signal intensity on T1-weighted images and decreases in signal intensity on T2-weighted images. After radiation, the pelvic sidewall muscles demonstrate high signal intensity on T2-weighted images. This change is identified most commonly in the subacute phase. Moreover, the involved muscles correspond to the radiation port used, as indicated in Figures 14.32 and 14.35. Differentiation between muscle radiation change and muscle abnormality due to infection relies on the uniform involvement of the whole muscle bulk and the absence of other clinical or imaging features of infection.

Bone marrow

MRI is excellent for evaluation of bone marrow changes. Normally the marrow is of medium signal intensity on T1-weighted images. After radiation therapy, however, it demonstrates high signal intensity (Figures 14.16, 14.20, 14.22, 14.26, 14.27 and 14.36). This change is considered to be related to increased fat content within the marrow space. The margins of bone marrow radiation change accurately correspond to the dimensions of the radiation port.

MRI in relation to other imaging modalities

Currently MRI is the most sensitive imaging modality for the detection of radiation-induced tissue injury and enables an appreciation of changes in organs and tissues which are difficult to assess clinically.

MRI appearance of recurrent tumor versus post-treatment fibrosis

The differentiation between residual or recurrent tumor and post-treatment fibrosis is an area of ongoing concern, since the clinical distinction may be extremely difficult and biopsy is often required. Both CT and MRI allow assessment of areas that are clinically inaccessible, thereby complementing clinical examination and allowing better overall patient evaluation. Although a soft tissue mass can be demonstrated on CT scans, the tissue characteristics or etiology of the mass cannot be identified. With MRI, however, there is some evidence to suggest that tumor recurrence can be differentiated from radiation fibrosis on the basis of signal intensity on T2-weighted imaging sequences.[26–30] As demonstrated in Figures 14.37–14.39, fibrosis is typically of low signal intensity on both T1- and T2-weighted images, whereas tumor is of high signal intensity on T2-weighted images. Differentiation is not precise, however, since an incorrect diagnosis of tumor may be made in the presence of acute radiation change which causes inflammation and edema, also demonstrating high signal intensity on T2-weighted images.[26,27] Such inflammatory postradiation changes may persist for up to 18 months.[31] The use of Gd-DTPA causes tumor enhancement (Figure 14.39), but enhancement is also seen in edematous, inflamed, irradiated tissues (Figures 14.26 and 14.33). In addition, infiltrative tumors which excite a desmoplastic response, for example rectal and breast carcinoma,

may mimic fibrosis and remain of low signal intensity on both T1- and T2-weighted images.[32]

References

1 BOYD ME, Myomectomy, *Can J Surg* (1986) **29**:161–3.

2 MONAGHAN JM, Myomectomy and management of fibroids in pregnancy. In: Monaghan JM, ed. *Bonney's Gynaecological Surgery*, (WB Saunders: Philadelphia 1986) 87–116.

3 MONAGHAN JM, Total abdominal hysterectomy. In: Monaghan JM, ed. *Bonney's Gynaecological Surgery*, (WB Saunders: Philadelphia 1986) 54–9.

4 HUSSENZADEH N, NAHHAS WA, VELKELEY DE, The preservation of ovarian function in young women undergoing pelvic radiation therapy, *Gynecol Oncol* (1984) **18**:373–9.

5 BASHIST B, FRIEDMAN WN, KILLACKEY MA, Surgical transposition of the ovary: radiologic appearance, *Radiology* (1989) **173**:857–60.

6 NEWBOLD R, SAFRIT H, COOPER C, Surgical lateral ovarian transposition: CT appearance, *AJR* (1990) **154**:119–20.

7 MCLAUGHLIN AP, Suprapubic and retropubic prostatectomy. In: Harrison JH, Gittes RF, Perlmutter AD et al, eds. *Campbell's Urology*, (WB Saunders: Philadelphia 1979) 2299–314.

8 MCLAUGHLIN AP, Radical retropubic prostatectomy. In: Harrison JH, Gittes RF, Perlmutter AD et al, eds. *Campbell's Urology*, (WB Saunders: Philadelphia 1979) 2315–26.

9 HENEY NM, PROUT GR, Open bladder surgery. In: Harrison JH, Gittes RF, Perlmutter AD et al, eds. *Campbell's Urology*, (WB Saunders: Philadelphia 1979) 2243–58.

10 SKINNER DG, RICHIE JP, Urointestinal diversion. In: Harrison JH, Gittes RF, Perlmutter AD et al, eds. *Campbell's Urology*, (WB Saunders: Philadelphia 1979) 2211–30.

11 VAN DE VELDE CJH, BLOEM RM, ZWAVELING A, Management of colorectal cancer, *Eur J Cancer Clin Oncol* (1986) **22(3)**:339–44.

12 STEELE G JR, RAVIKUMAR TS, BENOTTI PN, New surgical treatments for recurrent colorectal cancer, *Cancer* (1990) **65**:723–30.

13 LAWHEAD RA, CLARK DGC, SMITH DH et al, Pelvic exenteration for recurrent or persistent gynecologic malignancies: a ten year review of the Memorial Sloan-Kettering Cancer experience (1972-1981), *Gynecol Oncol* (1989) **33**:279–82.

14 HELLMAN S, Principles of radiation therapy. In: DeVita VT, Hellman S, Rosenberg SA, eds. *Cancer Principles and Practice of Oncology*, (JB Lippincott: Philadelphia 1989) 247–75.

15 FLETCHER GH, Parameters involved in radiotherapy complications. In: Libshitz HI, ed. *Diagnostic Roentgenology of Radiotherapy Change*, (Williams and Wilkins: Baltimore 1979) 1–2, 85–100, 123–35.

16 RUBIN P, CASARETT GW, *Clinical Radiation Pathology*, Vol 1. (WB Saunders: Philadelphia 1968) 1–61.

17 MAIER JG, Effects of radiation on kidney, bladder and prostate. In: Vaetg JM, ed. *Frontiers in Radiation Therapy and Oncology*, (University Park Press: Baltimore 1972) 196–227.

18 ORTON CG, Dose dependence of complication rates in cervix cancer radiotherapy, *Int J Radiat Oncol Biol Phys* (1958) **12**:37–44.

19 OHTOMO K, SHUMAN WP, GRIFFIN BR et al, CT manifestation in

the pararectal area following fast neutron radiotherapy, *Radiat Med* (1987) **5**:198–201.

20 ADALSTEINSSON B, PAHLMAN L, HEMMINGSON A et al, Computed tomography in early diagnosis of local recurrence of rectal carcinoma, *Acta Radiol* (1987) **28**:41–7.

21 SUGIMURA K, CARRINGTON BM, QUIVEY JM et al, Postirradiation changes in the pelvis: assessment with MR imaging, *Radiology* (1990) **175**:805–13.

22 ARRIVÉ L, CHANG YCF, HRICAK H et al, Radiation-induced uterine changes: MR imaging, *Radiology* (1989) **170**:55–8.

23 HRICAK H, CARROLL P, radiologic imaging in monitoring patients following therapy for prostate carcinoma. *Proceedings of the First International Workshop on Diagnostic Ultrasound of the Prostate*, Washington DC (1988).

24 TAVARES NJ, ARRIVÉ L, DEMAS BE et al, Bladder morphology following radiation therapy: assessment with MR imaging (abstr), *Radiology* (1988) **169**:169.

25 RAMSEY RG, ZACHARIAS CE, MR imaging of the spine after radiation therapy: easily recognizable effects, *AJR* (1985) **144**:1131–5.

26 EBNER F, KRESSEL HY, MINTZ MC et al, Tumor recurrence versus fibrosis in the female pelvis: differentiation with MR imaging at 1.5 T, *Radiology* (1988) **166**:333–40.

27 GOMBERG JS, FRIEDMAN AC, RADECKI PD et al, MRI differentiation of recurrent colorectal carcinoma from postoperative fibrosis, *Gastrointest Radiol* (1986) **11**:361–3.

28 KRESTIN GP, STEINBRICH W, FRIEDMANN G, Recurrent rectal cancer: diagnosis with MR imaging versus CT, *Radiology* (1988) **168**:307–11.

29 JOHNSON RJ, JENKINS JPR, ISHERWOOD I et al, Quantitative magnetic resonance imaging in rectal carcinoma, *Br J Radiol* (1987) **60**:761–4.

30 RAFTO SE, AMENDOLA MA, GEFTER WB, Case report: MR imaging of recurrent colorectal carcinoma versus fibrosis, *J Comput Assist Tomogr* (1988) **12(3)**:521–3.

31 JOHNSON RJ, CARRINGTON BM, JENKINS JPR et al, Accuracy in staging carcinoma of the bladder by magnetic resonance imaging, *Clin Radiol* (1990) **41**:258–63.

32 LANGE EE, FECHNER RE, WANEBO HJ, Suspected recurrent rectosigmoid carcinoma after abdominoperineal resection: MR imaging and histopathologic findings, *Radiology* (1989) **170**:323–8.

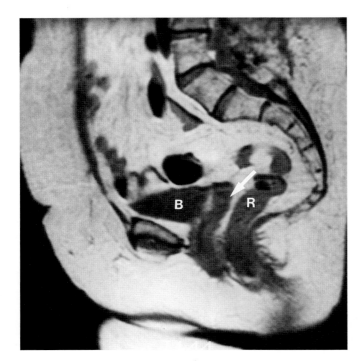

a

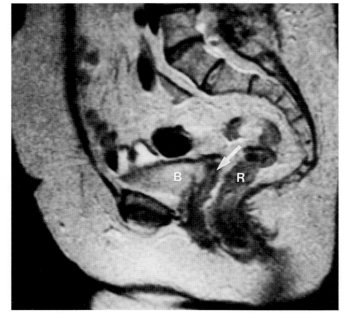

b

Figure 14.1

Total abdominal hysterectomy. Sagittal (**a**) proton density and (**b**) T2-weighted images showing a blind ending vaginal vault (arrows). (B)-urinary bladder; (R)-rectum.

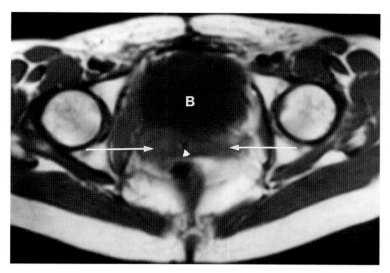

a

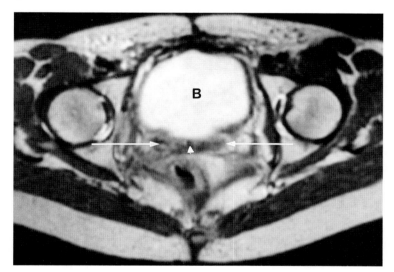

b

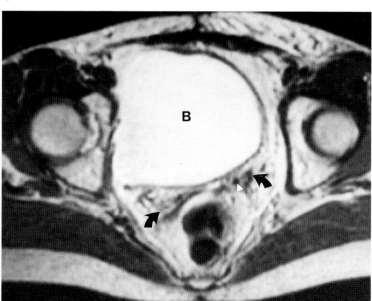

c

Figure 14.2
Vaginal appearance after hysterectomy. Transaxial (**a**) T1-weighted and (**b**) T2-weighted images at the same level, and (**c**) T2-weighted image 1 cm cranial to (**a**) and (**b**). The opposed vaginal fornices have a linear appearance (arrows) which is of low signal intensity on the T2-weighted image due to the presence of fibrosis. Surgical clips (arrowheads) can be identified. The lateral margins of the scar show some nodularity (curved arrows). (B)-urinary bladder.

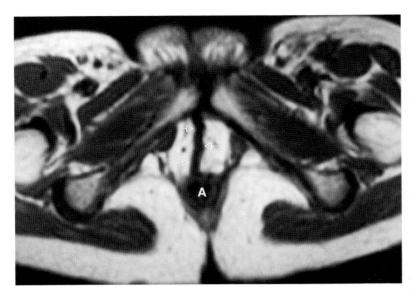

a

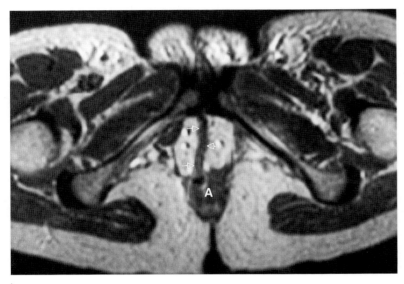

b

Figure 14.3

Neovagina in a patient following anterior exenteration. Transaxial (**a**) T1- and (**b**) T2- weighted images of the perineum showing the neovagina (arrows) within the anterior, or urogenital, triangle. The native vagina and urethra have been removed during the anterior exenteration but the anal canal (A) is normal in position.

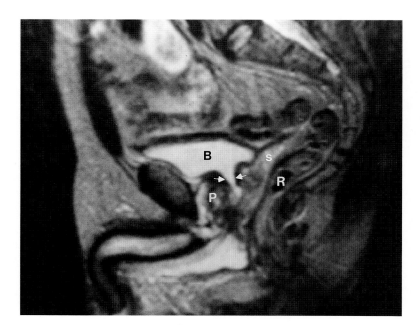

Figure 14.4

TURP defect. Sagittal T2-weighted image demonstrating the urine-filled TURP defect (arrows) at the base of the bladder (B). (P)-prostate; (S)-seminal vesicle; (R)-rectum.

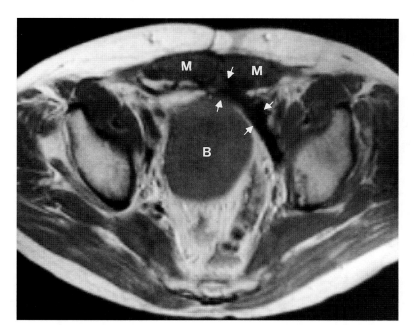

Figure 14.5

Anterior fibrosis after suprapubic prostatectomy. Transaxial proton density image demonstrating low signal intensity fibrosis (arrows) between the bladder (B) and the rectus abdominis muscles (M). (0.35 T.)

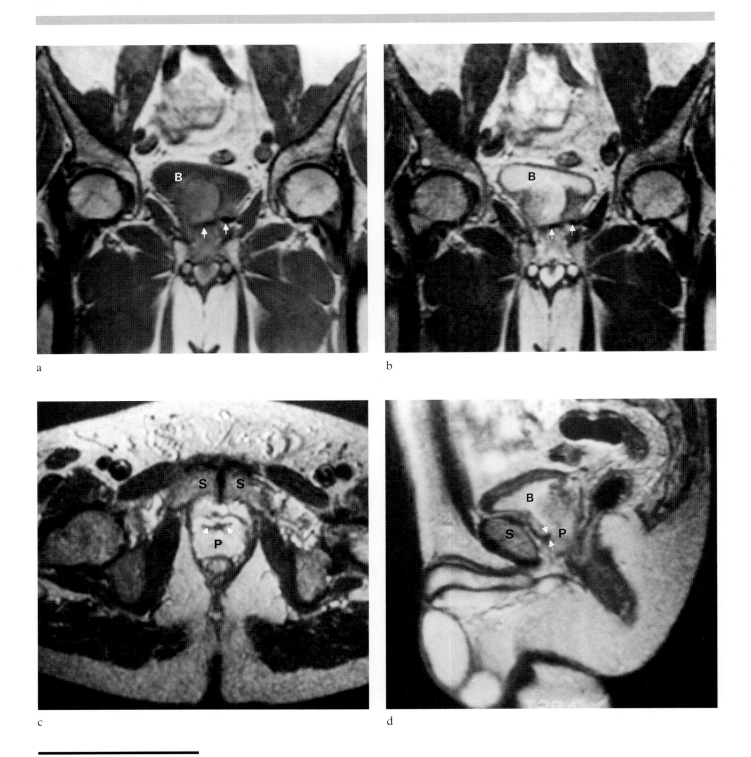

a

b

c

d

Figure 14.6

Retropubic prostatectomy. Coronal (**a**) proton density and (**b**) T2-weighted images, (**c**) transaxial and (**d**) sagittal T2-weighted images. The retropubic surgical scar (small arrows) is identified as a linear low signal intensity band within the anterior prostate (P) and posterior to the symphysis pubis (S). The surgical defect is small due to further prostatic hypertrophy. (B)-urinary bladder.

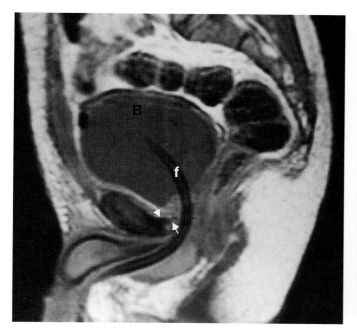

a

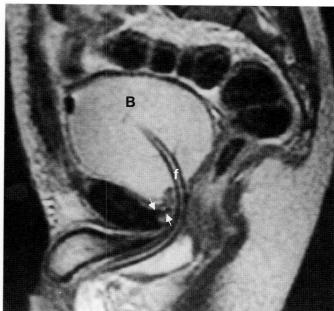

b

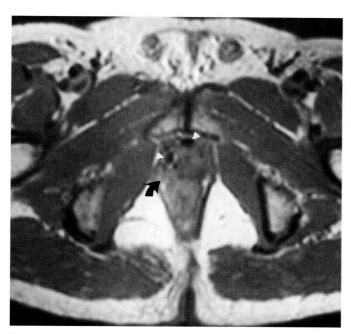

c

Figure 14.7

Radical prostatectomy. Sagittal (**a**) proton density and (**b**) T2-weighted images, (**c**) transaxial proton density image. The prostate and seminal vesicles have been resected. The base of the bladder (B) is low-lying behind the symphysis pubis and the site of anastomosis (small arrows) with the membranous urethra is of low signal intensity due to the presence of fibrous tissue and surgical clips. On the transaxial image, asymmetry at the anastomotic site (curved arrow) is due to recurrent tumor. There is signal void from surgical clips (arrowheads). A Foley catheter (f) is present in the bladder.

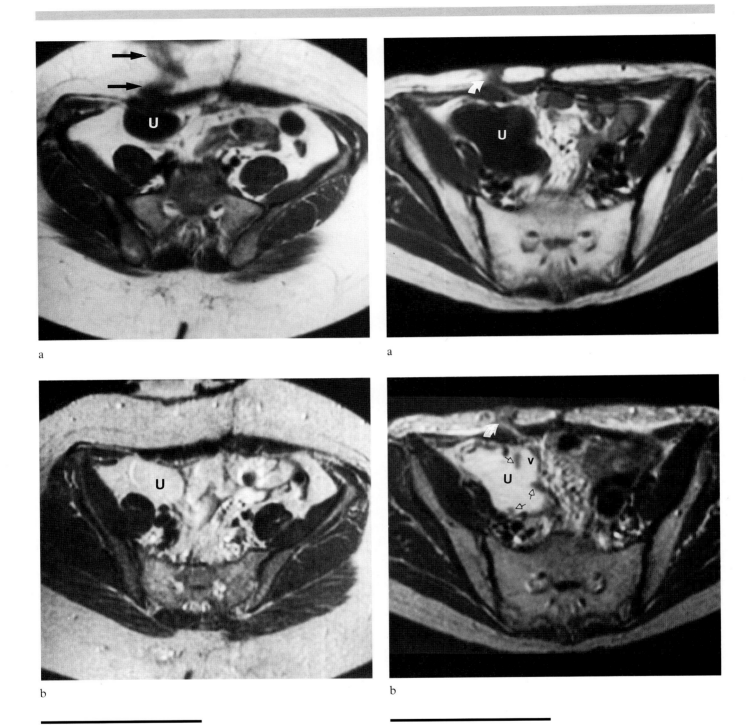

Figure 14.8

Urinary conduit. Transaxial (**a**) T1- and (**b**) T2-weighted images demonstrating the urinary conduit (U) in the right iliac fossa beneath the anterior abdominal wall. The bowel (arrows) passes through the rectus abdominis muscle to reach the skin.

Figure 14.9

Continent urinary reservoir. Transaxial (**a**) T1- and (**b**) T2-weighted images demonstrating a urinary reservoir (U) made from cecum with visible haustra (small arrows). The ileocecal valve (v) is the continence mechanism and ileum (curved arrows) is the link between cecum and skin.

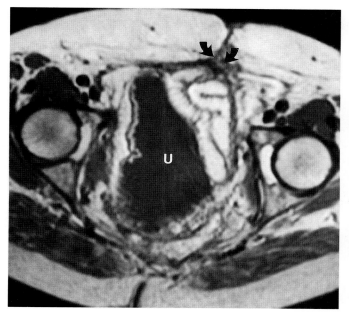

a

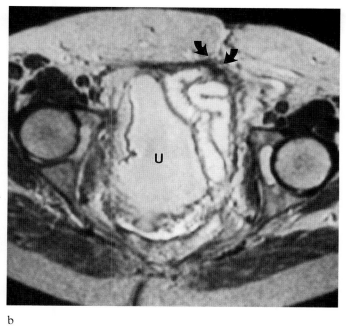

b

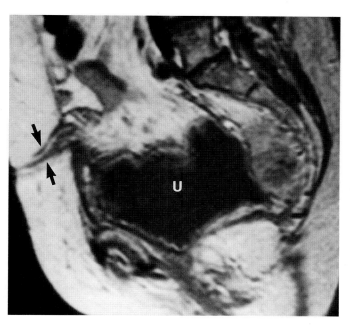

c

Figure 14.10

Bladder substitute. Transaxial
(**a**) T1- and (**b**) T2-weighted
images, and (**c**) sagittal T1-
weighted image. The urinary
bladder substitute (U) is
transposed cecum with a
lobulated margin due to
haustra. The track of a previous
suprapubic catheter can be
identified (arrows). (Curved
arrows)-laparotomy scar.

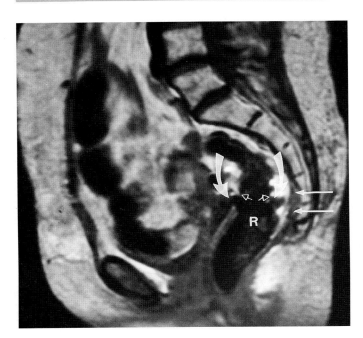

Figure 14.11

Prior anterior resection of rectum. Sagittal T1-weighted image showing the signal void and artifacts from metallic sutures (curved arrows) around the rectum (R) at the site of anastomosis. There is also a localized irregularity of the rectal wall (small open arrows) and minor reduction in caliber. There is low signal intensity fibrous tissue in the presacral space (straight arrows).

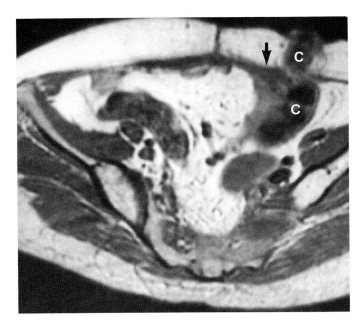

Figure 14.12

Sigmoid colostomy after AP resection. Transaxial proton density image illustrating the position of the colostomy in the left iliac fossa. Sigmoid colon (C) passes through the rectus abdominis muscle (arrow).

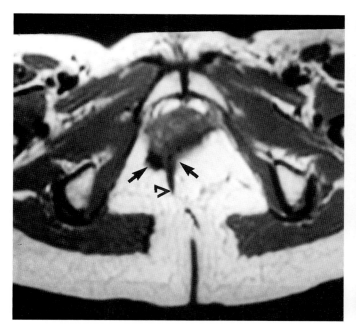

a

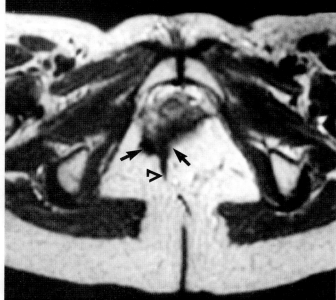

b

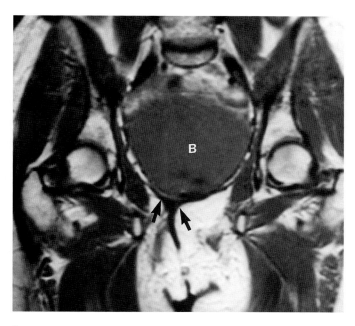

c

Figure 14.13

Appearance of levator ani muscles after AP resection. Transaxial (**a**) proton density and (**b**) T2-weighted images, and (**c**) coronal proton density image. The levator ani muscles (arrows) have been resutured asymmetrically and they are of very low signal intensity due to postsurgical fibrosis. The region of the anal canal (open arrows) has been oversewn. (B)-urinary bladder.

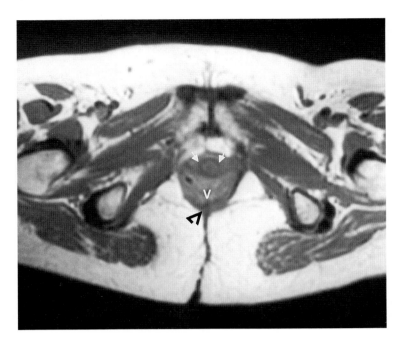

a

Figure 14.14
Perineum after AP resection. Transaxial (**a**) proton density and (**b**) T2-weighted images without the anal canal. The normal position of the anal canal is marked by low signal intensity fibrous tissue (open arrows) and there is a normal anterior urogenital triangle containing the urethra (small arrows) and the vagina (V).

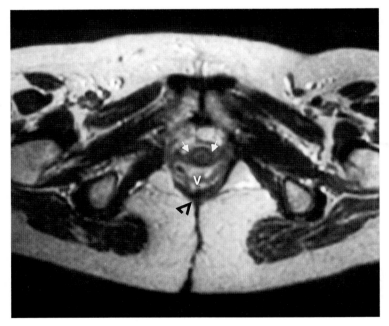

b

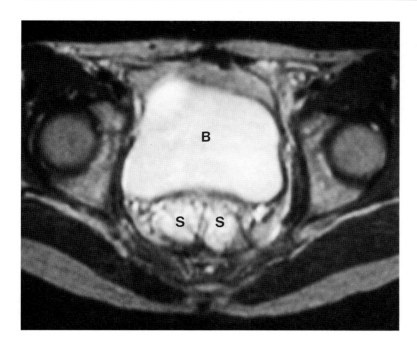

Figure 14.15

Altered position of the bladder and seminal vesicles after AP resection. Transaxial T2-weighted image depicting the more posterior position of both the bladder (B) and seminal vesicles (S) after AP resection.

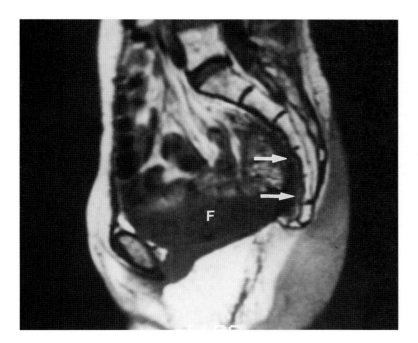

Figure 14.16

Total pelvic exenteration. Sagittal T1-weighted image demonstrating extensive low signal intensity fibrous tissue (F) within the pelvis and presacral space (arrows) and absence of all pelvic organs. There is high signal intensity within all the visualized vertebral bodies due to previous radiation therapy.

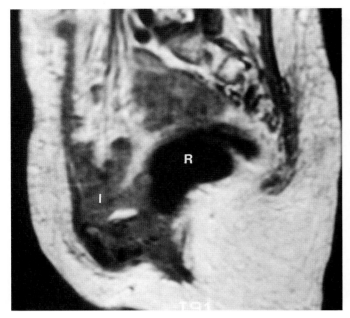

a

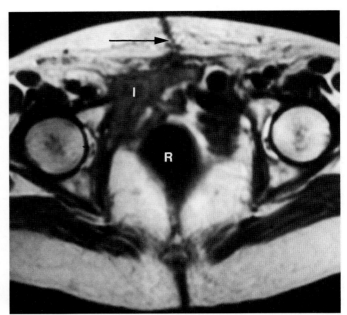

b

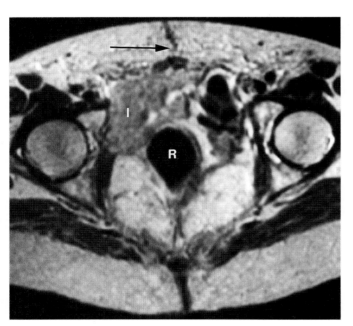

c

Figure 14.17

Anterior pelvic exenteration.
Sagittal (**a**) proton density
image, and transaxial (**b**) T1-
and (**c**) T2-weighted images
showing the more anterior
position occupied by the
rectum (R) after an anterior
exenteration. The potential
space left by the procedure is
also filled by small intestine (I).
(Arrows)-laparotomy scar.

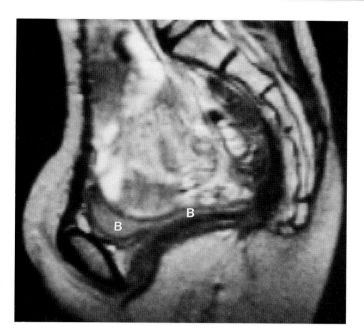

Figure 14.18

Posterior pelvic exenteration. Sagittal proton density image illustrating the more posterior position adopted by the bladder (B) after posterior exenteration. (0.35 T.)

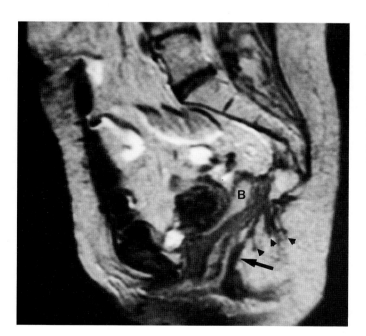

Figure 14.19

Posterior pelvic exenteration. Sagittal T2-weighted image showing posteriorly positioned bladder (B) and low signal intensity of the pelvic floor muscles (arrow) with multiple fibrotic strands radiating into the buttock (arrowheads).

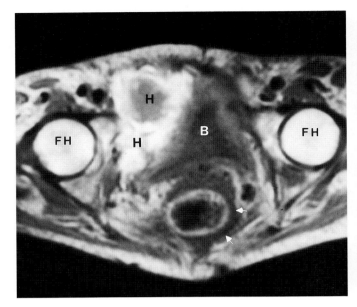

a

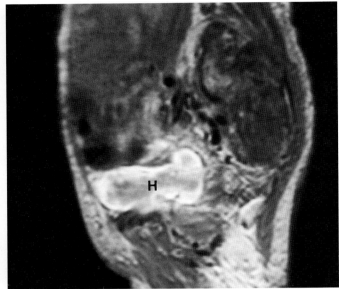

b

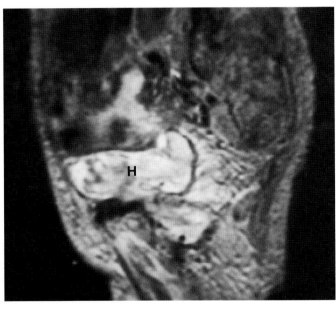

c

Figure 14.20

Subacute pelvic hematoma. Transaxial (**a**) T1-weighted image, and sagittal (**b**) proton density and (**c**) T2-weighted images. A large hematoma (H) demonstrates heterogeneous high signal intensity on all sequences. It is compressing the bladder (B), which is thick-walled due to radiation change. The femoral heads (FH) are of abnormal high signal intensity also due to radiation therapy. There is marked thickening of the perirectal fascia (arrows) from postsurgical and radiation effects.

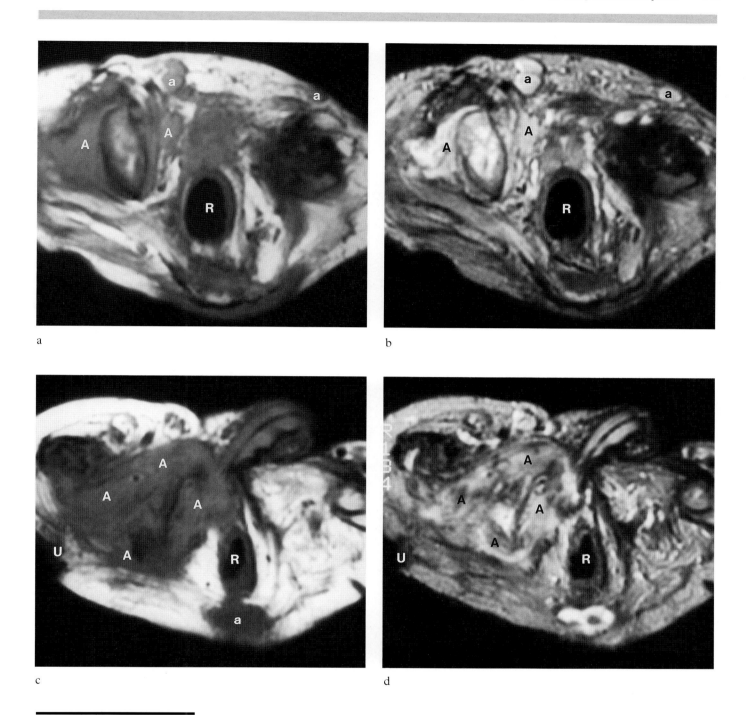

a

b

c

d

Figure 14.21

Extensive pelvic sepsis. Transaxial (**a**) T1- and (**b**) T2-weighted images, and (**c**) T1- and (**d**) T2-weighted images at different levels through the pelvis of a paraplegic patient. There is a huge abscess (A) involving the right hemipelvis which is of medium signal intensity on T1-weighted images and heterogeneous high signal intensity on T2-weighted images. Several smaller abscesses (a) are seen, in the presacral space and under the anterior abdominal wall. A right decubitus ulcer (U) may have been the original source for the infection. (R)-rectum.

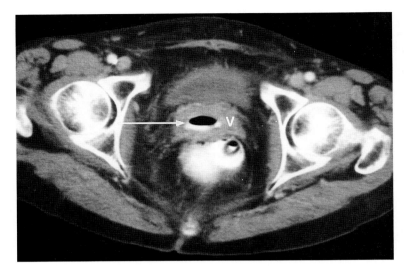

a

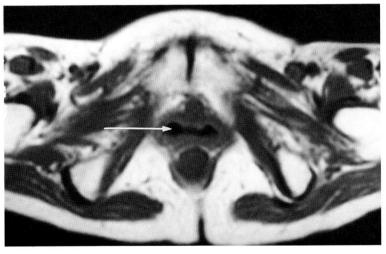

b

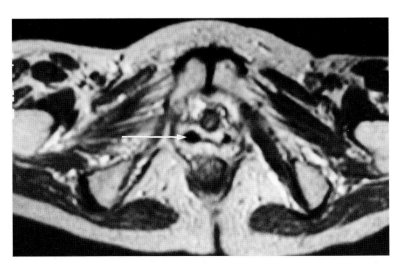

c

Figure 14.22

Rectovaginal fistula. (**a**) CT scan through the vaginal vault demonstrates an air/oral contrast level (arrow) in the thick-walled vagina (V). Transaxial (**b**) proton density and (**c**) T2-weighted images through the vagina with (**d**) proton density and (**e**) T2-weighted images at a lower level also show air (arrows) in the vaginal lumen. However, on the lower slice the fistula (small arrows) is identified as a linear tract of low signal intensity on both proton density and T2-weighted images. The patient had undergone both surgery and radiotherapy and the vagina is of very high signal intensity on the T2-weighted images due to radiation effect.

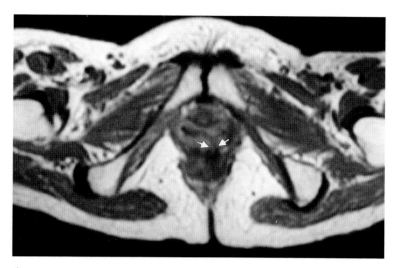

d

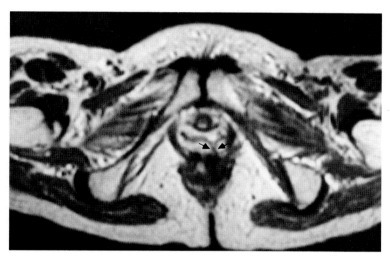

e

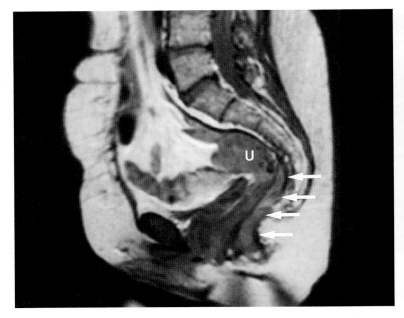

a

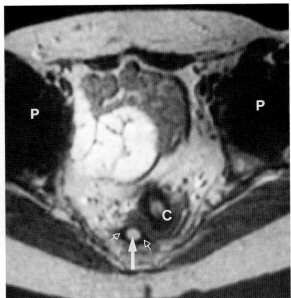

b

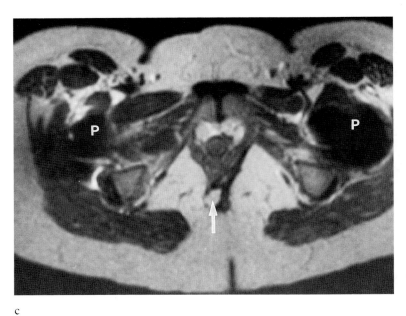

c

Figure 14.23

Pelvic sinus tract after AP resection. (**a**) Sagittal proton density image, (**b**) and (**c**) T2-weighted images showing a sinus tract (arrows) running longitudinally in the presacral space in the position previously occupied by the rectum. The tract is delineated by a rim of low signal intensity fibrous tissue (open arrows) and has a central high signal intensity component. The tract is immediately adjacent to the cervix (C). The position of the uterus (U) is posterior in the pelvis secondary to the AP resection procedure. (P)-hip prostheses causing signal voids.

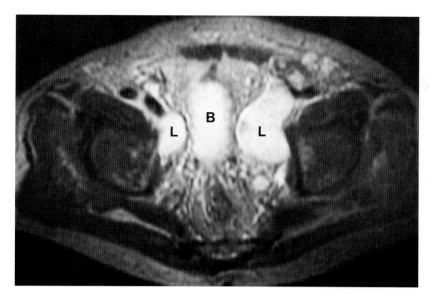

Figure 14.24

Bilateral pelvic lymphoceles. Transaxial T2-weighted image demonstrating high signal intensity, smooth-walled lymphoceles (L) on both pelvic sidewalls. (B)-urinary bladder.

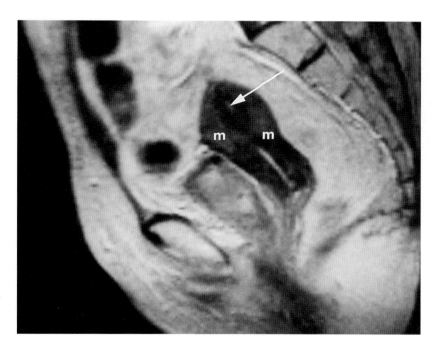

Figure 14.25

Radiation change affecting the uterus. Sagittal T2-weighted image showing loss of uterine zonal anatomy due to decreased signal intensity of the myometrium (m). The endometrium (arrow) is also of reduced width.

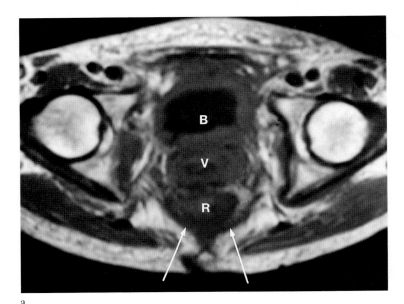

a

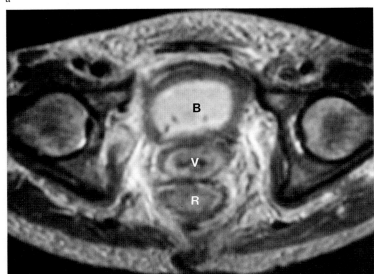

b

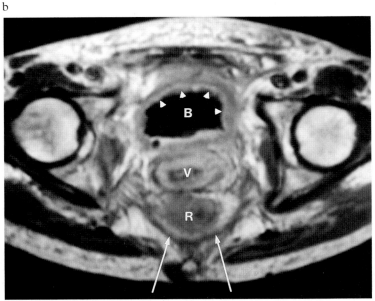

c

Figure 14.26

Radiation changes affecting the vagina, bladder and rectal tissues. Transaxial (**a**) T1-, (**b**) T2- and (**c**) Gd-DTPA-enhanced T1-weighted images illustrating a markedly thickened upper-third of the vagina (V), which enhances after Gd-DTPA administration. The bladder (B) is thick-walled and shows contrast enhancement, particularly of the mucosa (arrowheads). On the T2-weighted image the rectum (R) has a high signal intensity wall and there is thickening of the perirectal fascia (arrows). There is abnormal high signal intensity in the visualized bony pelvis on the T1-weighted images due to radiation-induced marrow changes.

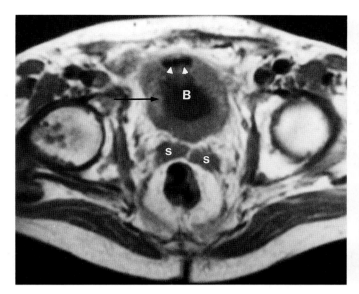

a

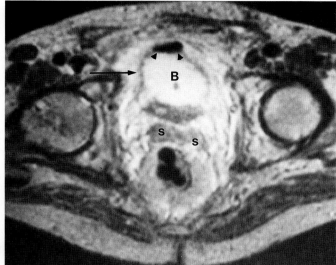

b

Figure 14.27

Radiation changes affecting the seminal vesicles and bladder. Transaxial (**a**) T1- and (**b**) T2-weighted images demonstrating small seminal vesicles (S) of abnormal medium-to-low signal intensity on the T2-weighted image due to radiation therapy. The bladder (B) is thick-walled and displays high signal intensity of its wall (arrows) on the T2-weighted sequence. Air is seen in the bladder wall (arrowheads). The bony pelvis is of high signal intensity on the T1-weighted image due to radiation effect and there are multiple medium signal intensity foci within the acetabulum and femoral heads due to metastases. The perirectal fascia is thickened.

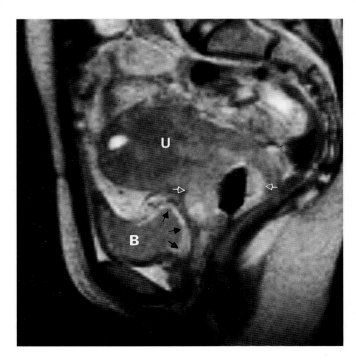

Figure 14.28

Early radiation change affecting the bladder. Sagittal T2-weighted image displaying early radiation bladder change with high signal intensity of the mucosa around the trigone and posterior wall (arrows). The uterus (U) is enlarged and there is a high signal intensity cervical tumor (open arrows) with air in its center. (B)-urinary bladder. (0.35 T.)

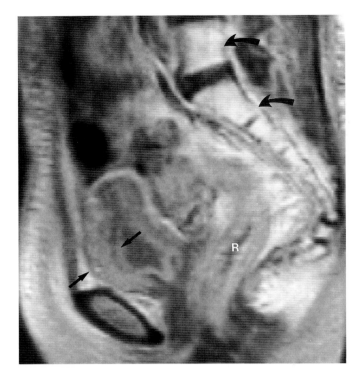

a

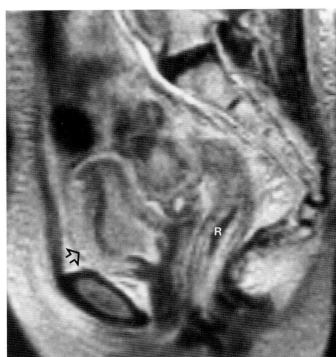

b

Figure 14.29

Radiation change affecting the bladder. Sagittal (**a**) proton density and (**b**) T2-weighted images showing the thickened bladder wall (straight arrows). Its outer portion demonstrates abnormal high signal intensity on the T2-weighted image (open arrow), whereas the inner portion is of low signal intensity. There is widening of the presacral space. Radiation changes in the rectum (R) and the lumbosacral spine (curved arrows) can also be observed. (0.35T.)

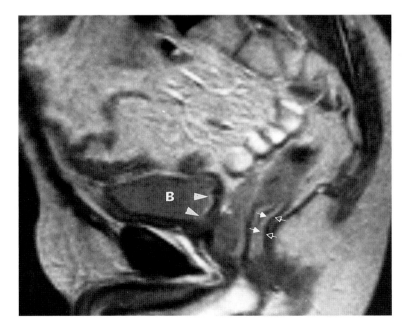

Figure 14.30

Early radiation change affecting the rectal mucosa. Sagittal T2-weighted image showing the high signal intensity rectal submucosa (small white arrows). The submucosa can be differentiated from the low signal intensity outer muscle wall (small open arrows). The bladder trigone demonstrates radiation-induced high signal intensity (arrowheads). (B)-urinary bladder.

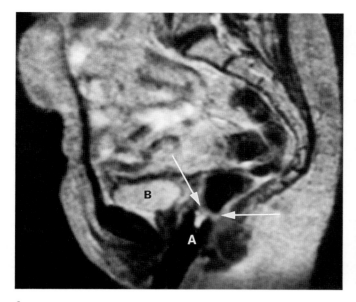

a

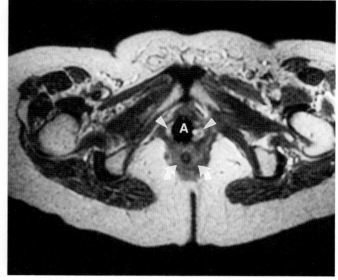

b

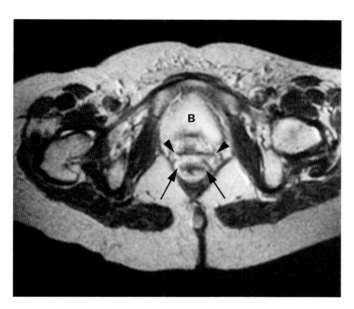

c

Figure 14.31

Radiation change affecting the rectum and vagina due to brachytherapy. (**a**) Sagittal T2-weighted image, (**b**) transaxial T2-weighted image at the level of the lower-third of the vagina, and (**c**) transaxial T2-weighted image at the level of the middle-third of the vagina. The metal applicator for intracavitary radiation (A) is seen as a tubular area of signal void within the vagina in (**a**) and (**b**). The vagina (arrowheads) is of very high signal intensity due to radiation effect. The rectum is normal inferiorly (curved arrows), but demonstrates thickening of the wall with loss of definition between the individual layers (straight arrows) immediately adjacent to the tip of the applicator, which had held the radioactive source. (B)-urinary bladder.

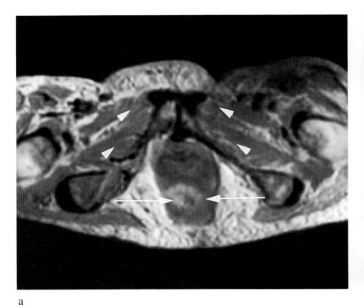

a

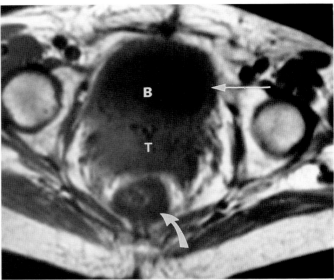

a

b

b

Figure 14.32

Radiation change affecting the rectum, pelvic musculature, and fat. Transaxial (**a**) proton density and (**b**) T2-weighted images showing uniform high signal intensity throughout the rectal wall (arrows) and loss of definition of the individual layers of the wall. Radiation changes affecting the obturator externus and pectineus muscles (arrowheads) lead to high signal intensity on the T2-weighted image. The right pectineus muscle shows an abrupt change from high to low signal intensity on the T2-weighted image corresponding to the edge of the radiation port. The pelvic fat is of heterogeneous appearance on both images.

Figure 14.33

Radiation change of rectum and bladder after Gd-DTPA administration. Transaxial (**a**) T1- and (**b**) Gd-DTPA-enhanced T1-weighted images showing thickening of the walls of both the bladder (straight arrows) and the rectum (curved arrows). After intravenous gadolinium there is enhancement of both rectum and bladder walls. There is a central pelvic ovarian mass (T) caused by a granulosa cell tumor recurrence. (B)-urinary bladder.

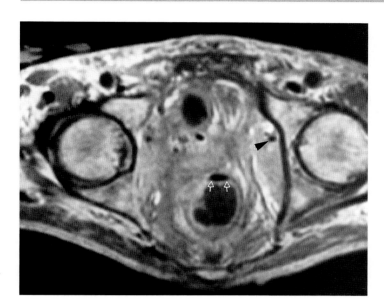

Figure 14.34

Severe radiation change affecting the rectum. Transaxial proton density image showing rectal wall necrosis with air trapped within the submucosa (open arrows) and diffuse pelvic sepsis resulting in air within the left obturator muscle (arrowhead). The patient had radiotherapy following a cystectomy.

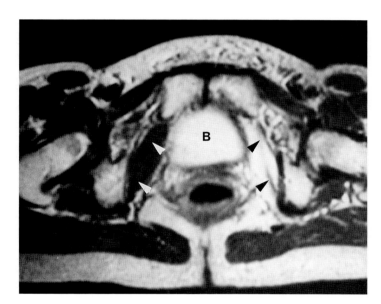

Figure 14.35

Radiation-induced muscle change. Transaxial T2-weighted image demonstrating marked asymmetry of the obturator internus muscles (arrowheads). The low signal intensity of the right obturator internus is normal. The uniformly high signal intensity of the left obturator internus is due to radiation injury. Previously the patient had brachytherapy to the left pelvic sidewall for recurrent tumor. (B)-urinary bladder.

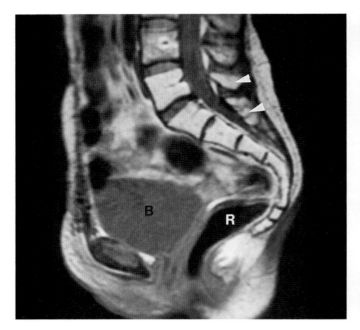

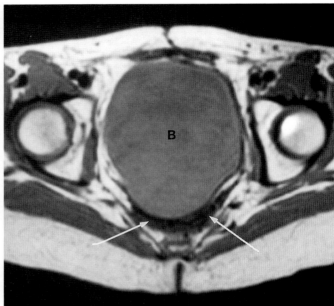

a

Figure 14.36

Radiation change affecting bone marrow. Sagittal T1-weighted image showing high signal intensity of the L5 vertebra, sacral vertebrae, and the coccyx. The vertebral bodies and the spinous processes (arrowheads) are seen to be involved. The L4 vertebra was above the radiation port and its marrow demonstrates normal medium signal intensity. The patient had a prior radical hysterectomy. (B)-urinary bladder; (R)-rectum.

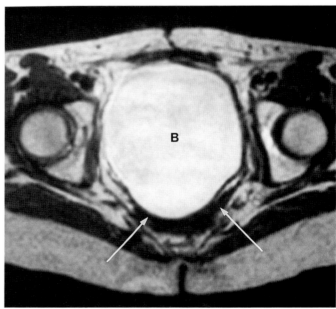

b

Figure 14.37

Postsurgical fibrosis. Transaxial (**a**) proton density and (**b**) T2-weighted images in a patient after AP resection. There is a crescentic band of tissue (arrows) in the presacral space, which is of low signal intensity on the proton density image and becomes of very low signal intensity on the T2-weighted image. The bladder (B) fills the potential space left by the rectum.

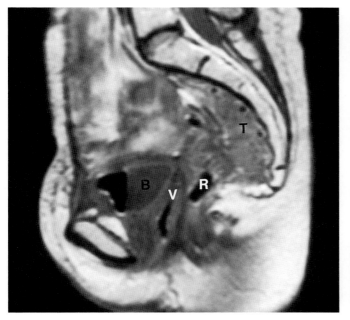

a

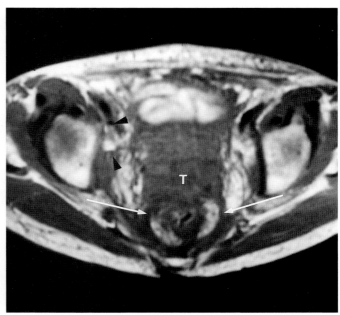

a

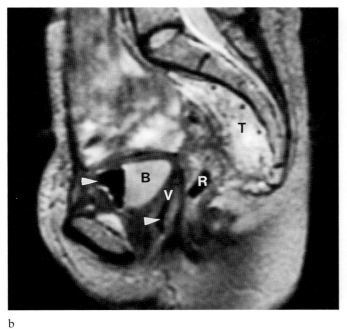

b

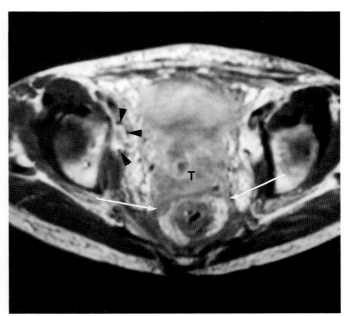

b

Figure 14.38

Recurrent tumor in the presacral space. Sagittal (**a**) proton density and (**b**) T2-weighted images showing the appearance of a large recurrent tumor (T) in the presacral space after anterior resection. The rectum (R) is displaced anteriorly by the tumor. There is air (arrowheads) in the bladder (B) and the vagina (V) due to the presence of a vesicovaginal fistula. Radiation-induced bone marrow change is seen in the spine on the proton density image.

Figure 14.39

Gadolinium-DTPA enhancement of recurrent tumor invading the uterosacral ligaments. Transaxial (**a**) T1- and (**b**) Gd-DTPA-enhanced T1-weighted images showing a central pelvic tumor recurrence (T). Tumor demonstrating medium signal intensity on the T1-weighted image with enhancement after gadolinium administration can be seen extending into the uterosacral ligaments (arrows) and presacral space. There are multiple low signal intensity surgical clips (arrowheads) from a prior radical lymph node dissection adjacent to the pelvic vessels.

Index